Radiology
Differential Diagnosis

Radiologic Differential Diagnosis

Satish K Bhargava

MBBS MD (Radiodiagnosis) MD (Radiotherapy)
DMRD FICRI FIAMS FCCP FUSI FIMSA FAMS
Professor and Head
Department of Radiology and Imaging
University College of Medical Sciences
(University of Delhi) and GTB Hospital
Delhi

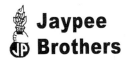

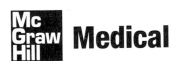

© 2007 Satish K Bhargava

First published in India by
Jaypee Brothers Medical Publishers (P) Ltd
EMCA House, 23/23B Ansari Road, Daryaganj
New Delhi 110 002, India
Phones: +91-11-23272143, +91-11-23272703, +91-11-23282021, +91-11-23245672
Fax: +91-11-23276490, +91-11-23245683   e-mail: jaypee@jaypeebrothers.com
Visit our website: www.jaypeebrothers.com

First published in USA by The McGraw-Hill Companies, 2 Penn Plaza, New York, NY 10121-2298.
Exclusively worldwide distributor except South Asia (India, Nepal, Sri Lanka, Bhutan, Pakistan,
Bangladesh).

NOTICE

Medicine is an ever-changing science. As new research and clinical experience broaden our knowledge, changes in treatment and drug therapy are required. The authors and the publisher of this work
have checked with sources believed to be reliable in their efforts to provide information that is complete
and generally in accord with the standards accepted at the time of publication. However, in view of the
possibility of human error changes in medical science, neither the editors nor the publisher nor any
other party who has been involved in the preparation or publication of this work warrants that the
information contained herein is in every respect accurate or complete, and they disclaim all respon-
sibility for any errors or omissions or for the results obtained from use of the information contained in
this work. Readers are encouraged to confirm the information contained herein with other sources. For
example and in particular, readers are advised to check the product information sheet included in the
package of each drug they plan to administer to be certain that the information contained in this work
is accurate and that changes have not been made in the recommended dose or in the contraindications
for administration. This recommendation is of particular importance in connection with new or infrequently used drugs.

ISBN   0-07-148574-0
ISBN 13 9780071485746

Dedicated to
My loving late wife
Kalpana
and my son
Sumeet
Whose inspiration and sacrifice
have made possible to
bring out this book

Contributors

Nidhi Bhargava
Ex. Senior Resident
Department of Radiology and Imaging
University College of Medical Sciences
(University of Delhi) and GTB Hospital
Delhi

Satish K Bhargava
Professor and Head
Department of Radiology and Imaging
University College of Medical Sciences
(University of Delhi) and GTB Hospital
Delhi

Sumeet Bhargava
LLR Medical College, Meerut, (UP)

Shuchi Bhatt
Senior Lecturer
Department of Radiology and Imaging
University College of Medical Sciences
(University of Delhi) and GTB Hospital
Delhi

Rajeev Chaturvedi
Ex. Senior Resident
Department of Radiology and Imaging
University College of Medical Sciences
(University of Delhi) and GTB Hospital
Delhi

Parul Garg
Senior Resident
Department of Radiology and Imaging
University College of Medical Sciences
(University of Delhi) and GTB Hospital
Delhi

Pushpender Gupta
Resident
Department of Radiology and Imaging
University College of Medical Sciences
(University of Delhi) and GTB Hospital
Delhi

Sarika Jain
Resident
Department of Radiology and Imaging
University College of Medical Sciences
(University of Delhi) and GTB Hospital
Delhi

Shashank Jain
Senior Resident
Maulana Azad Medical College and
Associated LNJP Hospital
New Delhi

Puneet Singh Kochar
Resident
Department of Radiology and Imaging
University College of Medical Sciences
(University of Delhi) and GTB Hospital
Delhi

Pardeep Kumar
Resident, Department of Radiology and Imaging
University College of Medical Sciences
(University of Delhi) and GTB Hospital
Delhi

Gaurav Luthra
Senior Resident
Department of Radiology and Imaging
Sanjay Gandhi Postgraduate
Institute of Medical Sciences
Rai Bareilly Road, Lucknow (UP)

Sapna Maheshwari (Somani)
Senior Resident, Department of Radiology
and Imaging, University College of Medical Sciences
(University of Delhi) and GTB Hospital
Delhi

Gopesh Mehrotra
Reader, Department of Radiology and Imaging
University College of Medical Sciences
(University of Delhi) and GTB Hospital
Delhi

Mamta Motla
Senior Resident, Department of Radiology
and Imaging, University College of Medical Sciences
(University of Delhi) and GTB Hospital
Delhi

Rajul Rastogi
Senior Resident, Department of Radiology
and Imaging, University College of Medical Sciences
(University of Delhi) and GTB Hospital
Delhi

Ruchi Rastogi
Senior Resident
Department of Cardiac Radiology
All India Institute of Medical Sciences
Ansari Nagar, New Delhi

Vinita Rathi
Associate Professor
Department of Radiology and Imaging
University College of Medical Sciences
(University of Delhi) and GTB Hospital
Delhi

Anubhav Sarikwal
Senior Resident
Department of Radiology and Imaging
University College of Medical Sciences
(University of Delhi) and GTB Hospital
Delhi

OP Sharma
Professor and Head
Department of Radiodiagnosis
Institute of Medical Sciences
Banaras Hindu University, Varanasi (UP)
University College of Medical Sciences
(University of Delhi) and GTB Hospital
Delhi

Ashish Verma
Senior Resident
Department of Radiodiagnosis and Imaging
Sanjay Gandhi Postgraduate
Institute of Medical Sciences
Rai Bareilly Road, Lucknow (UP)

Preface

The advancement in Radiology and subspecialties over a period of two decades has tremendously enhanced this course and in-depth knowledge of Image interpretation. This is particularly true in a developing country like ours where still majority of Radiologists practices in broader specialty and it is not always feasible to update the knowledge because of paucity of time and availability of literature/newer books at all places. However, interpretation of any radiograph is extremely essential for radiologist to arrive at a correct diagnosis keeping in view of various salient features of disease entity on various imaging modalities and to exclude other similar looking pictures. Thus it is more important for a trainee radiologist and radiologist in practice to have a book which should be and valuable primer and also the concise and handy reference to use in day-to-day practice. An attempt has been made to list out as many as important condition possible, enumerated their salient features and important differential diagnosis so as to arrive at a particular diagnosis.

Satish K Bhargava

Acknowledgements

I am grateful to my colleagues and friends who gave timely support and stood solidly behind me in our joint endeavor of bringing out this book which was required keeping in view of wide acceptability of ultrasound in developing countries like ours. My special heartfelt thanks are due to the sincere and hardworking staff of M/s Jaypee Brothers Medical Publishers (P) Ltd. particularly Shri Jitendar P Vij, Chairman and Managing Director, Mr Tarun Duneja, General Manager (Publishing), Mr PS Ghuman, Senior Production Manager, Ms Mubeen Bano and Mr Arun Sharma, DTP Operator. It is indeed the result of the hardwork of the staff of M/s Jaypee Brothers Medical Publishers (P) Ltd. and the contributors who have always been in keen desire to work with smiling faces and with polite voices as a result of which this book has seen the light of day.

Contents

1. Chest

1.1. **Lesions of Thoracic Inlet** *1*
   Satish K Bhargava, Rajeev Chaturvedi
1.2. **Mediastinal Masses** *15*
   Satish K Bhargava, Nidhi Bhargava
1.3. **Superior Mediastinal Masses** *25*
   Shuchi Bhatt, Sapna Maheshwari (Somani)
1.4. **Anterior Mediastinal Mass** *32*
   Shuchi Bhatt, Parul Garg
1.5. **Middle Mediastinal Masses** *38*
   Gopesh Mehrotra, Pardeep Kumar
1.6. **Posterior Mediastinal Masses** *45*
   Pushpender Gupta, Satish K Bhargava
1.7. **Chest Wall Abnormalities** *51*
   Shashank Jain, Vinita Rathi
1.8. **Superior Rib Notching** *55*
   Shuchi Bhatt, Pardeep Kumar
1.9. **Inferior Rib Notching** *60*
   Nidhi Bhargava, Satish K Bhargava
1.10. **Elevation of Diaphragm** *62*
   Nidhi Bhargava, Shuchi Bhatt
1.11. **Pneumomediastinum** *64*
   Nidhi Bhargava, Satish K Bhargava
1.12. **Lung Tumors** *66*
   Satish K Bhargava, Nidhi Bhargava
1.13. **Hilar Enlargement** *70*
   Nidhi Bhargava, Satish K Bhargava

1.14.   **Calcification on Chest Radiograph**   *72*
        Nidhi Bhargava, Satish K Bhargava

1.15.   **Air-Fluid Levels on Chest X-ray**   *74*
        Nidhi Bhargava, Satish K Bhargava

1.16A   **Cavitating Pulmonary Lesions**   *74*
        Nidhi Bhargava, Satish K Bhargava

1.16B   **Mass within Cavity**   *75*
        Nidhi Bhargava, Satish K Bhargava

1.17.   **Cavitating Pulmonary Lesions**   *76*
        Pardeep Kumar, Satish K Bhargava

1.18A   **Lucent Lung Lesions**   *83*
        Nidhi Bhargava, Satish K Bhargava

1.18B   **Solitary Pulmonary Nodule**   *85*
        Nidhi Bhargava, Shuchi Bhatt

1.19.   **Solitary Pulmonary Nodule**   *86*
        Rajeev Chaturvedi, Satish K Bhargava

1.20.   **Pulmonary Edema on the Opposite Side
        to a Preexisting Abnormality**   *99*
        Nidhi Bhargava

1.21A   **Miliary Shadowing**   *106*
        Parul Garg, Satish K Bhargava

1.21B   **Miliary Shadowing (0.5 to 2 mm)**   *111*
        Nidhi Bhargava, Gopesh Mehrotra

1.22.   **Multiple Pin Point Opacities**   *113*
        Nidhi Bhargava, Shuchi Bhatt

1.23.   **Complete Opaque Hemithorax**   *113*
        Nidhi Bhargava, Vinita Rathi

1.24.   **Opaque Hemithorax**   *114*
        Satish K Bhargava, Pushpender Gupta

1.25.   **Hypertransradiant Lung Field**   *120*
        Satish K Bhargava, Anubhav Sarikwal

1.26.   **Hypertranslucent Lung Field**   *128*
        Nidhi Bhargava

1.27A **Honeycomb Lung** *129*
    Nidhi Bhargava
1.27B **Honeycomb Lung** *132*
    Vinita Rathi, Sarika Jain
1.28. **Pleural Diseases** *137*
    Sapna Maheshwari (Somani),
    Gopesh Mehrotra
1.29. **Pleural Fluid** *144*
    Shuchi Bhatt, Nidhi Bhargava
1.30. **Pleural Tumors** *146*
    Nidhi Bhargava
1.31. **Pleural Calcification** *147*
    Rajeev Chaturvedi, Satish K Bhargava
1.32. **High Resolution CT—Pattern of**
    Parenchymal Disease *149*
    Nidhi Bhargava, Satish K Bhargava
1.33. **Cardiophrenic Angle Mass** *150*
    Satish K Bhargava, Pardeep Kumar

2. Breast—Mammographic Differential Diagnosis

Satish K Bhargava, Pushpender Gupta
2.1. **Circumscribed Radiolucent Lesion** *155*

3. Cardiovascular System

3.1. **D/D of Cardiovascular Disorders** *177*
    Satish K Bhargava, Parul Garg
3.2. **Invisible Main Pulmonary Artery** *178*
    Satish K Bhargava, Parul Garg
3.3. **Pulmonary Arterial Hypertension** *180*
    Satish K Bhargava, Parul Garg
3.4. **Enlarged Left Ventricle (ELV)** *182*
    Satish K Bhargava, Parul Garg
3.5. **Enlarged Left Atrium** *185*
    Satish K Bhargava, Parul Garg

3.6.	**Dilatation of Pulmonary Trunk**	*188*
	Satish K Bhargava, Parul Garg	
3.7.	**Enlargement Aorta**	*191*
	Parul Garg, Satish K Bhargava	
3.8.	**Small Aorta**	*193*
	Parul Garg, Satish K Bhargava	
3.9.	**Enlarged Right Atrium**	*195*
	Parul Garg, Satish K Bhargava	
3.10.	**Enlarged Right Ventricle**	*196*
	Parul Garg, Satish K Bhargava	
3.11.	**Right Aortic Arch**	*199*
	Parul Garg, Satish K Bhargava	
3.12.	**Pulmonary Venous Hypertension**	*201*
	Parul Garg, Satish K Bhargava	
3.13.	**Enlarged Superior Vena Cava**	*204*
	Parul Garg, Satish K Bhargava	
3.14.	**Cardiac Calcifications**	*204*
	Parul Garg, Satish K Bhargava	
3.15.	**Cardiac Valve Calcifications**	*205*
	Parul Garg, Satish K Bhargava	
3.16.	**Situs**	*206*
	Parul Garg, Satish K Bhargava	
3.17.	**Cyanotic Heart Disease**	*207*
	Parul Garg, Satish K Bhargava	

4. Soft Tissue Lesions

Parul Garg, Satish K Bhargava, Shuchi Bhatt

4.1.	**D/D of Soft Tissue Lesions**	*209*
4.2.	**Soft Tissue Ossification**	*211*
4.3.	**Linear Calcification of Soft Tissues**	*214*
4.4.	**Parasitic Calcification**	*215*
4.5.	**Areas of Decreased Density**	*216*
4.6.	**Periarticular Soft Tissue Calcification**	*217*

| 4.7. | Generalized Calcinosis | *217* |
| 4.8. | Sheet Like Calcification in Soft Tissue | *221* |

5. Abdomen, Gastrointestinal Tract and Hepatobiliary System

5.1.	Dilated Esophagus	*222*
	Satish K Bhargava, Rajeev Chaturvedi	
5.2.	Esophageal Carcinoma	*229*
	Rajeev Chaturvedi, Satish K Bhargava	
5.3.	Thickened Mucosal Folds Esophagus and Stomach	*235*
	Ashish Verma, Shuchi Bhatt	
5.4.	Thickened Gastric Folds	*256*
	Rajul Rastogi, Satish K Bhargava	
5.5.	Thickened Duodenal Folds	*258*
	Rajul Rastogi, Satish K Bhargava	
5.6.	Massively Dilated Stomach	*260*
	Satish K Bhargava, Rajul Rastogi	
5.7.	Target Lesions in Stomach on Barium Studies	*261*
	Satish K Bhargava, Rajul Rastogi	
5.8.	Gas in Gastric Wall	*263*
	Satish K Bhargava, Rajul Rastogi	
5.9.	Cobblestone Duodenal Cap on Barium Study	*264*
	Satish K Bhargava, Rajul Rastogi	
5.10.	Dilated Duodenum/Obstruction of Duodenum	*265*
	Rajul Rastogi, Satish K Bhargava	
5.11.	Dilated Small Bowel/Jejunal and Ileal Obstruction	*266*
	Rajul Rastogi, Shuchi Bhatt	

5.12. **Strictures Small Bowel** *268*
Rajul Rastogi, Gopesh Mehrotra

5.13. **Small Intestinal Strictures** *269*
Anubhav Sarikwal, Gopesh Mehrotra

5.14. **Thickened Folds in Small Bowel** *275*
Rajul Rastogi, Shuchi Bhatt

5.15. **Thickened Small Bowel Folds with Gastric Abnormality** *277*
Rajul Rastogi, Satish K Bhargava

5.16. **Nodular Appearance of Small Bowel** *278*
Rajul Rastogi, Satish K Bhargava

5.17. **Malabsorption** *279*
Satish K Bhargava, Rajul Rastogi

5.18. **Malabsorption** *279*
Pushpender Gupta, Shuchi Bhatt

5.19. **Protein Losing Enteropathy** *292*
Satish K Bhargava, Rajul Rastogi

5.20. **Pathologic Lesions in Terminalileum** *293*
Satish K Bhargava, Rajul Rastogi

5.21. **Colonic Polyps** *295*
Satish K Bhargava, Rajul Rastogi

5.22. **Colonic Polyps** *298*
Gaurav Luthra, Gopesh Mehrotra

5.23. **Colonic Strictures/Narrowing** *302*
Rajul Rastogi, Satish K Bhargava

5.24. **Pneumatosis Intestinalis** *304*
Rajul Rastogi, Satish K Bhargava

5.25. **Megacolon in Adults** *305*
Rajul Rastogi, Satish K Bhargava

5.26. **Thumb Printing in Colon** *306*
Rajul Rastogi, Satish K Bhargava

5.27. **Aphthous Ulcers** *307*
Rajul Rastogi, Satish K Bhargava

5.28. **Anterior Indentation of Rectosigmoid Junction** *308*
Rajul Rastogi, Satish K Bhargava

5.29. **Widening/Enlargement of Presacral/Retrorectal Space** *309*
Rajul Rastogi, Satish K Bhargava

5.30. **Cystic Mesenteric Masses** *310*
Rajul Rastogi, Satish K Bhargava

5.31. **Nonvisualization of Gall Bladder on US** *311*
Rajul Rastogi, Sumeet Bhargava

5.32. **Gas in Biliary Tree** *312*
Rajul Rastogi, Satish K Bhargava

5.33. **Gas in Portal Venous** *313*
Rajul Rastogi, Satish K Bhargava

5.34. **Diffuse Hepatomegaly** *314*
Rajul Rastogi, Satish K Bhargava

5.35. **Hepatic Calcification** *315*
Rajul Rastogi, Satish K Bhargava

5.36. **Primary Hepatic Masses** *317*
Rajul Rastogi, Satish K Bhargava

5.37. **Neonatal Obstructive Jaundice** *318*
Rajul Rastogi, Satish K Bhargava

5.38. **Fetal/Neonatal Hepatic Calcification** *320*
Rajul Rastogi, Satish K Bhargava

5.39. **Diffuse Hypoechoic Liver** *321*
Rajul Rastogi, Satish K Bhargava

5.40. **Diffuse Hyperechoic Liver (Bright Liver)** *321*
Rajul Rastogi, Satish K Bhargava

5.41. **Focal Hyperechoic Hepatic Lesions** *322*
Rajul Rastogi, Satish K Bhargava

5.42. **Focal Hypoechoic Hepatic Lesions** *322*
Satish K Bhargava, Rajul Rastogi

5.43. **Periportal Hyperechogenicity** *323*
Satish K Bhargava, Rajul Rastogi

5.44. **Thickened Gall Bladder Wall** *323*
Satish K Bhargava, Rajul Rastogi

5.45. **Focal Hypodense Lesion on
NECT Liver** *324*
Satish K Bhargava, Rajul Rastogi

5.46. **Hyperperfusion Abnormalities of Liver** *325*
Satish K Bhargava, Rajul Rastogi

5.47. **Hepatic Tumors with Vascular Scar** *326*
Satish K Bhargava, Rajul Rastogi

5.48. **Diffuse Hypodense Liver on NECT** *326*
Satish K Bhargava, Rajul Rastogi

5.49. **Splenomegaly** *327*
Sumeet Bhargava

5.50. **Splenic Calcification** *328*
Rajul Rastogi, Satish K Bhargava

5.51. **Hyperechoic Splenic Lesions** *329*
Rajul Rastogi, Satish K Bhargava

5.52. **Focal Hypoattenuating Lesions
in Spleen** *329*
Rajul Rastogi, Satish K Bhargava

5.53. **Pancreatic Calcification** *330*
Rajul Rastogi, Satish K Bhargava

5.54. **Pancreatic Masses** *331*
*Gopesh Mehrotra, Pushpender Gupta,
Pardeep Kumar, Puneet Singh Kocher*

5.55. **Focal Pancreatic Masses** *338*
Rajul Rastogi, Satish K Bhargava

5.56. **Adrenal Mass** *339*
Rajul Rastogi, Satish K Bhargava

5.57. **Adrenal Calcification** *340*
Rajul Rastogi, Satish K Bhargava

5.58. **Extraluminal Intra-abdominal Gas** *342*
Rajul Rastogi, Satish K Bhargava

5.59. **Pneumoperitoneum** *343*
Anubhav Sarikwal, Shuchi Bhatt

5.60. **Pneumoperitoneum** *346*
Rajul Rastogi, Satish K Bhargava

5.61. **Gasless Abdomen** *347*
Rajul Rastogi, Satish K Bhargava

5.62. **Ascites** *349*
Rajul Rastogi, Satish K Bhargava

5.63. **Abdominal Mass in Neonates** *352*
Rajul Rastogi

5.64. **Abdominal Mass in Child** *353*
Satish K Bhargava, Rajul Rastogi

5.65. **Intestinal Obstruction in Neonates** *356*
Rajul Rastogi, Satish K Bhargava

5.66. **Abnormalities of Bowel Rotation** *357*
Rajul Rastogi, Satish K Bhargava

5.67. **Intra-abdominal Calcification
in Neonates** *358*
Rajul Rastogi, Satish K Bhargava

5.68. **Hematemesis** *358*
Satish K Bhargava, Rajul Rastogi

5.69. **Dysphagia in Adults** *359*
Satish K Bhargava, Rajul Rastogi

5.70. **Neonatal Dysphagia** *362*
Satish K Bhargava, Rajul Rastogi

5.71. **Pharyngeal/Esophageal Diverticula** *363*
Satish K Bhargava, Rajul Rastogi

5.72. **Esophagitis/Esophageal Ulcers** *365*
Rajul Rastogi, Satish K Bhargava

5.73. **Esophageal Strictures** *369*
Satish K Bhargava, Rajul Rastogi

5.74. **Tertiary Contractions in Esophagus** *371*
Rajul Rastogi, Satish K Bhargava

5.75. **Gastric Masses with Filling Defects** *372*
Satish K Bhargava, Rajul Rastogi

5.76. **Linitis Plastica** *376*
Anubhav Sarikwal, Gopesh Mehrotra

5.77. **Linitis Plastica** *380*
Rajul Rastogi, Shuchi Bhatt

5.78. **Gastrocolic Fistula** *381*
Rajul Rastogi, Satish K Bhargava

5.79. **Retroperitoneal Fibrosis** *381*
Sapna Maheshwari (Somani),
Shuchi Bhatt, Satish K Bhargava

5.80. **Mass of Ilio-psoas Compartment** *386*
Satish K Bhargava, Ashish Verma

5.81. **Anatomy of Liver, Bile Ducts, and**
Pancreas *390*
Sumeet Bhargava

5.82. **Inflammatory Bowel Disease** *406*
Gopesh Mehrotra, Pushpender Gupta,
Shuchi Bhatt, Pardeep Kumar

6. Skeletal System and Joints

6.1. **Abnormal Skeletal Maturation** *418*
Satish K Bhargava, Rajul Rastogi

6.2. **Short-limb Skeletal Dysplasia** *420*
Satish K Bhargava, Rajul Rastogi

6.3. **Short Spine Skeletal Dysplasia** *423*
Satish K Bhargava, Rajul Rastogi

6.4. **Lethal Neonatal Dysplasia** *424*
Satish K Bhargava, Rajul Rastogi

6.5. **Dumb-bell Shaped Long Bones** *426*
Satish K Bhargava, Rajul Rastogi

6.6. **Mucopolysaccharidosis and Mucolipidosis** *427*
Satish K Bhargava, Rajul Rastogi

6.7. **Mucolipidosis** *427*
Satish K Bhargava, Rajul Rastogi

6.8. **Generalized Osteosclerosis** *429*
Satish K Bhargava, Rajul Rastogi

6.9. **Sclerotic Bone Lesions** *433*
Satish K Bhargava, Rajul Rastogi

6.10. **Bone Sclerosis Associated with Periosteal Reaction** *437*
Satish K Bhargava, Rajul Rastogi

6.11. **Solitary Sclerotic Lesions with Lucent Center** *439*
Satish K Bhargava, Rajul Rastogi

6.12. **Coarse Trabecular Pattern of Bone** *439*
Satish K Bhargava, Rajul Rastogi

6.13. **Relationship of Metastatic Lesions to the Primary Tumors** *440*
Satish K Bhargava, Rajul Rastogi

6.14. **Childhood Tumors Metastasizing to Bone** *441*
Satish K Bhargava, Rajul Rastogi

6.15. **Bubbly Bone Lesions** *443*
Satish K Bhargava, Rajul Rastogi

6.16. **Primary Bone Tumors—Clinical Features, Site of Predilection, Radiologic Presentation** *446*
Satish K Bhargava, Rajul Rastogi

6.17. **Radiological Characteristic of Benign and Malignant Bone Lesions** *454*
Satish K Bhargava, Rajul Rastogi

6.18. **Subarticular Bone Lesions** *455*
Satish K Bhargava, Rajul Rastogi

6.19. **Osteolytic Defect in the Medulla** *462*
Satish K Bhargava, Rajul Rastogi

6.20. **Lucent Bone Lesions Containing Bone/Calcium** *464*
Satish K Bhargava, Rajul Rastogi

6.21. **Common Lytic Bone Lesions** *465*
Satish K Bhargava, Rajul Rastogi

6.22. **Locations of Some Common Neoplasms/Lesions** *466*
Satish K Bhargava, Rajul Rastogi

6.23. **Septated Bone Lesions** *467*
Satish K Bhargava, Rajul Rastogi

6.24. **Moth-Eaten Bone** *467*
Satish K Bhargava, Rajul Rastogi

6.25. **Osteopenia** *468*
Satish K Bhargava, Rajul Rastogi

6.26A. **Periosteal Reaction—Types and Conditions** *474*
Satish K Bhargava, Rajul Rastogi

6.26B. **Periosteal Reaction** *478*
Satish K Bhargava, Rajul Rastogi

6.27. **Periosteal Reaction in Childhood** *480*
Satish K Bhargava, Rajul Rastogi

6.28. **Hypertrophic Osteoarthropathy** *486*
Satish K Bhargava, Rajul Rastogi

6.29. **D/D of Skeletal Lesions in Nonaccidental Injury** *488*
Satish K Bhargava, Rajul Rastogi

6.30. **Bone Dysplasias Associated with Multiple Fractures** *489*
Satish K Bhargava, Rajul Rastogi

6.31. **Excessive Callus Formation** *489*
Rajul Rastogi, Satish K Bhargava

6.32. **Bone within Bone Appearance** *490*
Rajul Rastogi, Satish K Bhargava

6.33. **Fatigue Fractures** *490*
Rajul Rastogi, Satish K Bhargava

6.34. **Pseudoarthrosis** *492*
Rajul Rastogi, Satish K Bhargava

6.35. **Irregular/Stippled Epiphysis** *492*
Rajul Rastogi, Satish K Bhargava

6.36. **Avascular Necrosis/Osteonecrosis/
Aseptic Necrosis** *494*
Rajul Rastogi, Satish K Bhargava

6.37. **Solitary Radiolucent Metaphyseal
Bands** *496*
Rajul Rastogi, Satish K Bhargava

6.38. **Solitary Dense Metaphyseal Bands** *496*
Rajul Rastogi, Satish K Bhargava

6.39. **Alternating Radiolucent/Dense
Metaphyseal Bands** *497*
Rajul Rastogi, Satish K Bhargava

6.40. **Dense Vertical Metaphyseal Lines** *497*
Rajul Rastogi, Satish K Bhargava

6.41. **Frayed Metaphysis** *498*
Rajul Rastogi

6.42. **Cupping Metaphysis** *498*
Rajul Rastogi, Satish K Bhargava

6.43. **Erlenmeyer Flask Deformity** *498*
Rajul Rastogi, Satish K Bhargava

6.44. **Erosion of Medial Metaphyses of
Proximal Humerus** *499*
Rajul Rastogi, Satish K Bhargava

6.45. **Abnormality Related to Clavicles** *500*
Rajul Rastogi, Satish K Bhargava

6.46. **Rib Lesions** *501*
Rajul Rastogi, Satish K Bhargava

6.47. **Rib Notching** *502*
Rajul Rastogi, Satish K Bhargava

6.48. **Abnormal Shape, Size and Density of Ribs** *503*
Rajul Rastogi, Satish K Bhargava

6.49. **Madelung Deformity** *504*
Rajul Rastogi, Satish K Bhargava

6.50. **Carpal Fusions** *505*
Rajul Rastogi, Satish K Bhargava

6.51. **Abnormal Digits** *506*
Rajul Rastogi, Satish K Bhargava

6.52. **Abnormal Thumb** *507*
Rajul Rastogi, Satish K Bhargava

6.53. **Lytic Lesions in Digits** *508*
Rajul Rastogi, Satish K Bhargava

6.54. **Acro-Osteal Changes** *509*
Rajul Rastogi, Satish K Bhargava

6.55. **Monoarthritis** *512*
Rajul Rastogi, Satish K Bhargava

6.56. **Arthritis with Periostitis** *513*
Rajul Rastogi, Satish K Bhargava

6.57. **Arthritis with Demineralization** *513*
Rajul Rastogi, Satish K Bhargava

6.58. **Arthritis without Demineralization** *513*
Rajul Rastogi, Satish K Bhargava

6.59. **Arthritis with Preserved/Widened Joint Space** *514*
Rajul Rastogi, Satish K Bhargava

6.60. **Enlarged Femoral Intercondylar Notch** *515*
Rajul Rastogi, Satish K Bhargava

6.61. **Plantar Calcaneal Spur** *516*
Rajul Rastogi, Satish K Bhargava

6.62. **Chondrocalcinosis** *516*
Rajul Rastogi, Satish K Bhargava

6.63. **Ankylosis of Interphalangeal Joints** *517*
Rajul Rastogi, Satish K Bhargava

6.64. **Enthesiopathy** *517*
Rajul Rastogi, Satish K Bhargava

6.65. **Sacroiliitis** *518*
Rajul Rastogi, Satish K Bhargava

6.66. **Protrusio Acetabuli** *519*
Rajul Rastogi, Satish K Bhargava

6.67. **Widening of Symphysis Pubis** *520*
Rajul Rastogi, Satish K Bhargava

6.68. **Fusion of Symphysis Pubis** *521*
Rajul Rastogi, Satish K Bhargava

6.69. **Radiographic Findings in Degenerative, Inflammatory and Neuropathic Arthritis** *522*
Rajul Rastogi, Satish K Bhargava

6.70. **Comparative Features of Seronegative Spondyloarthritides** *523*
Rajul Rastogi, Satish K Bhargava

6.71. **Dwarfism** *524*
Parul Garg, Satish K Bhargava

6.72. **Sclerotic Lesions of Bone** *531*
Ashish Verma

6.73. **Lytic Lesion in Bone** *543*
Sapna Maheshwari (Somani), Shuchi Bhatt

6.74. **Generalized Osteoporosis** *552*
Parul Garg, Satish K Bhargava

6.75. **Solitary Dense Vertebra** *561*
Pushpender Gupta, Gopesh Mehrotra

6.76. **Acro-Osteolysis** *564*
Vinita Rathi, Sarika Jain

6.77. **Sacroiliitis** *570*
Gopesh Mehrotra,
Sapna Maheshwari (Somani)

6.78. **Bone Cyst** *576*
Satish K Bhargava, Anubhav Sarikwal

7. Urogenital System

7.1. **Neonatal and Adult Kidney—Differences** *594*
Sumeet Bhargava, Satish K Bhargava

7.2. **Smooth, Small Kidneys** *594*
Rajul Rastogi, Satish K Bhargava

7.3. **Small, Smooth Kidneys** *601*
Shuchi Bhatt, Ashish Verma

7.4. **Small Irregular Kidneys** *605*
Satish K Bhargava, Rajul Rastogi

7.5. **Large Smooth Kidneys** *610*
Gopesh Mehrotra, Rajeev Chaturvedi

7.6. **Bilateral Large Smooth Kidneys** *616*
Rajeev Chaturvedi, Satish K Bhargava

7.7. **Nonvisualization of a Kidney During Excretion Urography** *626*
Sarika Jain

7.8. **Dilated Calyx and Dilated Ureter** *631*
Pardeep Kumar, Shuchi Bhatt

7.9. **Gas in Urinary Tract** *641*
Parul Garg, Gopesh Mehrotra

7.10. **Loss of Renal Outline on Plain Film** *644*
Satish K Bhargava, Parul Garg

7.11. **Renovascular Hypertension** *648*
Sarika Jain, Gopesh Mehrotra

7.12. **Renal Calcification** *653*
  Satish K Bhargava, Parul Garg

7.13. **Renal Mass** *659*
  Satish K Bhargava, Pushpender Gupta

7.14. **Cystic Diseases of Kidney** *675*
  Gaurav Luthra, Satish K Bhargava

7.15. **Carcinoma of Bladder** *686*
  Rajul Rastogi, Satish K Bhargava

7.16. **Bladder Outflow Obstruction** *690*
  Rajeev Chaturvedi, Shuchi Bhatt

7.17. **Testicular Tumors** *701*
  Rajeev Chaturvedi, Gopesh Mehrotra

7.18. **Seminal Vesicle Calcification** *708*
  Anubhav Sarikwal, Satish K Bhargava

7.19. **D/D of Abnormal Nephrogram** *711*
  Mamta Motla, Shuchi Bhatt

7.20. **Filling Defect in the Bladder** *712*
  Mamta Motla, Satish K Bhargava

7.21. **Carcinoma Prostate** *713*
  Satish K Bhargava, Anubhav Sarikwal

7.22. **The Prostate** *724*
  Ruchi Rastogi, Shuchi Bhatt

7.23. **D/D of Adrenal Mass** *735*
  Parul Garg, Satish K Bhargava

7.24. **Painless Hematuria** *741*
  Satish K Bhargava, Ashish Verma

8. Head, Neck and Spine

8.1. **Lucency in the Skull Vault—without Sclerosis** *749*
  Sapna Maheshwari (Somani)
  Satish K Bhargava

8.2. **Lucency in the Skull Vault—with Surrounding Sclerosis** *754*
Sapna Maheshwari (Somani), Satish K Bhargava

8.3. **Thickening of the Skull Vault** *756*
Vinita Rathi, Sarika Jain

8.4. **Generalized Increase in Density of Skull Vault** *760*
Sapna Maheshwari (Somani), Satish K Bhargava

8.5. **Localized Increase in Density of Skull Vault** *765*
Sapna Maheshwari (Somani), Satish K Bhargava

8.6. **Destruction of Petrous Bone (Apex)** *768*
Sapna Maheshwari (Somani), Satish K Bhargava

8.7. **Basilar Invagination** *771*
Sapna Maheshwari (Somani), Satish K Bhargava

8.8. **Hair on End Skull Vault** *774*
Sapna Maheshwari (Somani), Satish K Bhargava

8.9. **Multiple Wormian Bones** *778*
Sapna Maheshwari (Somani), Satish K Bhargava

8.10. **Posterior Fossa Cyst and Cyst Like Masses** *782*
Sapna Maheshwari (Somani), Satish K Bhargava

8.11. **Enlarged Sylvian Fissure/Middle Cranial Fossa of CSF Density** *785*
Sapna Maheshwari (Somani), Satish K Bhargava

8.12. **Skull Base and Cavernous Sinus** *788*
Sapna Maheshwari (Somani),
Satish K Bhargava

8.13. **Central Skull Base Lesions** *792*
Sapna Maheshwari (Somani),
Satish K Bhargava

8.14. **Cerebellopontine Angle Masses** *794*
Sapna Maheshwari (Somani),
Satish K Bhargava

8.15. **Major Apertures of the Skull Base** *801*
Sumeet Bhargava, Satish K Bhargava

8.16. **D/D Suprasellar Masses** *803*
Satish K Bhargava,
Sapna Maheshwari (Somani)

8.17. **Sellar and Suprasellar Masses** *810*
Satish K Bhargava,
Sapna Maheshwari (Somani)

8.18. **Expanded Pituitary Fossa** *819*
Satish K Bhargava,
Sapna Maheshwari (Somani)

8.19. **Ring Enhancing Lesion on CECT** *824*
Satish K Bhargava,
Sapna Maheshwari (Somani)

8.20. **Superior Orbital Fissure Enlargement** *828*
Satish K Bhargava,
Sapna Maheshwari (Somani)

8.21. **Temporal Bone Sclerosis** *838*
Satish K Bhargava,
Sapna Maheshwari (Somani)

8.22. **IV Disc Space Calcification** *844*
Satish K Bhargava,
Sapna Maheshwari (Somani)

8.23. **Ivory Vertebral Body** *847*
Satish K Bhargava,
Sapna Maheshwari (Somani)

8.24. **Atlanto Axial Subluxation** *850*
Satish K Bhargava,
Sapna Maheshwari (Somani)

8.25. **Posterior Scalloping of Vertebral Body** *851*
Satish K Bhargava,
Sapna Maheshwari (Somani)

8.26. **Anterior Scalloping of Vertebral Body** *854*
Satish K Bhargava,
Sapna Maheshwari (Somani)

8.27. **Anterior Vertebral Body Beaks** *857*
Satish K Bhargava,
Sapna Maheshwari (Somani)

8.28. **Block Vertebra** *860*
Satish K Bhargava,
Sapna Maheshwari (Somani)

8.29. **Enlarged Vertebral Body** *863*
Satish K Bhargava,
Sapna Maheshwari (Somani)

8.30. **Solitary Collapsed Vertebra** *866*
Satish K Bhargava,
Sapna Maheshwari (Somani)

8.31. **Multiple Collapsed Vertebral** *869*
Satish K Bhargava,
Sapna Maheshwari (Somani)

8.32. **Intra Spinal Mass** *871*
Satish K Bhargava,
Sapna Maheshwari (Somani)

8.33. **D/D of Posterior Fossa Cysts** *879*
Pardeep Kumar, Gopesh Mehrotra

8.34. **Enlarged Optic Foramen** *883*
Shashank Jain, Shuchi Bhatt

8.35. **Bare Orbit/Hypoplasia of Greater-Wing of Sphenoid** *886*
Sarika Jain, Gopesh Mehrotra

8.36. **Orbital Hyperostosis** *890*
Rajeev Chaturvedi, Satish K Bhargava

8.37. **Cephaloceles** *894*
Sarika Jain, Gopesh Mehrotra

8.38. **Pathological Intracranial Calcification** *896*
Sarika Jain

8.39. **J-Shaped Sella** *905*
Pardeep Kumar, Satish K Bhargava

8.40. **Cerebellar Malformations** *908*
Anubhav Sarikwal, Satish K Bhargava

8.41. **Demyelinating Disorders** *912*
Pushpender Gupta, Shuchi Bhatt

8.42. **Prevertebral Soft Tissue Thickening** *928*
Pardeep Kumar, Satish K Bhargava

8.43. **Nasopharyngeal Masses** *933*
Satish K Bhargava, Anubhav Sarikwal

8.44. **Laryngeal Masses** *939*
Rajul Rastogi, Satish K Bhargava

8.45. **Orbital Masses** *943*
Rajul Rastogi, Satish K Bhargava

8.46. **Intraorbital Calcifications** *954*
Satish K Bhargava, Rajeev Chaturvedi

8.47. **Inner Ear Masses** *959*
Satish K Bhargava, Ashish Verma, Shuchi Bhatt

8.48. **Middle Ear Masses** *965*
Rajul Rastogi, Satish K Bhargava

8.49. **External Acoustic Masses** *970*
Rajeev Chaturvedi, Satish K Bhargava

8.50. **Intramedullary Lesions** *975*
Satish K Bhargava, Pushpender Gupta

8.51. **Intradural Extramedullary Masses** *984*
Rajul Rastogi, Gopesh Mehrotra

8.52. **Extradural Extramedullary Masses** *991*
Pushpender Gupta, Satish K Bhargava

8.53. **D/D of Floating Teeth** *1000*
Ashish Verma, Satish K Bhargava

8.54. **Cysts of Jaw** *1005*
Sarika Jain, Vinita Rathi

8.55. **Loss of Lamina Dura of Teeth** *1010*
Rajul Rastogi, Satish K Bhargava

8.56. **Opaque Maxillary Antrum** *1016*
Rajul Rastogi, Gopesh Mehrotra

8.57. **Thyroid Lesions** *1019*
Satish K Bhargava, Pushpender Gupta

9. Obstetrics and Gynecology

9.1. **D/D Between Blighted Ovum and Pseudogestation of Ectopic Pregnancy** *1038*
OP Sharma

9.2. **D/D Between Ectopic Pregnancy, Abortion in Progress (Early Gestation) Nabothian Cysts** *1039*
OP Sharma

9.3. **DD Between Partial Mole, IUFD with Hydropic Placental Degeneration, Twin Pregnancy (Mole and Fetus)** *1039*
OP Sharma

9.4. **D/D between Pelvic Masses, Extruded Fetal Parts with Uterine Perforation; Ectopic Pregnancy (Postpartum/Intervention)** *1040*
OP Sharma, Rajul Rastogi

9.5 **D/D of a Presacral Fetal Mass** *1041*
OP Sharma, Rajul Rastogi

9.6 **Fetal Neck Masses** *1042*
OP Sharma, Rajul Rastogi

9.7   **D/D of Fetal Renal Cystic Diseases**   *1044*
OP Sharma, Rajul Rastogi

9.8   **D/D of Various Fetal Anterior Abdominal Wall Defects**   *1045*
OP Sharma

9.9   **D/D between Renal Cyst and Hydronephrosis**   *1047*
OP Sharma, Rajul Rastogi

9.10   **D/D of Cystic Adnexal Masses**   *1047*
OP Sharma, Rajul Rastogi

9.11   **D/D of Benign and Malignant Ovarian Masses**   *1048*
OP Sharma

9.12   **D/D of Cystic Abdominal Masses**   *1048*
OP Sharma

9.13.   **D/D of Non-Gynecological Pelvic Masses**   *1050*
Ashish Verma, Satish K Bhargava

9.14   **D/D of Non-Ovarian Adnexal Mass**   *1050*
Ashish Verma, Satish K Bhargava

9.15   **D/D of Ovarian Masses**   *1051*
Ashish Verma, Satish K Bhargava

9.16   **Sonographic Classification of Adnexal Masses**   *1056*
Ashish Verma, Satish K Bhargava

9.17   **Absent Intrauterine Pregnancy with Positive Pregnancy Test**   *1058*
Ashish Verma, Satish K Bhargava, Rajul Rastogi

9.18   **D/D of Thickened Placenta**   *1060*
Ashish Verma, Satish K Bhargava Rajul Rastogi

9.19 **Ultrasound Signs of Chromosomal Abnormality** *1063*
Ashish Verma, Satish K Bhargava, Rajul Rastogi

9.20. **D/D of Enlarged Uterus** *1066*
Ashish Verma, Satish K Bhargava, Rajul Rastogi

9.21 **Cystic Structures in Fetal Abdomen** *1067*
Satish K Bhargava, Ashish Verma, Rajul Rastogi

9.22 **D/D of Fetal Hydrops** *1069*
Satish K Bhargava, Ashish Verma Rajul Rastogi

9.23 **D/D of Fetal Brain and Head Abnormalities** *1072*
Satish K Bhargava, Ashish Verma, Rajul Rastogi

9.24 **D/D of Brain and Hand Abnormality** *1075*
Satish K Bhargava, Ashish Verma Rajul Rastogi

9.25 **D/D of Thickened Endometrium** *1076*
Satish K Bhargava, Ashish Verma

9.26 **USG Signs of Abortions** *1078*
Satish K Bhargava, Ashish Verma

9.27 **D/D of Fetal Causes of Abnormality in Liquor Volume** *1080*
Satish K Bhargava, Ashish Verma

9.28 **D/D of Gas in Genital Tract** *1085*
Satish K Bhargava, Ashish Verma

9.29 **D/D of Fetal Intra-abdominal Calcification** *1087*
Satish K Bhargava, Ashish Verma

9.30 **D/D of Fetal Thoracic Abnormalities** *1090*
Satish K Bhargava, Ashish Verma

Index *1095*

1

Chest

Anatomy of Thoracic Inlet

- Thoracic inlet/root of neck is a narrow space that serves as a junction between the neck and the thorax.
- Boundaries are
  Anteriorly:
  Manubrium
  Posteriorly:
  First thoracic vertebra.
  Laterally:
  First ribs.
- This area is further delineated by Sibson's fascia which extends from the transverse process of C7 vertebra to the medial border of first rib.
- Plane of the thoracic inlet, is tilted downward anteriorly and laterally on either side being highest medially and posteriorly (Fig. 1.1.1).

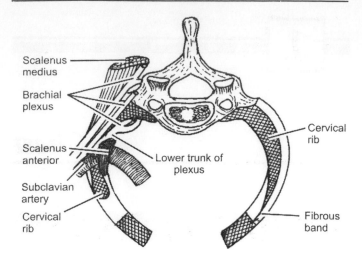

Fig. 1.1.1: Thoracic inlet as seen from above. Note presence of cervical ribs (gray area) on both sides. On right side of thorax, rib is almost complete and articulates anteriorly with first rib. On left side of thorax, rib is rudimentary but is continued forward as fibrous band that is attached to first costal cartilage. Note that cervical rib may exert pressure on lower trunk of brachial plexus and may kink subclavian artery.

Differential Diagnosis of Lesions at Thoracic Inlet

1. *Congenital lesions:*
   Lymphangioma
   Hemangioma
   Cervical extension of mediastinal thymus
   Thymic cyst
   Vascular anomalies.
2. *Inflammatory lesions:*
   Inflammatory adenopathy—TB, Mononucleosis, HIV infection, etc.
   Cervical abscess

Tubercular spondylitis with abscess
Retropharyngeal abscess with mediastinal extension.
3. *Benign tumors:*
   Lipoma
   Lipoblastoma
   Schwannomas and neurofibromas
   Fibromatosis.
4. *Malignant tumors:*
   Lymphoma
   Neuroblastoma
   Thyroid carcinoma
   Pancoast tumor
   Lymph node metastasis
   Liposarcoma
   Metastasis to thoracic vertebra and ribs.
5. *Traumatic lesions:*
   Pneumomediastinum
   Esophageal foreign body
   Cervicothoracic hematoma
6. *Miscellaneous:*
   Cervical rib
   – Thoracic outlet syndrome
   – Intrathoracic goiter.

Lymphangioma

Develops from congenital obstruction of lymphatic drainage.

Tends to surround and invade normal anatomical structures. Five percent occur in neck (posttriangle); 3-10% extend into mediastinum, asymptomatic and painless masses, 90% detected by 2 yrs of age.

Imaging: Multilocular transseptal masses of fluid attenuation, walls of septa-enhance (if history of surgery/infection).

Occasionally hemorrhagic areas and fluid-fluid levels are present.

Hemangiomas

Benign masses composed of proliferating endothelial cells characteristically increase in size and gradually involute. Most commonly occurs in 1st year of life.

Imaging: Calcified phleboliths within mass may be present. Enhance with adjacent vascular structure and fill with contrast over a short time.

MRI: Intermediate SI on T1WI and high SI on T2WI, fatty replacement may be present.

Cervical Extension of Mediastinal Thymus

- Due to incomplete mediastinal descent and manifests as solid midline thymus at thoracic inlet.
- Diagnosis is made on the basis of homogenous SI similar to that of the thymus with all MR imaging sequences or connection to the normally located thymus.

Thymic Cyst

- Caused by persistence or degeneration of the thymopharyngeal ducts.
- 50% of cervical thymic cysts are continuous with mediastinal masses. Most commonly on left side.

CT: Well marginated, unilocular/multilocular, attenuation is close to water.

MR: Decrease SI on T1WI and intermediate/high SI on T2WI.

SI on T1WI may increase if cyst contains blood/protein.

Then septa may be present.

When these cysts occur in neck they are located partially within the carotid sheath.

Most thymic cysts are congenital but they have also been reported with infection, neoplasms, radiation therapy, trauma and thoracotomy.

Vascular Anomalies

- Venous malformations and AVM are rarely seen in neck.
- Jugular vein thrombosis occurs after placement of a central catheter or in association with compressive lesion and is seen as luminal obstruction with thin rim of enhancement of the vasa vassorum.
- Cervical aortic arch—High positioned, usually right sided aortic arch. Occasionally associated with other cardiac and vascular anomalies, patient presents with respiratory problems/dysphagia.

  A pulsatile mass is found in the neck.

Cervical Abscess

- Cervical abscess seldom cross the thoracic inlet into the mediastinum.
- Infection in the visceral space may extend into the anterior mediastinum, whereas infection in the retropharyngeal and prevertebral spaces may extend into the posterior mediastinum.

  Imaging is required to distinguish cellulitis and suppuration adenopathy from abscess which require surgical treatment.

  In suppuration-focal hypoattenuating mass with an enhancing rim on CECT and a complete hypoechoic to anechoic mass with a variable thick rim of solid tissue is seen on ultrasound scans.

In fluid collection-SI on MR varies according to protein content, skin thickening and reticulated fat planes may be seen adjacent to the abscess margins in CT and MR.

Tuberculous Spondylitis with Abscess Formation

- Infection usually starts anteriorly in the vertebral body.
  In 90% cases at least 2 vertebra are affected.
  Skip lesions occur in 4% cases.
  Paraspinal abscess are present in 55-90% cases.
  Imaging features:
    - Vertebral body destruction.
    - Loss of disc space.
    - Paraspinal abscess
    - Prevertebral and epidural collections.
    - Paraspinal calcification.
  In neck—dysphagia, hoarseness and lymphadenopathy are accompanying features.

Retropharyngeal Abscess with Mediastinal Extension

Causes of Retropharyngeal Abscess

- Tonsillar infection
- Iatrogenic/traumatic
- Perforation of pharynx.

X-ray neck soft tissue: Retropharyngeal soft tissue thickening, Forward displacement of airway.

CT/MR: Retropharyngeal collection continuing into the post-mediastinum through the thoracic inlet.

Lipoma

- Most common cervical neoplasms of mesenchymal origin.
- Typically present as painless slowly growing masses, most commonly occurring in posterior triangle.

CT: Homogenous nonenhancing mass, isodense with subcutaneous fat, usually well-encapsulated lesions. (–10 to –100 HU).

MRI: SI similar to subcutaneous fat (increase on T1WI, intermediate SI on T2WI and loss of SI on fat suppressed MR images).

Lipoblastoma

Rare, usually encapsulated benign neoplasm of the embryonal fat. Composed of mature and immature fat and found almost exclusively in infants (90% <3 yrs) and children.

Most common site—Extremities → trunk → head → neck.

CT: Fat separated by septa of soft tissue which does not enhance.

MR: Heterogenous and have intermediate to high SI on T1WI according to the amount of immature fat. On fat suppressed images-areas of high SI is suggestive lipoblastoma.

Schwannomas and Neurofibromas

Common sites are—vagus nerve, ventral and cervical nerve roots, cervical sympathetic chains and brachial plexus.

Plexiform neurofibromas are pathognomic of Type I neurofibromatosis.

CT: Hypo to isoattenuating at CT. Contrast enhancement is more often seen with schwannomas.

MR: Low to intermediate SI on T1WI and intermediate to high SI on T2WI. Shows nonuniform enhancement. Plexiform neurofibromas usually involves cartilaginous soft tissue.

Malignant degeneration is seen in 15-30% cases.

Tumor arising in vagus nerve—displace the common carotid and internal carotid arteries. Anteromedially and the internal jugular vein posterolaterally.

Sympathetic chain tumors demonstrate a constant relationship with the longus colli muscle.

Brachial plexus tumors displace the anterior scalene muscle anteriorly.

Aggressive Fibromatosis

Characterized by proliferation of fibrous tissue with locally aggressive behavior and a tendency toward recurrence after resection.

Etiology is unknown.

Appearance on MR is often infiltrative and can suggest malignancy. Usually has decrease SI on T1 and T2WI which permits diagnosis.

Lymphoma

- Hodgkin's disease accounts for majority of lymphomatous anterior mediastinal masses and the neoplastic cells typically infiltrate the thymus.
  Thymic involvement is always accompanied by involvement of mediastinal lymph node.
- Lymphoma of neck involves cervical lymph node chain, Waldeyer's tonsillar ring and lymphoid tissue at the base of tongue. Such lymphoma is most often of the non-Hodgkin's type.
- Calcification and necrosis can be seen if lymphoma was treated previously.

Thyroid Carcinoma

- Papillary carcinoma accounts for 75-90% of all cases and is especially prevalent in younger patients.
- Medullary, follicular and anaplastic carcinoma accounts for 10-25%.
- Usually evaluated by ultrasound or scintigraphy. CT/MR is required to evaluate tumoral extent when malignant tumors are suspected.
- Difficult to distinguish benign from malignant nodule because the findings are nonspecific, however thyroid masses with infiltrating margins that obscure soft tissue plane and associated with adenopathy is suggestive of carcinoma.
- Cold' nodules on scintigraphy have a higher frequency of malignancy.
- MR is preferred as compared to CT because iodine administered during CT can cause iodine 131 therapy to be postponed for upto 6 months after removal of maximum tumor volume.

Neuroblastoma

- 10-15% neuroblastomas are located in posterior mediastinum. More than 5% neuroblastomas arise in neck.
- Arise from the renal cell rest blasts located in the adrenal gland or sympathetic chain.
- Osteochondritis and ipsilateral Horner's syndrome is related to lesion of cervical sympathetic nerve.
    - 50% neuroblastoma show calcification on X-ray.
    - 90% show calcification on CT.
    - MR imaging is the modality of choice for demonstrating the full extent of mass, chest wall invasion and extra-adrenal intraspinal involvement.

Metastatic Lymph Nodes

Head and neck squamous cell Ca	Renal cell Ca
Breast Ca.	Seminoma
Melanomas	Mucinous adeno Ca of GIT
Neuroblastomas	Nasopharyngeal Ca
Rhabdomyosarcomas	Thyroid Ca
Small cell Ca of lung	Ovarian and prostate Ca

Lymph nodes involved are deep cervical lymph node along internal jugular vein, supraclavicular lymph node, scalene nodes, highest lymph node in superior mediastinum.

Pancoast Tumor

- Pancoast syndrome consists of a constillation of signs and symptoms that include shoulder and arm pain in the distribution of C8, T1 and T2 nerve roots, Horner's syndrome and atrophy of hand muscle.
- This is caused by tumor in lung apex (Squamous cell carcinoma) which is causing invasion of the chest wall, and prevertebral sympathetic chain or the inferior or stellate ganglion.
- A Pancoast tumor should be ruled out if—unilateral pleural thickening or asymmetric thickening. > 5mm is noted on chest X-ray.

Metastases: (to rib and thoracic vertebra).

Usually has a mixed pattern:Breast/lung.

Blastic—Prostate.

Lytic—Thyroid, kidney.

Vertebra—Pedicles and vertebral body is involved.

Ribs—Lesions early recognized when rib is expanded.

Pneumomediastinum

Air can travel from the mediastinum along the fascial planes to the neck; subcutaneous tissue and chest wall.

Most common cause in children: are asthma, aspiration of foreign body, trauma.

Esophageal—foreign body granuloma.

- Most commonly seen in infants and children.
- Most common site of retention is the upper esophagus at the thoracic inlet.
- Long standing foreign body produces a granulomatous tissue reaction that manifests as mass.
- Mediastinites and abscess can be seen in this region as a complication of foreign body perforation.

Cervicothoracic Hematoma

Causes

Trauma
Faulty placement of central catheter.
Hematomas are usually transspatial lesion

CT

Hyperdense in acute phase
Hypodense in chronic phase
and on MR SI varies depending on the phase.

Cervical Rib

Seen in 1% of population.
Symptomatic in 10%
Unilateral in 50-80%
Cervical ribs vary in length and may be connected to the first rib by a fibrous band.

Cervical rib may affect the brachial plexus in one of two ways.

a. May narrow the space between the posterior aspect of 1st rib and anterior scalene muscle through which the nerve and subclavian artery passes.

Or

b. Cervical rib may be situated such that a portion of the brachial plexus must pass over it thereby stretching the lower trunks. Results in cervical rib syndrome—Sensory symptoms usually antedate motor involvement and occur along the ulnar border of forearm and hand. Muscle wasting of Thenar eminence.

Thoracic Outlet Syndrome

Because of compression of subclavian artery and C8/T1 nerve.

Usual Causes

- Cervical rib
- Elongated transverse process of C7.
- Fibrous band extending from transverse process of C7 to first rib.
- Low set shoulder gurdle.
- Pancoast tumor.

Intrathoracic Goiter

Characterized
- Continuity with cervical thyroid gland.
- Marked enhancement on CECT
- Well-defined margins
- Inhomogenity
- Focal calcification.

Flow Chart 1.1.1

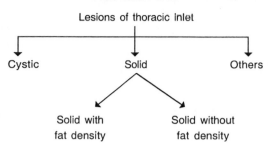

CYSTIC

Lymphangioma

Detected by 2 yrs of age, seen to extend from posterior triangle multilocular cystic mass.

Thymic Cyst

Unilocular/multilocular cystic mass seen in continuation with thymus.

Cervical Abscess

Hypodense collection with enhancing rim with adjacent reticulated fat plane.

Potts Spine with Abscess

Vertebral body destruction with loss of IVD space with adjacent collection and calcification.

SOLID WITH FAT DENSITY

Lipoma

- Painless progressive mass, well-encapsulated isointense to fat.

Liposarcoma

- Fast growing; Adults.
- Soft tissue admixed with fat.

Lipoblastoma

- 90% <3 yrs.
- Areas of increase SI on T2WI
- Fat separated by septa.

SOLID WITHOUT FAT

Schwannoma and Neurofibroma

- Plexiform neurofibroma associated with neurofibroma.

Neuroblastoma

- Arises from sympathetic chain
- Children
- Calcification present in 90%
- Horner's syndrome.

Thyroid Carcinoma

- Mass is contiguous with thyroid and has infiltrating margins and obscures soft tissue plane.

Pancoast Tumor

Mass lesion in lung apex with destruction of 1st rib.
- Patient presents with Pancoast syndrome.

Metastatic Lymph Node Mass

Primary lesion can be localized.

Others

Hemangioma

Compressible mass lesion, multiple small cystic spaces, phlebolith is present, vascular enhancement is present.

Cervical Rib

Extra rib is seen to arise from transverse process of C7.

1.2 MEDIASTINAL MASSES	
Common	*Rare*

Anterior

1. • Tortuous innominate artery	• Innominate artery aneurysm
• Lymph node	Parathyroid adenoma
• Retrosternal goiter	Lymphangioma
• Fat deposition	
2. • Lymph node enlargement	• Sternal mass
	• Lipoma
• Aneurysm of ascending aorta	• Hemangioma
• Thymoma	
• Teratoma	
3. • Epicardial fat pad	• Morgagni hernia
• Diaphragmatic hump	
• Pleuropericardial cyst	

Middle

4. • Lymph node enlargement	• Tracheal lesion
• Aortic arch aneurysm	• Cardiac tumor
enlarged pulmonary artery	
• Dilatation of SVC	
• Bronchogenic cyst	

Posterior

5. • Neurogenic tumor	
Pharyngoesophageal pouch	

Contd...

	Common	Rare
6.	• Aneurysm of descending aorta	• Neurenteric cyst
	• Esophageal dilatation	• Pancreatic pseudocyst
	• Azygous dilatation	• Sequestrated lung
	• Hiatus hernia	
7.	• Neurogenic tumor	• Bochdalek hernia
	• Paravertebral mass	• Extramedullary hemopoiesis

Mediastinum

Anterior Mediastinal Masses

Thyroid Tumor:-

1. Nontoxic enlargement of the gland
2. Thyrotoxicosis
3. CA thyroid
4. Hashimoto's disease

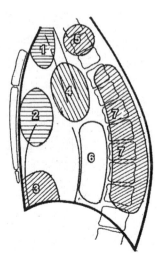

Fig. 1.2.1: Typical sites of the common and rare mediastinal masses

	Nontoxic enlargement of thyroid	*Thyrotoxicosis*	*CA thyroid*	*Hashimoto's disease*
A. Vocal cord involvement	–	–	+	–
B. SVC compression	–	–	+	–
C. Calcification	+/–	–	+/–	–
D. Rapid increase in size	hemo-rrhage cyst	-do-	++	–
E. Symptom severity	+/–	Clinical manifestation	+	–
F. Orbital lesion	–	+	–	–

Thymic Tumors

Normal thymic shadow	: Triangular soft tissue mass which projects to one side of the mediastinum.
Prominent	: • On expiratory film. • Slightly rotated film.
Disappears	: • Severe neonatal infection. • After major surgery. • Use of steroids.

Commonest Tumors

1. Thymoma
    a. Benign
    b. Malignant 30%
2. Hyperplasia of the gland
3. Thymic cyst
4. Thymolipoma
5. Lymphoma
6. Germ cell tumor
7. Carcinoids

Flow Chart 1.2.1

	Thymoma a. benign b. Malignant (30%)	Hyperplasia of the gland	Thymic cyst	Thymo-lipoma	Lymphoma	Germ cell tumors	Carcinoids
A. Asymptomatic	+/-	+/-	+	+	+/-	+/-	-
B. Associated with myasthenia gravis	+	+	-	-	-	-	+
C. Associated with thyrotoxicosis	-	+	-			-	-
• Addison's disease							
• Acromegaly							
• SLE							
• Rheumatoid arthritis							
D. Associated with Cushing syndrome, HPT	-	-	-	-	-	-	+
E. Calcification	Peripheral or rim like	-	-	-	Postchemotherapy	Large nodular Calcifica-tion (more)	-
F. Radiographic density	Soft tissue with calcification	ST	ST	Fat (Low)	-	Calcifica-tion (more)	-
G. Alters shape on respiration	-	-	-	+	-	-	-

Teratodermoid Tumors

- Dermoid cyst
- Teratoma
  - Benign
  - Malignant
- All arise from primitive germ cell nests in the urogenital ridge.
- Dermoid cyst contains mainly ectodermal tissues.
- Solid teratoma contains tissues of ectodermal, mesodermal and endodermal origin.

Dermoid cyst appears as a round or oval soft tissue mass, which may show peripheral rim or central nodular calcification. A fat fluid level or a rudimentary tooth is diagnostic radiological sign. Teratoma appears as a lobulated soft tissue mass which on CT shows a mass of mixed attenuation containing soft tissue, cyst fluid, fat, calcification or bone.

PLEUROPERICARDIAL CYST

- Anterior mediastinal mass.
- 75% occur in right anterior cardiophrenic angle.
- Cysts have thin walls, which contain clear fluid.
- These changes shape with respiration.

D/D OF SOFT TISSUE LESIONS IN RIGHT ANTERIOR CARDIOPHRENIC ANGLE

(See Flow Chart next page).

Morgagni Hernia

- Persistent developmental defect in the diaphragm anteriorly.
- Anterior mediastinal mass.
- May contain omentum or transverse colon.

Flow Chart 1.2.2

	Change shape with respiration	Density	Content	Separate from pericardium	Silhouette sign
A. Pleuroperi-cardial cyst	+	Soft tissue	Fluid	+	+
B. Epicardial fat pad	–	Fatty	Fat	+	+
C. Partial eventration of right hemi-diaphragm	+	Soft tissue	Diaphragm contour	+	–
D. Right middle lobe pathology	–	Soft tissue	Lung	+	+
E. Morgagni hernia	–	Fat if Omentum +	Omentum	+	+
F. Right atrial tumor	–	Soft tissue	Soft tissue	+	–
G. Pericardial lesion	–	-do-	Soft tissue fluid	–	+

- Appears as a soft tissue mass
- Containing either gas or air-fluid level or fat.
- Diagnosis is confirmed by barium meal and follow through or barium enema.

MIDDLE MEDIASTINAL MASSES

Lymph Node Enlargement

Metastatic

- Intrathoracic
  - Bronchial CA
  - Esophageal CA
- Extrathoracic
  - Breast, renal
    Adrenal, Testicular
    Tumor of pharynx and larynx.
- Lymphoma
- Leukemia
- *Sarcoidosis*: Bilateral hilar masses with well-defined outline. These show egg shell calcification.
- Primary tuberculous infection produces an area of consolidation in one of the lobes with unilateral hilar mass and an associated pleural effusion.
- Low attenuation areas due to cyst formation or necrosis are seen in lymph nodes involved with Hodgkin's disease and metastatic testicular or squamous cell tumors. Particularly after treatment with radiotherapy or chemotherapy.

Aortic Aneurysm

These produce either widening of the mediastinum or a round or oval soft tissue mass in any part of the mediastinum with well-defined outline. Curvilinear or peripheral calcification may be due to syphilitic aortitis or atherosclerosis. May cause pressure erosion defect of the sternum or anterior scalloping of one or two vertebral bodies. The subintimal flap and false lumen of a dissecting aneurysm can be demonstrated by CT.

Tortuous Innominate Artery

It occurs in 20% of the elderly patients with hypertension and produces widening of the superior part of the mediastinum on the right without displacement of the trachea to the left.

Bronchogenic Cyst

- Middle or posterior mediastinal mass.
- Majority occur around the carina in the paratracheal, tracheobronchial or subcarinal region.
- Can alter in shape on respiration.
- Pericardial defect may occur in association.

Tracheal Tumors

Tracheal tumors include carcinoma, plasmacytoma. They narrow the tracheal lumen and appear as soft tissue mass.

POSTERIOR MEDIASTINAL MASSES

Neurogenic Tumors

Adults

Neurofibroma
Neurilemmoma.

Children

Neuroblastoma
These may be asymptomatic or may produce back pain and may even extend through an intervertebral foramen into the

spinal canal (dumb-bell tumors) to produce spinal cord compressions.

	Shape	*Calcification*	*Dumb-bell*
Neurofibroma	Rounded	+/−	+
Neurilemmoma	-do-	−	−
Neuroblastoma	elongated	Central spicules or peripheral rim	+

Involvement of the posterior ribs or adjacent thoracic vertebrae – produce ribs splaying, localized pressure erosion defect of one or two vertebral bodies and ribs notching.

HIATUS HERNIA

- Commonest cause of a mediastinal mass on a chest radiograph in an elderly patient. Soft tissue mass with an air-fluid level.
- Lies to the left of the midline.
- Contents could be liver, omentum and small intestine.

ESOPHAGEAL LESIONS

Present with dysphagia.

Pharyngoesophageal pouch: Soft tissue mass with an air-fluid level, lies in the midline, displaces trachea forwards.

Carcinoma/leiomyoma: Soft tissue mass with an air-fluid level, behind the heart.

Achalasia: Large soft tissue mass with air-fluid level with barium flowing in spurts. Pulmonary consolidation/Bronchiectasis may be present.

PARAVERTEBRAL LESIONS

Involves the thoracic vertebrae or intervertebral disk space.

They appear as an elongated or lobulated soft tissue mass with a well-defined outline.

D/D would be:

- Hematoma
- Pyogenic abscess
- Tubercular abscess
- Multiple myeloma
- Lymphoma
- Metastasis
- Extramedullary hematopoiesis.

Bochdalek Hernia

Persistent develop mental defect in the diaphragm posteriorly.

Occurs in the left hemidiaphragm.

Small hernias usually contain retroperitoneal fat, kidney or spleen, which appears as a soft tissue mass in the posterior costophrenic angle.

Larger hernias may contain jejunum, ileum and colon.

Neurenteric Cysts

Result due to partial or complete persistence of the neurenteric canal or its incomplete resorption include, gastrointestinal duplication, enteric cyst, neurenteric cyst, anterior meningocele and cysts of the canal.

Pancreatic Pseudocyst

- Posterior mediastinal mass.
- Round/oval soft tissue mass behind the heart.
- A left basal pleural effusion or atelectasis in the lower lobes may result.

- Extramedullary hemopoiesis.
  Appears as lobulated paravertebral soft tissue mass behind the heart.

1.3 SUPERIOR MEDIASTINAL MASSES—DIFFERENTIAL DIAGNOSIS

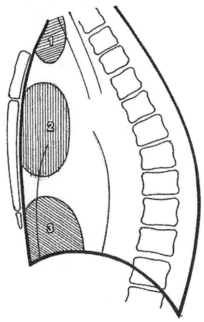

Fig. 1.3.1

Contents→
1. Trachea and esophagus
2. Muscles – sternohyoid, sternothyroid and lower ends of longus colli.

3. Anterior arch of aorta, brachiocephalic artery. ICC and left subclavian artery.
4. Veins—Right and left brachiocephalic vein, upper half of SVC.
5. Nerves—Vagus, phrenic, cardiac nerve, right laryngeal nerve.
6. Thymus
7. Thoracic duct
8. LNs-paratracheal, brachiocephalic, TB

Criteria for Superior Mediastinum Widening→

>8cm in the transverse diameter
>25% of the thoracic diameter at that level.
1. *Retrosternal goiter*: Less than 5% of enlarged thyroid in neck. Extend into mediastinum due to nontoxic enlargement, thyrotoxicosis, Carcinoma Hashimoto's disease.
   - Soft tissue swelling that moves on swallowing
   - Dysphagia, stridor if benign, vocal cord paralysis or SVC compression-malignancy
   - Patients present soft tissue mass in anterior part; extend down from the neck
   - Outline well-defined in mediastinum but fades off into neck
   - Displacement and compression of trachea to left, 20% are retrotracheal
   - Ca++ nodules, linear or crescent pattern
   - CT mass of mixed attenuation extending from one of lower pole of thyroid
   - Radionucleide scan 99 Tc per technetate on 123 I NaI
   - MRI – Diagnostic
2. Thymus – Normal thymus—most common in infants
   Most common in adult benign and malignant thymoma. Associated with myasthenia gravis, red cells aplasia or decreased granulocytes.

Plain X-ray chest –Ve

CT – Grossly asymmetrical lobular configuration.

– Homogenous with mild contrast enhancement

– Less commonly decreased attenuation areas-Hemorrhage/Necrosis/cyst Ca++-occasionally

MRI = T1 = Med. SI, T2 = > fat

Thymic Hyperplasia

Seen in 2/3rd of myasthenia gravis

CT = symmetric diffuse enlargement

MR = same signal as normal gland

Enlargement of thymus may also be seen in thymic cyst, thymolipoma, lymphoma, germ cell tumor and carcinoid.

3. Teratodermoid tumors/germ cell tumor – Extragonadal germ cell tumor located within or adjacent to thymus.

Most common germ cell tumor in sup. mediastinum is dermoid cyst and benign and malignant teratoma. CxR round or oval soft mass with well-defined border and may contain peripheral rim or central nodules of Ca++.

III CT fat fluid level, Ca++ well-defined border and soft tissue attenuation highly S/O germ cell tumor.

Malignancy – more solid component and aggressive features.

4. Lymph node enlargement

Widened mediastinum may have lobulated margins in case of LN enlargement.

Hodgkin/NonHodgkin disease – paratracheal and Tracheobronchial, asymmetrical widening of middle part of superior mediastinum

– Associated feature—parenchymal lung disease

– Ca++ in LN seen after irradiation

TB-U/L paratracheal lymph adenopathy without obvious mediastinum or pleural involvement seen in immunocompromised patients.

In adult/children area of consolidation/caseation

Fungal disease histoplasmosis, coccidioidomycosis, blastomycosis
- Enlargement of Hila or paratracheal LN
- Ca++ in healing histoplasmosis

Sarcoidosis—B/L lobulated hilar mass

Metastasis

Primary tumor is usually intrathoracic – Esophagus/ Bronchus

Benign— in adult
   papilloma
   chordoma - Ca^{++} Smooth, well-defined and
   Fibroma   < 2 cm in diameter
   Hemangioma

Mucus plug - decreased alternation, mixed with air and will change in position and resolve after coughing.

Malignant - sq cell Ca and adenoid cystic Ca_2. – Most common a smooth or irregular intraluminal mass with asymm. Narrowing of tracheal lumen is seen.

5. *Aneurysm and dissection of arch of aorta*—true, pseudo, post-traumatic atherosclerotic, post-traumatic elderly, fusiform.

Younger, contained by adventitia only, saccular

c.presentation→Asymptomatic

 Symptoms—enlarged compresses adjacent structure

C×R = Widening with or without Ca++

CT = Saccular and fusiform dilatation of segment of aorta. –>4cm; use short axis diameter

- Ca++ in aortic wall, peripheral
- Intraluminal thrombus-crescentic/circumferential
- Displacement of adjacent structure = Trachea, bronchus and pul artery, Sup. Vena cava, esophagus, bony erosion, growth rate 5.6 cm/year

Aortic dissection emergency situation:

Peak 7th–8th Decade

Most common predisposing condition is hypertension–congenital heart disease, coarctation, bicuspid AV

Intimal tear → blood enter into the aortic wall and creates a false and true lumen.

CXR wide mediastinum aortic contour displaced, intimal Ca++.

CT = Internal displacement or intimal Ca++

Visible internal flap increased in attenuation

High density thrombus in false lumen if actue hemorrhage.

CECT—Contrast filled true and false lumen separated by intimal flap

Delayed enhancement of false lumen because of slow flow.

MR—very well-demonstrate the intimal flap

Aortography—Highly accurate.

6. Dilatation of SVC and other veins

Dilatation of SVC seen in raised CVP

CCF

Tricuspid valve disease

Mediastinal mass

Constrictive pericarditis

TAPVD—Supracardiac variety. All the pulmonary veins open into large ascending vein on left side which is a remnant of embryonic. Left SVC. This connects into the left brachiocephalic vein which then passes into the right sided SVC and into the RA.

7. A pharyngoesophageal pouch/Zenker's diverticulum

CXR = Soft tissue mass in posterior part of superior mediastinum which contain an air-fluid level

Soft tissue mass lies in the midline and displaces the trachea forward.

Ba-esophagogram—Confirm the diagnoses.

Flow Chart 1.3.1

Widening of Sup. Mediastinum

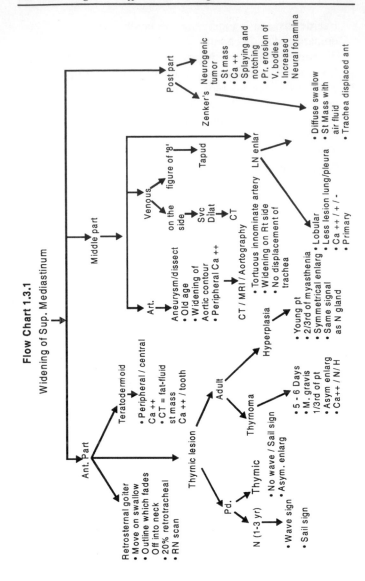

Widening of Sup. Mediastinum

Ant. Part

Retrosternal goiter
• Move on swallow
• Outline which fades
• Off into neck
• 20% retrotracheal
• RN scan

Teratodermoid
• Peripheral / central
• Ca ++
• CT = fat-fluid st mass
• Ca ++ / tooth

Thymic lesion

Adult

Hyperplasia
• Young pt
• 2/3rd of myasthenia
• Symmetrical enlarg
• Same signal as N gland

Thymoma
• 5 - 6 Days
• M. gravis
• 1/3rd of pt
• Asym enlarg
• Ca ++ / N / H

Pd.

Thymic
• No wave / Sail sign
• Asym. enlarg

N (1-3 yr)
• Wave sign
• Sail sign

Middle part

Art.

Aneurysm/dissect
• Old age
• Widening of Aortic contour
• Peripheral Ca ++

CT / MRI / Aortography
• Tortuous innominate artery
• Widening on Rt side
• No displacement of trachea

Venous

on the side
Svc Dilat
CT

figure of '8'
Tapud

LN enlar
• Lobular
• Less lesion lung/pleura
• Ca ++ / + / -
• Primary

Post part

Neurogenic tumor
• St mass
• Ca ++
• Splaying and notching
• Pr. erosion of V. bodies
• Increased Neural foramina

Zenker's
• Diffuse swallow
• St Mass with air fluid
• Trachea displaced ant

8. Fat deposition—superior mediastinum widening and epicardial fat pad seen in obese adult patient, Cushing disease, steroid therapy.

   CT = shows an excessive amount of mediastinal fat

9. Tracheal Mass—positive with nonspecific symptoms like cough, dyspnea, stridor, wheezing.

   CXR = Not very helpful.

   Benign – in adult

   Papilloma

   Chordoma Ca++ ⎫ Smooth well-defined and

   Fibroma ⎬ < 2cm in diameter

   Hemangioma ⎭

   Mucus plug-decrease attenuation, mixed with air and will change in position and resolve after coughing.

   Malignant-Sq cell Ca and adenoid cystic Ca = Most common

   A smooth or irregular intraluminal mass with asymmetric narrowing of tracheae lumen is seen

10. Neurogenic tumor.

    Adult—NF and schwannoma—peripheral intercostal nerve children—ganglioneuroma and neuroblastoma - which arise is thoracic sympathetic ganglia.

    CXR—A round or oval soft tissue mass in paravertebral gutter which usually project to one side of mediastinum.

    Neuroblastoma—central spicules or peripheral rim Ca^{++} splaying of post ribs.

    Pressure erosion, defect of vertebral-bodies

    Rib notching

    Enlargement of an intervertebral foramen

    CT = solid mass of soft tissue attemation, may contain Ca^{++} and involve the adjacent bone.

    MRI = intraspinal extension.

    MRI = Transaxial SE

    GRF/phase velocity mapping

1.4 DIFFERENTIAL DIAGNOSIS OF ANTERIOR MEDIASTINAL MASS

Anterior mediastinum lies anterior to anterior pericardium and trachea. For ease of differential diagnosis it can be divided into 3 areas.

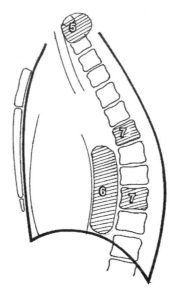

Fig. 1.4.1

Region 1	Region 2	Region 3
1. Tortuous innominate artery	• L N enlargement	• Epicardial fat pad
2. Lymph nodes	• Aneurysm of aorta	• Diaphragmatic hump
3. Retrosternal goiter	• Thymoma	• Pleuropericardial cyst
	• Teratodermoid tumors	

Contd...

Contd...

Region 1	Region 2	Region 3
4. Fat deposition		• Morgagni's hernia
5. Aneurysm of innominate artery	• Sternal mass Lipoma	
6. Parathyroid adenoma	• Hemangioma	
7. Cystic hygroma or lymphangioma		

Salient Features

Region 1

1. *Thyroid tumor (Retrosternal Goiter)*
   - Less than 5% goiters extened into the mediastinum.
   - Mostly females presenting with soft tissue swelling, dysphagia, stridor.
   - Chest X-ray shows oval soft tissue mass in superior part of anterior mediastinum fading off into neck.
   - Well-defined smooth or lobulated.
   - Central nodular, linear calcification.
   - Displacement and compression of trachea.
   - CT shows mass of mixed attenuation with cysts and calcifications, contiguous with one of the poles of thyroid.
2. *Lymph node enlargement.*
   May be due to lymphoma, metastasis or infection.
   - Widening of mediastinum on chest X-ray.
   - Lobulated soft tissue mass due to indentation by ribs.
   - Calcification may be present.
   - Lymphadenopathy else where in body.
   - CT shows discrete round or slightly irregular densities of various sizes +/- enhancement and necrosis.

3. *Fat deposition*
   - Cushing's disease, corticosteroid therapy.
   - Widening of superior mediastinum on chest X-ray.
   - CT shows excessive amount of mediastinal fat with density – 50-100 HU.

4. *Tortuous innominate artery or aneurysm*
   - Common in elderly.
   - Widening of superior mediastinum.
   - CT shows dilatation of innominate artery

5. *Lymphangioma/cystic hygroma*
   - Mainly in children.
   - Transilluminating soft tissue swelling in root of neck.
   - Chest X-ray shows: Oval soft tissue mass extending into neck.
   - Alters shape on respiration but does not displace trachea.
   - U/S and CT shows cystic septated mass.

6. *Parathyroid adenoma*
   - Hypercalcemia with hyperparathyroidism.
   - Usually small with normal chest X-ray.
   - Confirmed by radionuclide scan with 201 Tl chloride with increased activity.

Region 2

1. *Thymoma*: usually adults.
   - Can present with myasthenia gravis (10-15%)
   - Round oval and smooth or lobulated.
   - May have nodular or rim calcification.
   - CT shows mixed attenuation mass with calcification and cysts.

2. *Teratodermoid Tumor*: Commonly dermoid cysts and benign and malignant teratomas.

- Anterior mediastinal mass in young adult patient dyspnea, cough, chest pain.
- Round or oval soft tissue mass, projects to one side.
- Calcification especially rim, fragments of bone and teeth are diagnostic.
- Fat with fat-fluid level.

3. *Lymph node enlargement*
4. *Aneurysm of ascending aorta*
   - Widening of mediastinum or mediastinal mass
   - Well-defined outline
   - Peripheral rim of calcification.
   - Pulsatile mass on fluoroscopy.
   - Pressure erosion of sternum.
   - CT shows dilated aorta with blood of higher attenuation.
5. *Sternal mass*
   Metastasis, plasmocytoma, chondrosarcoma, osteomyelitis.
   - Soft tissue mass with sternal destruction.
   - Tumor new bone formation or lytic expansion of sternum.
   - Collection in anterior mediastinum with sternal destruction in osteomyelitis.
6. *Lipomas*
   - Round or oval soft tissue density mass with low density.
   - Alters shape on respiration.
   - CT shows solid mass of fatty attenuation.
7. *Hemangioma*
   Widening of mediastinum, round or oval soft tissue mass, phleboliths are diagnostic.

Region 3

1. *Epicardial fat pad*

- Especially in obesity.
- Triangular opacity in cardiophrenic angle.
- Less dense due to fat.
- CT shows fat density and is diagnostic.

2. *Diaphragmatic hump*
   - Localized eventration
   - Common on anteromedial portion of right dome.
   - Portion of liver extends into it.
   - Can be confirmed by U/S.

3. *Pleuropericardial cyst*
   - Spring water cyst or pericardial diverticulum.
   - 75% in Rt. anterior cardiophrenic angle.
   - Round/oval/triangular soft tissue mass.
   - Alters shape on respiration.
   - U/S or CT shows transsonic or cystic mass adjacent to pericardium with density 0-20 HU.

4. *Morgagni's hernia*
   - 90% in Rt anterior cardiophrenic angle.
   - Round or oval soft tissue mass.
   - Lower radiographic density than expected for its size.
   - Larger hernias contain transverse colon which appear as soft tissue mass with air-fluid level.
   - Diagnosis by u/s, confirmed by barium meal examination or CT.

ANTERIOR MEDIASTINAL MASS

Children

Congenital

- Normal thymus
  - Sail sign +ve
  - Wave sign +ve
  - Notch sign +ve

- Cystic hygroma
  - Cystic septated mass in neck and mediastinum
- Morgagni's hernia.
  - Soft tissue density in cardiophrenic angle.
- Neoplastic
- Soft tissue density mass.
  - With discrete L.N. +/- enhancement
  +/- calcification.
  - L.N elsewhere

Lymphoma

- With calcifications fat, tooth, cyst.
- Teratodermoid tumor.
- Inflammatory
  - Lymph nodes with rim enhancement.
  - Collection or abscess.

ANTERIOR MEDIASTINAL MASS

Adults

Widening of mediastinum on X-ray with lobulated soft tissue density mass on CT.

Lymphoma

Multiple discrete or matted L.N +/- enhancement, calcification, LN elsewhere.

Thymoma

Soft tissue calcification cysts
Associated with myasthenia gravis
Teratodermoid
Cyst calcification
Tooth, fat, young adult.

Thyroid

Mixed attenuation contiguous with thyroid pole.
Widening with fat density on CT
Epicardial fat pad
Lipoma
Widening with cystic density
Pleuropericardial cyst.
• Abscess

Vascular

• Aortic aneurysm
• Hemangioma
• Mass

1.5 MIDDLE MEDIASTINAL MASSES

Children

1. Lymph nodes
   – Neoplastic
   – Inflammatory
2. Foregut duplication cysts
   – Bronchogenic cyst
   – Esophageal duplication cyst
   – Neurenteric cyst
3. Cystic hygroma
4. Vascular
   – Vena cava enlargement

Adult

1. Lymph nodes
   – Neoplastic

- – Inflammatory
- = Inhalation disease
2. Primary tumors
   - – Carcinoma of trachea
   - – Bronchogenic carcinoma
   - – Esophageal tumor
     - – Leiomyoma, carcinoma
   - – Mesothelioma
3. Vascular lesions
   - – Aortic aneurysm
   - – Distended arteries or veins
4. Bronchogenic cyst.

LYMPH NODES

- 90% of masses in the middle mediastinum are malignant.
- Paratracheal, tracheobronchial, subcarinal and broncho-pulmonary groups. Middle mediastinal lymph node groups.
- Often asymptomatic, may produce cough, dyspnea and wt. loss.
- It appears as widening of right paratracheal stripe, bulge in aortopulmonary window, lateral displacement of azygo-esophageal line, lobulated widening of mediastinum and unilateral or bilateral lobulated hilar soft tissue mass.

Neoplastic

- Hodgkin's disease, non-Hodgkin's disease and the lymphatic leukemias produce middle mediastinal lymphadenopathy which is often unilateral.

Hodgkin's Disease

On CT, nodal involvement ranges from enlarged discrete lymph nodes to large conglomerate masses.

- Thymic involvement is seen in 70% of cases.
- Involvement of superior mediastinal lymph node was seen in 98% of patients with intrathoracic disease.

Non-Hodgkin's Disease

- Noncontiguous spread, more advanced disease, other sites involvement more common.
- Involvement of superior mediastinum in <75% cases.
  Parenchymal involvement of lungs also occurs and calcification occasionally develops in Hodgkin's disease after radiation.
- Fungal infections like histoplasmosis, coccidioidomycosis, blastomycosis produce hilar or paratracheal mediastinal adenopathy with or without pulmonary involvement.
- Other infective and inflammatory causes include infectious mononucleosis, measles, whooping cough, mycoplasma, adenóvirus and lung abscess.

Inhalation Disease

- Silicosis-egg-shell calcification
- Coal worker's pneumoconiosis
- Berylliosis

Foregut Duplication Cyst

Bronchogenic cyst—is a thin-walled foregut cyst lined by ciliated columnar epithelial cells of respiratory origin. Which contains viscid mucoid material.

- Usually seen as an incidental mass in a young adult.
- Rarely the cyst can become affected in children and rupture into the bronchial tree and hemorrhage into the cyst can also occur.
- Majority occur around carina in subcarinal region but can occur in right paratracheal or posterior mediastinum.
- Appear as well-defined round or oval soft tissue mass which can alter in shape on respiration.

Diagnosis is confirmed by CT or MRI. CT shows a thin-walled cyst containing fluid of either low attenuation (0 20 HU) or mucinous material containing cysts (20-50HU).

Esophageal Duplication Cyst

- Less common than bronchogenic cysts, usually larger and usually situated to the right of the midline extending into the posterior mediastinum.
- May be incidental finding or produce symptoms related to esophageal or respiratory compression. May contain ectopic gastric mucosa causing ulceration, hemorrhage or perforation.

Neurenteric Cyst

- Located in middle or posterior mediastinum
- Contain neural tissue and maintain a connection with spinal canal.
- Commonly right sided and associated with vertebral-body anomalies like hemivertebrae, butterfly vertebrae, and scoliosis which are usually superior to it.
  CT, MRI-for defining extent, relationship to other structure and defining intrinsic contents which may be watery or viscous.

Cystic Hygroma

- 5% cases extend into the mediastinum from the neck.
- Most present at birth.
- Cystic with septation and some solid components on all imaging modalities.

Thoracic Aortic Aneurysm

- Usually seen as an incidental mediastinal abnormality on a chest radiograph in elderly patients.

- It appears as either widening of the mediastinum or as a well-defined round or oval soft tissue mass in any part of the mediastinum often with curvilinear calcification in its wall.
- Displacement of rim of calcification—Aortic dissection.
- Pressure erosion of sternum or vertebral bodies.
- Diagnosis confirmed by CT or MRI which shows—aorta >4cm and containing contrast-enhanced blood in its lumen with surrounding mural thrombus of lower attenuation and calcification in its wall.

Other Arterial Abnormalities

- Dilatation of the main pulmonary artery due to pulmonary artery hypertension, pulmonary valve stenosis with post-stenotic dilatation or a pulmonary artery aneurysm also produces an apparent left hilar mass.
- A tortuous innominate artery produces widening of the superior mediastinum on the right and an aneurysm of the innominate or subclavian arteries produce widening of the mediastinum on the left often simulating a left hilar mass.

Venous Abnormality

- Dilated superior vena cava produces slight widening of the mediastinum on the right usually caused by congestive, cardiac failure, tricuspid valve disease, etc.
- A persistent left sided superior vena cava produces slight widening of the mediastinum on left side.
- A dilated azygous vein—oval soft tissue mass in the right tracheobronchial angle.

Metastasis

- Most mediastinal lymph node metastasis arise from a primary thoracic neoplasm, most commonly bronchogenic carcinoma.
- Generally the lymph node are on the same side.
- In patient with central sq. cell Carcinoma or small cell carcinoma the hilar/mediastinal mass may be the only abnormality on plain X-ray or CT.
- In patients with extrathoracic neoplasms, intrapulmonary metastasis are 10 times more common than nodal metastasis.
- Most common tumors associated with nodal metastasis are—
  - Genitourinary (renal and testicular)
  - Head and neck
  - Breast
  - Melanoma
- Isolated lymph node involvement seen in 60% cases.
- Hilar and right paratracheal are most common involved.

Inflammatory

Tuberculosis: Primary tuberculosis produces an area of consolidation in one lobe with unilateral enlargement of the bronchopulmonary, paratracheal, and subcarinal lymph node.
- Pleural effusion also occurs and complete calcification of the lymph node may develop as healing occurs.

Sarcoidosis

- Enlargement of the bronchopulmonary and paratracheal lymph node, which usually are bilateral.
- Enlarged lymph node in locations like subcarinal, anterior and posterior mediastinum may be seen particularly if CT is performed.

Flow Chart 1.5.1

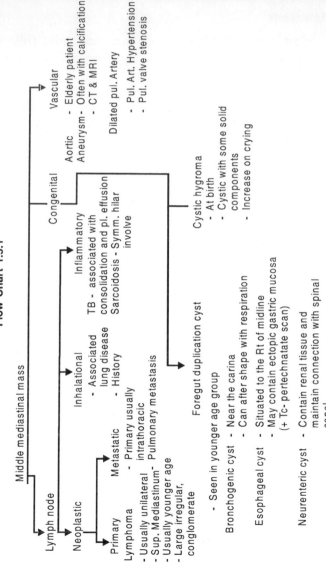

Middle mediastinal mass

Lymph node

Neoplastic

Primary

Lymphoma
- Usually unilateral
- Sup. Mediastinum
- Usually younger age
- Large irregular, conglomerate

Metastatic
- Primary usually intrathoracic
- Pulmonary metastasis

Inhalational
- Associated lung disease
- History

Inflammatory

TB - associated with consolidation and pl. effusion
Sarcoidosis - Symm. hilar involve

Congenital

Foregut duplication cyst
- Seen in younger age group

Bronchogenic cyst
- Near the carina
- Can after shape with respiration

Esophageal cyst
- Situated to the Rt of midline
- May contain ectopic gastric mucosa (+ Tc- perfechnatate scan)

Neurenteric cyst
- Contain renal tissue and maintain connection with spinal canal

Cystic hygroma
- At birth
- Cystic with some solid components
- Increase on crying

Vascular

Aortic Aneurysm
- Elderly patient
- Often with calcification
- CT & MRI

Dilated pul. Artery
- Pul. Art. Hypertension
- Pul. valve stenosis

1.6 D/D POSTERIOR MEDIASTINAL MASSES

Mediastinum

- Anterior—in front of the anterior pericardium and trachea
- Middle—within the pericardium including the trachea
- Posterior—lies behind the posterior pericardium and trachea

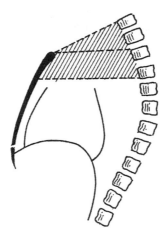

Fig. 1.6.1

DD's

Region 5	• Neurogenic tumors	
	• Pharyngoesophageal pouch	
6	• Hiatus hernia	• Neurenteric cyst
	• Aneurysm of descending aorta	• Sequestrated lung segment
	• Esophageal dilatation	

- Dilatation of azygous vein
7.
   - Neurogenic tumors
   - Paravertebral mass
   - Bochdalek's hernia
   - Extramedullary hemopoiesis

Neurenteric Cyst

- Partial or complete persistence of the neurenteric canal or its incomplete resorption.
  - Gastrointestinal reduplication
  - Enteric cysts
  - Neurenteric cysts
  - Anterior meningocele
  - Cysts of the cord
- Associated spinal anomalies
  - Block vertebra
  - Hemivertebra
  - Butterfly vertebrae
  - Spina bifida
- Usually present in infants.
- Respiratory distress
- Feeding difficulties
- Cysts—appears as oval or rounded soft tissue mass in posterior mediastinum.
- Anterior meningocele: diagnosed by CT–myelo, prone scan
- Esophageal duplication cyst – Barium swallow – ectopic gastric mucosa – Tc 99m positive

Pertechnetate Scan

- Neurenteric cyst can be diagnosis by USG/CT/MRI/— usually right sided

Dilated Azygous Vein

- Oval soft tissue mass in right tracheobronchial angle.
- Caused by – increased central venous pressure.
  - Superior or inferior vena cava obstruction
  - Portal hypertension
  - Congenital azygous continution of IVC
  - D/D- Enlarged azygous lymph node
  - Azygous vein – decrease in size – in erect position
  - On deep inspiration
  - During maneuver

Esophageal Lesions

- Pharyngoesophageal pouch or Zenker's diverticulum:
  - Round mass containing air-fluid level in the superior part of posterior mediastinum usually in the midline displaying the trachea anteriorly.
- Leiomyoma/Leiomyosarcoma – soft tissue mass
- Lower esophageal diverticulum – rounded mass with air-fluid level behind the heart
- *Dilated esophagus* – Widening of the posterior mediastinum on right side from thoracic inlet to diaphragm with lateral displacement of azygoesophageal line. Dilated esophagus displaces the trachea anteriorly.
- Air-fluid level with nonhomogenous mottled appearance of food mixed with air diagnosis confirmed by barium swallow or CT.

Paravertebral Lesions

- Traumatic wedge compression fracture of vertebral body with paraspinal hematoma – H/o trauma.
- Pyogenic/tubercular paravertebral abscess – narrowing of disk space with involvement of vertebral endplates.
- Smooth fusiform bilateral or unilateral soft tissue mass
- Metastasis – bone destruction with pathological fracture

- Extramedullary hematopoiesis – Lobulated mass in chronic hemolytic anemia
- Lymphoma

Bochdalek's Hernia

- Developmental defect in posterolateral part of left hemidiaphragm
- Contents of the hernial sac includes retroperitoneal fat, kidney, spleen, splenic flexure.

Large or small intestine, stomach, colon may also herniate
- Mediastinal shift/ipsilateral hypoplastic lung
- Thirteen pair of ribs may be associated.

Neurogenic Tumors

- Peripheral nerves

I. Nerve sheath tumor
- Neurofibroma
- Schwannoma or neurilemmoma
- Neurofibrosarcoma
- Malignant schwannoma

II. Ganglion cell tumors
- Ganglioneuroma benign (> 10 yr)
- Ganglioneuroblastoma (5-10 yr)
- Neuroblastoma (<5 yr) (Most malignant)

III. Paraganglionic nerve tissue tumors

  ↓ -(rarest)
- Chemodectomas
- Pheochromocytomas
  – 30% malignant
  – Childhood or young adult patient
  – Asymptomatic, back pain, spinal cord compression.

– Can be multiple in the setting of neurofibromatosis—association with lateral thoracic meningocele.

Radiological features – Well-defined oval soft tissue mass in paravertebral gutter

Nerve sheath tumors – Circular, calcification – rare.

Ganglion cell tumors – Elongated, central spicules or nodules of calcification, enlargement of intervertebral foramen, scoliosis.

Hiatus Hernia

- Usually an incidental findings in an elderly patient
- Often asymptomatic

Clinical features – Dyspnea, retrosternal chest pain, epigastric discomfort, iron deficiency anemia.

CXR – Round soft tissue mass with air or air-fluid level, behind heart usually to the left of midline

Flow Chart 1.6.1

Region 5

Neurogenic tumors → Well-defined oval to round soft tissue mass in paravertebral gutter

Pharyngo-esophageal pouch

Round mass containing air or air-fluid level in the superior part of posterior mediastinum in midline displacing trachea anteriorly

PNST
- In adults
- Elongated
- Calcification rare
- Extension through intervertebral foramen (dumb-bell tumor)

GCT
- In children
- Rounded
- Central spicules or nodules of calcification

Paraganglioma
Mass rare

Flow Chart 1.6.2
Region 6

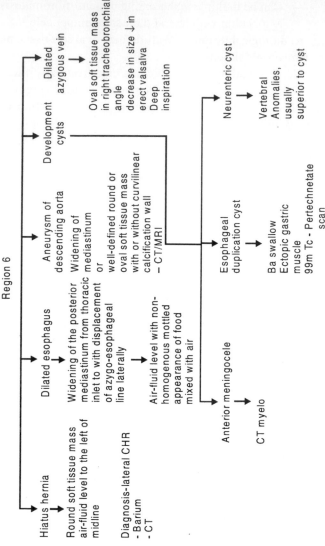

Hiatus hernia → Round soft tissue mass air-fluid level to the left of midline → Diagnosis-lateral CHR - Barium - CT

Dilated esophagus → Widening of the posterior mediastinum from thoracic inlet to with displacement of azygo-esophageal line laterally → Air-fluid level with non-homogenous mottled appearance of food mixed with air

Aneurysm of descending aorta → Widening of mediastinum or well-defined round or oval soft tissue mass with or without curvilinear calcification wall – CT/MRI

Development cysts

Dilated azygous vein → Oval soft tissue mass in right tracheobronchial angle decrease in size ↓ in erect valsalva Deep inspiration

Anterior meningocele → CT myelo

Esophageal duplication cyst → Ba swallow Ectopic gastric muscle 99m Tc - Pertechnetate scan

Neurenteric cyst → Vertebral Anomalies, usually superior to cyst

Flow Chart 1.6.3
Region 7

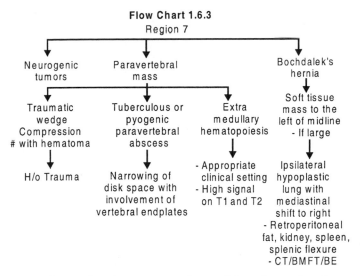

– Larger hernias may contain small intestine, colon, liver
– Diagnosis – confirmed by lateral chest X-ray, barium or CT.

1.7 CHEST WALL ABNORMALITIES

Congenital and developmental anomalies

- Pectus excavatum
- Pectus cavinatum
- Poland syndrome
- Cervical rib
- Cleidocranial dysplasia

Inflammatory and infectious

- Pyogenic
- TB

Tumors
Soft tissue tumors

- Lipomas
- Neurogenic tumors
- Hemangiomas
- Desmoid tumors
  – Lymphomas
- Sarcomas
  – Osseous tumors
- Osteochondroma
- Enchondroma

- Actinomycosis
- Aspergillosis

- Osteoblastoma
- Chondrosarcoma
- Myeloma
- Plasmacytoma
  Nonneoplastic osseous
- Fibrous dysplasia
- Paget's disease
- Giant cell tumor
- Aneurysmal bone cyst

PECTUS EXCAVATUM

- Most common congenital anomaly of sternum.
- Decrease prevertebral space—left hand deviation of heart with axial rotation
  - Increased parasternal soft tissue in right inferomedial hemithorax.
  - Lateral chest X-ray and CT quantify the severity.

PECTUS CAVINATUM

- Protrusion of sternum anterioly
- May be seen in isolation or with cyanotic congenital heart disease.

CERVICAL RIB

- Supernumerary rib that articulates with cervical type of transverse process.

CLEIDOCRANIAL DYSOSTOSIS

- Incomplete ossification of ribs with defective development of pubic bones, vertebral column and long bones.

POLAND SYNDROME

- Partial/total absence of greater pectoral muscle and ipsilateral syndactyly.
- Atrophy of ipsilateral fifth ribs, absence of smaller pectoral muscle, aplasia of ipsilateral breast/nipple, simian crease of affected extremity.

Inflammatory and Infectious Disease

- Primary infection rare and seen in diabetes mellitus, immunosuppression, trauma and i.v drug abuses.
- Secondary infection due to disease processes in lung or to pleurae, empyema more common.
- May produce parenchymal infection, pleural effusion, chest wall masses, rib destruction and even cutaneous fistula, air-fluid levels may be seen in soft tissues. Patient usually have febrile cause.

TUMORS OF CHEST WALL

- Primarily soft tissue tumors are rare.
- In adults, most common benign soft tissue neoplasm is lipoma and most common malignant neoplasms are fibrous sarcoma and MFH.

  In children, PNET(Askan) tumor, rhabdomyosarcoma and extraosseous Ewing's are most common malignant soft tissue tumors.
- Secondary tumors are more common in thoracic skeleton.
- Majority of osseous lesions are in ribs, large numbers are metastatic.
- Osteochondroma is most common benign tumor of cartilage bone. Most common malignant tumor is chondrosarcoma.

- Majority of lesions arising from sternum are malignant and represent chondrosarcoma most often.
- Lesions of thoracic vertebrae are invariably metastatic.
- Most common tumors to produce pattern of chest wall mass with bone destruction are metastases and small round cell tumors (multiple myeloma), Ewing's tumor and neuroblastoma. The differential diagnosis in adults is mets v/s myeloma, while in a child pattern in more s/o Ewing's tumor or metastatic neuroblastoma.

Radiologic Differentiation of Chest Wall Tumors

Benign

Imaging findings	*Tumor type*
• Fat attenuation/intensity	• Lipoma
• Calcification	
– Skeletal	
• Amorphous	• Fibrous dysplasia
• Cartilaginous apical cap	• Osteochondroma
– Extraskeleton, punctate	• Cavernous hemangioma
• Cortical thinning-fluid-fluid levels	• ABC or GCT
• Cortical expansion, sclerotic band	• Ossifying fibromyxoid tumor or chondromyxoid fibroma
• Rib erosion, well-defined contours, extraskeletal location	• Schwannoma or nonossifying fibroma
• Location at costochondral junction	• Osteochondroma
• Location in paravertebral region	• Ganglioneuroma or paraganglioma
• Location in shoulder region	• Spindle cell lipoma

Malignant

Imaging	*Tumor*
• Fat component	• Liposarcoma
• Calcification	
– Skeletal	
– Rings and arcs	• Chondrosarcoma
– Flocculent or stippled	
– Centrally dense	• Osteosarcoma
• Extraskeletal	
– Heterogeneous	• Ganglioneuroma or neuroblastoma
– Speckled	• Proximal type epitheliod sarcoma
• Diffuse osteolytic changes	• Myeloma
• Ill-defined mass	
– Eccentric growth, in children and young adults	• Ewing sarcoma
– Fluid-fluid levels and calcification in adolescents and adults	• Synovial sarcoma
– Chronic lymphedema	• Angiosarcoma
– Infiltrative growth	• Malignant lymphoma
• Nonspecific findings	• LMS, RMS, MFH,etc.

1.8 SUPERIOR RIB NOTCHING

CLASSIFICATION (Sargent et al)

1. *Normal*
2. *Disturbance of osteoblastic activity with decreased or deficient bone formation.*

- Paralytic poliomyelitis
- Collagen diseases
  - Scleroderma
  - Rheumatoid arthritis
  - Systemic lupus erythematosus (SLE)
- Exostosis
- Neurofibroma
- Surgery
- Osteogenesis imperfecta
- Coarctation of aorta
- Marfan's syndrome
- Radiation damage
- Quadriplegia

3. *Disturbance of osteoclastic activity with increased bone resorption.*
   - Hyperparathyroidism
   - Hypovitaminosis - D

4. *Idiopathic*

SALIENT FEATURES

Poliomyelitis

- Limb deformities and muscle atrophy seen particularly involving the pectoral muscles and shoulder girdle.
- Rib notching seen in chronic cases usually involving 3rd-9th ribs.
- Unilateral hypertransradiant hemithorax
- Scoliosis

Rheumatoid Arthritis

- More common in females.
- Symmetrical arthritis especially involving the MCP and PIP joints of hands and feet and wrist.

- Absence of lateral end of clavicle or pencil pointing may be seen.
- Caplan syndrome—Multiple nodules in lung
- Subcutaneous nodules.

Systemic Sclerosis

- Raynaud phenomenon
- Subcutaneous calcification-especially in the fingertips
- Esophageal abnormalities—dilatation, atonicity, poor or absent peristalsis
- Symmetric erosions on superior surface, predominate along the posterior aspect of 3-6 ribs.
- Terminal phalanx resorption
- Skin thickening.

SLE (Systemic Lupus Erythematosus)

- Mostly females, butterfly rash
- *Polyarthritis*: Bilateral and symmetrical involving the small joints of the hand, knee, wrist.
- MCP and PIP joint involvement—No erosions.
- Recurrent pleural effusion often with pleurisy resulting in elevation of a hemidiaphragm and plate atelectasis at base.

Osteochondroma

- 10-20 yrs of age
- Well-defined protrusion with the parent cortex and trabeculae continuous with that of parent bone. Cartilage cap.
- Most common distal femur, proximal tibia
- Lesions arising from ribs and scapulae cause rib notching
- Diaphyseal achalasia—Multiple lesions.

Neurofibromatosis

- One or more primary relatives with neurofibromas
- Café au lait spots
- Optic gliomas
- Typical bone lesions—sphenoid dysplasia
  (absent greater wing or lesser wing, absent posterolateral wall of orbit)
  Tibial pseudoarthrosis.
- Rib notching, twisted ribbon ribs, splaying of ribs.
- Cerebral and cerebellar calcification, heavy calcification of choroid plexus.

Marfan's Syndrome

- Tall stature, long slim limbs
- Arachnodactyly
- Joint laxity-dislocation of sternoclavicular joint and hip joint
- Scoliosis and kyphosis
- Pectus excavatum and cavinatum
- Aortic sinus dilatation and aortic regurgitation

Osteogenesis Imperfecta

- Osteoporotic, fragile bones often with deformities secondary to fractures and mechanical stress.
- Often in infant or child with blue sclerae.
- Flattened or biconcave vertebrae
- Wormian bones
- Rapid fracture healing with exuberant callus.
- Wavy, thin, ribbon-like ribs with notching.

Hyperparathyroidism

- Subperiosteal bone erosion—particularly affecting the radial side of middle phalanx of middle finger, medial proximal tibia, lateral end of clavicle.
- Diffuse cortical damage—Pepper-pot skull
- Brown tumors—mandible, ribs, pelvis
- Ribs
    - Characteristically show random notching
    - Coarse sclerosis of trabecular pattern of clavicles and ribs.

Flow Chart 1.8.1

Superior margin rib erosions

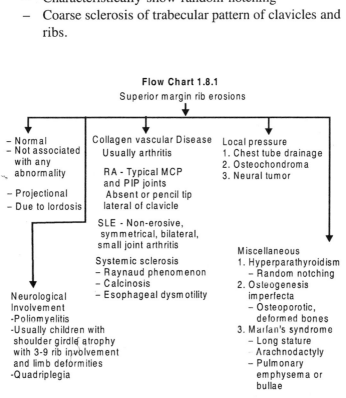

- Normal
- Not associated with any abnormality
- Projectional
- Due to lordosis

Collagen vascular Disease
Usually arthritis

RA - Typical MCP and PIP joints
Absent or pencil tip lateral of clavicle

SLE - Non-erosive, symmetrical, bilateral, small joint arthritis

Systemic sclerosis
- Raynaud phenomenon
- Calcinosis
- Esophageal dysmotility

Local pressure
1. Chest tube drainage
2. Osteochondroma
3. Neural tumor

Miscellaneous
1. Hyperparathyroidism
   - Random notching
2. Osteogenesis imperfecta
   - Osteoporotic, deformed bones
3. Marfan's syndrome
   - Long stature
   - Arachnodactyly
   - Pulmonary emphysema or bullae

Neurological Involvement
-Poliomyelitis
-Usually children with shoulder girdle atrophy with 3-9 rib involvement and limb deformities
-Quadriplegia

1.9 INFERIOR RIB NOTCHING

Unilateral
- Blalock-Taussig operation
  Subclavian artery occlusion
  Aortic coarctation left subclavian artery or anomalous right subclavian artery

Bilateral
- Aorta coarctation, occlusion, aortitis
  Subclavian
  – Takayasu disease, atheroma
  Pulmonary oligemia
  – Fallot's tetralogy
  – Pulmonary atresia
  – Stenosis
  Venous
  – SVC, IVC obstruction
  Shunts
  – Intercostal-pulmonary fistula
  – AV fistula
  Others
  – HPT
  – Neurogenic
  – Idiopathic

Pleural Effusion

	U/L, B/L	Biochemical derangement	Consolidation
Transudate			
Cardiac failure	B/L	+	–
Hepatic failure	B/L	+	–
Nephrotic syndrome	B/L	+	–
Meigs' syndrome	U/L	–	–

Contd...

Contd...

	U/L, B/L	Biochemical derangement	Consolidation
Exudate			
Infection	U/L, B/L	–	+
Malignancy	U/L, B/L	–	+
Pulmonary infarction	U/L	–	+
Collagen vascular disease	–	–	
Subphrenic Abscess	U/L	–	+
Pancreatitis	U/L	–	+
Hemorrhagic			
CA bronchus	U/L, B/L	–	+/–
Trauma	U/L	–	–
Pulmonary infarction	–	–	+
Bleeding disorders	–	–	–
Chylous			
Obstructive thoracic duct	–	–	–

Small Hilum

Apparent rotation, scoliosis	Vol. loss	Soft tissue	Consolidation
Unilateral			
Normal or left side			
Lobar collapse, lobectomy	+	–	–
Hypoplastic pulmonary artery	–	+	–
Macleod's syndrome	–	–	+
Unilateral pulmonary embolus	–	–	–
Bilateral			
Cyanotic congenital heart disease	–	–	–
Central pulmonary embolus	–	–	+

1.10 ELEVATION OF DIAPHRAGM

Unilateral

- Causes above the diaphragm
    - Phrenic nerve palsy
    - Pulmonary collapse
    - Pulmonary infarction
    - Pleural disease
    - Hemiplegia
        - Diaphragmatic cause
    - Eventration
        - Causes below the diaphragm
    - Gaseous distension of stomach/splenic flexure
    - Subphrenic inflammation of diaphragm
    - Scoliosis
    - Decubitus

Bilateral

- Poor inspiratory effort
- Obesity

    Above the diaphragm
    - B/L basal pulmonary collapse
    - Small lungs

    Below the diaphragm
    - Ascites
    - Pregnancy
    - Pneumoperitoneum
    - Hepatosplenomegaly
    - Intra-abdominal tumor
    - B/L subphrenic abscess

Unilaterally Elevated Diaphragm

Phrenic nerve palsy: Smooth hemidiaphragm, no movement on respiration. Paradoxical movement on snuffing.

Pleural disease: Especially old pleural disease, e.g. Hemothorax, empyema, tuberculosis, thoracotomy.

Splinting of the diaphragm: Associated with rib fracture or pleurisy due to any cause.

Hemiplegia: Associated with an upper motor neuron lesion.

Eventration: More common on the left side.
Heart is shifted to the contralateral side.
Paradoxical movement on snuffing.

Gaseous distension of stomach or splenic flexure: Only the left hemidiaphragm.

Subphrenic inflammatory disease: Subdiaphragmatic abscess or infection, inflammation

Scoliosis: Raised hemidiaphragm on the side of the concavity.

Decubitus: Raised hemidiaphragm is on the dependent side.

Bilaterally Elevated Diaphragm

- *Bilateral basal pulmonary collapse*: Which may be secondary to infarction or subphrenic abscess.
- Small lung due to fibrotic lung disease.
- Hepatosplenomegaly in patients of lymphoma, anemia and many infectious pathologies.
- Large intra-abdominal tumors either located in the midline or in any of the superior abdominal quadrant. Ascites in ovarian tumor can also cause this.

Pneumothorax

- Spontaneous
- Iatrogenic

- Traumatic
- Sec to mediastinal emphysema
- Sec to lung disease
  - Emphysema
  - Honeycomb lung
  - Pneumonia
  - Bronchopleural fistula
- Pneumoperitoneum

Pneumomediastinal

- Lung tear
- Perforation of esophagus, trachea, bronchus, perforation of hollow viscera

Pleural calcification	*Local pleural mass*
Old empyema	Loculated pleural effusion
Old hemothorax	Metastasis
Asbestosis inhalation	Malignant mesothelioma
Silicosis	Pleural fibroma
Talc exposure	

1.11 PNEUMOMEDIASTINUM

May be associated with pneumothorax and subcutaneous emphysema.

1. *Lung tear*: A sudden rise in the intra-alveolar pressure, often with airway narrowing, causes air to dissect through the interstitium to the hilum and then to the mediastinum.
   - *Spontaneous*: Following severe bout of cough or a severe strenous exercise.
   - *Asthma*: Usually not before 2 years of age.

- Diabetic ketoacidosis: Secondary to severe and protracted vomiting.
- Childbirth—due to repeated Valsalva maneuvers
- Artificial respiration
- Chest trauma
- Foreign body aspiration.

2. *Perforation of esophagus, trachea or bronchus*:
   - Spontaneous
   - Boerhaave's syndrome
   - Following severe and protracted vomiting
   - Trauma
   - Foreign body aspiration or inhalation

   Ruptured esophagus also produces left sided pneumo-thorax, hydropneumothorax.

3. Perforation of a hollow abdominal viscus with extension of gas via the retroperitoneum.

Right Sided Diaphragmatic Humps

At any site

- Collapse/consolidation of the adjacent lung
- Localized eventration
- Loculated effusion
- Subphrenic abscess
- Hepatic abscess
- Hydatid cyst
- Hepatic metastasis.

Medially

- Pericardial fat pad
- Aortic aneurysm.
- Pleuropericardial cyst
- Sequestrated segment

Anteriorly

- Morgagni's hernia

Posteriorly

- Bochdalek hernia.

1.12 LUNG TUMORS

Carcinoma: Approximately 50% of lung cancers arise centrally, i.e. in or proximal to segmental bronchi.

- Obstruction of lumen leads to collapse and often infection.
- Peripheral tumors appear as soft tissue nodules or irregular masses and invade the adjacent tissues. Signs of collapse and consolidation may occur.
- Peripheral tumors may arise in the scar. These mass lesions may present as hilar enlargement, airway obstruction, peripheral mass lesion, mediastinal involvement, pleural and bone involvement.

  Alveolar cell CA: Arises more peripherally, probably from the type II pneumocysts. It arises within the alveoli and produces areas of consolidation.

Metastasis

- *Hematogenous*: Breast, skeleton, urogenital
- *Lymphatic*: Less common, breast
- *Endobronchial spread*: Alveolar cell carcinoma

Metastasis is usually bilateral, affecting both lung equally, with basal predominance. They are often peripheral and may be subpleural.

Cavitatory Met

- Squamous cell CA
- Sarcoma

Calcifying Met

- Osteogenic sarcoma
- Chondrosarcoma
- Mucinous adenocarcinoma

Endobronchial Met

- Carcinoma kidney, breast
- Large bowel.

Lymphangitis Carcinoma

Commonest sites—Lung, breast, stomach pancreas, cervix, prostate.

It is usually bilateral, but lung and breast cancers may cause unilateral lymphangitis.

Hodgkin's/Non-Hodgkin's Lymphoma

Present as nodal enlargement, which is usually bilateral, asymmetric and involves anterior mediastinal glands. These may calcify following therapy. Pulmonary infiltration may appear as areas of consolidation or areas of miliary nodules. Pleural effusion may be present in 30% of cases.

Leukemia

Mediastinal lymph node enlargement and pleural effusion are the commonest radiologic abnormalities.

Sarcoma

Kaposi's sarcoma may appear as segmental or lobar consolidation.

Other primary pulmonary sarcomas include fibrosarcoma, leiomyosarcoma—which appear as solitary pulmonary masses, radiographically indistinguishable from a carcinoma of the lung.

Adenoma

Carcinoid account for approximately 90% of bronchial adenomas and adenoid cystic tumors for about 10%. These appear as well-circumscribed round or ovoid solitary nodules. On CT, calcification may be seen within the tumor.

Hamartoma

They are seen in childhood as solitary pulmonary nodule. Thirty percent of these show calcification, often with a characteristic 'popcorn' appearance.

Lung Abscess

Radiographically, an abscess may or may not be surrounded by consolidation. Appearance of an air-fluid level indicates that a communication with the airway has developed. It show thick irregular wall, which shows postcontrast enhancement.

Bronchiectasis

It is the irreversible dilatation of one or more bronchi and is usually the result of severe, recurrent and chronic infection. It is frequently basal but in tuberculosis and cystic fibrosis, it usually involve the upper zone. Dilated bronchi produce tramline shadows or ring shadows, and dilated, fluid filled bronchi may cause 'gloved friger' shadows.

Asthma

During an attack, the chest X-ray may show signs of hyperinflation, with the depression of the diaphragm and expansion of the retrosternal air space. The peripheral pulmonary vessels appear normal, but if the central pulmonary arteries are enlarged, the irreversible pulmonary arterial hypertension is probably present.

Chronic Bronchitis

Fifty percent of these patients may have normal chest X-ray. In patients, with a plain film abnormality, the signs are due to emphysema, superimposed infection or possibly bronchiectasis. 'Dirty chest' appearance is seen.

Emphysema

With emphysema, air trapping is present, the lung volumes increase, the diaphragm become flattened, and the retrosternal air space increases. The no. and size of the peripheral vessels decreases. Central pulmonary arteries may enlarge s/o corpulmonale.

Bronchiolitis

Results due to infection (often in childhood) or due to inhalation of toxic fumer, drug therapy and rheumatoid disease. Radiologically, the appearance are most frequently of hyperinflation of lungs and perihilar prominence and indistinctness.

1.13 HILAR ENLARGEMENT

Unilateral

	Egg shell calcification	Air broncho-gram	LN	Angio
Lymph Node				
Carcinoma	–	–	+	–
Lymphoma	–	+	+	–
Infective				
TB	–	–	+	–
Histoplasmosis	–	–	+	–
Coccidioidomycosis	–	–	+	–
Sarcoidosis	+	–	+	–
Pulmonary Artery				
Poststenotic dilatation	–	–	–	+
Pulmonary embolus	–	–	–	+
Aneurysm	+	–	–	+
Mediastinal mass—superimposed on a hilum				
	–	–	–	–
Perihilar pneumonia		+	+/–	–

Bilateral

	Symmetrical	Occupational	Lobulated
Idiopathic	+	–	+
Sarcoidosis			
Neoplastic			
Lymphoma	–		+
Lymphangitis carcinomatosis		–	–
Infective			
Viruses	–		–
Primary TB	+/–		+
Histoplasmosis	–	–	–
Coccidioidomycosis	–	–	–

Contd...

Contd...

	Symmetrical	Occupational	Lobulated
Vascular			
Pulmonary arterial hypertension	–	–	–
Immunological			
Extrinsic allergic alveolitis	–	+	–
Inhalation			
Silicosis			
Berylliosis	–	+	–

Unilateral Hilar Enlargement

Carcinoma bronchus: The hilar enlargement may be due to the tumor itself or due to the involved lymph nodes.

Lymphoma	:	Unilateral is very unusual.
	:	Anterior mediastinal nodes are also involved.
Infective	:	Due to the nodal enlargement
Poststenotic dilatation of the pulmonary artery	:	Usually on the left side.
Pulmonary embolus	:	Peripheral oligemia is characteristic
Aneurysm	:	In chronic pulmonary arterial hypertension. Calcification may also be present.
Mediastinal mass	:	Middle mediastinum masses may superimpose.

Perihilar pneumonia, ill-defined borders with presence of air bronchogram.

Bilateral Hilar Enlargement

Sarcoidosis	:	Symmetrical, lobulated. Associated bronchotracheal and paratracheal lymphadenopathy.

Lymphoma	:	Asymmetrical, but multiple sites
Infective	:	Viral mainly is children
		TB - B/L is rare
		Histoplasmosis pulmonary nodules (multiple) accompany.
Pulmonary arterial hypertension	:	B/L is rare
Peripheral oligemia is characteristic		
Silicosis	:	Symmetrical
		Pin point multiple pulmonary nodules are present.

Apical Shadows

	U/L, B/L	Ellis curve	Pleural outline seen	Rib destruc-tion	Symmetry
Pleural caps	U/L	–	–	–	+/–
Pleural fluid	U/L or B/L	+	–	–	+/–
Bullae	U/L	–	+	–	–
Pancoast tumor	U/L	–	–	+	–
Infections – TB	U/L or B/L	–	–	–	
Pneumothorax	U/L	–	+	–	–
Soft tissue	B/L	–	–	+	+

1.14 CALCIFICATION ON CHEST RADIOGRAPH

Intrapulmonary

Granuloma, infection
Chronic abscess
Tumor - Metastases
Hamartoma
AVM

Hematoma
Infarct
Broncholith
Alveolar microlithiasis
Idiopathic

Lymph Nodes

TB, histoplasmosis, sarcoidosis, silicosis

Pleural

TB, asbestosis, talcosis
Hemothorax, empyema

Mediastinal

Cardiac
Vascular
Tumors

Pulmonary Artery

Hypertension
Aneurysm
Thrombus

Chest Wall

Costal cartilage
   Breast
Bone tumor, callus
   Soft tissues

1.15 AIR-FLUID LEVELS ON CHEST X-RAY

Intrapulmonary	
Hydropneumothorax	Trauma
	Bronchopleural fistula
Esophageal	Pharyngeal pouch, diverticula
	Obstruction – tumor, achalasia
	esophagectomy
Mediastinal	Infections
	Perforation – esophageal
Pneumopericardium	Diagnostic, trauma
Chest wall	Infection
Diaphragm	Hernia, eventration, rupture

Cresent Sign

- Fungal ball
- Blood clot in tubercular cavity
- Bronchial adenoma, carcinoma
- Hamartoma
- Hydatid cyst
- Pulmonary infarct.

1.16A CAVITATING PULMONARY LESIONS

Infection

- Staphylococcus
- Klebsiella
- Tuberculosis
- Histoplasmosis
- Amebic
- Hydatid
- Fungal

Malignant

- Primary
- Secondary
- Lymphoma

Abscess

- Blood borne
- Aspiration

Pulmonary infarct
Pulmonary hematoma
Pneumoconiosis

Collagen Diseases

- Rheumatoid nodules
- Wegener's granulomatosis

Developmental

- Sequestrated segment
- Bronchogenic cyst
- Congenital cystic adenomatoid malformation

Sarcoidosis
Bullae, blebs
Pneumatocele
Traumatic lung cyst

1.16B MASS WITHIN CAVITY

1. Mycetoma - Aspergilloma
2. Tissue fragment from carcinoma
3. Necrotic lung within abscess

4. Disintegrating hydatid cyst
5. Intracavitatory blood clot.

	1	2	3	4	5
• Thick, irregular walled cavity	+	+	+	−	+
• Adjacent lung parenchymal reaction	+	+/−	+	+/−	+/−
• Clinical history	of infection	of wt. loss	Infection	Infection	+/−
• Mobile	+	+/−	+/−	+	+
• Contrast enhancement in CT of mass	+	+	−	+/−	−
• Calcification	−	+/−	−	−	+/− if chronic.

1.17 CAVITATING PULMONARY LESIONS

Causes

- Malignant
  - Primary
  - Secondary
  - Lymphoma
- Infections
  - Tuberculosis
  - Staphylococcus
  - Klebsiella
  - Amebic
  - Hydatid
  - Fungal

- Abscess
  - Aspiration
  - Blood borne
- Pulmonary infarct
- Hematoma
- Pneumoconiosis
  - Pulmonary massive fibrosis
  - Rheumatoid nodular
  - Collagen diseases
  - Wegener's granulomatosis
- Developmental
  Sequestration
  Bronchogenic cyst
  Congenital cystic adenomatoid malformation
- Sarcoidosis
- Bullae, blebs
- Traumatic lung cyst
- Pneumatocele

Carcinoma

Primary

Very frequently cavity nodules turn out to be malignant.

Mechanism

Obstruction of an artery
(Infection of a nodule)
- In 2-10%, especially peripheral upper lobe involvement
- Most cavities are thick-walled, irregular inner surface
- Thickness > 15 mm – 85-90% malignant
- Cavitation—Centric or eccentric
- Multiple cavitation
- More common in squamous cell carcinoma and then may be thin-walled.

Metastasis—Cavitation less than

- More common in upper lobe, may involve few nodules
- Thin or thick-walled
- Seen especially in squamous cell carcinoma—head and neck
     (Uncommon in adenocarcinoma—esp colon)
  Sarcoma—osteosarcoma

Hodgkin's Disease

- Thick or thin-walled
- Typically in an area of infiltration
- Hilar or mediastinal LN

Tuberculosis

- Thick-walled and smooth, sometimes fluid level
- Mainly affects upper lobes and apical segment of lower lobe
- Usually surrounded by consolidation and fibrosis
- Typical there is large cavity surrounded by smaller satellite cavities
- Cavity walls are lined by tuberculous granulation tissue
- Cavities traversed by fibrotic remnants of bronchi and vessels
- Rasmussen aneurysm

Staphylococcus Aureus

- Mostly children, multiple
- Thick-walled cavities with a ragged inner lining
- No lobar predilection
- Associated with effusion and empyema

Hydatid Cysts

- Complicated hydatid cyst
- Rupture into a bronchus-air cresent sign/air cap
- Water lily sign

Aspergillosis

- Any pulmonary cavity—TB, histoplasmosis, sarcoidosis
- Forms a ball which changes position, ball is seen to be mobile
- Almost always pleural thickening related to mycetoma
- Vascular granular tissue-bleeding may occur.

Abscess (Aspiration)

- Multiple or single
- Usually thick-walled
- Following aspiration
- Postsegment or apical segment-UL
- In sitting-right lower lobe

Pulmonary Infarct

(Infection—may be)

Primarily–
1. Septic embolus
Secondary to–
2. Initially sterile, infarct, infection
Tertiary to–
3. As aseptic cavitating infarct infected
   Aseptic cavitation is usually solitary and arises in a large area of consolidation after about 2 weeks.
- Cavity has scalloped inner margins and cross cavity band shadows/effusion.

Cystic Bronchiectasis

- Thin- walled. Lower lobes
- Air-fluid levels, peribronchial thickening and retained secretions
- Crowded vessels and retained secretions

Sequestered Lung

- Thin- or thick-walled
- 66% in left lower lobe, 33% in right lower lobe
- Air-fluid level, surrounding pneumonia

Wegener's Granulomatosis

- B/L and widely spread
- Nodules, cavitation in some nodules (1/3rd)
- Cavities are thick-walled, shaggy/irregular lining
- Become thinner with time
- After therapy may disappear

Rheumatoid Nodules

- Thick-walled with a smooth inner lining and well-defined
- Lower lobes and peripherally
- Become thinner with time

Progressive Massive Fibrosis

- Predominantly in mid and upper zone
- Begin peripherally and move centrally
- Nodule formation which cavitate into thick and irregular walled cavities in a background nodularity of pneumoconiosis.

Sarcoidosis

- In early disease, necrosis of coalescent granuloma and check valve mechanism beyond partial obstruction

- Thin-walled cavities
- B/L hilar lymph nodes

Infected Emphysematous Bullae

- Thin-walled, air-fluid level
- Usually seen in emphysema particularly paraseptal and scar associated
- Apical asymptomatic and those associated with scarring (throughout the lungs-COPD)
- Associated changes of inflammation in surrounding lung

TRAUMA

Hematoma—peripheral

- Air-fluid level—communication with bronchus

Traumatic Lung Cyst

- Single or multiple
- Peripheral and thin-walled
- Uni- or multilocular
- Within hours of injury

Bronchogenic Cyst

- Medial 1/3 of lower lobes
- If ruptures into a bronchus, thin-walled, air-fluid level and surrounding pneumonia

Cystic Adenomatoid Malformation

- Causes neonatal respiratory distress.
- Cavities of various shapes and sizes scattered in an area of opaque lung with well-defined margins.

Flow Chart 1.17.1

Cavitary Lesions of Lung

Malignant
- Upper lobes, squamous cell Ca
- Eccentric or multiple cavitation
- Nodular inner or outer margin
- Thick-walled

Lymphoma
- Thick or thin wall
- Typically in area of infiltration
- Hilar and mediastinal LN

Infective
TB—Large cavity with satellite cavities in UL or apical seg. of LL.
- Smooth and thick-walled
- Fibrotic vessels and bronchus

Staph or Klebsiella
- Thick and irregular walls
- Klebsiella - UL and single
- Assoc. with empyema or effusion

Hydatid
Complicated hydatid, RLZ
- Air crescent/air cap
- Water lily sign

Aspergillosis
- Fungal ball in a cavity
- Meniscus sign
- Mobile, calcification

Pneumoconiosis
Weg. Granulomatosis
- B/L, widespread
- Shaggy and thick-walled
- Completely disappear
- Other S/S

PMF- Mid and upper zones
- Begin peripherally
- Background nodularity

Rheumatoid Nodules
- Lower lobes peripherally
- Thick-walled and smooth
- Thinner with time

Trauma
Hematoma
- Peripheral
- Air-fluid level
T. lung cyst
- Within hours
- Peripheral and thin-walled

Bullous Lesion
- Usually with emphysema
- Infected with fluid level
- Infected changes in surrounding lung

1.18A LUCENT LUNG LESIONS

MULTIPLE LUCENT LUNG LESIONS

Cavities

Infection

Bacterial pneumonia
Granulomatous infection
Parasites

Neoplasm

Vascular

Wegener granulomatosis
Rheumatoid arthritis
Thromboembolic or septic infarct
    Cystic fibrosis
    Tuberculosis
    ABPA
    Rec. bacterial pneumonia

Cysts

Cystic bronchiectasis
Pneumatoccle
Congenital lesions—multiple bronchogenic cysts
    Intralobar sequestration
    CCAM Type I
    Diaphragmatic hernia
Centrilobar emphysema
Honeycomb lung disease

Differential Features are same as Localized Lucent Defects

Cyst	Cavity
Thin-walled	Thick-walled
	> 1 cm
Clear, smooth	Irregular, ragged wall
Well-defined wall	Adjacent lung parenchyma
	May show reactive changes
+/–	
+/–	Air-fluid level +/–

Localized Lucent Defect

Infection	Location	Air-fluid level	Cong/acq.	Uni/multi-cystic	Specific points
Bacterial	Any zone	+	Acquired	Multi cystic with areas of break-down	
Granulomat-tous	Apical	+	-do-	+ve	Fibrosis and cavita-ting
Fungal	Less likely To be apical	Fungal ball	-do-	uni	
Sarcoidosis	Upper zone	–	-do-	–	B/L hilar and R para-tracheal LNs

Contd...

Contd...

Infection	Location	Air-fluid level	Cong./ acq.	Uni/ multi-cystic	Specific points
Cystic bron-chiectasis	Lower lobes	Air-fluid level	Cong./ Acquired	+	
Pneumato-cele	In area of	+/–	Acquired	+	Staph. infect-ion Sequela
	Previous pneumonia/ post trau-matic hema-toma				
Intralobar sequestration	Lower lobes	+/–	Cong.	+	Vascular Drain-age is altered
Honeycomb Lung	Any zone	–	Acq./End state disease	+	
CCAM		+/–	Cong.	Multi-cystic	Cartilage Deve-lopment is defec-tive

1.18B SOLITARY PULMONARY NODULE

Malignant
    Primary
    Secondary
    Lymphoma
    Plasmacytoma
    Alveolar cell carcinoma

Benign
    Hamartoma
    Adenoma
    Connective tissue tumor

Granuloma	Tuberculosis
	Histoplasmosis
	Sarcoidosis
Infection	Round pneumonia
	Abscess
	Hydatid
	Amebic
	Fungal
Pulmonary infarct	
Pulmonary hematoma	
Collagen disease	Rheumatoid arthritis
	Wegener's granulomatosis
Congenital	Bronchogenic cyst
	Sequestration segment
	Cong. bronchial atresia
	AVM
	Impacted mucus
Amyloidosis	
Intraparenchymal lymph node	
Pleural	Fibroma
	Tumor
	Loculated fluid
Nonpulmonary	Skin and chest wall lesions
	Artefacts

1.19 SOLITARY PULMONARY NODULE

Definition

Single round intraparenchymal opacity, at least moderately well-marginated and no greater than 3 cm in maximum diameter.

Neoplasm

Benign – Hamartoma, inflammatory pseudotumor
    Malignant-Bronchogenic carcinoma, carcinoid tumor, metastasis.

Infection

Granuloma—Tuberculoma
    Fungal—Histoplasmoma
Abscess
Round pneumonia
Parasites—Echinococcus

Inflammatory

Connective tissue-Wegener's granulomatosis
    Rheumatoid nodule
    Sarcoidosis (Rare)

Vascular

Arteriovenous malformation
Hematoma
Pulmonary infarct
Pulmonary artery aneurysm

Airway

Congenital lesion-Bronchogenic cyst
Mucocele
Infected bulla
Pseudonodules
• ECG pads
    Cutaneous lesions
    Mole

Nipple shadow
Hemangiomas
Neurofibromas
Lipomas

Characteristics of SPN

1. Size
   - No size criteria that clearly distinguishes benign from malignant SPN
   - 80% of benign SPN <2 cm in diameter
   - 15% of malignant SPN <1 cm in diameter.
   - 42% of malignant SPN <2 cm in diameter.
2. Growth
   - Benign lesions - <30 days or <450 days (doubling time) SPN with doubling time between 30-450 days require further evaluation
   - Doubling time for spherical lesions is defined as 25% increase in diameter.
3. Calcification
   - Approximately 1/3rd of non calcified SPN's have calcification on CT
   - Complete/central/laminated: Granulomas
     Popcorn : Hamartoma
     Amorphous/Eccentric calcification : Malignancy.
4. Fat
   Fat within a smooth/lobulated SPN is suspected benignity of hamartoma – 50% show presence of fat.
5. Cavitation
   Cavity with greatest wall thickness <5mm are benign >15 mm are malignant
6. Air bronchogram/bubbly lucencies
   Presence of air bronchogram within SPN is s/o adenocarcinoma particularly bronchoalveolar cell Ca.

Other causes – Lymphoma, organizing pneumonia, pulmonary infarcts and mass like sarcoidosis
7. Margins
   - Smooth, well-defined margins s/o benign nodule although 21% of malignant nodules smooth margin.
   - Lobulated / ill-defined / spiculated s/o malignant nodule 25% of benign nodules may have undefined margins.
   - Presence of a small satellite nodule surrounding the periphery of a smooth SPN is s/o granulomatosis infection.

CT Nodule Enhancement

- Enhancement <15 HU s/o benign nodule.
  False +ve : Central necrosis, mucin producing malignant neoplasm
- Enhancement > 15 HU-Non-specific.

Pulmonary Hamartomas

Consist of masses of cartilage with clefts lined by bronchial epithelium which may contain large calcification (popcorn) of fat; Age group : 45-50 yrs
Triad: * Pulmonary chondromas
(Carney's triad): Gastric epitheloid leiomyosarcomas
- Functioning extra adrenal paragangliomas
  90% peripheral and 10% within a major bronchus.
- Spherical lobulated SPN with popcorn calcification, size <4 cm, fat density positive.

Inflammatory Pseudotumor (Plasma Cell Granuloma)

- Caused histology by mixture of fibroblasts, histiocytes, lymphocytes and plasma cells.

- Age range is wide and includes children.
- SPN (2-5cm) or as an area of consolidation, calcification is occasionally present.

Endobronchial tumor can cause obstructive pneumonitis.

Bronchial Carcinoid

Bronchial carcinoids can invade locally, may metastasize to hilar and mediastinal lymph nodes as well as to brain, liver and bone.

Age: Age range is wide; Peak-5 decade.

Clinical features-Wheeze, Cushing's syndrome (ectopic ACTH secretion) Carcinoid syndrome

Hilar / parahilar mass

80-90% Central (endobronchial)

10-20% Peripheral with feature of bronchial obstruction, pneumonia, Calcification +/-.

Spherical/lobular SPN (2-4 cm) smooth well-defined margin calcification +/-

Bronchial Carcinoma

Sq Cell Ca (30-50%)

Adeno Ca (30-50%)

Undefined Small cell Ca (20-30%)

Large cell Ca (10-15%)

Peak incidence: 50 to 60 yrs

Radiological features: Size > 2cm

Undefined margins

Umbilicated/notched margin

Corona radiata / speculations (+)

Pleural tail sign (+)

Doubling time between 30 to 450 days

Lesion crosses fissure

Cavitation: (>15 mm thick wall)
Calcification rare if present-eccentric
Associated findings—Hilar/mediastinal lymph nodes, bony mets, pleural effusion, visceral mets (+)
Bronchoalveolar Carcinoma: Air bronchogram/bobby lucencies

Grows slowly
Cavitation is unusual.

Metastasis

Pulmonary metastasis is usually from breast, GI tract, kidney, testes, head and neck tumors or from a bone and soft tissue sarcomas.

Site: Usually in the outer portions of lung.
Radiological features (R/f) Solitary/multiple
Spherical well-defined, occasionally irregular edge.
Calcification—unusual except-mets from osteosarcoma, chondrosarcoma
Rate of growth: variable-explosive in choriocarcinoma and osteosarcoma.
Cavitation-unusual (sq cell Ca+).

Tuberculoma

* Occurs in the setting of primary or postprimary TB and is considered to represent localized parenchymal diseases that alternatively activates and heals.
  Nodule is 10-15 mm in diameter.
  Situated most commonly in the right upper zone.
  Single or multiple (confined to a single segment)
  Margins well-defined
  Satellite lesions(+)
  Calcification frequent
  Cavitation +/-

Hydatid Cyst

Caused by tapeworm (*E. granulosus* or *E.alveolaris*)
Humans are accidental host.
Infection occurs by ingestion of ova by fomites/contaminated water.

R/F Unruptured cyst: Homogenous spherical/oval, well-defined lesion. Size 1 to 10 cm occurs particularly in middle zone/lower zone.

Ruptured cyst: Usually associated with secondary infection
1. Meniscus sign-Pericyst–ruptures ecto and endocyst intact appearance is that of an intracavitary body.
2. Disruption of inner layers.
   a. Air-fluid level
   b. Floating membranes (water lily, camalote sign)
   c. Double wall appearance
   d. Dry cyst with crumpled membranes lying at its bottom (rising sun, serpent sign)
   e. Cyst with all its content expectorated (empty cyst sign).

Histoplasmoma

Caused by histoplasma capsulatum which is a fungus found in moist soil and in bird or bat excreta.
Histoplasma represents a small necrotic focus of infection surrounded by a massive fibrous capsule consisting of concentric lamination, some or all of which may calcify.
Sharply defined nodular shadow
<3 cm in diameter
Most common site is in the lower lobe
Satellite lesions (+)
Calcification (+) central/eccentric

Target lesion is pathognomic—Homogenous density with central punctate deposit of calcium.

Associated findings – Calcified hilar/mediastinal lymph nodes.

Pneumonia

Round pneumonias are usually pneumococcal which are usually seen in children, air bronchogram.

Lung Abscess

Cavitation secondary to necrosis is seen in
Bacterial pneumonias – Staphylococcus aureus
Gram negative bacteria—*Klebsiella pneumoniae, Proteus pseudomonas*
Anaerobes
Amebic and fungal infection.

Cavitary Lesion with Adjacent Consolidation

Size-2 to 12 cm
Wall thickness < 15 mm
Inner aspect of cavity is smooth.

Wegener's Granulomatosis

- Necrotizing granulomatous vasculitis
- Lungs involved in 95% cases and late renal involvement is seen in 85% cases
- Men>Women
  Single/multiple nodules
  Size = 1 cm to several cm
  Well-defined margins
  Wax and wane
  Frequently cavitate

Associated findings—Granulomas in upper respiratory tract and glomerulonephritis.

Rheumatoid Nodules

Pleuropulmonary is seen in 5 to 54% cases of rheumatoid arthritis.

Pulmonary, necrobiotic nodules are uncommon features of rheumatoid arthritis.

Associated with subcutaneous nodules.

Single/multiple

Variable in size

Wax and wane in size

Cavitation (+) / (-) more common in lower lobe and in periphery.

Similar nodule may be seen in patients of rheumatoid arthritis who have been exposed to silica. Known as Caplan's syndrome.

Pulmonary A-V Fistula

Congenital – 50% have hereditary hemorrhagic telangiectasia (Osler-Weber-Rendu disease).

Acquired – Liver diseases (cirrhosis), schistosomiasis and metastatic thyroid cancer.

Round/lobulated nodule

Prominent adjacent vascular shadow

Most common site—Lower lobe

Variation in size with Valsalva (size)

CT and pulmonary angio shows the feeding artery and vein and vascular nature of nodule.

Pulmonary Artery Aneurysm

Most pulmonary artery aneurysms are acquired as a result of

septic embolization or an extension from a pulmonary parenchymal calcification.

- Peripheral aneurysms may mimic a SPN pulsations of
  mass seen on fluoroscopy.
  Confirmation done by CT or pulmonary angiography.

Pulmonary Hematoma

H/o trauma (+); usually appears following resolution of
contusion.

Peripheral in location
Smooth and well defined
Slow resolution over several weeks
A pocket of air or fluid level (+).

Pulmonary Infarct

- Becomes visible 12-24 hrs after embolic episode
  Lesions are more frequent in the lower lobe
- Hump shaped opacity with its base applied to the pleural
  surface because of partial collapse, hemorrhagic conges-
  tion.
- Cavitation is rare
- Matched defect is seen on ventricular perfusion scan.
- Associated pleural effusion (+).

Bronchogenic Cyst

- Peak incidence is in 2nd and 3rd decade.
- 2/3rd are intrapulmonary and occur in the medial 1/3rd
  of the lower pulmonary region.
- Round to oval
- Smooth-walled and well-defined
  CT shows thin-walled water density cyst.

Clinical and Radiographic Criteria for Differentiating Benign and Malignant SPN

Clinical	Benign	Malignant
• Age	<40 yrs except hamartomas	>45 yrs
• Sex	Female	Male
• History	• High incidence of granuloma in area	• Primary lesion elsewhere
	• Exposure to TB	• H/o smoking
• Skin test	Positive with specific infectious organism	Negative/positive
Radiographic		
• Size	Small (< 2 cm)	Large (>2 cm)
• Location	No predilection except for TB	Predominantly on upper lobes except for lung mets
• Definition and contour	Well-defined and smooth	Ill-defined, lobulated umbilicated
• Calcification	Central, laminated Popcorn, complete	Eccentric (very rare)
• Satellite lesion	More common	Less common
• Doubling time	< 30 to >450 days	30 to 450 days
• Presence of fat	(+) S/o hamartoma	—

Flow Chart 1.19.1
Investigative algorithm for evaluation of SPN

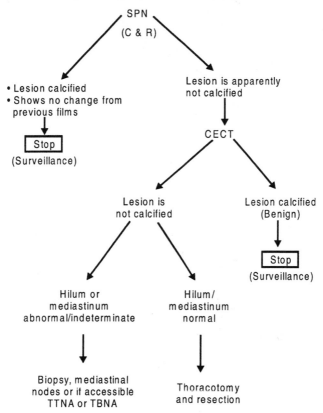

Flow Chart 1.19.2

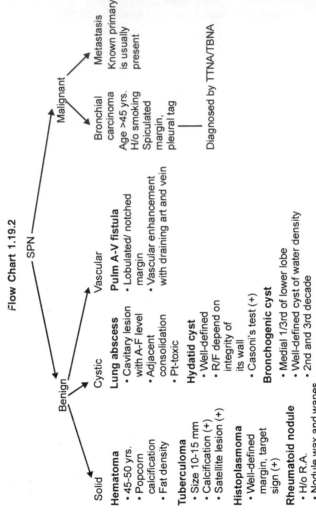

SPN

Benign

Malignant

Solid

Hematoma
• 45–50 yrs.
• Popcorn calcification
• Fat density

Tuberculoma
• Size 10–15 mm
• Calcification (+)
• Satellite lesion (+)

Histoplasmoma
• Well-defined margin, target sign (+)

Rheumatoid nodule
• H/o R.A.
• Nodule wax and wanes
• Most common lower lobe and periphery

Cystic

Lung abscess
• Cavitary lesion with A-F level
• Adjacent consolidation
• Pt-toxic

Hydatid cyst
• Well-defined
• R/F depend on integrity of its wall
• Casoni's test (+)

Bronchogenic cyst
• Medial 1/3rd of lower lobe
• Well-defined cyst of water density
• 2nd and 3rd decade

Vascular

Pulm A-V fistula
• Lobulated/ notched margin
• Vascular enhancement with draining art and vein

Bronchial carcinoma
Age >45 yrs.
H/o smoking
Spiculated margin, pleural tag

Diagnosed by TTNA/TBNA

Metastasis
Known primary is usually present

1.20 PULMONARY EDEMA ON THE OPPOSITE SIDE TO A PREEXISTING ABNORMALITY

1. Congenital absence or hypoplasia of a pulmonary artery
2. Macleod's syndrome
3. Thromboembolism
4. Unilateral emphysema
5. Lobectomy
6. Pleural disease

(See Table next page)

Localized Air Space Disease

- Pneumonia
  Infarction
  Contusion
  Edema
  Radiation
  Alveolar cell CA.
  Differential features are discussed in alveolar shadowing.

Unilateral Pulmonary Edema

- Pulmonary edema on the same side as a preexisting abnormality
  Prolonged lateral decubitus
  Unilateral aspiration
  Pulmonary contusion
  Rapid thoracocentasis of air or fluid
  Bronchial obstruction
  Clinical history is most important in the differential diagnosis of all the above entities.
Bronchial obstruction
- Respiratory distress +/-
- e/o occulsion seen in the form of luminal obstruction, atelectasis, fissural displacement.

Flow Chart 1.20.1

	Congenital absence or hypoplasia of a pulmonary artery	Macleod's syndrome	Thromboem- bolism	Unilateral emphysema	Lobectomy	Pleural disease
Lack of soft tissue outline	+	+	–	–	–	–
Prominent hilum	–	–	+	–	–	–
Subpleural consolidation	–	–	+	–	–	–
Elevated diaphragm	–	–	+	–	+	–
Pleural reaction	–	–	+	–	–	+
Cavitation	–	–	+	–	–	–
Mediastinal shift	–	–	–	+	+	–
Linear outline of pleura	–	–	–	+	–	+

	Location	Duration	Effusion	LNs	Air broncho-gram			
Infection	Any	Rapid Resolution	+/-	+/-	+/-	Reticulono-dular pattern	Peripheral, central	
Hyaline Memb disease	Whole lung	"	+/-	-	+	-	Any	Usually presents with un-usual features
Aspiration	Right UL in Erect Right LL in Supine	"	-	-	+/-	During resolu-tion	Any	White out lung
Hemo-rrhage/ Contusion	Any	-	-	-	-	-	-	Clinical h/o
Alveolar cell CA	Any	Nonresol-ving Pneumonia	++	-	+	-	-	Clinical h/o
Lymphoma	Any	"	+	++	-	-	Any	
Embolism/ infarct	Any	1-2 day posttrauma resolves in 1-4 wks	-	-	-	-	Any	

Contd...

Contd...

	Location	Duration	Effusion	LNs	Air broncho-gram	
Sarcoidosis	UL		–	+	–	Peripheral
Löffler's	UZ	Rapid	–	–	–	Central
Metastasis	Any	No show	+/–	+/–	–	Peripheral
Consolida-tion	Follow the exposure history	show	+/–	–	+ in acute-in chronic	P/C usually from chronic CA

Alveolar Shadowing

Acute

Pulmonary Edema
Cardiac
    Noncardiac
        Hypoproteinemia
        Fluid overload
        Drowning
        Aspiration
        Inhalation
        ARDS, uremia
        Infection
    At birth
    Aspiration
    Hyaline membrane disease
    Alveolar
    Blood pulmonary hemorrhage
    In hematoma
    Goodpasture's syndrome
    Pulmonary infarction

Chronic

Tumors
Alveolar cell carcinoma
Lymphoma
Alveolar proteinosis
    Microlithiasis
Radiation pneumonitis
Sarcoidosis
Eosinophilic lung.

Characteristics

4-10 mm diameter
Ill-defined margins
Coalescence
Nonsegmental

Air Bronchogram

Common

1. Consolidation pneumonic
2. Pulmonary edema
3. Hyaline membrane disease

Rare

4. Lymphoma
5. Sarcoidosis
6. Alveolar proteinosis
7. Alveolar cell carcinoma
8. Adult respiratory distress syndrome

	1	2	3	4	5	6	7	8
Location	Any zone	Peri -hilar	Any zone	Any	UL	Any	Any	Any
Pleural effusion	+/–	+	+/–	+/–	–	–	+/–	+
Hilar enlargement	+/–	–	–	+	+	–	+/–	–
Silhouette with cardiac	+/–	+	+	+/–	–	–	+/–	+
Diaphragm	+/–	–	+	+/–	–	–	+/–	+
LNs.	+/–	–	–	+	+	–	+/–	–
Crazy pavement pattern	–	–	–	–	–	+	–	–
White out lung.	–	–	+	–	–	–	–	+
Vascular markings visualized	–	+	–	–	+	–	–	–
Resolution	+	+	+	–	+	+	–	+

Mesothelioma

Asymmetrical, irregular
Thickening
Calcification +/-
U/L

Pneumonectomy

Rib resection +/-
Thoracoplasty asymmetrical bony contour
H/o present

Pulmonary Agenesis

Cong. anomaly
Resp. distress +
Status of diaphragm

D/D Diaphragmatic Hernia

N.	–Scaphoid Abd.
Absent	Bowel loops with air +/-
Opaque thorax	A few lucencies +

Consolidation

Air bronchogram
Confined to one segment
Air alveologram.

Collapse

Vessels not seen
Crowding of fissure and ribs
Hilar and diaphragmatic
displacement

Fibrosis

e/o vol. Loss +

Cardiomegaly

Cardiac contour conforming of uni/multichamber enlargement.

1.21A MILIARY SHADOWING

D/D Miliary Shadowing

Disseminated pulmonary opacities
1. Acinar
2. Interstitial
Acinar—poorly defined, round, parenchymal opacities
- 4-8 mm in diameter
- Represent an anatomical acinus filled with fluid.

Interstitial

Pulmonary interstitium is a network of connective tissue fibers that supports the lung. It includes alveolar walls, interlobular septa and peribronchovascular interstitium.

Interstitial nodules may take various patterns.
- Linear and septal lines
  Miliary shadows
  Reticulonodular shadows
  Honeycomb shadows
  Peribronchial cuffing and ground glass pattern.

Alveolar	Interstitial
1. Pluffy ill-defined	Sharply defined
2. 4-8 mm	2-4 mm

3. Coalescent	Discrete
4. Segmental/lobei	Widespread
5. Air brochogram	usually 1 week
6. Time from onset of nodules is a small	
7. Higher density	Lower density

Miliary Shadowing

Is the presence of small, discrete, rounded pulmonary nodules of almost similar size measuring 2-4 mm in the interstitium.

Causes

1. Infectious Diseases
   a. Tuberculosis
   b. Fungal infections—Histoplasmosis, coccidioido-mycosis, blastomycosis
   c. Chickenpox.
2. Inhalational Disease
   a. Silicosis
   b. Barytosis
   c. Stannosis
   d. Coal miner's pneumoconiosis
   e. Berryliosis
3. Granulomatous Diseases
   a. Sarcoidosis
   b. Histiocytosis-X
4. Metastases
5. Secondary hyperparathyroidism
6. Oil embolism
7. Alveolar microlithiasis

8. Hemosiderosis
9. Bronchiolitis obliterans

Miliary Tuberculosis

- Due to hematogenous spread of infection
- May be seen in both primary and post primary disease
- Small discrete nodules 1-2 mm in diameter, evenly distributed throughout both lungs
- These are of soft tissue density and are well-defined
- Other tubercular manifestations as consolidation, pleural effusion, lymphadenopathy may be present.

Histoplasmosis

- Due to infection with histoplasma capsulatum
- Infection is usually subclinical and heal spontaneously leaving small calcified nodules or calcified mediastinal nodes
- Infection in immunocompromised may produce multiple nodules scatterred throughout the lung resulting in miliary shadowing.
- Hilar nodes enlargement is common
- Consolidation, fibrosis and cavitation may occur.

Silicosis

- Multiple nodular shadows 2-5 mm in diameter
- Affects mainly mid and upper zones, relatively sparing the bases
- Hilar adenopathy which may calcify, fibrosis, cavitation may occur.

Coal Miner's Pneumoconiosis

- Small faint, nodules 1-5 mm in diameter appear in mid zone spreading to whole lung
- Progressive massive fibrosis-mid and upper zones-in complicated cases
- Emphysematous bullae may appear.

Sarcoidosis

- Multisystem granulomatous disorder affecting young adults
- 75-90% patients show small, rounded or irregular nodules 2-4 mm in diameter, bilaterally symmetrical with upper and mid zone preponderance
- Bilateral symmetrical lymphadenopathy, hilar and para-tracheal
- Air trapping, pleural thickening and effusion may be positive.

Histiocytosis X

- Granulomatous disorder affecting young or middle-aged adults
- Pulmonary involvement is bilateral symmetrical
- Chest X-ray shows diffuse nodular pattern in upper and mid zones, 1-5 mm in size. Progress of disease leads to ring shadows, honeycombing and linear shadows.

Miliary Metastasis

- Rare cause of miliary shadowing

- Primary tumors most likely to provide miliary nodulation are thyroid, renal carcinoma, bone sarcomas and chorio-carcinomas.

Hemosiderosis

In patients with heart disease which elevates left atrial pressure, e.g. in mitral stenosis, there is permanent miliary stippling due to focal nature of bleeding.

Alveolar Microlithiasis

- Multiple fine sand like calculi in the alveoli
- Produce widespread dense opacities on chest X-ray.
- Clinically there is relative lack of symptoms.

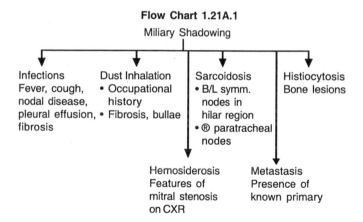

Flow Chart 1.21A.1

Miliary Shadowing

Infections
Fever, cough,
nodal disease,
pleural effusion,
fibrosis

Dust Inhalation
• Occupational
  history
• Fibrosis, bullae

Sarcoidosis
• B/L symm.
  nodes in
  hilar region
• ® paratracheal
  nodes

Histiocytosis
Bone lesions

Hemosiderosis
Features of
mitral stenosis
on CXR

Metastasis
Presence of
known primary

1.21B MILIARY SHADOWING (0.5 TO 2 MM)

Soft tissue densities
Miliary TB
Fungal disease
Pneumoconiosis
Sarcoidosis
Extrinsic allergic alveolitis
Fibrosing alveolitis

Greater than Soft Tissue Density

Hemosiderosis
Silicosis
Siderosis
Stannosis
Barylosis

Multiple Opacities (2-5mm)

Remaining discrete	LN	Location	Size
Carcinomatosis	+/−	Any	Variable
Lymphoma	+	Any	Same
Sarcoidosis	+	Mid zone	Variable
Tending to confluence and varying rapidly			
Multifocal pneumonia	+/−	Any	Variable
Pulmonary edema	−	Perihilar	Variable
Extrinsic allergic alveolitis	−	Basal	Same
Fat emboli	−	Peripheral	Same

Pneumoconiosis

These are diseases caused by inhalation of inorganic dusts.
The diagnosis depends on a history of exposure to the dust

and an abnormal chest radiograph and respiratory function tests.

Silicosis

Gold mining, sand blasting, foundry ceramic and pottery workers.
Multiple, nodular shadows 2-5 mm in diameter mid and upper zones.
Linear lines and septal lines may also be seen.

Coal Workers

Pneumoconiosis

Small, faint, indistinct nodules 1-5 mm in diameter appear in the mid zones.
Coalescence of these nodules is common
Develop bilaterally
Fibrotic masses may calcify.

Asbestosis

Asbestosis mining and processing.
In construction and demolition workers ship building.
- Lower zones nodules
- Pleural plaque, calcification, diffuse thickening and effusion – mid zone, bilaterally.
- Pulmonary fibrosis is marked.
- Initially reticulonodular pattern results – which with progression becomes coarser and there is loss of clarity of the diaphragm and heart.

Berylliosis

In acute stage produces noncardiogenic pulmonary edema, while in the chronic stage produces widespread noncavitating granulomas.

1.22 MULTIPLE PIN POINT OPACITIES

1. Post lymphogram
2. Silicosis
3. Stannosis
4. Barylosis
5. Alveolar microlithiasis

	1	2	3	4	5
At the termination of the thoracic duct	+	–	–	–	–
In gold miners	–	+	–	–	–
Inhalation of tin oxide	–	–	+	–	–
Distribution	Near thoracic duct	–	–	Bases and apices spared	–
Kerley lines	–	–	+	–	–
Inhalation of barytes	–	–	–	+	–
Miliary	+	+	+	–	+
Negative shadows	–	–	–	–	+

Septal Lines

Pulmonary edema
Mitral valve disease
Pneumoconiosis
Lymphangitis carcinomatosa
Sarcoidosis
Infection
Lymphoma.

1.23 COMPLETE OPAQUE HEMITHORAX

Causes

Technical   Rotation, scoliosis

Pleural	Hydrothorax, lung effusion thickening, mesothelioma
Surgical	Pneumonectomy, thoracoplasty
Congenital	Pulmonary agenesis
Mediastinal	Gross cardiomegaly, tumors
Pulmonary	Collapse, consolidation fibrosis

Diaphragmatic Hernia

Scoliosis
- Lucency on   Vertebral
- Concave side   anomaly
- Rotated   Clavicular
  side   Asymmetry

Effusion

- Blunted cardiophrenic angle
- Fluid along the lateral chest wall
- Silhouette with cardiac and diaphragm
- Changes with change of posture
- Thickening
  - Does not follow
    Ellis curve

1.24 OPAQUE HEMITHORAX

Causes
- Technical   Rotation, scoliosis
- Pleural   Pleural effusion
  - Pleural thickening
  - Mesothelioma
- Surgical   Pneumonectomy
  - Thoracoplasty

- Congenital   Pulmonary agenesis
- Mediastinal   Gross cardiomegaly, tumors
- Pulmonary   Collapse, consolidation, fibrosis
- Diaphragmatic hernia

Rotation

- In well-centered film medial ends of clavicle are equidistant from spinous process of T4/5 level.
- Lung nearest to the film, less translucent.

Pleural Effusion

- A massive effusion may cause complete radiopacity of a hemithorax
- Mediastinal shift to contralateral side
- Inversion of diaphragm
- If effusion without mediastinal shift collapse of underlying lung.

Exclude Carcinoma Bronchus

- Ultrasound reveals fluid in pleural cavity. In AP-CXR-with patient supine a small effusion gravitates posteriorly – generalized increased density with apical cap.
  Erect or decubitus film confirms the diagnosis.
  Pulmonary agenesis/aplasia/hypoplasia.

Agenesis

- Complete absence of the lobe as well as its bronchus.
- Absent vascular supply.

Aplasia

- No lung tissue
- Rudimentary bronchus

Hypoplasia

- Bronchi and alveoli are present, but the lobe is under-developed.
- More common on right side.
- Mediastinal shifts present. Absence of a lobe is more common than absence of whole lung.
- Loss of silhouette on the right side of the heart and ascending aorta due to deposition of extrapleural alveolar tissue.
- If whole lung absent—completely opaque hemithorax with mediastinal shift and diaphragmatic shift.
- Unlike acquired pneumonectomy, gross loss of lung volume, external diameter is not considerable less than normal side in congenital absence.
- Bronchography—diagnostic.
- Scintigraphy—absent ventilation and perfusion on affected site.
- Angiography—absent/hypoplastic pulmonary artery.

Diaphragmatic Hernia

- L > R more common in left side
- If large hernia in early neonatal period may lead to opaque hemithorax.
- Bochdalek hernia – posterolaterally due to persistent pleuroperitoneal canal.
  May contain fat, omentum, spleen, kidney, bowel – Associated with pulmonary hypoplasia and contralateral mediastinal shift.
  - In older age group—hemithorax not opaque due to gas in bowel loops.

Consolidation

- Parenchymal opacification caused by replacement of air in the distal air spaces by fluid (transudates, exudate or blood) or tissue (e.g. bronchoalveolar cell carcinoma, lymphoma) is defined as consolidation.
- Usually no volume loss
- Expansile consolidation   Pneumococcal and
  Klebsiella pneumonia
  - Neoplasms
  - Air bronchogram

Pleural Thickening

If extensive – may lead to opaque hemithorax
- Previous thoracotomy
- Empyema
- Hemithorax
- Viewed an profile–appears as a band of soft tissue density.
- An face—ill-defined veil like shadowing
- USG – not so sensitive pleural thickening not reliably detected unless 1 cm in thickness
- CT – very sensitive
- May calcify, involve visceral pleura
- If entire lung is surrounded by fibrotic pleura – Fibrothorax

Fibrothorax is Defined by Criteria

- If uninterrupted pleural density that extends over at least a forth of the chest wall
- On CT - > 8 cm craniocaudal
  - 5 cm laterally
  - 3 mm thick
- No mediastinal shift

- Reduced ventilation due to decreased by volume
  If on X-ray—Decreased vascularity, significant ventilatory restriction is present.
  Surgical decortication is required.

Mesothelioma

More common primary pleural malignancy

- Prolonged exposure to asbestos dust – crocidolite (M.C)
- Nodular pleural thickening ± hemorrhagic pleural effusion around all or part of lung.

With central mediastinum
Volume loss due to ventilatory restriction

Bronchial stenosis by tumor compression at hilum.
Malignant pleural thickening is nodule and extends into fissures or over the mediastinal surface, may surround whole lung.

- MRI better than CT in assessing involvement of mediastinum and chest wall. Signal intensity slightly more than muscles on both T1 and T2 WI.

Postpneumonectomy

- 2-3 months after surgery
- H/o of pneumonectomy
- ± Rib resection
- ± opaque bronchial sutures.

Flow Chart 1.24.1

Opaque hemithorax

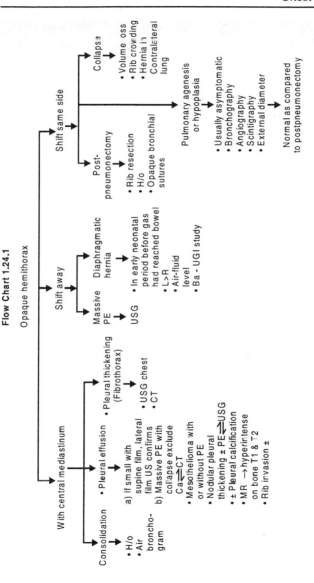

Opaque hemithorax

With central mediastinum

Consolidation
• H/o
• Air broncho-gram

Pleural effusion
a) If small with supine film, lateral film US confirms Massive PE with collapse exclude
Ca ⇌ CT
b) Massive PE with collapse exclude
Ca ⇌ CT
• Mesothelioma with or without PE
• Nodular pleural thickening ± PE ⇌ USG
± Pleural calcification
• MR → hyperintense on bone T1 & T2
• Rib invasion ±

Pleural thickening (Fibrothorax)
• USG chest
• CT

Shift away

Massive PE
→ USG

Diaphragmatic hernia
• In early neonatal period before gas had reached bowel
• L > R
• Air-fluid level
• Ba - UGI study

Shift same side

Post-pneumonectomy
→ • Rib resection
• H/o
• Opaque bronchial sutures

Collapse
• Volume oss
• Rib crowding
• Hernia in Contralateral lung

Pulmonary agenesis or hypoplasia
→ • Usually asymptomatic
• Bronchography
• Angiography
• Scintigraphy
• External diameter
→ Normal as compared to postpneumonectomy

1.25 HYPERTRANSRADIANT LUNG FIELD

Bilateral

A. *Faulty radiologic technique*
  - Over penetrated films
B. *Decreased soft tissues*
  - Thin body habitus
  - Bilateral mastectomy
C. *Cardiac causes of decreased pulmonary blood flow*
  - Right to left shunts (Tetralogy of Fallot, Ebstein's malformation, Tricuspid atresia)
  - Eisenmenger physiology
D. *Pulmonary causes of decreased pulmonary blood flow*
  - Pulmonary embolism
  - Air trapping
  - Emphysema
  - Bulla
  - Bleb
  - Interstitial emphysema

Unilateral

A. *Faulty radiologic technique*
  - Rotation of patient
B. *Chest wall defects*
  - Mastectomy
  - Poland syndrome (absence of pectoralis major)
C. *Air trapping*
  - Extrinsic compression of main bronchus
  - Endobronchial obstruction
  - Bronchiolitis obliterans
  - Macleod syndrome

- Emphysema
- Pneumothorax

D. *Vascular causes*
  - Pulmonary arterial hypoplasia
  - Pulmonary embolism
  - Congenital lobar emphysema
  - Compensatory over-aeration

Tetralogy of Fallot

- Congenital disease presenting as left to right shunt with four components VSD, infundibular narrowing of the right ventricular outflow tract, right ventricular hypertrophy, overriding aorta.

Plain Skiagram Chest

- Boot shaped heart
- Hypoplasia of pulmonary artery
- Pulmonary oligemia leading to translucent lungs
- Right sided aortic arch

ECHO

- Discontinuity between anterior aortic wall and IV septum due to overriding aorta
- Small left atrium
- RV hypertrophy with small outflow tract
- Doppler USG can quantify severity of VSD and pulmonary stenosis.

Ebstein's Anomaly

- Congenital disease with left to right shunt with atrialization of right ventricle due to downward displacement of the dysplastic incompetent tricuspid valve leading to a small right ventricle. There is associated ASD or PDA.

- Patient presents early reversal of the shunt from right to left leading to cyanosis.

Plain Skiagram Chest

- Massive globular "funnel like" cardiomegaly with small pedicle due to hypoplastic aorta and pulmonary trunk (the only CHD with this feature)
- Extreme RA enlargement
- Dilated IVC and azygous vein
- Severe pulmonary oligemia leading to translucent lung fields
- Calcification of tricuspid valve may occur.

ECHO

- Large sail like tricuspid valve
- RA enlargement
- Doppler USG can quantify tricuspid regurgitation.

Tricuspid Atresia

- Congenital disease with atresia of the tricuspid valve and pronounced cyanosis at birth. Associated with ASD and a small VSD. Pulmonary stenosis may or may not be present. May present with or without transposition of great vessels.

Plain Skiagram Chest

- Left ventricular contour of the heart with rounding due to both enlargement and hypertrophy of left ventricle.
- RA enlargement
- Concave pulmonary bay
- Pulmonary oligemia leading to translucent lung fields.

Eisenmenger Physiology

- Occurs when there is reversal of left to right shunt as a consequence of pulmonary arterial hypertension

Plain Skiagram Chest

- Pronounced dilatation of central pulmonary arteries
- Pruning of peripheral pulmonary arteries leading to increased translucency
- Enlargement of RV
- Return of LA and LV to normal size
- Normal pulmonary venous pressure.

Pulmonary Embolism

- The embolism is usually a result of DVT in the lower limbs
- There is a classic traid seen in 33% of cases of hemoptysis, pleural rub and thrombophlebitis
- Hypertranslucency is seen bilaterally in cases presenting with acute massive embolic episode, which blocks the main pulmonary artery before the development of infarction. The development of infarction leads to segmental, lobar or wedge shaped areas of consolidation. Pleural effusion is usually present.
- Unilateral hypertranslucency may occur in cases where the embolus block one of the major pulmonary artery.

Air Trapping

- There is trapping of air in the lungs due to valve mechanism acting at the level of the trachea or major bronchi
- In children this usually due to a foreign body. In adults an endotracheal or endobronchial growth of extrinsic pressure is the usual cause.
- On plain skiagram chest there is hypertranslucency with evidence of increased volume like splaying of ribs, long

tubular heart, barrel-shaped chest due to increase AP diameter of the chest and depressed domes of diaphragm. These findings may be unilateral or bilateral depending on the etiology. However in unilateral increase in volume these findings are unilateral except for the contralateral shift of mediastinum and largely normal cardiac contour.

Bulla, Blebs and Pneumatoceles: When very large may compress the surrounding normal lung and may lead to either unilateral or bilateral hypertranslucency.

Bronchiolitis obliterans: Also known as constrictive bronchiolitis or obliterative bronchiolitis is a result of inflammation of bronchioles leading to obstruction of bronchial lumen.

- Chest X-ray may be normal
- Hyperinflated lungs leading to increased lucency may be seen in upto 60% of cases
- There is decrease in pulmonary blood flow
- On HRCT there is mosaic perfusion and lobular air trapping may be seen, bronchial wall thickening and bronchiectasis may also be seen.

Macleod syndrome: Also known as Swyer-James syndrome is result of acute viral bronchiolitis in infancy, leading to constrictive bronchiolitis.

- There is increased translucency of the affected lung
- Small hemithorax with decreased or normal volume of the lung
- Air trapping during expiration
- Small ipsilateral hilum
- Reduced pulmonary vasculature with pruning of vessels.

Emphysema: This term is broadly used to define pulmonary diseases characterized by permanently enlarged air spaces distal to terminal bronchioles accompanied by destruction of alveolar walls and local elastic fiber network.

Plain Skiagram Chest

- Hyperinflated translucent lungs
- Low or flat hemidiaphragms
- Increased retrosternal air space
- Barrel chest
- Pulmonary vascular pruning
- Right heart enlargement
- Bullae

Compensatory Emphysema or over-aeration is a distinct clinical entity where there is unilateral findings of emphysema seen due to diseased nonfunctional contralateral lung.

Pneumothorax

- Can be unilateral or bilateral and is a result of collection of air in the pleural cavity.

Plain Skiagram Chest

- There is increased translucency with loss of broncho-vascular markings
- There is contralateral shift of mediastinum in the unilateral types
- In tension pneumothorax there may be inversion of diaphragm.

Congenital Lobar Emphysema

- Result of congenital insult leading to constriction of bronchi supplying one lobe leading to air trapping and increase in volume.
- The enlarged lobe compresses the remaining normal lobes
- Contralateral mediastinal shift.

Pulmonary Arterial Hypoplasia

- Small or absent main pulmonary artery
- Concave pulmonary bay
- Pulmonary oligemia.

Flow Chart 1.25.1

Bilateral Causes of Hypertransradiancy

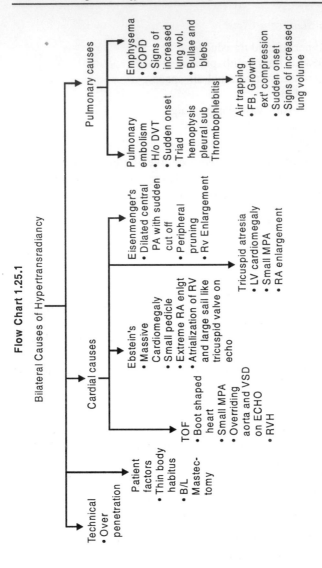

- Technical
  - Over penetration

- Patient factors
  - Thin body habitus
  - B/L Mastectomy

Cardial causes

- TOF
  - Boot shaped heart
  - Small MPA
  - Overriding aorta and VSD on ECHO
  - RVH

- Ebstein's
  - Massive Cardiomegaly
  - Small pedicle
  - Extreme RA enlgt
  - Atrialization of RV and large sail like tricuspid valve on echo

- Eisenmenger's
  - Dilated central PA with sudden cut off
  - Peripheral pruning
  - Rv Enlargement

- Tricuspid atresia
  - LV cardiomegaly
  - Small MPA
  - RA enlargement

Pulmonary causes

- Emphysema
  - COPD
  - Signs of increased lung vol.
  - Bullae and blebs

- Pulmonary embolism
  - H/o DVT
  - Sudden onset
  - Triad hemoptysis pleural sub Thrombophlebitis

- Air trapping
  - FB, Growth ext' compression
  - Sudden onset
  - Signs of increased lung volume

Flow Chart 1.25.2

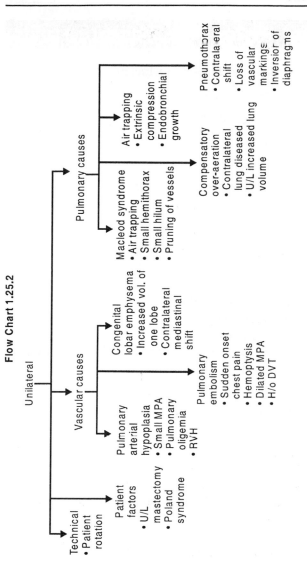

Unilateral

Technical
- Patient rotation

Patient factors
- U/L mastectomy
- Poland syndrome

Vascular causes

Pulmonary arterial hypoplasia
- Small MPA
- Pulmonary oligemia
- RVH

Pulmonary embolism
- Sudden onset chest pain
- Hemoptysis
- Dilated MPA
- H/o DVT

Congenital lobar emphysema
- Increased vol. of one lobe
- Contralateral mediastinal shift

Pulmonary causes

Macleod syndrome
- Air trapping
- Small hemithorax
- Small hilum
- Pruning of vessels

Compensatory over-aeration
- Contralateral lung diseased
- U/L increased lung volume

Air trapping
- Extrinsic compression
- Endobronchial growth

Pneumothorax
- Contralateral shift
- Loss of vascular markings
- Inversion of diaphragms

1.26 HYPERTRANSLUCENT LUNG FIELD

Causes of Bilateral Hypertranslucency

Faulty Radiologic Technique

- Over penetrated film

Decreased Soft Tissues

- Thin body habitus
- Bilateral mastectomy

Cardiac Cause

- Right to left shunt
- Eisenmengerization of left to right shunt

Pulmonary Cause

- Decreased vascular bed
  - Pulmonary embolus.
- Increase in air space
  - Air trapping—asthma, acute bronchitis, emphysema
  - Bullae, blebs
  - Interstitial emphysema.

Localized Lucent Lung Defect

- Cavity
  - Infection
  - Neoplasm
  - Vascular occlusion
  - Inhalational – Silicosis with coal worker's pneumoconiosis.
- Cyst
  - Cystic bronchiectasis

- Pneumatocele
- Centrilobular/bullous emphysema
- Honeycomb lung
- Diaphragmatic hernia
- CCAM Type I, CLE, bronchogenic cyst.

Hyperlucent lung :	(Unilateral)
Normal	Increased density contralateral lung
	Over penetrated film
Technical	Over penetrated film
	Rotation, scoliosis
Soft tissue	Mastectomy
	Cong. Absence of pectoralis major poliomyelitis (Poland's syndrome)
Emphysema	Compensatory: Lobar collapse
	Lobectomy
	Obstructive : Foreign body, tumor
	Macleod's syndrome.
	CLE.
	Bullous.
Vascular	Absent/hypoplastic pulmonary artery, obstructed pulmonary artery
	< Tumor embolus
Pneumothorax	Macleod's syndrome.

1.27A HONEYCOMB LUNG

Common	Rare
Histiocytosis-X	Tuberous sclerosis
Scleroderma	Amyloidosis
Rheumatoid disease	Neurofibromatosis
Fibrosing alveolitis	Lymphangiomyomatosis
Pneumoconiosis	

Sarcoidosis
Similar appearance

Bronchiectasis	Connection with bronchus +
Cystic fibrosis	Pancreatic anomalies +
	Achlorhydria

Location	Upper zones	Extrinsic allergic alveolitis
	Upper and midzones bases	Histiocytosis
		Rheumatoid
		Scleroderma
		Cystic bronchiectasis
		Cryptogenic fibrosing alveolitis
	Mid and bases	Sarcoidosis

Multiple Pin Point Opacities

Postlymphogram	:	Iodized oil emboli. Contrast medium is seen at the site of termination of the thoracic duct.
Silicosis	:	Located in upper and mid zones, seen in gold miners.
Stannosis	:	Evenly distributed throughout the lung with Kerley A and B lines
Barylosis	:	Inhalation of barytes
		Very dense, discrete opacities
		May be slightly larger in size
		Bases and apices are spared
Alveolar microlithiasis	:	Familial, black pleura, enlarged heart size is positive.

Lobar Pneumonia

Consolidation involving the air spaces of an anatomically recognizable lobe. The entire lobe may not be involved and there may be a degree of associated collapse.

1. *Streptococcus pneumonia*: Commonest cause, unilobar in distribution. No cavitation. Little or no collapse. Pleural effusion is uncommon.
2. *Staphylococcus*: Especially in children. Sixty percent develop pneumatocele. No lobar predilection, effusion, empyema and pneumothorax and bronchopleural fistulae are common.
3. *Klebsiella pneumoniae*: Multilobar involvement, cavitation and lobar enlargement is common.
4. *Tuberculosis*: Associated collapse is common.
   Right lung is more frequently involved.
   Anterior segment of the upper lobe and the medial segment of the middle lobe are the commonest sites.
5. *Streptococcus pyogenes*: Lower lobe predominates, often associated with pleural effusion.

Consolidation with Bulging Fissures

Homogeneous or inhomogeneous air space opacification with bulging of the bounding fissures.

1. Infection with abundant exudates
   Klebsiella, *Streptococcus pneumoniae*, Tubercular bacilli
2. *Abscess*: When air-area of consolidation breaks down.
   Common organism include *Staph. aureus*, klebsiella and other gram –ve organism
3. CA of the bronchus.

LUNG DISEASE ASSOCIATED WITH HONEY COMBING

Collagen Disorders

Rheumatoid lung : Basal predominance
                   Infiltrates and effusion are common

Scleroderma basal

Preceded by fine, linear basal streaks.

Extrinsic allergic alveolitis upper zones

Sarcoidosis sparing of extreme apices

• Hilar lymph adenopathy

• Egg shell calcification.

Pneumoconiosis : Mainly due to asbestosis

Cystic bronchiectasis lower and middle zones

Bronchial wall thickening

Localized areas of consolidation

Histiocytosis-mid and upper zones.

Disseminated nodules followed by honeycomb pattern

Tuberous sclerosis : Rare

Neurofibromatosis : Rib notching +

Ribbon ribs +

Scoliosis

1.27B HONEY COMB PATTERN

1. A generalized reticular pattern or miliary mottling which when summated produces the appearance of air containing 'cysts' 0.5-2 cm in diameter.
2. Obscured pulmonary vasculature.
3. Late appearance of radiological signs after the onset of symptoms.
4. Complications
   a. Pneumothorax is frequent
   b. Cor pulmonale later in the course of the disease.

Causes

1. Collagen diseases-Rheumatoid arthritis
   Scleroderma

2. Extrinsic allergic alveolitis
3. Sarcoidosis
4. Pneumoconiosis
5. Cystic bronchiectasis
6. Cystic fibrosis
7. Drugs—nitrofurantion busulfan, cyclophosphamide, bleomycin and melphalan
8. Langerhans cells histiocytosis
9. Lymphangio leiomyomatosis
10. Tuberous sclerosis
11. Idiopathic interstitial fibrosis (cryptogenic fibrosing alveolitis)
12. Neurofibromatosis

Rheumatoid Arthritis

- Most pronounced at the bases.
- It's severity does not parallel to that of joint involvement.
- In the earlier stages it is characterized by radiologic appearance of patchy area of air space consolidation (multifocal ill-defined densities).
- In the intermediate stage there are fine reticular pattern or reticulonodular pattern.
- As the disease progress there is appearance of cystic spaces of honeycomb lung.
- All the above features may be preceded by basal infilterate ± small effusion.

Scleroderma

- Predominantly basal
- Less regular 'honeycomb' pattern which is preceded by fine, linear, basal streaks cor pulmonale is unusual.

- Other clinical signs which include skin changes, soft tissue calcification, disturbances of esophageal motility and dilatation of the esophagus.
- Radiologically, an upper GIT series may demonstrate. Both esophageal dilatation and decreased motility as well as small bowel dilatation.

ASBESTOSIS

- It produces a basilar distribution that may progress from a fine reticular interstitial pattern to a coarse interstitial pattern with honeycombing.
- The basilar reticular or honeycomb pattern is also frequently associated with pleural thickening, pleural calcification.

Silicosis

- It has predominant upper lobe distribution.
- It may be associated with hilar or mediastinal lymphadenopathy with pleural thickening. The fine reticular pattern is seen which progresses to honeycomb lung.

Extrinsic Allergic Alveolitis

- Predominantly seen in the upper lobes of the lung.

Sarcoidosis

Sparing of extreme apices

- Honeycombing of the lung is usually proceded by some classic finding including hilar adenopathy and an interstitial nodular or fine reticular interstitial pattern.

- As the interstitial disease progresses there is regression of hilar adenopathy.

Langerhans Cell Histiocytosis

- 'Honeycomb' pattern preceded by disseminated nodules.
- May be predominantly in the mid and upper zones.
- Cor pulmonale is uncommon.

Usual Interstitial Pneumonitis/Cryptogenic Fibrosing

Alveolitis

- More marked in the lower lobes of the lungs initially and progresses to involve the whole of the lungs.
- In HRCT there is honeycombing and fibrosis. It shows a uniform and patchy distribution.

Tuberous Sclerosis

- Symptoms when they appear, usually first appear in adult life.
- Pneumothorax, pulmonary insufficiency and cor pulmonale may complicate the syndrome.
- The clinical and radiological manifestation of the disease in the brain, kidneys and skin readily establish the diagnosis.

Neurofibromatosis

- Honeycomb lung ± rib notching ribbon ribs and/or scoliosis. In 10% but not before adulthood.

Flow Chart 1.27B.1

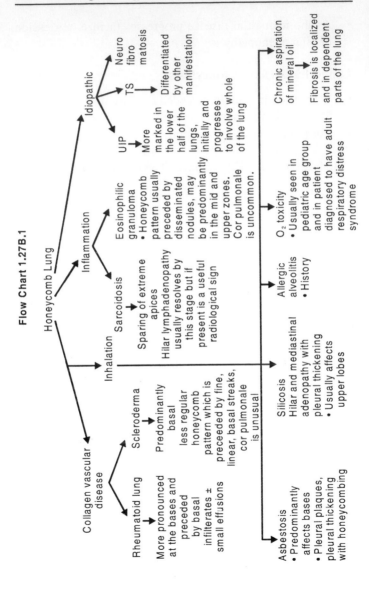

1.28 PLEURAL DISEASES

- Serous membrane which covers the surface of lung and lines the inner surface of chest wall.

Common conditions are:
- Pleural effusion
- Pleural thickening
- Pneumothorax
- Pleural masses
- Pleural calcification

Pleural Effusion

May be transudate, exudate, pus, blood or chyle.

Transudate

Contain < 3 gm/dl of protein, usually bilateral
a. Increase hydrostatic pressure
   Main cause is congestive cardiac failure (CCF)—1st on right side and then bilateral, constrictive pericarditis.
b. Decrease colloidosmotic pressure
   – Decrease protein product—cirrhosis with ascitis
   – Protein loss/hypervolemia
     Nephrotic syndrome
     Overhydration
     Peritoneal dialysis
c. Meig-Salmon syndrome
   Ovarian fibroma, thecoma, GCT, Brennet T, etc.
   – Ascitis
     Pleural effusion resolve with tumor removal.

Exudate

Increased permeability of abnormal pleural capillaries with release of high protein fluid into pleural space.
> 3 gm/dl of protein.

A. *Infection*
   1. *Empyema*—Pleural effusion with presence of pus.
      +/– positive culture.
      Microorganism are anaerobic bacteria
      Gross pus (WBC >15000/cm^3)
   2. *Parapneumonic effusion*—Less with pneumonia,
      abscess, bronchiectasis.
   3. *TB*—Increase protein content >75 gm/dl
   4. *Fungi and parasite*—amebiasis, secondary to liver
      abscess.
B. *Malignant disease*- Lung Ca, lymphoma, breast, ovarian
   Ca and malignant mesothelioma. Positive cytological result.
C. *Vascular*—Pulmonary embolism (15-30%)
D. *Abdominal disease*

Pancreatitis-	Left side pleural effusion (68%), right side (10%).
Boerhaave's syndrome-	Left side
Subphrenic abscess-	Pleural effusion—79% Elevation and restriction of diaphragmatic movement
Endometriosis	Plate-like atelectatic or pneumonia.

E. *Connective tissue disorder.*
   RA—UL(R>L) recurrent alternating sides relatively
   unchanged in size for months.

SLE

B/L in 50% (L>R), increase cardiac size.

Wegener's Granuloma

Hemothorax

Bleeding into the pleural space may be trauma.
Hemophilia or excessive anticoagulation—Rare
Pulmonary infarction – Blood stained
• Lung carcinoma-blood stained.

Chylothorax

Chyle is milky fluid high in neutral fat and fatty acid.

Secondary to damage or obstruction of the thoracic lymphatic vessels

Causes   Most common cause—trauma—surgery.
          Carcinoma of lung, lymphoma, filariasis.

Radiological Features

Plain film: Frontal view less sensitive < Lateral view < lat. decubitus view.

- Moderate effusion with mediastinum, is shifted towards the side of collapse-likely due to carcinoma of bronchus.
- Empyema may be suspected by the appearance of a fluid level.
- Septations.

USG

Very sensitive, can detect few ml of fluid.

Transudate—Clear fluid separating the visceral and parietal pleura

Moving lung suspended within the pleural space.

Exudate—Echogenic fluid, containing floating particulate material, septations or fibrin strands may be associated with pleural nodule or thickening > 3 mm

CT—Simple pleural effusion—Sickle shaped disease in the most dependent part of thorax posteriorly

- In regard to tissue density—CT is rarely helpful, however
- Exudate- >water density septation.
- Parietal pleural thickening on CECT
- Extrapleural fat thickening of >2 mm
- Chylous—Decrease density than H_2O

     Acute hemorrhage—Increase density of fluid with presence of fluid-fluid level.

PLEURAL THICKENING

- Nonpathological
  B/L apical pleural thickening, symmetrical
  Elderly patient
  Probably ischemia is the cause
- *Trauma*: If the entire lung is surrounded by the fibrotic
  Fibrothorax secondary to organized effusion, hemothorax
  or pyothorax.
- Dense fibrous layer of 2 cm thickness almost always on
  visceral pleura.
- Frequent calcification on inner aspect of pleura.

INFECTION

Chronic empyema—H/O pneumonia parenchymal scars.
Usually seen over the bases.

Frequently a thickened layer of extrapleural fat can be
seen separating the parietal and visceral layer.

Calcification may be seen.

TB

Lung apex
Can be associated with apical cavity
Calcification may be seen

Inhalation Disorder

Asbestos exposure involves the lower lateral chest wall, basilar
interstitial disease.

Pleural plaque: Involves the parietal pleura with sparing of
visceral pleura.

Neoplasm

Asymmetric apical pleural thickening may represent Pancoast
tumor destruction of adjacent ribs and spine penetrated film
will be helpful.

- Metastasis—often nodular

PLEURAL CALCIFICATION

Has the same causes as pleural thickening.

U/L pleural calcification—result of previous empyema, hemothorax or pleurisy and also occur in visceral pleura associated with pleural thickening.

Calcification may be in a continuous sheet or in discrete plaque.

B/L calcification seen in asbestos exposure, more delicate frequently visible over the diaphragm and adjacent to axilla located in parietal pleura.

PLEURAL MASSES

- Incomplete border and tapered superior and inferior borders.
- Usually make obtuse angle with chest wall.
- Displacement of adjacent lung parenchyma with compressive atelectasis and blowing of bronchi and pulmonary vessels around the mass.
- Vanishing tumor and encysted pleural effusion fluid may become loculated in interlobar fissure seen in heart failure lateral film typical lenticular configuration. Encysted pleural effusion-often associated with free pleural effusion.
- Water density.
- Neoplasm.

Benign

- *Lipoma*—CT detect the origin of mass of fat density. Benign lipoma confirm fat density with few fibrin strands.
- Thymolipoma, angiolipoma, teratoma, characterized by islands of soft tissue density, interspersed with fat.
- Fibroma/benign fibrous mesothelioma—Most common benign tumor may be associated with hypoglycemia and HPOA solitary lobulated non-calcification mass.

If pedicle is seen—diagnostic, shape change with the change in patient's position.

Malignant Pleural Thickening

Bronchogenic Carcinoma: Most common cause.

When a bronchogenic carcinoma involves the pleura diffusely with resultant pleural effusion, the tumor is considered unresectable.

Malignant Mesothelioma

- Rare tumor.
  70% of cases—H/O asbestos exposure
  Nodular pleural thickening around all or part of lung with pleural effusion
  Pleural—plaque
  Metastatic disease—Breast and GIT
  Most common manifestation is malignant pleural effusion. Pleural thickening is nodular and frequent. Encase the entire lung including mediastinum.
- Pleural lymphoma.
- Pleural effusion.
  CT= localized broad based lymphomatous pleural plaque.

PNEUMOTHORAX

Spontaneous—Most common type
M:F: 8:1, young male with tall thin stature

Due to rupture of a congenital pleural bleb such blebs are usually in the lung apex may be B/L.

Iatrogenic— For example postoperative, after chest aspiration during artificial ventilation, after lung biopsy.

Traumatic—result of a penetrating chest wound, closed chest trauma, associated finding like rib fracture.

Hemothorax

Surgical/mediastinal emphysema

Secondary to lung disease—

* Emphysema
* Chronic bronchitis
  Common factor in elderly patient
  Rupture of a tension cyst in *Staph. pneumoniae*
  Rupture of a subpleural TB focus
  Rupture of a cavitating subpleural mets.
  Pneumoperitoneum—air passes through a pleuroperitoneal foramen.
  Generalized
* Localized—If pl. adhesion are present.

Open

If air can move freely in and out of pleural space during respiration.

Closed

If no movement.

Valvular: If air enters the pleural space on inspiration but does not leave on expiration it is valvular-as intrapleural pressure increase it leads to development of tension pneumothorax.

Radiological features: Small pneumothorax in an erect patient collects at the apex.
Expiratory film—useful in closed pneumothorax.
Lat. decubitus film with affected side uppermost.
Tension Pneumothorax: Massive displacement of mediastinum.

* Kinking of great veins
* Acute cardiac and resp. embarrassment.
* Ipsilateral lung may be squashed against the mediastinum and herniate across the midline.

- Depression of ipsilateral diaphragm.

Loculated pneumothorax = pleural adhesion may result in loculated pneumothorax.

D/D—subpleural bullae, thin-walled pulmonary cavity/cyst.

Few linear strands can be seen in these but not in pneumothorax.

Hydropneumothorax containing a horizontal fluid level.

(See Flow Chart 1.28.1 Next Page)

1.29 PLEURAL FLUID

Radiological Appearances of Pleural Fluid

- Most dependent recess of the pleura is the posterior costophrenic angle (100-200 ml of fluid is required to fill this). Small effusions are hence seen earlier on a lateral film and now on ultrasound.
- Decubitus views with a horizontal beam is the most sensitive view.
- The effusion casts a homogeneous opacity spread upwards. Typically, this opacity has a fairly well-defined, concave upper edge, which is higher laterally than medially and obscures the diaphragmatic shadow.
- A massive effusion may cause complete radiopacity of a hemithorax.
- In the presence of a large effusion, lack of displacement of the mediastinum suggests that the underlying lung is completely collapsed.
- Lamellar effusion are shadow collection between the lung surface and the visceral pleura.
- Large effusions may accumulate between the diaphragm and the undersurface of a lung—this is called sub-pulmonary pleural effusion. The apex is more lateral than normal. This collection moves fully with changes of posture.

Flow Chart 1.28.1

Pleural Lesions

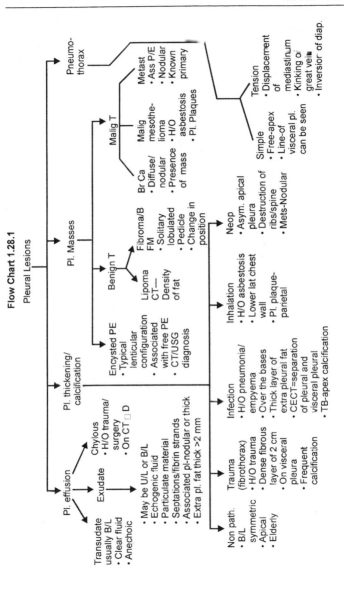

Pl. effusion

- Transudate
  - usually B/L
  - Clear fluid
  - Anechoic

- Exudate
  - May be U/L or B/L
  - Echogenic fluid
  - Particulate material
  - Septations/fibrin strands
  - Associated pl-nodular or thick
  - Extra pl. fat thick >2 mm

- Chylous
  - H/O trauma/ surgery
  - On CT□D

Pl. thickening/ calcification

- Non path.
  - B/L symmetric
  - Apical
  - Elderly

- Trauma (fibrothorax)
  - H/O trauma
  - Dense fibrous layer of 2 cm
  - On visceral pleura
  - Frequent calcification

- Infection
  - H/O pneumonia/ empyema
  - Over the bases
  - Thick layer of extra pleural fat
  - CECT=separation of pleural and visceral pleural
  - TB-apex calcification

- Inhalation
  - H/O asbestosis
  - Lower lat chest wall
  - Pl. plaque-parietal

Pl. Masses

- Encysted PE
  - Typical lenticular configuration
  - Associated with free PE
  - CT/USG diagnosis

- Benign T
  - Lipoma CT— Density of fat
  - Fibroma/B FM
    - Solitary lobulated
    - Pedicle
    - Change in position

- Neop
  - Asym. apical pleura
  - Destruction of ribs/spine
  - Mets-Nodular

- Malig T
  - Br Ca
    - Diffuse/ nodular
    - Presence of mass
  - Malig mesothe-lioma
    - H/O asbestosis
    - Pl. Plaques
  - Metast
    - Ass P/E
    - Nodular
    - Known primary

Pneumo-thorax

- Simple
  - Free-apex
  - Line-of visceral pl. can be seen

- Tension
  - Displacement of mediastinum
  - Kinking of great vein
  - Inversion of diap.

- Empyema usually has a lenticular shape, irregular thick walls and may compress the underlying lung.
- Loculated effusions tend to have comparatively little depth, best considerable width, rather like a biconvex lens.

Pneumothorax

It collect in a free pleural space in an erect patient at the apex. On the frontal film, sharp white line of the visceral pleura will be visible, separated from the chest wall by the radiolucent pleural space, which is devoid of lung markings.

An expiratory film will make a closed pneumothorax easier to see since on a full expiration, the lung volume is at its smallest, while the volume of pleural air is unchanged.

In tension pneumothorax, the ipsilateral lung may be squashed against the mediastinum, or herniate across the midline, and the ipsilateral hemidiaphragm may be depressed.

Nodular extension into the fissures, pleural effusion, volume loss of the ipsilateral lung all suggest malignancy.

Metastatic: The most frequent primary tumors being of the bronchus and breast.

1.30 PLEURAL TUMORS

Benign:　　　　Mesothelioma: Well-defined, lobulated mass adjacent to chest wall, mediastinum, diaphragm.

Lipoma: Well-defined, lobulated mass may change shape with respiration on CT, presence of fat is diagnostic.

Malignant:　　　Mesothelioma: Due to prolonged exposure to asbestosis.

Nodular pleural thickening with pleural effusion. Rib involvement may occur but is rare.

1.31 PLEURAL CALCIFICATION

The common conditions are:
1. Old empyema
2. Old hemothorax
3. Asbestos inhalation
4. Silicosis

Old Empyema and Old Hemothorax

- Calcification is irregular, resembles a plaque or sheet and is contained within thickened pleura.
- Enface it is hazy and veil like but inprofile it is dense and linear, paralleling the chest wall
- Usually unilateral
- Most common site: Lower posterior half of chest
- In tuberculous empyema—both visceral and parietal pleura may be calcified which are sometimes separated by a soft tissue opacity which may contain fluid.

Asbestos Inhalation

Features of asbestosis is pleural plaque which is a well-defined soft tissue sheet orginating in the parietal pleura (latent period is 10 yrs.)
- Latent period for calcification to develop is 20 yrs.
- Lesions are usually bilateral, lying in the middle zone, lower zone and diaphragm.
  When calcified – 'holly leaf pattern' with sharp and often angulated outlincs and often follow the margins of the ribs.
- Usually <1 cm thick
  Diffuse pleural thickening: Unlike pleural plaques the margins are well-defined and tapered; may reach several cm in thickness.
  Pleural effusion—Uncommon

Malignant Mesothelioma

Latent period: 40 yrs
Pulmonary changes : (peripheral lower zone)
- Fibrosis
- Bronchial carcinoma
- Pseudotumor (fibrotic atelectasis)

Extrathoracic Manifestation

Peritoneal mesothelioma, malignancy of upper GIT.

Silicosis

- Inhalation of silica (SiO_2)
- Pleural calcification is similar to asbestosis .

Other Features

- Multiple small nodules in upper zone and middle zone.
- Hilar lymph nodes with egg shell calcification
- Progressive massive fibrosis
- Caplan's syndrome also occurs in patients with rheumatoid arthritis and silicosis.

Flow Chart 1.31.1
Pleural Calcification

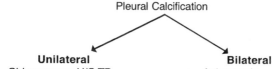

Unilateral
- Old empyema H/O TB
- Old hemothorax-H/O trauma

Calcification along the
inner surface of thickened pleura

Bilateral
- *Asbestosis*
- Pulmonary changes are in middle and lower.

Silicosis
- Pulmonary changes in upper and middle zone, egg shell calcification of lymph nodes.

Calcification of parietal pleural with holly leaf pattern and occurs along margins of ribs.

1.32 HIGH RESOLUTION CT-PATTERN OF PARENCHYMAL DISEASE

Peripheral, Base

1. Cryptogenic fibrosing alveolites
Early	:	Ground glass appearance
		Subpleural reticular shadows
Later	:	Reticulations extend centrally
Chronic	:	Small cyst formation, commencing at subpleural site.

2. Asbestosis
Early	:	Changes are seen at the lung base. Posteriorly.
		Thickened curvilinear, subpleural lines are seen.
		Thickened subpleural septal lines, coarse parenchymal lines extending centrally.
Chronic	:	Honey combing
		Rounded atelectasis with comet tail sign.

Central Upper Fluid Zones

Sarcoidosis	:	Thickened bronchovascular markings with perivascular beading present centrally.

Patchy alveolar opacification.
Subpleural and peribronchovascular nodules.

Peripheral and Central

Lymphangitis:		Bronchovascular markings and septal line thickening.
		No alveolar opacification is seen.

Widespread

> *Lymphangio-*
> *leiomyoma-*
> *tosis*   :   Characteristic widespread distribution.
>   More common in women.
>   Uniform sized well-defined cysts with
>   normal parenchyma surrounding them.

Tuberous Sclerosis

Variable sized cyst
No feminine predilection.

1.33 CARDIOPHRENIC ANGLE MASS

A. Solid
  i. *Fat Density*
      1. Epicardial Fat Pad
          – Obese, Cushing's syndrome
          – Uncapsulated, homogeneous extrapleural fat
      2. Lipoma
          – Uncommon, well-defined, encapsulated thin
            fibrous septae
      3. Liposarcoma
          – Ill-defined
          – Inhomogeneous
      4. Morgagni hernia
  ii. *Soft Tissue*
      Lymph Nodes
      – Lymphoma
      – Carcinoma—breast, lung, colon

Traumatic-Diaphragmatic Hernia
– H/O trauma
– Mostly left sided

- Single entry and exit
- Barium or other studies—useful in diagnosis

Diaphragmatic Hump
- Herniation of liver through the gap
- Liver scan or USG

Fibrous Tumors of Pleura
- Pleura based, well-defined, homogeneously enhancing, stalked.

Primary or Secondary Malignancy
- Well-defined smoothly marginated lung based.

B. **Cystic or Vascular**
- Pericardial cyst
- Well-defined, round to oval, fluid density, non-enhancing, right CP angle.

Hydatid Cyst
- Unilocular, associated with hepatic cyst or may be bilateral.
- Meniscus sign, water lily sign.
- Loculated pleural effusion.
- USG—makes the diagnosis
- Varices
- Delayed phase scanning is needed
- Portal hypertension, more on right.
- Scimitar syndrome
- Abnormal vessel draining into IVC or hepatic vein
- Lobar agenesis or aplasia
- Accessory diaphragm, pulmonary sequestration.

Pericardial Cyst
- Etiology—embryogenesis, parietal recess, diverticulum, sequelae.
- 30-40 yrs, asymptomatic

Plain film chest—well-defined, round to oval mass
- Cardiophrenic angle mass usually right
- Changes shape with respiration and body position.

US

Well-defined, anechoic to hypoechoic, No septae

CT

3-8 cm in size
- May extend into fissures
- No enhancement, no perceptible wall

Hydatid Cyst

- Three layers—Adventitia, friable ectocyst, inner germinal layer.
- Lung cyst—Unilocular, 20% bilateral, 10% associated with hepatic cyst.
- Well-defined, round-oval, homogenous masses upto 10 cm in diameter.
- Calcification is rare.
- Meniscus sign, water lily sign.

Morgagni Hernia

- Defect between septum transversum and right and left costal margins of diaphragm.
- Usually asymptomatic, more common in obese people.
- Right sided, small lesions may only have omental fat, then it may be difficult to distinguish from epicardial fat pad.
- Large lesion—colon, liver, stomach or small intensive may herniate.
  Ba study—tenting of colon or loop above the diaphragm.
  CT—Omental fat, omental vessels and abdominal viscera seen in the mass.

Diaphragmatic Hump and Hernia

- Trauma—Hernia mostly seen on Lt side (post central)
- Colon or less commonly stomach are the contents.

Ba—Entry and exit through the defect are closely apposed.
- Obstruction is frequent probably because of angular margins of the defect but are detected late because of subtle changes in plain film.

On Rt side—Liver may herniate in severe trauma
- A liver scan is helpful.

Congenital Hernia

More common on right
It has a hernial sac.

Scimitar Syndrome

- Presence of partial anomalous pulmonary venous return below the diaphragm, mostly right side.
- Lobar agenesis or aplasia, other systemic artery from aorta in lower thorax or upper abdomen.
- Pulmonary artery may be small or entirely absent, accessory diaphragm, hepatic herniation, pulmonary sequestration.

Fibrous Tumors of Pleura

- Solitary, sharply defined, sometimes lobulated soft tissue pleural based mass without evidence chest wall invasion, homogeneous enhancement.
- Pedicle or stalk—pathognomonic and indicator of benign lesion, mobility.
- May grow very large than obtuse or acute angle may be formed with pleura.

Primary or Secondary Carcinoma

- Well-defined, smoothly marginated
- Lung based
- Multiple

Flow Chart 1.33.1

Cardiophrenic Angle Masses

Solid
- Epicardial fat pad
- Lymphadenopathy
- Lipoma
- Carcinoma
- Solitary fibrous tumor of pleura

Cystic
- Pericardial cyst
- Bronchogenic cyst
- Hydatid cyst
- Loculated pleural effusion

Diaphragmatic
- Morgagni hernia
- Diaphragmatic hump
- Diaphragmatic hernia
- Nodes

Vascular lesions
- Dilated RA
- Varices
- Scimitar syndrome

Epicardial Fat Pad

- Excessive deposition of fat in mediastinum
- Obese patient
- Cushing syndrome or excessive corticosteroid intake
- Uncapsulated and extrapleural fat.

Lipoma

- Uncommon
- Well-defined, encapsulated, generally homogeneous
- May contain thin fibrous septae
- Inhomogeneous, poorly defined.

Lymph Nodes

- Anterior diaphragmatic group of L.N. - 2 nodes, < 5 mm- is normal.

Causes of enlargement are:

- U/L or B/L
  - Lymphoma
  - Lung, breast or colon cancer—metastasis.

2

Breast– Mammographic Differential Diagnosis

2.1 CIRCUMSCRIBED RADIOLUCENT LESION

Lipoma

- Usually solitary, presents usually in older women.
- Usually have a thin capsule.
- Frequently large at diagnosis.
- Difficult to palpate due to soft consistency.

Oil Cyst

- Single or multiple.
- Usually small 2-3 cm.
- H/o trauma.
  - Surgical.
  - Seat belt injury.
- +/- mural calcification.

Galactocele

- During lactation = Milk containing cyst caused by obstruction of a duct by inspissated milk in a women who has abruptly stopped breastfeeding 2-3 cm in diameter.
- Lucent or mixed density mass.

- Characteristic fat-fluid level when imaged with horizontal beam.

Mixed Density Lesions

- Fibroadenolipoma (hamartoma)—Mammographic appearance is determined by the relative amount of fat and glandular tissue.
- Uncommon benign tumor composed of normal or dysplastic mammary tissue, including adipose and fibrous tissues and ducts and lobules in varying amount.
- Often large at diagnosis often 6 cm in diameter at the time of diagnosis.
- Lack of normal architecture with lack of orientation of glandular tissue towards the nipple results in an appearance resembling a "slice of sausage".
- There may be a thin soft tissue density capsule visible.

Galactocele

Discussed above.

Hematoma

- H/o trauma - Blunt/or surgical.
- H/o anticoagulant intake.
- H/o clotting abnormalities.
- Medium to high density mass, often having irregular margins.
- Overlying skin edema present in acute stage.
- Gradual decrease in size or disappearance of the lesion on follow-up.

Lymph Node

- Medium to low-density lesion with a fatty notch or center.
- Often B/L and multiple.
- Almost always located in the superolateral quadrant.

- Pathological nodes have +/- loss of central fatty hilum. +/- enlargement.

Causes

- *Rheumatoid arthritis:* (after gold treatment ± fine dense gold deposits.
- *Sarcoidosis*: (+/- punctate calcification).
- *Infection*: Tuberculosis-(coarse calcification +/-)
- *Malignancy*
  – Leukemia
  – Lymphoma
  – Metastasis from carcinoma breast carcinoma ovary. (+/- irregular microcalcification).

Radiopaque(Soft Tissue Density Lesion)

Simple Cyst

- Most common cause of a circumscribed mass arising in a female 40 years or > in age.
- Sharply circumscribed low soft tissue density mass +/- radiolucent halo (halo sign).
- Often multiple and bilateral.
- Most commonly 1-3 cm in diameter.
- Calcification-Uncommon rarely peripheral thin egg shell calcification may be present.
- Cyst may develop quickly prior to menses and diminish in size just as rapidly.
- USG - oval or round echo free lesion with smooth well-defined walls.

Strict sonographic criteria for simple cysts are:
- Well-circumscribed margins.
- A bright posterior wall.

- Round or oval contour.
- Absence of internal echoes.
- Through transmission.

Fibroadenoma

- Common benign estrogen sensitive tumor composed of fibrotic and glandular tissues in varying proportion that usually appears in adolescent and young women before the age of thirty years.
- Usually solitary, round, ovoid or smoothy lobulated mass of medium density.
- Calcification, which is coarse, popcorn like or primarily peripherally distributed is characteristic.
- USG-Typical appearance is of a well circumscribed, round or oval mass showing posterior acoustic enhancement and with a homogenous internal echo pattern-usually of low reflectivity compared to the surrounding breast tissue.

Papilloma

- Usually occurs in the retroareolar region.
- May cause a serous or serosanguineous nipple discharge.
- Usually the lesion is several millimeters in size. The mammogram may show a slight bulging of a retroareolar duct or may appear normal.
- Crescent, rosette or egg shell calcification may occur.

Phylloides Tumor (Cystosarcoma Phylloides)

- Fibroepithelial tumor which is usually large when diagnosed.
- On mammography solitary large, round, oval or polylobulated sharply outline lesion.

- May develop plaque like calcification.
- Can recur, if not completely excised.

Metastasis

Lymphoma, and other hematologic malignancies, melanoma and lung cancer are the three most common blood borne hematologic sources, followed by ovarian cancer, soft tissue sarcomas and other gastrointestinal and genitourinary cancer.

- Seen on mammograms as discrete nodules, usually solitary (85%) and less often multiple (15%).
- Unilateral in 75% and bilateral in 25% cases.
- Diffuse involvement is much less frequent.
- Majority are found in upper outer quadrant.
- Cannot be differentiated from other benign nodules, such as cysts or fibroadenomas. However, the presence of one or more nodules in patient with known primary should alert one to the possibility of blood borne metastasis.
- A spiculated mass indicates the presence of a second primary breast cancer and not metastasis.
- With the exception of psammomatous calcification in metastatic ovarian carcinoma, metastases to the breast do not calcify.

Lymphoma

- Primary lymphoma of the breast is rare.
- Secondary involvement of the breast with lymphoma is more frequent.
- The most common form of involvement is a circumscribed mass that is well defined or shows minimal irregularity.
- Moderate to marked spiculation may or may not be present.
- In the absence of known or suspected lymphoma, the mammographic findings are non-specific.

- Bilateral axillary lymphadenopathy suggests the possibility of lymphoma.

Circumscribed Malignant Lesions:
(Circumscribed Carcinoma)

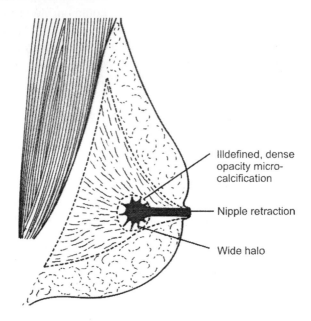

Illdefined, dense opacity micro-calcification

Nipple retraction

Wide halo

Fig. 2.1.1: Typical carcinoma

- Circumscribed carcinoma is a descriptive term referring to any ductal carcinoma, that appears as a circumscribed mass on mammogram.
- Circumscribed malignant lesions are most commonly medullary, mucinous, papillary or intracystic carcinoma, and rarely invasive ductal carcinoma.
- Medullary carcinomas may grow rapidly and most occur in women less than 50 years old.

- Mucinous and papillary carcinomas have a favorable prognosis and most occur in women over 50 years.
- Medullary carcinoma exhibit, varying degrees of lobulation. Invasive papillary carcinoma frequently appears as a cluster of smooth or irregular nodules, nodules in several quadrants or as a solitary nodule.
- The outline of malignant circumscribed lesion is usually less sharply defined than benign circumscribed masses and malignant lesion are typically of high soft tissue density.

Spiculated Breast Masses

Invasive Carcinoma

- Approximately 95% of spiculated masses are due to invasive breast cancer.
- On mammography there is evidence of a distinct irregular, central tumor mass from which dense spicules radiate in all directions.
- Spicules that reach the skin or muscles cause retraction and localized skin thickening.
- This sunburst appearance is most commonly seen in scirrhous infiltrating ductal carcinoma.
- A web-like pattern of spicules may be seen with invasive lobular carcinoma.
- Most spiculated carcinomas of 1 cm diameter or more can be demonstrated by ultrasound. The typical ultrasound features are of an echo-poor mass, with poorly defined margins and posterior acoustic shadowing.

Post-surgical Scar

- Surgical scar can be diagnosed from the appropriate clinical history and physical examination, showing the position of incision site corresponds to the position of the stellate lesion, if necessary by carrying out mammogram with skin marker on the incisional skin scar.

- Post-surgical scarring usually will regress with time-whereas spiculated carcinoma usually will grow.
- Post-surgical scarring will characteristically lack a central density and will appears different on the craniocaudal and oblique lateral views. It will have a planar configuration corresponding to the incisional plane rather than a three-dimensional one.
- A central lucency due to fat necrosis, when present is a reliable sign, that a lesion is due to previous surgery.

Fat Necrosis

- Fat necrosis may assume any one of several mammographic appearances, stellate mass circumscribed mass, amorphous density or architectural distortion.
- When present central lucency in the mass or lipid cysts seen as a round lucent areas surrounded by a thin fibrotic capsule, suggests the correct diagnosis.
- Fat necrosis may occur secondary to blunt trauma, surgical procedures or on an idiopathic basis, especially in older women who have pendulous, fatty breasts.

Radial Scar(Complex Sclerosing Lesion)

- It is characterized histologically by a fibroelastic center surrounded by ducts and lobules arranged in a radiating fashion.
- On mammograms the lesion is fairly small, 10 to 15 cm in diameter. Some appears solid in the center, but in most, there is a radiolucent center or no solid central core.

- Although seen on both mammographic views, the lesion tends to occur in one plane, both on mammogram and histologic sections. It typically varies in appearance from one projection to another.
- All patients have normal physical findings. Skin thickening and retraction over the lesion are infrequent.
- Even when the mammographic findings are suggesting a radial scar they are not diagnostic. Thus biopsy is required.

Breast Abscess

- Usually caused by staphylococcus and Streptococcus.
- May also appear as a spiculated or poorly defined mass.
- The clinical diagnosis is usually clear, there is pain, swelling and erythema.
- Usually retroareolar and occurs in young primiparous women during lactation.

Sclerosing Adenosis

- It may also appear as a small stellate tumor, which may be difficult to distinguish from radial scar or cancer on mammography.
- *Extra-abdominal dermoid (fibromatosis)* is a rare benign condition that can appears as a spiculated or poorly defined mass an mammography.
- *Granular cell myoblastoma*: Is a rare benign tumor that produces a palpable lump with ill-defined stellate margins on mammography, suggestive of malignancy.

Pseudomass (Summation Shadows)

- Overlapping glandular tissue may simulate a mass on one projection, but no similar mass is seen on an orthogonal view.

- Therefore an area of asymmetric tissue must be identified on two views before it can be considered abnormal.

The Edematous Breast

The mammographic features are:
- Skin thickening, initially affecting mainly the lower part of the breast.
- Diffuse increased density.
- Coarse trabecular pattern.
- Enlargement of the breast.

D/D,s

1. *Carcinoma of the breast*: An edematous breast may be caused either by an advanced primary tumor, lymphatic spread from a primary tumor or inflammatory carcinoma.
   - Extension of tumor into lymphatic vessels can produce focal skin thickening and increased density of the subcutaneous tissue. In inflammatory carcinoma, intense edema causes rapid enlargement and tenderness of the affected breast with diffuse skin thickening.
2. *Axillary lymphatic obstruction*: Axillary lymphatic obstruction can occur secondary to metastasis from ipsilateral breast or contralateral breast or from non-breast. Primary advanced gynecologic malignancies (ovarian, uterine), rarely may block primary lymphatic drainage in the lesser pelvis, causing lymph flow through thoraco-epigastric collaterals and overloading the axillary and supraclavicular lymphatic drainage.
3. *Postoperative axillary lymph node removal or dissection*: It may also lead to edematous breast. Edema of the breast may persist mammographically even when it is not obvious clinically.

- If axillary lymph node dissection has been performed for metastatic disease and skin thickening occurs it may be impossible to determine whether this appearance represents metastatic involvement of the breast or impaired lymphatic drainage from surgery.

4. *Radiation therapy*: The features of edema develop progressively following radiotherapy treatment, reaches maximum at about 6 months and has resolved approximately 18 months following treatment.
   - If skin thickening and breast edema recur after the initial edema has resolved or decreased, recurrent carcinoma should be considered.

5. *Mastitis or breast abscess*: Focal or diffuse skin thickening may be related to lactation, skin or nipple infection with extension into the breast or hematogenous spread of infection.

   Fluid overload state: Edematous breast may develop in patients with cardiac failure, renal failure, cirrhosis and hypoalbuminemia. It is usually bilateral. The thickening occurs mostly in the dependent aspect of the breast. In a bedridden patient lying on one side, the skin thickening may be unilateral and involve only the dependent breast.

BREAST CALCIFICATIONS

A. Characteristically Benign Calcification

- *Egg shell calcification*: It represents hollow spherical structure with a thin calcific rim.
- Can occur in
  Idiopathic fat necrosis- Small, several centimeters across.
                                  Common in large fatty breast.
- Post-traumatic or post-surgical -Larger.

- Rarely in the wall of the "garden variety", type of breast cysts which occur in fibrocystic disease.
- *Tram tracks calcification*: (Rail road track calcification).
- The typical appearance of vascular calcification is that of two parallel calcific lines, along the vessel walls.
- These calcification may be seen to be continuous with non-calcified soft tissue shadows of the vessels.
- *Large rod like calcification*: These follows the course of the ducts branching out in a series of orderly areas which radiate from the retroareolar area.
- These occur in the duct lumen as solid cores, and are due to benign secretory involvement.
- These are distinguishable from malignant linear calcification by being longer, wider and more variable in width, and being more frequently bilateral.
- *Popcorn calcification*: It is characteristic of fibro-adenoma.
- *Dystrophic calcification*: Dystrophic calcification resulting from surgery and/or radiation therapy often has a bizarre or plaque like shape and is frequently large.
- *Milk of calcium*: It represents calcium that layers out in the dependent portion of tiny microcysts.
- Best seen on horizontal beam lateral view-which demonstrates a calcium-fluid level or meniscus (the tea-cup sign) while a craniocaudal view will show a round smudge shadow often, but not always bilateral.
- *Skin calcifications:* There may be punctate or tiny hollow spheres of 1-2 mm diameter each.
  - These occur in sebaceous glands.
  - Most common location are in the periareolar, axillary and medial breast areas.

- Some times may present as localized cluster of punctate calcification, rather than diffuse calcification.

  In these cases, findings that raise the possibility that clustered calcification may be in the skin and do not require biopsy, in comparison to clustered parenchymal calcification that do require biopsy, include a peripheral location, (frequently in the subcutaneous tissue) or a location in the periareolar region, axillary area or medial breast. The presence of one or more tiny hollow spherical calcification with in the cluster also suggests skin calcifications.
- True nature can be confirmed by tangential view, which projects the cluster in the skin.
- *Pseudocalcification*: These include aluminium chloride deodrant seen in the axilla or talcum powder seen in the inframammary area or in the medial side of breasts.
- Confirmation can be obtained when necessary, by repeating the appropriate view, after the area has been cleaned.

Calcification Suspicious for Malignancy

- *Characteristics required for suspicion of malignancy*:
  - Linear(casting shape).
  - Linear distribution.
  - Segmental distribution.
  - Markedly clustered distribution.
- *Characteristics not specific for malignancy but increasing degree of suspicion.*
  - Variation in shape (pleomorphism).
  - Variation in size.
  - Irregular margins of individual particles.
  - Irregular boundaries of areas of calcification.

Flow Chart 2.1.1
Circumscribed radiolucent lesion

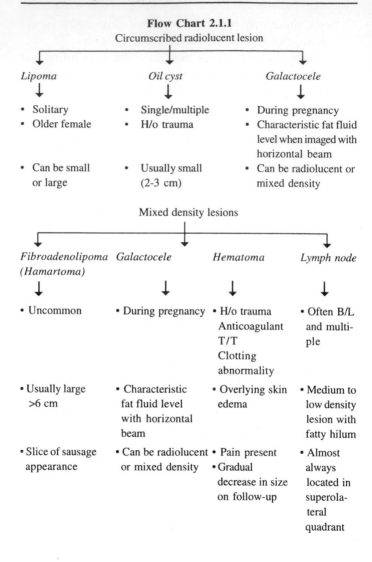

Lipoma	*Oil cyst*	*Galactocele*
• Solitary	• Single/multiple	• During pregnancy
• Older female	• H/o trauma	• Characteristic fat fluid level when imaged with horizontal beam
• Can be small or large	• Usually small (2-3 cm)	• Can be radiolucent or mixed density

Mixed density lesions

Fibroadenolipoma (Hamartoma)	*Galactocele*	*Hematoma*	*Lymph node*
• Uncommon	• During pregnancy	• H/o trauma Anticoagulant T/T Clotting abnormality	• Often B/L and multiple
• Usually large >6 cm	• Characteristic fat fluid level with horizontal beam	• Overlying skin edema	• Medium to low density lesion with fatty hilum
• Slice of sausage appearance	• Can be radiolucent or mixed density	• Pain present • Gradual decrease in size on follow-up	• Almost always located in superolateral quadrant

Flow Chart 2.1.2

Soft tissue density lesions

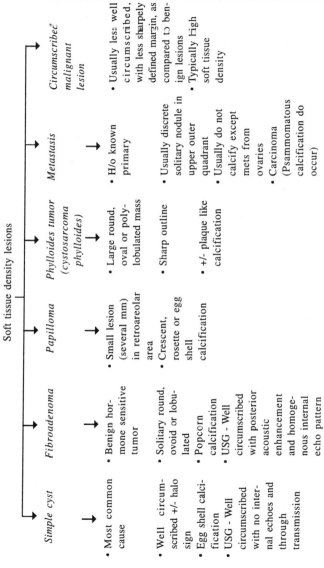

Simple cyst	Fibroadenoma	Papilloma	Phylloides tumor (cystosarcoma phylloides)	Metastasis	Circumscribed malignant lesion
• Most common cause	• Benign hormone sensitive tumor	• Small lesion (several mm) in retroareolar area	• Large round, oval or poly-lobulated mass	• H/o known primary	• Usually less well circumscribed, with less sharply defined margin, as compared to benign lesions
• Well circumscribed +/- halo sign	• Solitary round, ovoid or lobulated	• Crescent, rosette or egg shell calcification	• Sharp outline	• Usually discrete solitary nodule in upper outer quadrant	• Typically high soft tissue density
• Egg shell calcification	• Popcorn calcification		• +/- plaque like calcification	• Usually do not calcify except mets from ovaries	
• USG - Well circumscribed with no internal echoes and through transmission	• USG - Well circumscribed with posterior acoustic enhancement and homogenous internal echo pattern			• Carcinoma (Psammomatous calcification do occur)	

Flow Chart 2.1.3
The edematous breast

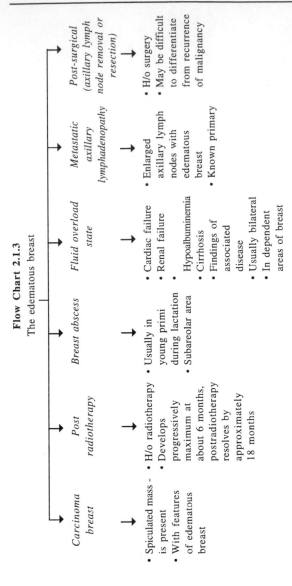

Carcinoma breast	Post radiotherapy	Breast abscess	Fluid overload state	Metastatic axillary lymphadenopathy	Post-surgical (axillary lymph node removal or resection)
• Spiculated mass - is present • With features of edematous breast	• H/o radiotherapy • Develops progressively maximum at about 6 months, postradiotherapy resolves by approximately 18 months	• Usually in young primi during lactation • Subareolar area	• Cardiac failure • Renal failure • Hypoalbuminemia • Cirrhosis • Findings of associated disease • Usually bilateral • In dependent areas of breast	• Enlarged axillary lymph nodes with edematous breast • Known primary	• H/o surgery • May be difficult to differentiate from recurrence of malignancy

Flow Chart 2.1.4
Spiculated breast masses

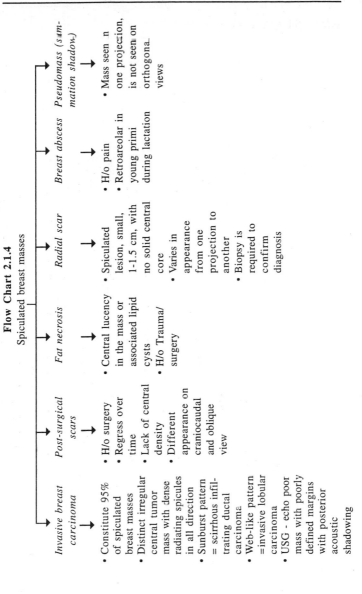

Invasive breast carcinoma

- Constitute 95% of spiculated breast masses
- Distinct irregular central tumor mass with dense radiating spicules in all direction
- Sunburst pattern = scirrhous infiltrating ductal carcinoma
- Web-like pattern =invasive lobular carcinoma
- USG - echo poor mass with poorly defined margins with posterior acoustic shadowing

Post-surgical scars

- H/o surgery
- Regress over time
- Lack of central density
- Different appearance on craniocaudal and oblique view

Fat necrosis

- Central lucency in the mass or associated lipid cysts
- H/o Trauma/ surgery

Radial scar

- Spiculated lesion, small, 1-1.5 cm, with no solid central core
- Varies in appearance from one projection to another
- Biopsy is required to confirm diagnosis

Breast abscess

- H/o pain
- Retroareolar in young primi during lactation

Pseudomass (summation shadow)

- Mass seen in one projection, is not seen on orthogonal views

BREAST CALCIFICATION

1. Arterial

2. Smooth ± lucent center
widely separated

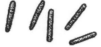

3. Linear, thick, rod-like
± lucent centers

4. 'Egg-shell'

5. 'Pop-corn'

6. Large calcific opacity

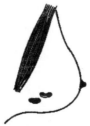

7. Floating calcification

Microcalcification, mixture of sizes
shapes, cluster, haphazard arrangement,
linear branching pattern

Fig. 2.1.2

Flow Chart 2.1.5
Breast calcification

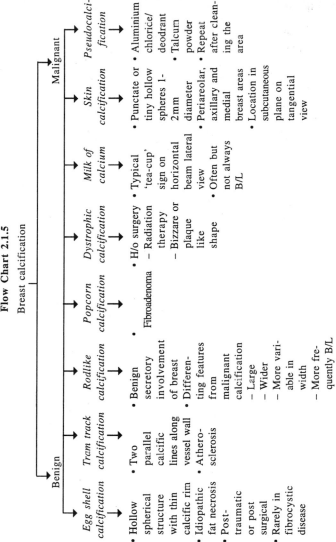

Benign

Egg shell calcification →
- Hollow spherical structure with thin calcific rim
- Idiopathic fat necrosis
- Post-traumatic or post surgical
- Rarely in fibrocystic disease

Tram track calcification →
- Two parallel calcific lines along vessel wall
- Atherosclerosis

Rodlike calcification →
- Benign secretory involvement of breast
- Differentiating features from malignant calcification
  - Large
  - Wider
  - More variable in width
  - More frequently B/L

Popcorn calcification →
- Fibroadenoma

Dystrophic calcification →
- H/o surgery
  - Radiation therapy
  - Bizzare or plaque like shape

Milk of calcium →
- Typical 'tea-cup' sign on horizontal beam lateral view
- Often but not always B/L

Malignant

Skin calcification →
- Punctate or tiny hollow spheres 1-2mm diameter
- Periareolar, axillary and medial breast areas
- Location in subcutaneous plane on tangential view

Pseudocalcification →
- Aluminium chloride/deodorant
- Talcum powder
- Repeat after cleaning the area

Malignant

- Linear (casting type).
- Linear distribution.
- Segmental distribution.
- Markedly clustered distribution.
- Pleomorphism in size and shape.
- Irregular margins of individual particles.
- Irregular boundaries areas of calcification.

CALCIFICATION

1. Microcalcification is defined as individual calcific opacities measuring < 0.5 mm diameter.
2. Macrocalcification: Opacities > 0.5 mm diameter.
3. Microcalcification is not specific to carcinoma.
4. Microcalcification is seen in 30-40% of carcinomas on mammography.
5. Macrocalcification may be found in carcinoma.

Definitely Benign

1. Arterial – tortuous, tramline.
2. Smooth, widely separated, some with radiolucent center.
3. Linear thick, rod-like, widespread, some with radiolucent center.
4. 'Egg shell' curvilinear: Margin of cyst, fat necrosis.
5. 'Popcorn' in fibroadenoma.
6. Large individual calcific opacity > 2 mm, e.g. involutional fibroadenoma.
7. 'Floating' calcification – seen as calcific/fluid level seen on lateral oblique projection in 'milk of calcium' cysts.

Probably Benign

1. Widespread – all one/both breasts.
2. Macrocalcification of one size.
3. Symmetrical distribution.
4. Widely separated opacities.
5. Superficial distribution.
6. Normal parenchyma.

Possibly Malignant – Biopsy Indicated

(see microcalcification figure)

1. Microcalcification – particularly segmental, cluster distribution (> 5 particles in 1.0 cm^3 space; of these 30% will be malignant).
2. Mixture of sizes and shapes – linear, branching, punctate.
3. Associated suspicious soft tissue opacity.
4. Microcalcification eccentrically located in soft tissue mass.
5. Deterioration on serial mammography.

Benign Conditions that Mimic Malignancy

1. Microcalcification
   a. Sclerosing adenosis: One/both breasts, widely separated opacities.
2. Suspicious soft tissue opacity
   a. Fibroadenoma – when one margin ill-defined.
   b. Fat necrosis – ill-defined, sometimes with radiolucent center.
   c. Post biopsy scar.
   d. Radial scar.
   e. Plasma cell mastitis.
   f. Hematoma.
   g. Summation of normal tissues.
   h. Irregular skin lesion, e.g. wart.

CARCINOMA

Primary Features

1. Opacity – ill-defined, spiculated outline, comet tail. Usually dense.
2. Microcalcification – mixture of sizes, shapes; linear, branching, punctate cluster arrangement. Eccentric to and/ or outside soft-tissue opacity.

Secondary Features

1. Distortion – adjacent tissues, obliteration subcutaneous, retromammary spaces.
2. Skin, nipple retraction.
3. Edema – all or part of breast.
4. Halo – wide around primary opacity.
5. Duct dilatation.
6. Venous engorgement.

Note: Approximately 10% of palpable carcinomas in premenopausal women are not diagnosable on mammography.

3

Cardiovascular System

3.1 D/D OF CARDIOVASCULAR DISORDERS

1. Pericardial effusion
   - pericardial fluid >50 ml.

Causes

1. *Malignancy*
   - Secondaries normally from breast, lung.
   - May cause tamponade.
   - Usually hemorrhagic.
2. *Inflammatory*
   Bacterial, viral, tuberculous infection.
   Exudative in nature.
3. *Heart diseases*
   Cardiac failure—Transudative in nature.
   Myocardial infarction—Known as Dressler's syndrome.
4. *Endocrine diseases*
   Myxoedema causes substantial pleural effusion, often asymptomatic.
5. *Collagen diseases*
   All collagen diseases may cause pericardial effusion (SLE causes large pericardial effusion).

6. *Uremia*
   18% in acute uremia.
   51% in chronic uremia.
   May lead to tamponade.
7. *Hemopericardium*
   – Traumatic.
   – Rupture of heart in course of MI.
   Dissecting aneurysm leading into pericardium.
         (See Flow Chart 3.1.1 Next Page)

3.2 INVISIBLE MAIN PULMONARY ARTERY

A. Underdeveloped Main Pulmonary Artery

1. *Tetralogy of Fallot*
   – Obstruction of right ventricular outflow tract due to pulmonary stenosis.
   – Associated VSD and right ventricular hypertrophy.
   – Overriding of aorta.
2. *Pulmonary stenosis*
   – Due to reduced flow.
   – Associated right ventricular hypertrophy.
   – Decreased pulmonary vascularity.
3. *Tricuspid stenosis*
   – Due to reduced blood flow into the right ventricle and pulmonary artery.
   – Enlarged right atrium.
   – Hepatic congestion-anasarca.

B. Misplaced Pulmonary Artery

1. Complete transportion of great vessels.

Flow Chart 3.1.1

Pericardial effusion

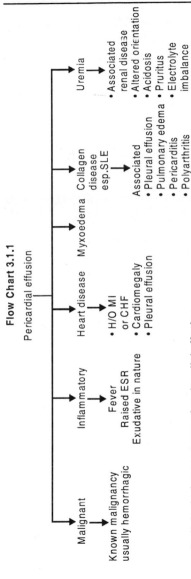

Malignant	Inflammatory	Heart disease	Myxoedema	Collagen disease esp.SLE	Uremia
Known malignancy usually hemorrhagic	Fever Raised ESR Exudative in nature	• H/O MI or CHF • Cardiomegaly • Pleural effusion		Associated • Pleural effusion • Pulmonary edema • Pericarditis • Polyarthritis	• Associated renal disease • Altered orientation • Acidosis • Pruritus • Electrolyte imbalance

Radiological appearance of pericardial effusion

1. Enlarged heart shadow — water bottle configuration
2. Rapid change in heart size on serial films
3. Inward displacement of epicardial stripe
4. Loss of retrosternal clear space in lateral view
5. Differential density sign – increase in lucency at heart margin

- Pulmonary trunk is absent in 99%—Pulmonary artery is located posteriorly in midline
- "Egg on its side" appearance of heart with narrow superior mediastinum

2. Persistent truncus arteriosus-single artery giving rise to pulmonary and systemic AS.
   - Cardiomegaly with enlarged left atrium.
   - Large aortic shadow.
   - Markedly increase pulmonary blood flow.
     (See Table 3.2.1 Next Page)

3.3 PULMONARY ARTERIAL HYPERTENSION

Sustained pulmonary artery pressure >30 mmHg

1. Primary
   - Idiopathic, 3rd decade M<F dyspnea, syncope.
2. Secondary
   a. Parenchymal pulmonary disease:
      - Cor pulmonale, COPD, chronic bronchitis, asthma, emphysema, interstitial fibrosis.
      - Alveolar hypoxia and hypercapnia–pulmonary vasoconstriction – pulmonary arterial hypertension.
   b. Congenital heart disease:
      - Large left to right shunt (Eisenmenger's syndrome) ASD, VSD, PDA lead to increase pulmonary blood flow leading to increase pulmonary resistance—PA hypertension.
      - Tetralogy of Fallot.
   c. Pulmonary thromboembolism
      Thrombus impacted in pulmonary arteries–rise in pulmonary arterial pressure – pulmonary arterial hypertension.

Table 3.2.1

Causes of underdeveloped pulmonary artery	Clinical features	Main pulmonary artery	Heart shadow	Pulmonary flow	Associated features
• Tetralogy of Fallot	• Cyanosis, fainting spells on exertion	• Underdeveloped	• RVH concave pulmonary bay, upward prominence of cardiac apex, cor-En-sabot appearance	• Decreased	• Pulmonary stenosis, VSD, Rt aortic arch
• Pulmonary stenosis	• Mostly asymptomatic, cyanosis, heart failure	• Underdeveloped	• Right ventricular hypertrophy	• Decreased	• Cor pulmonale
• Tricuspid atresia	• Progressive cyanosis from birth	• Underdeveloped	• Right atrial enlargement, enlarged LV small pulmonary bay	• Decreased	• ASD, small VSD
• Complete transposition of great arteries	• Cyanosis, symptomatic 2 wks. After birth	• Located in midline posteriorly	• Right heart enlargement, "egg on side" appearance	• Increased	• PDA + patent forman ovale, VSD in 50%
• Truncus arteriosus	• Cyanosis, CHF systolic murmur	• Arising from single trunk along with systemic arteries		• Markedly increased	• Rt aortic arch in 35%, forked ribs

- Modest increase in heart size.
- Pulmonary oligemia.
- Right ventricular enlargement.
d. Arteritides, e.g. Polyarteritis nodosa.
  Narrowing of pulmonary arteries causes increase in pressure – PHT.

Radiographic appearance of pulmonary arterial HT
1. Large triangular heart.
2. Large main and central pulmonary artery.
3. Pruning of pulmonary arteries.
4. Calcification of central pulmonary vessels.

(See Flow Chart 3.3.1 Next Page)

3.4 ENLARGED LEFT VENTRICLE (ELV)

A. Volume Overload

1. *Ventricular Septal Defect (VSD)*
   Most common congenital heart disease.

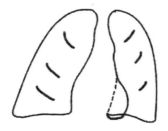

PA view: Chest shows prominent LT heart border (inferior part).
Rounding of LT heart border (apex of heart).
Fig. 3.4.1: Apex displaced inferiorly – ventricular septal defect

Flow Chart 3.3.1

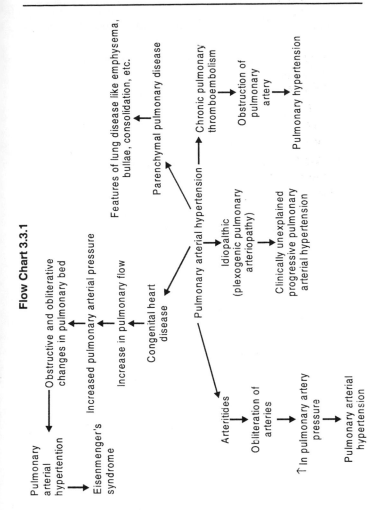

Bouts of respiratory infection, feeding problems, failure to thrive.

Increased pulmonary vascular resistance causes LV enlargement.

2. *Patent Ductus Arteriosus (PDA)*

Mostly asymptomatic.

Congestive heart failure usually by 3 months of age.

Continuous murmur.

Enlarged RV, LV and LA, enlarged pulmonary artery segment and enlarged aorta.

3. *Mitral Incompetence*
   - Backward flow of blood from LV into LA during systole with consequent increase in LV volume.
   - LA + LV enlargement, mitral annular calcification.

4. *Aortic Incompetence*
   - Water hammer pulse with systolic ejection and high pitched diastolic murmur.
   - LV enlargement with dilatation of aorta.

B. Pressure Overload

1. *Aortic Stenosis*
   - Angina, syncope, heart failure with systolic murmur.
   - Calcification of aortic valve.
   - Enlarged LV with post stenotic dilatation of ascending aorta in 90% cases.

2. *Coarctation of Aorta*
   - Shelf like narrowing of aorta usually beyond the origin of left subclavian artery.
   - Small irregular contour of upper descending aorta on X-ray.
   - Rib notching.

3. *Systemic Hypertension*
   - Due to increased resistance to blood flow.
   - May lead to congestive heart failure.
   - Dyspnea on exertion, headache.

C. High Output States

1. Anemia.
2. AV fistula.
3. Hyperthyroidism.

D. Myocardial Causes

1. Cardiomyopathy
   - Cardiomegaly with poor contractility of ventricular wall.
   - Global heart enlargement.
2. Ischemic heart disease.
   Coronary artery calcification.
   Left ventricular aneurysm may be present.

(See Table 3.4.1 Next Page)

3.5 ENLARGED LEFT ATRIUM

A. Volume Overload

Mitral Regurgitation

| VSD | Refer to cause of enlargement left |
| PDA | ventricle for salient features. |

ASD with shunt reversal.

Table 3.4.1

	Clinical features	Chamber enlargement	Pulmonary artery	Pulmonary veins	Pulmonary vasculature	Associated features
1. Mitral incompetence	Fatigue, exertional dyspnea orthopnea	LA + LV	Normal	Mild pulmonary venous HT	Normal	Frequent mitral annular calcification
2. Aortic incompetence	Collapsing pulse, early diastolic murmur	LV enlargement dilated aorta	Normal	Pulmonary venous HT	Normal	Dilatation + calcification of ascending aorta
3. VSD	Dyspnea, syncope, chest pain, hemoptysis	LA + LV + RV	Enlarged	Pulmonary venous HT in shunt reversal	Pulmonary plethora	Small aorta
4. PDA	CHF by 3 months of age	LV + LA + RV	Enlarged	–	Increased	Enlarged ascending aorta and arch
5. Aortic stenosis	Angina, syncope, systolic murmur	LV hypertrophy	Normal	Pulmonary venous congestion	Normal	Post-stenotic dilatation of aorta
6. Coarctation of aorta	Lower extremity cyanosis, headache, cold extremities	LV hypertrophy, dilated left subclavian artery and dilated ascending aorta	Normal	Normal	–	Enlarged pulsatile collateral in intercostal spaces
7. Cardiomyopathy	Congestive cardiac failure	LV enlargement or globular heart	Normal	Prominent	–	Rib notching

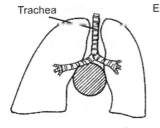 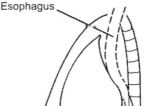

PA view: 1. Obliteration of concavity on LT heart border. 2. Double RT cardiac border. 3. Elevated LT carinal angle more than 70° and splaying of carina. 4. Prominent LT atrial appendage and straigtening of LT heart border.

In RAO view: Barium swallow shows LT atrial enlargement shadow or impression

Fig. 3.5.1: Mitral valvular disease

B. Pressure Overload

1. *Mitral Stenosis*
   - History of rheumatic fever.
   - Shortness of breath on exertion.
   - Left atrial enlargement with universal enlargement of left atrial appendage.
   - Changes in pulmonary circulation with pulmonary venous hypertension.
2. *Left Atrial Myxoma*
   - Dyspnea, chest pain, fever, myalgia, weight loss, raised ESR.
   - Enlargement of LA, no enlargement of atrial appendage.

C. Secondary to Left Ventricular Failure

Radiographic features of enlarged left atrium.
1. Straightening of left heart border or discrete bulge below the pulmonary conus.

2. Double heart shadow progressing to form the Rt heart border.
3. Displacement of barium filled esophagus backwards (in Lat. view)
4. Splaying of carina and elevated left main bronchus.

(See Table 3.5.1 Next Page)

3.6 DILATATION OF PULMONARY TRUNK

1. *Idiopathic*
   Unexplained dilatation of main pulmonary artery.
2. *Pulmonary Regurgitation*
   – High pitched diastolic blowing murmur.
   – Enlarged RV.
3. *Post Stenotic Dilatation in Pulmonary Valve Stenosis*
   – Mostly asymptomatic.
   – Enlarged pulmonary trunk and left pulmonary artery.
   – Hypertrophy of RV with elevation of cardiac apex.
4. *Congenital L-R shunts*
   – Due to volume overload in RV and pulmonary artery.
   – RV enlargement.
5. *Pulmonary Artery Hypertension*
   – Large and often triangular heart.
   – Main and central pulmonary arteries are large.
   – Prunning of pulmonary arteries, i.e. tapering to periphery.
6. *Pulmonary Artery Aneurysm*
   – Can be traumatic or mycotic.
   – Focally dilated main pulmonary artery with convex pulmonary bay.

Table 3.5.1

	Clinical features	Chamber enlargement	Pulmonary artery	Pulmonary veins	Aorta	Associated features
Mitral stenosis	Dyspnea, cough orthopnea	Esp. left atrial appendage RV enlargement LV enlargement	Prominent	Prominent with pulmonary venous HT	Small	Ossific nodules in lung, Kerley's lines
Mitral regurgitation	Fatigue, exertional dyspnea	LA + LV	Normal	Prominent but mild venous HT then MS	Enlargement	Kerley's lines, less frequent
VSD	Dyspnea, syncope chest pain hemoptysis	LA, LV, RV	Enlarged pulmonary plethora	Pulmonary venous HT occurs in Eisenmenger's syndrome	Small	–
PDA	CHF by 3 months of age	LA, RV + LV	Enlarged	–	Enlarged	Obscured aorto pulmonary window
Myxoma	Dyspnea, weight loss, fever, increase ESR	LA, No enlargement of left atrial appendage	–	Pulmonary venous HT	Small	–

Table 3.6.1

	Clinical features	Chamber enlargement	Pulmonary artery	Pulmonary veins	Pulmonary vasculature	Associated features
1. Pulmonary regurgitation	High pitched diastolic murmur	Right ventricular enlargement + RA enlargement	Enlarged due to RV volume overload	–	Increased pulmonary vascularity	–
2. Post-stenotic dilatation	Mostly asymptomatic heart failure	RV hypertrophy with reduced size of chamber	Prominent pulmonary conus	–	Diminished due to reduced flow	–
3. Congenital L-R shunts (Eisenmenger's syndrome)	Cardiorespiratory symptoms, fainting spells in children, chest pain	Common-RV dilatation with Rt heart failure later leading to pulmonary artery hypertension	Prominent due to volume overload	–	Pulmonary plethora	Eisenmenger's syndrome due to ↑ pulmonary resistance leading to pulmonary arterial HT with pronounced dilatation of central pulmonary arteries
4. Pulmonary arterial HT	Syncope, angina shortness of breath	RV enlargement with large and triangular heart	Enlarged central pulmonary arteries with peripheral prunning		Clear lung fields	
5. Pulmonary artery	Asymptomatic or chest pain and hemoptysis	Normal	Rounded shadow in hilum with curvilinear calcification in its wall	–	Normal	Angiography may show clot lining the wall

3.7 ENLARGEMENT AORTA

1. *Volume overload*
   a. Aortic regurgitation
      - Water hammer pulse, diastolic murmur.
      - LV enlargement.
   b. Patent ductus arteriosus (PDA)
      - Continuous murmur.
      - Enlargement RV, LV and LA. Enlargement pulmonary artery segment, pulmonary plethora.
2. *Post-stenotic dilatation in aortic stenosis*
   Angina, syncope.
   Calcification of aortic valve.
   Left ventricular enlargement.
   Enlarged ascending aorta.
3. *Pressure overload*
   a. Coarctation of aorta
      - Shelf like narrowing of aorta beyond the origin of left subclavian artery.
      - Small irregular contour of upper descending aorta on X-ray with rib, notching.
   b. Systemic hypertension
      - May lead to left ventricular failure.
      - Dyspnea on exertion.
4. *Aneurysm of Aorta*
   Congenital
   Mycotic
   Syphilitic — There is widening of mediastinum.
   Atherosclerotic or round or oval soft tissue mass.
   Traumatic in mediastinum with or without.
   Dissecting aneurysm peripheral rim of calcification.

Table 3.7.1

	Clinical features	Chamber enlargement	Pulmonary artery	Pulmonary veins	Pulmonary vasculature	Associated features
1. Aortic regurgitation	Collapsing pulse, early diastolic murmur	LV enlargement dilated aorta	Normal	Pulmonary venous HT	Normal	Dilatation and calcification of ascending aorta
2. Post-stenotic dilatation	Angina, syncope, chest pain, systolic murmur due to AS	LV hypertrophy	Normal	Pulmonary venous congestion	–	Discrete enlargement without correlation with stenosis
3. Patent ductus arteriosus	CHF by 8 months of age	LV + RV + LA	Enlarged	–	Increased	Enlarged associated aorta and arch
4. Coarctation of aorta	Lower extremity cyanosis, headache cold extremities	LV hypertrophy dilated left subclavian artery dilated ascending aorta	Normal	Normal	–	Enlarged pulsatile collaterals in intercostal spaces with rib notching
5. Aortic aneurysm						
6. Systemic hypertension	Headache angina, cardiac failure	LV hypertrophy and dilatation	–	–	–	–

3.8 SMALL AORTA

1. *Aortic Stenosis*
   - Angina, syncope, heart failure with systolic murmur.
   - Calcification of aortic valve.
   - Left ventricular hypertrophy.

2. *Mitral Stenosis*
   - History of rheumatic fever.
   - Shortness of breath on exertion.
   - Left atrial enlargement with universal enlargement of left atrial appendage.
   - Pulmonary venous hypertension with pulmonary ossific nodules.

3. *Left to Right Shunts*
   - Most of the blood flows into right sided chambers and into the pulmonary circulation causing pulmonary plethora.
   - Left ventricle recovers less blood and aorta is small.

4. *Hypertrophic Obstructive Cardiomyopathy*
   - Asymmetrical hypertrophy of the left ventricle with difficulty in filling of LV.
   - Shortness of breath, angina, arrhythmias, jerky pulse.
   - Left ventricle has a chunky outline.

5. *Long Segment Coarctation of Aorta (Infantile or Tubular Hypoplasia)*
   - Hypoplasia of long segment of aortic arch after origin of innominate artery.
   - Coexistent cardiac anomalies are common.
   - CHF in neonatal period (in 50%).

Table 3.8.1

	Clinical features	Chamber enlargement	Pulmonary vasculature	Pulmonary arteries	Pulmonary veins	Associated features
1. Aortic stenosis	Angina, syncope, systolic murmur	LV hypertrophy	–	Normal	Pulmonary venous congestion	Post-stenotic dilatation, calcification of valve
2. Mitral stenosis	Dyspnea, cough, orthopnea	Left atrial appendage enlargement, RV enlargement, LV not enlarged	Redistribution of pulmonary blood flow to upper lobes	Prominent	Prominent with pulmonary venous hypertension	Ossific nodules in lung, Kerley's lines
3. Left to right shunt	Cardio-respiratory symptoms, fainting spells, chest pain	RV enlargement with Rt heart failure	Pulmonary plethora	Enlarged due to increase blood flow	–	–
4. Hypertrophic obstructive cardiomyopathy	Congestive heart failure	LV enlargement or globular heart	–	Normal	Prominent	–
5. Long segment coarctation of aorta	Lower extremity cyanosis, left ventricular failure	LV hypertrophy, figure 3 sign, i.e. indentation of left lateral margin of aortic arch in region of aorto-pulmonary window	Increased if associated with L to R shunt	–	Pulmonary venous hypertension	Cardiac malformation

3.9 ENLARGED RIGHT ATRIUM

1. *Volume Overload*
   a. Tricuspid regurgitation
      – There is systemic venous congestion and reduction of cardiac output.
      – Right sided heart failure, hepatomegaly, ascites, anasarca.
      – RV and RA enlargement.
   b. ASD
      – Most common congenital heart defect in subjects > 20 yrs of age.
      – Usually presents > 40 yrs.
      Mildly symptomatic, dyspnea, fatigue, palpitations.
      – Chest X-ray hilar dance (increased pulsations of central pulmonary arteries).
      – RA and RV enlargement and pulmonary plethora.

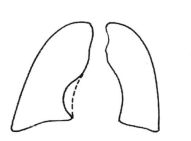

PA view : Prominent Rt heart border.

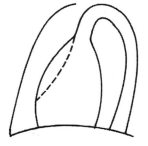

Lateral view: Anterosuperior part of cardiac outline is prominent.

Fig. 3.9.1: Enlarged right atrium

c. Total/Partial anomalous pulmonary venous return.
   – Pulmonary veins drain blood into right atrium.
   – Increased pulmonary blood flow.
   – ASD restores oxygenated blood to left side.
   – Volume overload to RV.
   Cyanosis, Rt ventricular heave (i.e. increased contact of RV with sternum)
   – Figure of '8' or Snowman configuration of cardiac silhouette

2. *Pressure Overload*
   a. Tricuspid stenosis/Atresia.
      – Pulmonary oligemia, small pulmonary bay.
      – Rt atrial enlargement, bulging the heart shadow to right.
   b. Myxoma of Rt atrium.
      – Causes occlusion of tricuspid valve and RA enlargement.
      – Systemic symptoms of fever, increase ESR, weight loss.

3. *Secondary to Right Ventricular Failure*
   Congestive hepatomegaly, anasarca and systemic venous distension.

(See Table 3.9.1 Next Page)

3.10 ENLARGED RIGHT VENTRICLE

A. *Volume Overload*
   1. ASD
      – Increase amount of blood entering the right atrium and hence right ventricle.
      – Increased pulmonary flow with prominent pulmonary arteries.
      – Rt atrial and Rt ventricle enlargement.

Table 3.9.1

	Clinical features	Chamber enlargement	Pulmonary vasculature	Pulmonary arteries	Pulmonary veins	Associated features
Tricuspid regurgitation	Systemic venous congestion hepatomegaly, ascites	RV and RA	Normal or diminished	Normal or small	Normal	Rt heart failure, pleural effusion edema, systolic pulsations of liver
ASD	Respiratory infections, feeling difficulties, arrhythmias	RA + RV	hilar dance due to ↑ pulsations of pulmonary arteries	Prominent	–	Loss of visualization of SVC
Total anomalous pulmonary venous return	Cyanosis Rt ventricular heave	RA + RV figure of 8 appearance, dilated SVC	Increased pulmonary flow	–	Absent connection of pulmonary veins to LA	Neck veins undistended
Tricuspid stenosis	Fatigue refractory edema, ascites, hepatomegaly	RA and SVC enlargement	Oligemia	Small with flat concave pulmonary segment	Normal	–
Rt atrial myxoma	Systemic venous congestion	Enlarged RA, SVC, IVC and azygous vein	Decreased	Normal	–	Pulmonary emboli may arise
Secondary to LVF	Dyspnea, orthoprea,PND → fatigue edema, ascites	LV, LA → RV and RA → Congestive heart failure	Redistribution of flow to upper lobes	Elevated pulmonary arterial pressure with PHT	Dilatation of pulm. veins	Pleural and interlobar effusion

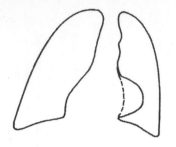 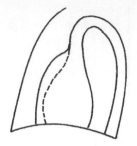

PA view : Left apex
of heart is prominent
and elevated.

Lateral view: Whole anterior
part of cardiac shadow is
prominent.

Fig. 3.10.1: Enlarged right ventricle

2. Total/Partial anomalous pulmonary venous return
   - Pulmonary vein drain blood to right atrium.
   - Volume overload of Rt ventricle with pulmonary overcirculation.
3. Tricuspid regurgitation
   - Increased amount of blood entering RV during diastole.
   - Rt heart failure with systemic venous congestion.
4. Pulmonary regurgitation
   - High pitched diastolic murmur.
   - Enlarged RV.
5. VSD
   - Flow of blood from LV to RV – Increased output of RV – increased size.
   - Enlarged RV, pulmonary artery.
   - Pulmonary plethora.

B. *Pressure Overload*
1. Pulmonary stenosis.
   – Increased contractility of RV – RVH.
   – Pulmonary oligemia, small pulmonary bay.
2. Pulmonary hypertension.
   – Increased resistance to right ventricular out flow – RVH.
   – Prunning of pulmonary arteries with enlarged proximal part.
3. Tetralogy of Fallot.
   Due to associated pulmonary stenosis.
4. VSD.
C. *Secondary to Left Heart Disease/Mitral Stenosis*
   – Increased left atrial pressure – pulmonary venous hypertension–Pulmonary arterial hypertension–RVH.

(See Table 3.10.1 Next Page)

3.11 RIGHT AORTIC ARCH

1. *Mirror Image Type* – Brachiocephalic branches being the mirror image of normal.
   a. Tetralogy of Fallot ⎱ Refer to previous section for
   b. Truncus arteriosus ⎰ features.
   c. Transposition of great vessels.
   d. Tricuspid atresia
   e. Large VSD — Refer to previous section for salient features.

Transposition of Great Vessels

- Rt aortic arch in 3%.
- Pulmonary artery originating from LV and aorta from RV.

Table 3.10.1

	Clinical features	Chamber enlargement	Pulmonary vasculature	Pulmonary arteries	Pulmonary veins	Associated features
ASD	Respiratory infections, feeding difficulty	RA + RV	Over circulation	Prominent	–	Loss of visualization of SVC due to clockwise rotation of heart due to RVH
Total anomalous pulmonary venous return	Cyanosis, R ventricular heave	RA + RV "figure of 8" appearance of heart	Increased flow	–	Absent connection of pulmonary veins to LA	Neck veins undistended
Tricuspid regurgitation	Systemic venous congestion	RV + RA	Normal or diminished	Normal or small	Normal	Rt heart failure, pleural effusions
Pulm. regurgitation	High pitched diastolic murmur	RV + RA	Increased	Enlarged	–	–
VSD	Dyspnea, syncope, chest pain	LA, LV, RV	Pulmonary plethora	Enlarged	Pulmonary venous hypertension in reversal of shunt	Small hyper-aorta
Pulmonary stenosis	Angina syncope	RV, RA	Oligemia	Small with concave pulm. bay.	–	–
Pulmonary hypertension Tetralogy of Fallot	Syncope, angina shortness of breath	RV enlargement with large triangular heart	Clear lung fields	Enlarged central pulmonary artery with peripheral prunning	–	–
Left heart disease	Dyspnea, orthopnea fatigue edema, ascites	LA, LV, RV, RA and congestive heart failure	Redistribution of flow to upper lobes	Elevated pulm. arterial pressure with PHT	Dilatation of pulmonary veins	Pleural and interlobar effusion

- Egg on its side appearance of heart with narrow superior mediastinum.
- Rt heart enlargement.
2. *Right Aortic Arch with Anomalous. Left Subclavian Artery*
   - Bulbous configuration of origin of LSA – retro esophageal aortic diverticulum (from descending aorta).
   - Small rounded density left lateral to trachea.
   - Right aortic impression on tracheal air shadow.

Causes

a. Tetralogy of Fallot–

b. ASD ± VSD
c. Coarctation
} Refer to previous sections for salient features.

3.12 PULMONARY VENOUS HYPERTENSION

Increased pulmonary venous pressure.
Pulmonary capillary wedge pressure > 15 mmHg.

Causes

A. *Left Ventricular in Flow Tract Obstruction*
   1. *Proximal to mitral valve* – Normal left atrium
      a. *Total anomalous pulmonary venous return* (below the diaphragm)
         - Pulmonary venous return into portal vein/IVC/ ductus venousus/left gastric vein with constriction of descending pulmonary vein by diaphragm enroute through esophageal hiatus – pulmonary venous hypertension.

- Pulmonary edema + pulmonary venous congestion.

  b. *Constrictive pericarditis*
     - Fibrous thickening of pericardium interfering with filling of ventricular chambers.
     - Dyspnea, peripheral edema, neck vein distension.
     - Dilatation of SVC, azygos vein, and pulmonary venous hypertention.

  c. *Fibrosing Mediastinitis*
     - Widening of upper mediastinum
     - Compression of SVC + pulmonary veins.

  d. *Primary pulmonary veno-occlusive disease*
     - Fibrous narrowing of intrapulmonary veins
     - Pulmonary edema, pleural effusion

2. *At Mitral Valve Level* – Enlarged left atrium

   a. *Mitral stenosis*
      - Redistribution of pulmonary blood flow to upper lobes due to back pressure.
      - Interstitial pulmonary edema and alveolar edema.

   b. *Left atrial myxoma*
      Obstructs the mitral valve with pulmonary back pressure similar to MS.

3. *Ball Valve Thrombus*

B. *Left Ventricular Failure*
   - Increase preload, increased after load, high output failure.
   - Transmission of backpressure to left-atrium – Pulmonary veins-pulmonary venous hypertension.

Table 3.12.1

	Clinical features	Chamber enlargement	Pulmonary vasculature	Associated features
Total anomalous pulmonary venous return subdiaphragmatic	Cyanosis, respiratory distress	RA + RV low anterior indentation to barium filled esophagus	Increased	Pulmonary edema
Constrictive pericarditis	Dyspnea, hepatomegaly, ascites, edema, neck veins distended	Normal or small sized heart dilatation of SVC azygos vein small atria	Normal	Straightening of left and right heart borders Linear or plaque like pericardial calcifications
Fibrosing mediastinitis	Cough, dyspnea hemoptysis, SVC syndrome	–	Pulmonary arterial hypertension due to compression of pulmonary arteries and veins	Widening of upper mediastinum lobulated paratracheal/hilar mass
Primary pulmonary veno-occlusive disease	Fibrosis, narrowing of intrapulmonary veins in presence of N left heart	RV	–	Pulmonary edema, pleural effusions delayed filling of normal main pulm. veins+ left heart
Mitral stenosis	Dyspnea, cough orthopnea	Left atrial appendage enlargement + RV enlargement	Upper lobe blood diversion	Ossific nodules in lung Kerley's lines
Left atrial myxoma	Dyspnea, weight loss fever – ESR	LA. No enlargement of atrial appendage	–	Small aorta
Left ventricular failure	Dyspnea, fatigue edema, ascities	LA, LV, RV, RA	Redistribution of blood flow to upper lobes	Pleural and interlobar effusion, pulmonary arterial hypertension

3.13 ENLARGED SUPERIOR VENA CAVA

A. *Increased Volume of Blood Flow*
  1. *Tricuspid regurgitation*
     - Systemic venous congestion and reduction of cardiac output.
     - Right sided heart failure.
     - RV and RA enlargement.
     - Congestive hepatomegaly and anasarca.
  2. *Supracardiac total anomalous pulmonary venous return*
     - Pulmonary veins drain into superior vena cava.
     - Superior vena cava is dilated.
B. *Obstructive Causes* (Superior vena cava syndrome)
  1. *Bronchogenic carcinoma*
     Lymphoma
     Mediastinitis
     Constrictive pericarditis
     Retrosternal goiter.
     Ascending aortic aneurysm.
     - Head and neck edema.
     - Cutaneous enlarged venous collaterals.
     - Superior mediastinal widening.
     - Encasement/compression/occlusion of SVC.

3.14 CARDIAC CALCIFICATIONS

A. *Pericardial Calcifications*
  1. *Idiopathic Pericarditis*
     - Calcification occurs at front and sides', not at back as fluid does not collect here.
     - There may be pleuro pericardial adhesions roughning the outline of heart.

2. *Rheumatoid arthritis*
   - Pericarditis occurs in 20 to 50% cases.
   - Features of bones involvement – osteoporosis, erosions.
   - Pleural effusion, interstitial fibrosis.
3. *Tuberculosis*
   - Most important infectious cause.
   - Causes constrictive pericarditis.
4. *Viral infection*
5. *Chronic renal failure*
   - Associated pleural effusion, ascites, pericardial effusions.
6. *Radiotherapy to mediastinum*
   - May lead to pericarditis, pericardial fibrosis and calcification.
B. *Myocardial Calcifications.*
   1. *Infections*—viral or bacterial.
      This can be suspected when CHF occurs in relation to viral pyrexia and bacterial sepsis.
   2. *Myocardial aneurysm*—may show wall calcification.
   3. *Rheumatic fever*—causes myocarditis.
      May produce pericardial effusion, pleural effusion.
C. *Intracardiac*
   1. *Valvular*—See in valvular calcifications.
   2. *Cardiac tumors*—Atrial myxoma, rhabdomyoma and fibroma.

3.15 CARDIAC VALVE CALCIFICATIONS

1. Aortic valve.
   Indicates significant aortic stenosis.
   a. Congenitally bicuspid valve = 70 to 85%
   b. Atherosclerotic degeneration.

c. Rheumatic AS.
d. Syphilis.
2. Mitral valve
a. Rheumatic heart disease.
b. Mitral valve prolapse.
3. Pulmonary valve
a. Tetralogy of Fallot.
b. Pulmonary stenosis.
c. ASD.
4. Tricuspid valve
a. Rheumatic heart disease.
b. ASD
c. Infective endocarditis.

3.16 SITUS

Term describing position of atria, tracheobronchial tree, pulmonary arteries, thoracic and abdominal viscera.

A. *Situs solitus-Normal situs.*
1. *Abdominal*
   – Liver and IVC are right sided.
2. *Cardiac*
   – Morphologic Rt atrium is Rt sided.
     Morphologic Lt atrium is left sided.
B. *Situs Inversus*
   Mirror image of normal.
1. *Abdominal*
   – Mirror image position of abdominal organs.
2. *Cardiac*
   – Morphologic Rt atrium is left sided.
   – Morphologic Lt atrium is right sided.

C. *Situs Intermedius/Ambiguous*
   1. *Abdominal*
      - Liver may be midline.
      - Bowel malrotations.
   2. *Cardiac*
      - Indeterminate atrial morphology.
      - Bilateral right atria/Bilateral left atria.

3.17 CYANOTIC HEART DISEASE

A. *Cyanotic Heart Disease*
   1. *Increased pulmonary flow*
      - Complete transposition of great arteries.
      - Truncus arteriosus.
      - Total anomalous pulmonary venous connection.
      - Common atrium.
      - Double outlet right ventricle.
      - Single ventricle without pulmonic stenosis.
   2. *Normal or decreased pulmonary blood flow*
      - Tricuspid atresia.
      - Tetralogy of Fallot.
      - Pulmonary arteriovenous fistula.
      - Pulmonary atresia with intact interventricular septum.
      - Pulmonary stenosis with Rt to Lt atrial shunt.
      - Double outlet Rt ventricle with pulmonic stenosis.
B. *Acyanotic Heart Disease* (with left to right shunt)
   1. *Atrial level*
      - Atrial septal defect.
      - ASD with mitral stenosis (Lutembacher's syndrome).
      - Partial anomalous pulmonary venous return.

2. *Ventricular level*
   - Ventricular septal defect.
   - VSD with aortic regurgitation.
   - VSD with LV to RA shunt.
3. *Aortic root to right heart shunt*
   - Ruptured sinus of valsalva aneurysm.
   - Coronary AV fistula.
   - Anomalous origin of left coronary artery from pulmonary trunk.
4. *Aortopulmonary shunt*
   - Patent ductus arteriosus.
   - Aortopulmonary window.
5. *Multiple level shunts*
   - ASD with VSD.
   - VSD with PDA.
   - Common atrioventricular canal.
C. *Acyanotic without shunt*
   1. *Left heart malformations*
      - Congenital left atrial inflow obstruction
        a. Pulmonary vein stenosis.
        b. Mitral stenosis.
        c. Cor triatriatum.
      - Mitral regurgitation
        a. Congenitally corrected transposition of arteries.
        b. Atrioventricular septal defect.
        c. Primary dilated endocardial fibroelastosis.
        d. Aortic stenosis/Regurgitation.
        e. Coarctation of aorta.
   2. *Right heart malformations*
      - Acyanotic Ebsteins anomaly.
      - Pulmonic stenosis.
      - Congenital pulmonary regurgitations.
      - Idiopathic dilatation of pulmonary trunk.

Soft Tissue Lesions

4.1 D/D OF SOFT TISSUE LESIONS

1. *Increased Heel Pad Thickness*
   Males > 23 mm
   Females > 21.5 mm
   a. *Acromegaly*
      Osseous enlargement, flared ends of long bones.
      Spade like hands, widening of terminal tufts, prognathism, enlargement of paranasal sinuses, sellar enlargement.
      Posterior scalloping of vertebrae.
   b. *Myxoedema*
      - Clinical features—fatigue, lethargy, constipation, cold intolerance, stiffening of muscles.
      - Dull, expression less facies, periorbital puffiness.
      Calvarial thickening, wedging of dorsolumbar vertebrae, coxa vara.
   c. *Peripheral edema*
      Edema due to any cause will cause thickening of heel pad.

    d. *Obesity*
       Especially in children-heel pad is thick, because of fat deposition.
    e. Epanutin therapy.
       Erythematous eruptious, gingival hyperplasia may occur.
    f. Infection/Injury
       Due to pus collection or hematoma formation, heel pad thickness may be increased.

Increased Heel Pad Thickness (Flow Chart)

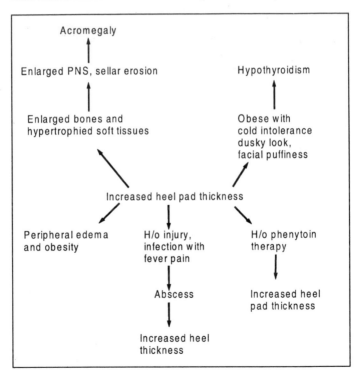

4.2 SOFT TISSUE OSSIFICATION

Formation of Trabecular Bone

1. Myositis ossificans
2. Burns
3. Paraplegia
4. Liposarcoma
5. Parosteal osteosarcoma
6. Congenital myositis ossificans progressiva
7. Tumoral calcinosis
8. Surgical scar

Myositis Ossificans

- Benign solitary self limiting ossifying soft tissue mass typically occurring in skeletal muscle.
- Adolescents, young atheletic adults.
- Located in large muscles of extremities in 80%.
- Well defined partially ossified soft tissue mass after 6-8 weeks.
- Radiolucent zone separating lesion from bone.
- Periphery more dense than center.

Liposarcoma

- Second most common soft tissue sarcoma in adults
- Age 5th-6th dccade
- Usually pain less, mass located in trunk, lower extremity upper extremity, head and neck.
- Amorphous calcification.

Parosteal Osteosarcoma

- Large lobulated cauliflower like homogenous ossific mass extending away from cortex.

- Large soft tissue component with osseous and cartilagenous elements.
- Periphery less dense than center.
- Located commonly at posterior aspect of distal femur, either end of tibia, proximal humerus, fibula.

Burns

- Ossification in relation to joints, commonly hips, elbows and shoulders.
- May occur at sites distal to injury.
- The cause is unknown.

Paraplegia

- Occurs in adults with spinal lesions and children with spinal dysraphism.
- Particularly in relation to pelvis.
- Wooly appearance.

Congenital Myositis Ossificans Progressiva

- Autosomal dominant or primary mutation.
- Ossification in perimuscular fascia, not in muscles.
- Sheets of bone in neck, thorax and limb.
- Abnormally short metacarpal of thumb and metatarsal of big toe.

Tumoral Calcinosis

- Masses of bones in soft tissue near joints.
- May cause discomfort and limitation of movement.

Surgical Scar

- True bone may form away from any pre-existing bone structure or periosteum.

Table 4.2.1: Soft tissue ossification

Features	Myositis ossificans	Paraplegia	Burns	Parosteal osteosarcoma	Cong. myo. oss. pro.	Tumoral calcinosis
1. Age	Adolescents, young adult athletics	Adults with spinal lesion and children spinal dysraphism	—	12-58 years	Early childhood	1st and 2nd decade
2. Type of calcification	Well defined partially ossified soft tissue mass	Woolly appearance	—	Large lobulated cauliflower like mass with soft tissue component	Sheet like	Large calcified masses
3. Location	Large muscles of extremities in 80%	Particularly in relation to pelvis	In relation to joints commonly hips > elbows and shoulders	Posterior aspect of distal femur tibial ends, proximal humerus and fibula	In perimuscular fascia not in muscles. Neck, thorax and limbs commonly	Periarticular hips > elbow > shoulder > feet newer bones
4. Specific feature	Periphery more dense than center	—	May occur at site distal to burns	Periphery less dense than center	Abnormal short metacarpal of thumb and metatarsal of big toe	Overlying ulceration and sinus, diaphyseal, periosteal reaction

4.3 LINEAR CALCIFICATION OF SOFT TISSUES

1. *Arterial*
   a. *Diabetes*
      - Occurs commonly in calf region.
      - Associated diabetic nephropathy or cystopathy.
   b. *Hyperparathyroidism*
      - Calcification in arterial tunica media.
      - Cornea, vessels, periarticular region.
      - Chondrocalcinosis.
      - Associated bone erosions, brown tumors.
   c. *Werner's syndrome*
   d. *Atheroma*
      - Plaque like calcification, linear calcification of walls.
      - Commonly femoral and popliteal arteries.
2. *Venous*
   a. *Thrombosed veins.*
      Phleboliths are present.
   b. *Varicose veins.*
3. *Nerves*
   a. *Leprosy*
      - Areas of decalcification, reticulated pattern.
      - Joint space preserved.
      - Absorption of nasal spine, alveolar ridge.
      - Neurotropic joints.
   b. *Neurofibromatosis*
      - Soft tissue masses.
      - Optic nerve gliomas.
      - Ribbon ribs, sphenoid dysplasia, pseudoarthrosis.
4. *Ligamentous*
   a. *Tendinitis*
      - Pellegrini-Stieda lesion - Calcification of medial collateral ligament of knee.

b. *Ankylosing spondylitis*
   – Posterior longitudinal/anterior long-ligament calcification.
c. *Fluorosis*
   – Sacrotuberous and sacrospinous ligamentous calcification, increased bone density.
   – Interosseous membrane calcification.
d. *Alkaptonuria*
   – Calcification in paravertebral soft tissues and tendon insertion.
   – Disc calcification.
   – Massive osteophytosis.

4.4 PARASITIC CALCIFICATION

1. *Cysticercus cellulosae*
   – Calcified cysts produce oval shadow 10-15 mm long and 2-3 mm broad with a translucent center.
   – Number of cysts usually in hundreds.
   – Arranged in direction of muscle fibers.
   – May be associated with cysts in brain.
2. *Loasis (Calabar swelling)*
   – Caused by microfilaria.
   – Found in subcutaneous tissues and undergoes calcification after death.
   – Commonly in hands, in web spaces.
   – Coiled thread like opacities with amorphous calcification.
3. *Guinea worm*
   – Calcifies after its death.
   – Elongated or coiled strip of calcium density.
   – May be crushed by muscle action into a round irregular mass.

4. *Armilifer armillatus*
   - Curved in one plane (comma shaped)
   - Chest and abdomen.

4.5 AREAS OF DECREASED DENSITY

1. *Fat*
   a. *Lipomas*
   b. *Normal sites*
      - In front of lower end of humerus, below patella, in front of Achilles tendon.
   c. *Lipohemarthrosis*
      - Following fractures.
      - Particularly around knees and shoulders.
2. *Gas*
   a. *Hernias*
      - Containing intestine.
      - Seen below inguinal ligament or in scrotum.
   b. *Air entering from outside.*
      i. Air bubbles near compound fractures.
      ii. Fractures of PNS - air in facial soft tissues.
      iii. Soft tissues of chest from lungs - after rib fractures, laceration of lung, thoracocentases or after surgery.
      iv. From mediastinum.
   c. *Lower abdominal wall or thigh*—following rupture of pelvic abscess or after perforation of a hollow viscus.
   d. Gas formed in tissues.
      i. Infection in diabetes, by *Clostridium welchii.*
      ii. Anaerobic myositis.

4.6 PERIARTICULAR SOFT TISSUE CALCIFICATION

1. *Inflammatory*
   a. Scleroderma
   b. Dermatomyositis
   c. Gout
2. *Degenerative*
   Calcium pyrophosphate dihydrate deposition disease.
3. *Renal failure*
   – Secondary hyperparathyroidism
4. *Hypercalcemia*
   a. Sarcoidosis
   b. Hypervitaminosis D
   c. Milk alkali syndrome
5. *Neoplastic*
   a. Synovial osteochondromatosis
   b. Synovioma
6. *Idiopathic*
   Tumoral calcinosis

(See Table 4.6.1 Next Page)

4.7 GENERALIZED CALCINOSIS

a. *Collagen vascular disorders*
   1. Scleroderma
   2. Dermatomyositis
b. *Idiopathic tumoral calcinosis*
c. *Idiopathic calcinosis universalis*

Scleroderma

• Calcinosis of skin
• Raynaud's phenomenon

Table 4.6.1: Periarticular soft tissue calcification

Features	Gout	Sarcoidosis	Secondary HPT	Hypervitaminosis D	Synovial osteo-chondromatosis	Synovioma
1. Age	> 40 years	20-40 years	–	–	20-50 years	20-50 years
2. Type of calcification	Large nodular calcification in gouty tophi	–	Periarticular, arterial walls, chondrocal-cinosis, viscera	Metastatic calcinosis in periarticular areas - putty like premature falx calcifica-tion	Multiple cal-cified bodies	Large sphenoid well defined soft tissue mass with amorphous calcification
3. Site	Hands and feet, 1st MTP most common ear > bones, ten-dons and bursae	Small bones of hands and feet	Around hip, knee, shoulder, wrist	Periarticular + arterial walls + neph-rocalcinosis	Large joints knee > elbow > hip > shoulder > ankle	Knee most common, hip ankle, elbow wrist hands, feet
4. Bone changes	Punched out lytic bone lesions, mouse bite erosions with overhang-ing margins joint space is preserved	Reticulated lace like trabecular pattern in middle and distal phalanges with cystic lesions acro-osteolysis	Osteosclerosis especially axial skeleton, pelvis ribs, clavicles, Rugger-Jersey spine	Cortical+ trabecular dense calvaria widening of provisional zone of calci-fication	Pressure erosion of bone or secondary dege-nerative changes due to press-widening of joint space and accu-mulation of loose bodies	Periosteal reaction, bone remodelling due to press-ure invasion of cortex and juxta-articular osteopenia

For Dermatomyositis
Scleroderma
Tumoral
Calcinosis
} Refer to generalized calcinosis

- Esophageal dysmotility
- Sclerodactyly
- Telangiectasia

Dermatomyositis

Inflammatory myopathy with linear and confluent calcifications in soft tissues.
- Pointing and resorption of terminal tufts
- Respiratory muscle weakness
- Dysphagia

Idopathic Tumoral Calcinosis

- Progressive large nodular juxta-articular calcified soft tissue masses.
- Normal serum calcium and phosphorus and no metabolic/renal or collagen disease.
- Diaphyseal periosteal reaction with patchy areas of calcification in medullary cavity.
- Calcinosis cutis.

Idiopathic Calcinosis Universalis

- Children and young adults
- Plaque like calcium deposits in skin and subcutaneous tissues.
- Sometimes in tendons and muscles
- No true bone formation.

Table 4.7.1: Generalized calcinosis

Features	Scleroderma	Dermato-myositis	Tumoral calcinosis	Calcinosis universalis
1. Age	30-50 years	5-15 and 50-60 years	1st and 2nd decade	Children and young adults
2. Sex	M:F = 1:3	M:F = 1:2	M:F = 1:1	–
3. Inheritance	Autoimmune	Inflammatory myopathy	Autosomal dominant	Unknown origin
4. Calcification	Punctate soft tissue calcification	Large, confluent, sheet like	Large soft tissue mass with overlying ulceration/sinus	Plaque like
5. Location	Axilla, ischial tuberosity, finger tips, elbows, lower, leg, around tendons, bursae and joints	Extremities, elbows hands, Abd and chest wall, knees	Periarticular hips > elbow > shoulder > feet, nearer knees	Skin, subcutaneous tissues, sometimes tendons and muscles
6. Bone changes	Acro-osteolysis, arthritis of small joints	Acro-osteolysis	Diaphyseal periostitis patchy calcification in medullary cavity	–
7. GI changes	Esophageal dysmotility, dilatation of stomach and bowel	Dysphagia, dilatation and atony of esophagus, small intestine and colon	–	–
8. Respiratory changes	Interstitial lung disease	Pulmonary infiltrate and respiratory muscle weakness	–	–
9. Others	Thickened waxy skin	Myocardial weakness	Skin calcifications vascular calcification	–

4.8 SHEET LIKE CALCIFICATION IN SOFT TISSUE

1. Congenital myositis ossificans progressiva
2. Dermatomyositis

Table 4.8.1: Sheet like calcification

Features	Congenital myositis ossificans progressiva	Dermatomyositis
1. Type	Autosomal dominant	Inflammatory myopathy
2. Calcification	In perimuscular fascia and not in muscles	Necrosis, fibrosis and calcification in muscles
3. Parts commonly affected	Sheets of bone in neck thorax and limbs	Extremities, elbows, knees, hands abdominal wall and chest wall
4. Age	Early childhood	5-15 yrs and 50-60 yrs
5. Bone changes	Short metacarpal of thumb and metatarsal of big toe + abnormality of vertebrae	Pointing and resorption of terminal tufts

5

Abdomen and Gastro-intestinal Tract and Hepatobiliary System

5.1 DILATED ESOPHAGUS

NORMAL VS ABNORMAL APPEARANCE OF ESOPHAGUS

Normal wall thickness – 3 mm when adequately distended
      – 5 mm when incompletely distended

Abnormal – Greater or eccentric thickness
    AP diameter esophagus   – > 16 mm
    Lateral diameter oesophagus – > 24 mm

Abnormal – Air filled level   ┐ Obstructive
    Fluid filled lumen   ├ or
    Lumen calibre > 10 mm ┘ Motility disorders

Strictures

Smooth	Irregular
Inflammatory	*Neoplastic*
Peptic, Barrett's	Carcinoma
Scleroderma	Leiomyosarcoma
Corrosive	Carcinosarcoma
	Lymphoma
Neoplastic	*Inflammatory*
Carcinoma	Reflux (rarely)
Mediastinal tumors	Crohn's disease
– Ca bronchus	
Leiomyoma	*Iatrogenic*
	Radiotherapy
	Fundoplication
Others	
Achalasia	
Iatrogenic-	Prolonged use of nasogastric tube
Skin disorders	• Epidermolysis bullose
	• Pemphigus

Peptic Stricture

- Situated most frequently in the distal esophagus near the G-E junction.
- Associated with reflux and hiatus hernia.
- Most peptic strictures are circumferential. Occasionally may be asymmetrical with radiating folds or a pseudo-diverticular appearance.
- If luminal diameter < 13 mm - Associated with dysphagia 14-19 mm - 50% cases - dysphagia

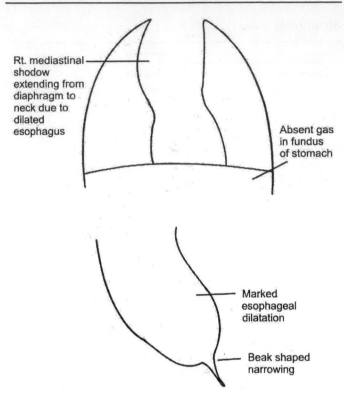

Rt. mediastinal shodow extending from diaphragm to neck due to dilated esophagus

Absent gas in fundus of stomach

Marked esophageal dilatation

Beak shaped narrowing

Fig. 5.1.1: Achalasia cardia - on barium study

Barrett's Esophagus

- The normal squamous epithelium is replaced by columnar epithelium. This usually begins in distal esophagus and progresses proximally.
- Esophagogram—(nonspecific)—reflux, hiatus hernia, stricture, thickened folds, shallow ulcers and erosions.

- More specific finding—(Double contrast) fine reticular mucosal pattern distal to a stricture (seen in < 1/3rd cases).

  In Barrett's esophagus—strictures usually develops at the junction of squamous and columnar epithelium.

Scleroderma

- Esophageal involvement seen in 75-85% cases.
- Caused by atrophy of smooth muscle and it's replacement by connective tissue.
- *Radiological features*: Dilatation, atonicity, poor or absent peristalsis of gastroesophageal reflux through a widely open G-E junction - stricture.

Other Associated Features:

- Raynaud's phenomenon.
- Skin thickening.
- Terminal phlalanx resorption with soft tissue atrophy.
- Erosions of distal interphalangeal, 1st carpometacarpal, metacarpophalangeal and metatarsophalangeal joints.
- *Respiratory system*: Aspiration pneumonitis, interstitial lung diseases and fibrosis in left lower zone.
- Small bowel-dilated, atonic with thickened folds and pseudosacculations.

Corrosives

- Ingestion of sodium hydroxide/acid ingestion.
- Site of involvement—Aortic arch, left main bronchus and above diaphragmatic hiatus.
- Acute phase—Edema, spasm, ulceration, loss of mucosal pattern at hold up points.
- After several weeks—smooth stricture develops—symmetrical and longitudinal.

Achalasia

Esophageal motor disturbance caused by—Failure of lower esophageal sphincter to relax.
* Loss of primary and secondary peristalsis
* Intermittent emptying.

Causes

Idiopathic (absence of smooth muscle ganglionic cells)
Secondary to Chaga's disease.
   Malignancy—with invasion of myanteric plexus, chest X-ray—dilated esophagus with air-fluid level. Barium examination—dilated sigmoid shaped esophagus.
* "Bird Beak" appearance of distal esophagus.
* Loss of primary and secondary peristalsis in distal 2/3rd of esophagus.
* Feature of esophagitis
* Intermittent spurting of barium into the stomach, stricture classically occurs below diaphragm.

Leiomyomas

* Commonest benign esophageal neoplasm, are usually intramural in origin.
* *Barium examination*: Sharply defined smooth/lobulated defect with superior and inferior margins that form right angles with the luminal wall.
   CT—shows the intraluminal and extrinsic component.

Carcinoma Esophagus

Incidence seen in—Plummer-Vinson syndrome, Barrett's, cardiac disease, asbestosis and dye-ingestion.
(10-20%) Adenocarcinoma—Distal 1/3rd
(80-90%) Sq. cell Ca—Middle 1/3rd

Types

Polypoidal, infiltrative, ulcerative and superior spreading.

Radiological features:
Irregular filling defects—

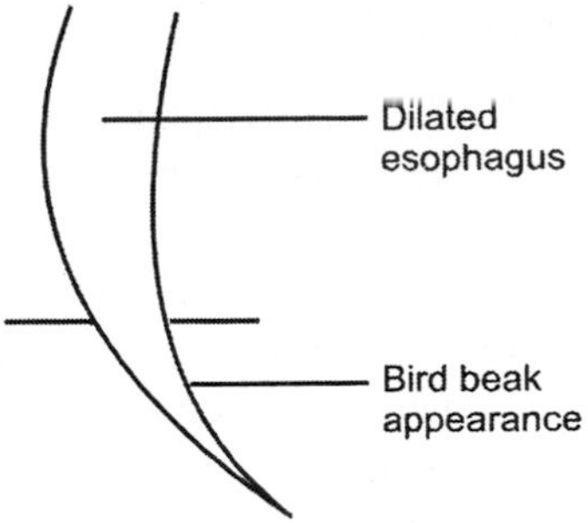

Annular/Eccentric

- Extraluminal soft tissue mass.
- Proximal and distal shouldering.
- Proximal dilatation.
- Mucosal destruction/ulcerations.
- Satellite lesions in esophagus.

Fig. 5.1.2: Achalasia cardia

Chest X-ray

- Mediastinum widening.
- Tracheal deviation, anterior bowing of posterior tracheal wall.
- Widened retrotracheal stripe (> 3 mm)
- Air-fluid level in esophagus.

CT

For extent of involvement
Tracheobronchial, aortic, pericardial invasion, mediastinal lymphadenopathy.

Esophageal Lymphoma (Rare)

Both non-Hodgkin's and less commonly Hodgkin's lymphoma may involve esophagus.

Invasion

1. Mediastinal lymph nodes with esophageal invasion.
   - Extrinsic compression with irregular. Serrated margins.
2. Contiguous spread of lymphoma from gastric fundus (cannot be differentiated from Carcinoma).
3. Synchronous development of lymphoma in the wall of esophagus.
   • Submucosal nodules, enlarged folds, polypoidal masses, strictures.

Secondary Esophageal Neoplasms

• Most common neoplasm that spread directly to esophagus are—gastric and bronchial carcinoma.

Others

Hypopharyngeal, thyroid and primary mediastinal.
• Esophageal invasion from neoplastically laden adjacent lymph node is more common than direct metastasis to the esophagus. (Most common primary sites are—lungs in males and breast in females).

Radiological Features

Extrinsic impression with regular/irregular margins. Displacement of esophagus.

Radiation Esophagitis

• Occurs when dose exceeds. 20 Gy (2000 rad) leading to ulceration, stricture and rarely perforation.

Flow Chart 5.1.1

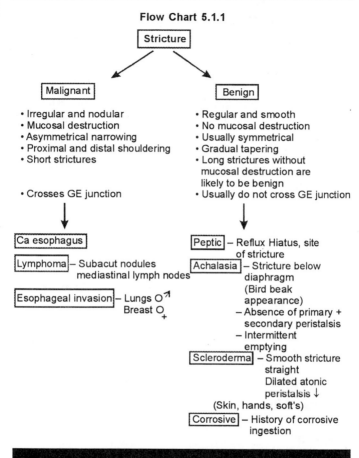

Stricture

Malignant

- Irregular and nodular
- Mucosal destruction
- Asymmetrical narrowing
- Proximal and distal shouldering
- Short strictures

- Crosses GE junction

Ca esophagus

Lymphoma – Subacut nodules mediastinal lymph nodes

Esophageal invasion – Lungs O♂
Breast O♀

Benign

- Regular and smooth
- No mucosal destruction
- Usually symmetrical
- Gradual tapering
- Long strictures without mucosal destruction are likely to be benign
- Usually do not cross GE junction

Peptic – Reflux Hiatus, site of stricture
Achalasia – Stricture below diaphragm (Bird beak appearance)
– Absence of primary + secondary peristalsis
– Intermittent emptying
Scleroderma – Smooth stricture straight Dilated atonic peristalsis ↓ (Skin, hands, soft's)
Corrosive – History of corrosive ingestion

5.2   ESOPHAGEAL CARCINOMA

Predisposing Factors

1. Achalasia 2 to 8% cases of long standing achalasia undergo malignant degeneration because of chronic stasis induced esophagitis.

2. Like strictures (2-16%)
3. Head and neck tumors (2-8%)
4. Celiac disease
5. Plummer-Vinson syndrome (4-16%)
6. Radiation (> 20 to 50 gray; Latent period -20 yrs)
7. Tylosis autosomal dominant condition characterized by hyperkeratosis of palms and soles (95% cases >65 yrs)
8. Smoking and Alcohol
9. Barrett's esophagitis (15%) predisposing factors for Adeno Ca.
10. Scleroderma.

Pathology

Gross

1. *Infiltrating*: Most common, irregular narrowing and constriction of lumen.
2. *Polypoidal*: Lobulated/Fungating mass protrudes into the lumen.
3. *Superficial Spreading*: Spreads superficially without invading deeper layers.
   Ulcerative: Flat masses in which the bulk of the tumor is replaced by ulceration.

Histology

Sq. Cell Ca- 80-90%
Adeno Ca- 10-20%

Japanese Society of Esophageal Disease

• Early esophageal Carcinoma-Mucosa and Submucosae involved.

- Superficial esophageal carcinoma—Mucosal and submucosal involvement with lymph node metastasis.
  Small esophageal Ca: Growth < 3.5 cm regardless of depth of invasion of lymph node metastasis.

Distribution

- Sq cell carcinoma have a relatively even distribution in the upper, middle and distal third of esophagus.
- 75% of adenocarcinoma arise in the distal 1/3rd at or adjacent to the gastroesophageal junction.

Routes of Spread

1. *Direct Extension*: Esophagus lacks mucosa therefore Carcinoma spread readily into adjacent structures—thyroid, larynx, trachea, bronchus, lungs, aorta, pericardium and diaphragm.
2. *Lymphatic Extension*: "Jump" metastasis can occur in the neck, mediastinal lymph nodes in the absence of segmental lymph node involvement because of rich interconnecting lymphatics in esophagus.
   - Subdiaphragmatic lymph nodes—Pericardial, lesser curvature and celiac lymph node.
   - Lymphatic metastasis can also occur within the esophagus which presents as submucosal nodules.
3. *Hematogenous metastasis*: Lung, liver, adrenal, kidney pancreas, peritoneum and bones.

Clinical Aspects

Dysphagia, odynophagia, anorexia, weight loss, persistent substernal chest pain, hoarseness of voice and chronic cough (aspiration and tracheoesophageal fistula), hematemesis.

Radiographic Findings

- *Early esophageal carcinoma*: Double contrast esophagography is the best radiological technique and has increased sensitivity but less specificity.
  Early esophageal Ca is seen as.

Small protrusions < 3.5 cm which may appear as:
- Plaque like with central ulceration
- Sessile polyp with smooth/lobulated contour.
- Focal irregularity/nodularity.
- Superficial spreading carcinoma extend longitudinally in the wall without invading beyond the mucosa/submucosa. Seen radiographically as tiny coalescent nodules or plaques causing nodularity/granularity.

Advanced Carcinoma

- Chest X-ray shows: mediastinal widening.
- Hilar/retrohilar/retrocardic mass
- Tracheal deviation, anterior bowing of posttracheal wall Widened retrotracheal stripe.
  Air-fluid level in esophagus.
- Barium studies
  - Irregular narrowing, nodular or ulcerated mucosa, proximal and distal shouldering, proximal dilatation.
- Lobulated/fungated mass (intraluminal) usually >3.5 cm with areas of ulceration.
- Well-defined meniscoid ulcer with a radiolucent rim of tumor surrounding the ulcer.
- Thickened, tortous or serpiginous long filling defects because of submucosal spread which are known as varicoid carcinoma.
  - Smooth extrinsic impression with gently sloping

obtuse borders because of-mediastinal lymphadenopathy.
- Satellite lesions in esophagus and stomach because of lymphatic metastasis.
• Detection of complications on barium study.
  - Esophago airway fistula-Lat. Film.
  - Necrotic tumor containing cavity in lung/mediastinum communicating with the esophagus.

Table 5.2.1: Differentiating features
squamous and adenocarcinoma

Sq.cell carcinoma	Adenocarcinoma
• Equal distribution in the upper, mid and lower esophagus	• Most common, situated in distal esophagus
• Rarely extends subdiaphragmatically to involve stomach	• Frequently extends and invades cardia/fundus
• Most common type—Infiltrating	• Most common type—Polypoidal and mixed polypoidal-infiltrative

CT

Best imaging modality for staging patients (Mediastinal invasion, mediastinal adenopathy and distant metastasis)
• *Criteria for tracheobronchial invasion*:
  - Displacement of trachea/bronchus from the spine
  - Indentation on the posterior wall of trachea/bronchus.
  - Bowing of posterior wall of trachea/bronchus.
  (Absence of fat plane between the trachea and/or bronchus and esophagus cannot be used to predict invasion)
• *Criteria for aortic invasion*:
  - Area of contact >90% or 1/4th of aortic circumference.

- – Obliteration of the triangular fat space between aorta, spine and esophagus suggests of invasion.
- *Criteria of pericardial invasion*:
  - – Presence of mass effect with concave deformity of the heart associated with loss of normal fat plane in this region.
- *Mediastinal Adenopathy*
  Limitations-CT cannot demonstrate lymph node metastasis that has not caused significant lymphadenopathy.
- Enlarged periesophageal lymph node cannot be detected because they are inseparable from the primary cancer.
- CT cannot differentiate benign from malignant lymphadenopathy.

Subdiaphragmatic Lymphadenopathy

Frequently the lymph node at or above the celiac axis are involved (>8 mm-Enlarged)

MRI

Superior to CT in detecting mediastinal invasion.

Endoscopic Ultrasound

Advantage: Evaluates the depth of tumor invasion. Periesophageal lymph node can also be identified.

Disadvantage: Esophageal ultrasound probe is unable to pass through a malignant stricture.

Differential Diagnosis of Esophageal Carcinoma

Early Esophageal Carcinoma

- *Sqamous papilloma*: Small, sessile lobulated polyp.

- *Candidae esophagitis*: Multiple plaque like defects with intervening normal mucosa.
- Pseudomembranes/inflammatory exudates-multiple plaque like defects are present.

Advanced Carcinoma

- *Benign stricture*
  - Smooth, no mucosal destruction
  - No shouldering.
- *Esophageal varices*
  - On full column film the varicoid appearance disappears, Valsalva increases the varicoid appearance.
- *Leiomyoma*: Submucosal mass lesion with smooth margins which forms right angle.

5.3 THICKENED MUCOSAL FOLDS ESOPHAGUS AND STOMACH

Q. What are mucosal folds?

Folds are convolutions of mucosa, made so in order to ↑ the functional assimilative capacity of gut keeping the structural needs to minimum. The total surface area thus increases greatly but the length of intestine is kept to a minimum. It consists of epithelium, lamina propria, muscularis mucosa.

Q. Why is their demonstration so important?

Because this is the basic functional layer of GIT and most diseases either originate or involves this layer early on.

Q. How are they radiologically demonstrated?

a. Mucosal relief.
b. Full barium.
c. Double contrast.

a and c are techniques of choice to demonstrate early involvement and diseases of mucosa, submucosa and even distal layers may be shows, through their effects on mucosa and submucosa.

Thickened Esophageal Folds

Causes

1. Varices
2. Esophagitis
3. Varicoid carcinoma
4. Lymphoma

1. Varices
   → Due To →
   1. Portal hypertension: k/a Uphill Varices.
   2. SVC obstruction: k/a Downhill Varices.
   3. Idiopathic: due to congenital wall weakness.

→ 1. Up Hill
   2. Down Hill

	Superior i/c; Superior Thyroid;
Above	Bronchial; Mediastinal ↓
Azygous	SVC → Heart ↑
Below/At Azygous	Azygous + Hemiazygous Periesophageal Plexus

→ CF Up Hill → Bleeding Anemia
   Down Hill → SVD Syndrome; Bleed Rare.
→ Imaging:-Plain X-ray → Dilated Azygous; ± Show As posterior mediastinal mass.

→ Barium
  › Prone (RAO).
  → ± Buscopan.
  → Wait/watch.
  → Mucosal relief.
  → Irregular serpiginous filling defects.
  → Faintly merge (D/D Ca).
→ CT → Nodular enhancing Streaks in Wall.
→ Angiography → Celiac, SMA, Portal, Splenic
  · → Change with Respiration, Deglutition, Valsalva, Position.
→ TES/Doppler → Abnormal Dilated Vascular Channels Seen.

2. *Esophagitis*
   Infectious → Candida; HSV; HIV; CMV; TB; Actino-mycetes.
   Noninfectious → Drugs; Caustic; RTT; NG Tube; Crohn's; Skin Diseases; Alcohol; GVHD.
→ Fold thickening is nodular and scalloped.
→ Associated specific findings seen:
   CMV → Giant Ulcers.
   Candida → Plaques
   HIV, HSV → Multiple Aphthoid Ulcers.
   TB → Strictures.
   Actinomyces → Sinus.
   Doxycycline Tetracyclines → Temporary superficial ulcers.
   Caustic → Long segment stricture.

3. *Varicoid Carcinoma*
   – is basically a morphological varient seen radiologically as fold thickening.
   – it's etiology, histopathology and management protocol is nearly the same.
     · usually involves the lower esophagus.

Flow Chart 5.3.1

Thick esophageal folds

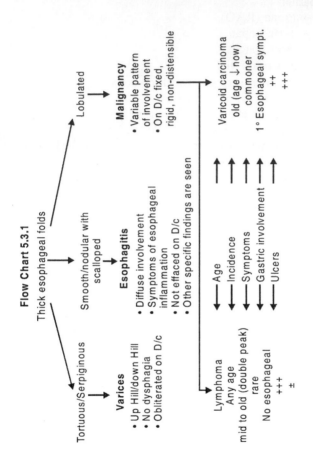

Tortuous/Serpiginous

Varices
- Up Hill/down Hill
- No dysphagia
- Obliterated on D/c

Smooth/nodular with scalloped

Esophagitis
- Diffuse involvement
- Symptoms of esophageal inflammation
- Not effaced on D/c
- Other specific findings are seen

Lobulated

Malignancy
- Variable pattern of involvement
- On D/c fixed, rigid, non-distensible

	Lymphoma	Varicoid carcinoma
Age	Any age, mid to old (double peak)	old (age ↓ now) commoner
Incidence	rare	
Symptoms	No esophageal	1° Esophageal sympt.
Gastric involvement	+++	++
Ulcers	±	+++

4. *Lymphoma*
   - MC secondarily involvement from mediastinal nodes.
   - Radiologically
     → Smooth Extrinsic Impression
     Intrinsic
     → Smooth Tapered Stricture with Achalasia.
     Large Mass
     Varicoid (Rare)

Thickened Gastric Folds

1. Normal varient
2. Gastritis — alcoholic
   - Hypertrophic
   - Antral
   - Corrosive
   - H. pylori and other infections
   - Postradiation
   - Postfreezing
3. Peptic ulcer disease.
4. ZES.
5. Ménétrier's disease.
6. Lymphoma.
7. Pseudolymphoma.
8. Carcinoma.
9. Varices and antral vascular ectasia.
10. Infiltrative process
    - Eosinophilic gastritis
      Crohn's disease
      Sarcoidosis
      TB
      Syphilis
      Amyloidosis

11. Adjacent pancreatic disease
    - Acute pancreatitis
      Extension of Ca pancreas.

1. *Alcoholic Gastritis*
   - Due to prolonged use of large volume; corrected by cessation.
   - MCC of acute exogenous gastritis.
   - Sometimes folds become so bizarre as to mimick malignancy.
   - Due to mucosal and submucosal edema.
   - May progress to atrophic gastritis.

2. *Hypertrophic Gastritis*
   - idiopathic local/diffuse hypertrophy of mucosa and glands without their destruction.
   - ? neuromuscular disorder, ? increase acid output, ? chr. inflammation.
   - increased secretions, poor coating.
   - thick (4-5 mm; N—1-2mm), Polygonal and angular area gastricae seen.
   - associated peptic ulcer commonly present.

3. *Antral Gastritis*
   - Misnomer
   - H. Pylori, Alcohol, tobacco, coffee.
   - ± a part of the spectrum of ulcer disease.
   - ± associated with antral spasm, with ± persistent/transient (Seen as loss of prepyloric shoulders).
   - Antral granulations seen.
   - Radiological features may not be corrected by ++

4. *Corrosive Gastritis*
   - Thick folds with ulcer, atony, rigidity.
   - Usually severe disease seen.
   - Fixed and gaping pylorus seen due to damaged muscles.

- ± gas in the wall.
- Antrum, body and L.C most affected.
- Acids more dangerous for stomach, alkalie for esophagus.

5. *Helicobacter Pylori: (and other infections)*:
   - Antrum and body affected more.
   - If fundus also involved d/d L_A and Ménétrier's disease.
   - On CT circumferential or focal thickening is seen points that need differentiation from malignancy.
   - CMV gastritis in AIDS leads to diffuse fold thickening and decreased distensibility.
   - Other infective process causing similar changes are Toxoplasmosis, Cryptococcosis.

6. *ZES and Ulcer Disease*
   - Body and antrum (never fundus).
   - Increase acid output.
   - In ZES fundic mucosa is seen in antrum.
   - In ulcer disease only perilesional thickening seen.
   - In ZES large amount of gastric fluid seen despite adequate fasting.

7. *Ménétrier's Disease: (k/a Giant-hypertrophic Gastritis)*
   - Whole stomach esp fundus and body; diffuse or focal; ESP greater curve.
   - Abrupt transition B/W normal and abnormal folds.
   - Massive hypertrophy and hyperplasia of folds (i.e. glands) leading to brain like appearance.
   - Decrease acid.
   - Polypoidal appearance when seen end on.
   - Mottle/reticular appearance due to excess mucus.
   - Overall wall is thick and hypoperistalsis seen.

- May be associated with or lead to adeno Ca.
- 'Pediatric Hypertrophic Gastropathy' that presents as hypoalbuminemia in absence of any cause, thick mucosa and following viral infection is a distinct but related entity.

8. *Lymphoma and Pseudolymphoma:*
   - Pseudolymphoma is a benign proliferation of lymphoid tissue.
   - Gastric lymphomas are usually nodular in type however other varieties may be ulcerative, polypoidal, infiltrative (that leads to fold thickening) and mixed types.
   - May lead to an associated ulcer, loss of wall 'pliability, lymphadenopathy (increased retrogastric space), splenomegaly, predominant involvement of distal stomach.

9. *Carcinoma:*
   - As usually misunderstood it is not the linitis plastica malignancies (diffuse infiltrative adeno Ca) that lead to fold thickening.
   - Malignancy leading to fold thickening is colloid Ca or mucinous adeno Ca which also have specks of calcification.
   - Fold thickening with normal volume and pliability is seen.
   - Peristalsis is normal.

10. *Varices:*
   - In PHT are associated with esophageal varices but if isolated gastric varices are seen then splenic vein thrombosis should be suspected.
   - Multiple, curvilinear, cresentric, smooth, lobulated filling defects with splenic impression.

- Seen mainly in fundus extending to LC.
- Charge in appearance.
- Varices in antrum and body are due to obstruction of splenic vein proximal to patent coronary veins.
- Watermelon stomach is a distinctive form of gastric antral vascular ectasia radiating to pylorus.

11. *Infiltrative Processes:*
    - Conditions like eosinophilic gastroenteritis (eosinophilia with eosinophilic infiltration and exudation), Crohn's disease, amyloidosis, sarcoidosis, TB, syphilis cause diffuse rugal thickening.

12. *Adjacent—Pancreatic Disease:*
    - Due to enzymatic mural irritation/spasm and due to perigastric inflammation.
    - Posterior wall and L.C more.
    - Is an indicator of severe pancreatic inflammation.
    - Malignant infiltration causes distorted fold thickening.

Flow Chart 5.3.2

Thickened Gastric Folds

Fundus with Body
- Lymphoma
- Carcinoma
- Hypertrophic gastritis
  - Increase secretion—poor coating
  - Large area gastricae
- Ménétrier
  - Excess mucus
  - No ulcer/true rigidity
  - Stop short - of incisura
  - Spares L.C.
- ZES
  - Near fundus
  - Large amount of fluid despite fasting

Antrum
- Lymphoma
- Carcinoma
- Infiltrations
- Watermelon stomach
  - Folds radiating to pylorus
- Caustic Ingestion
  - History
  - LC more
- Radiation
  - History

		Lymphoma	Carcinoma
1.	Age	— Bimodal	— Mid-Old
2.	CF	— Mass	— Mass + Bleed
3.	No.	— Multicentric +	— Rare
4.	Epicenter	— S/M	— Mucosa
5.	Distensibility	— N A/E H.D	— ($\downarrow\downarrow\downarrow$)
6.	Calibre	— N or $\downarrow$	— ($\downarrow\downarrow\downarrow$)
7.	Loss of area Gastricae	— +	— –
8.	Enhancement	— $\uparrow$	— ($\uparrow\uparrow\uparrow$)
9.	Perigastric fat	— N	— Involved
10.	Wall thickness	— $\uparrow\uparrow\uparrow\uparrow$ (>3cm)	— $\uparrow\uparrow$
11.	HSM	— +	— ±/–
12.	Lymph node $\uparrow$	— + (Above and below kidney)	— ±
13.	Ext. to Duodenum-Esophagus	— ++	— ±
14.	Hemorrhage and necrosis	— ±	— +++
15.	Contour	— Regular	— Irregular
16.	Adj. organ involvement	— +	— +++

Thickened Duodenal Folds

1. *Inflammatory disease*
   - Peptic ulcer disease
   - Brunner's gland hyperplasia
   - ZES (Zollinger-Ellison syndrome)
   - Duodenitis
   - Pancreatitis
   - Cholecystitis

- Uremia
- TB
- Crohn's disease (CD)
- Parasitoses (Giardia strongyloids)
- AIDS
- Non-tropical sprue
2. *Neoplastic*
   - Metastasis to peripancreatic nodes
   - Lymphoma
   - AIDS related malignancies
3. *Diffuse Infiltrative Disorders*
   - Amyloidosis
   - Whipple's disease
   - Mastocytosis
   - Eosinophilic enteritis
   - Intestinal lymphangiectasia

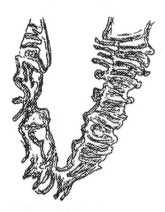

Fig. 5.3.1: Nodular and serpiginous thickening of duodenal mucosal fold involving 2nd port of duodenum

4. *Vascular Disorders*
   - Varices
   - Mesenteric arterial collaterals
   - Intramural hemorrhage
   - Chronic duodenal congestion
5. *Cystic Fibrosis (Mucoviscodosis)*
   - Peptic Ulcer Disease
     - Most common cause
     - May lead to Brunner's gland hyperplasia seen as nodular thickening of folds known as Cobble-stone appearance.
     - These do not disappear on compression as compared to simple mucosal thickening.
   - ZES
     - Non beta is let cell tumor of pancreas
     - Increase gastrin hyperstimulation of parietal cells and hypertrophy of rugae, hyperacidity and hypervolemic gastric secretions.

Ulcer Disease

Most common in bulb and stomach but also may occur in 2nd and 4th port of duodenum, jejunum.

Also Giant ulcers due to excess acids that over whelms the pancreaticobiliary secretions.

Also associated dilution and dilatation.

Disease may continue even after removal of primary and secondary or ectopic masses in stomach, duodenum, splenic hilum.

   - Duodenitis
     - Basically an endoscopic diagnosis
     - Thick (>5mm) duodenal folds are very sensitive but poorly specific indicator

- Hyperacidity leads to nodularity, deformity and spiculation
- Increased peristalsis is noted.
- However differentiation between different causes is not possible.
- Pancreatitis/cholecystitis
  - Very important causes in everyday practice.
  - Hyperirritable; poor filling; Narrow lumen; widened sweep;
  - Thickening in periampullary and proximal 2nd parts.
- Uremia and chronic dialysis
  - First and second part of duodenum shows thick and irregular folds; rigid.
  - ? Due to associated pancreatitis; ? due to associated ulcer.
- Crohn's disease/TB
  - Associated ulcers and stenosis.
  - In TB associated antral/Pyloric disease seen.
- Other infection
  Giardiasis—Increased fluid, increase peristalsis, jejunal involvement
  Strongyloidosis—CD like.
  HIV related cryptococcosis, MAIC, CMV- dilatation.
  Non-tropical sprue—Bizarre thickening with erosions in D1 and D2
- Neoplastic
  Lymphoma—Coarse, nodular, irregular.
  Metastasis to lymph nodes—Extrinsic impression mimicking thickfolds.
  Kaposi sarcoma-submucosal infiltration.

- Varices
  - Extrahepatic portal vein obstruction, intrahepatic portal vein obstruction, splenic vein obstruction.
  - Other associated varices.
    1. Vertical compression on duodenum bulb 1cm distal to pylorus by dilated posterior superior pancreaticoduodenal vein.
    2. Small variceal dilatation leading to Cobble-Stone
    3. Large serpiginous varices.
    4. An isolated varix on medial descending duodenal wall.
- Mesenteric arterial collaterals
  - Atherosclerotic occlusive disease leading to blocked celiac trunk, SMA or both is the cause.
  - Basically from pancreaticoduodenal arcade and gastroduodenal artery which are close to medial duodenal wall
    1. Serpiginous filling defects
    2. C-loop widening
    3. Nodular defects may be seen.
  - Sharp impression on superior aspect of D1 due to Aberrant right hepatic artery may be seen.
- Intramural bleed/congestion
  - STACKED COIN appearance
  - Bleeding disorder, trauma, anticoagulants.
  - Congestion is due to cirrhosis and CHF
- Cystic fibrosis
  - Thick, coarse mucosa
  - Nodules may be seen.
  - Smudging of coating.
  - Altered duodenal contour

- D1, D2 rarely jejunum.
  basically decrease HCO_3, increase H+ leading to irritation.

Flow Chart 5.3.3

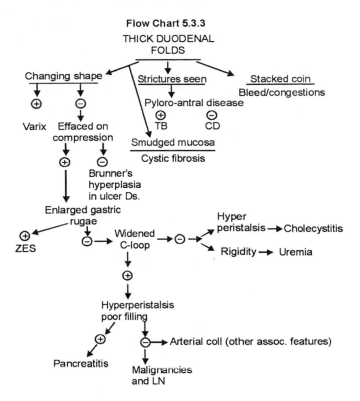

THICKENED SMALL BOWEL

Folds

1. Thickened small bowel folds with dilatation- ZES; Vascular insufficiency; infections; amyloidosis; abetalipoproteinemia; lymphoma; hypoalbuminemia; Disease of intestinal wall and mesentery (secondaries, TB, CD).
2. Thickened small bowel folds with gastric involvement—lymphoma; CD; eosinophilic enteritis; ZES; Ménétrier's; amyloid; Whipple's; varices.
3. Thickened small bowel folds which are regular with no other feature.
   Fold thickened: Jejunum > 2.5 mm
                      Ileum > 2.0 mm

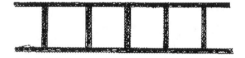

Fig. 5.3.2: Small bowel folds

Hemorrhage in bowel wall: Anticoagulants, ischemic bowel disease with infarction; vasculitis as thromboangiitis obliterans, Henoch-Schönlein purpura, collagen vascular disease hemophilia, idiopathic thrombocytopenic purpura; trauma; secondary clotting disorders as secondaries, myeloma, lymphoma, leukemia, hypofibrogenemia.

Intestinal edema: Hypoproteinemia—Cirrhosis, protein loosing enteropathy, nephrotic syndrome.

Lymphatic block: Tumor, fibrosis, lymphangiitis angioneurotic edema.

Intestinal lymphangiectasia: Primary or secondary.

Abetalipoprotcinemia.

Amyloidosis.

Vasculitis.

Pneumatosis intestinalis.

Xanthomatosis.

Eosinophilic gastroenteritis.

1. Vascular insufficiency:
   - Acute catastrophic
     - Length
     - Collaterals
     - Severity
     - Chronic

   Arterial/veno-occlusive disease.

   Systemic hypovolemia.

   Thickening of folds—hemorrhage+edema.

   Dilatation - adynamic ideus.

2. Disease of wall with mesentery

   Thickening: Due to infiltration + Edema (Venous/lymphatic block)

   (Metastatic, granulomatous, inflammatory)

   Dilatation: Mesenteric involvement leading to areas of obstruction.

   Crohn's disease (CD), a disease that may involve any part of GIT from mouth to anus, has certain specific associated features like ulcer, stricture, fistula, sinus (also TB).

   CD however shows a poorly distensible stomach having irregular tubular narrowing and poor peristalsis esp Antral. If both sides of pyloric canal are involved a characteristic Pseudo-Bilroth I deformity results.

3. Infectious enteritis
   Nonspecific fold thickening and dilatation is seen in salmonella, strongyloidosis, candida, CMV, cryptococcus, MAIC.
4. Hypoalbuminemia
   - Liver and kidney disease.
   - Infiltration free of cells.
   - Dilatation + thickening
   - Gastric fundal rugae +–
   - ALBUMIN THRESHOLD >2.7 gm%
5. Abetalipoproteinemia (Flow Chart see below)
6. Amyloidosis and Whipple's disease
   - Show dilatation (late) with symmetric fold thickening and thickened gastric rugae
   - In amyloidosis deposition is in between muscle fibers and in perivascular areas.

Flow Chart 5.3.4

Abetalipoproteinemia:-

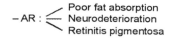

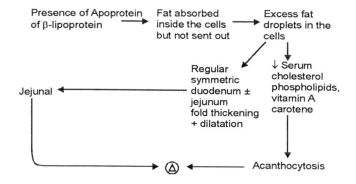

7. *Lymphoma*: Submucosal infiltration.
   1. Infiltrative
      - Dilatation
        - Due to distal narrowing
        - Due to neural involvement known as aneurysmal dilatation
        - Fold thickening
        - Slow passage
        - Most common.
   2. Exo-endoenteric- large mass with ulcer, displaced loops and fistula.
   3. Multinodular.
   4. Polypoidal.
   5. Mesenteric
8. Ménétrier's disease
   - PLE with giant gastric folds.
   - Regular intestinal folds
   - Altered surface metabolism.
9. Eosinophilic gastroenteritis
   - Immune/allergy.
   - Jejunum+distal stomach.
   - Initially regular but late irregular due to spreading of edema.
   - Eosinophilia+Eosinophilic infiltration + Eosinophilic Exudation.
   - Mural thickening may be associated with obstruction.
   - Good response to STEROIDS [Only definite D/D to Crohn's disease].
   - Folds are:
     a. Distorted   d. Saw toothed
     b. Irregular   e. Rigid
     c. Angulated   f. Separated
10. Xanthomatosis
    - Multicentric proliferation of lipid laden cells in bowel wall.

- Regular fold thickening
- Narrowing of stomach and colon.

11. Pneumatosis
    - A mimicker and not true wall thickening.

12. Intestinal lymphangiectasis
    Primary
    Secondary
    Obstruction
    - Giant foam cells in walls.
    - Diffuse regular fold thickening + loss of protein rich exudate in GIT+absent liver, kidney, heart disease.
    Lymphangiectasis
    - Thickening due to edema+lymphatic obstruction.

13. Angioneurotic edema
    - AD; multifocal mucosal edema attacks.
    - Focal changes, temporary during crisis, family history.
    - Regular fold thickening + mesenteric edema separated loops.

14. Vasculitis
    - Lead to infarcts, bleed, perforation, strictures associated with fold thickening.
    - HSP—Circumferential colonic wall thickening with luminal narrowing.

15. Hemophilia
    - Short-long segment fold thickening of bleed
    - Colon may be involved.

16. Idiopathic Thrombocytopenic Purpura
    Acute: healthy Young child, 1-2 week after sore throat
    Chronic: Young adult female, insiduous onset menorrhagia
    - Petechiae at GUT, GIT, skin, etc.
        (Flow chart See Next Page)

Flow Chart 5.3.5

Thickened small bowel folds

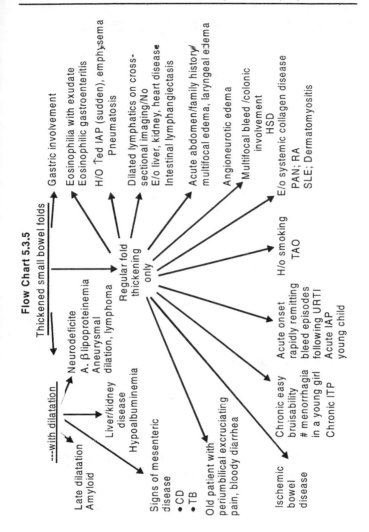

Gastric involvement

Eosinophilia with exudate
Eosinophilic gastroenteritis

H/O ↑ed IAP (sudden), emphysema
Pneumatosis

Dilated lymphatics on cross-
sectional imaging/No
E/o liver, kidney, heart disease
Intestinal lymphangiectasis

Acute abdomen/family history
multifocal edema, laryngeal edema

Angioneurotic edema

Multifocal bleed /colonic
involvement
HSD

E/o systemic collagen disease
PAN; RA
SLE; Dermatomyositis

H/o smoking
TAO

Acute onset
rapidly remitting
bleed episodes
following URTI
Acute IAP
young child

Chronic easy
bruisability
menorrhagia
in a young girl
Chronic ITP

Ischemic
bowel
disease

Old patient with
periumbilical excruciating
pain, bloody diarrhea

Signs of mesenteric
disease
• CD
• TB

Neurodeficite
A. β lipoproteinemia
Aneurysmal
dilation, lymphoma

Liver/kidney
disease
Hypoalbuminemia

Late dilatation
Amyloid

---with dilatation

Regular fold
thickening
only

Difference B/W TB and CD (Crohn's Disease)

		TB	CD
1.	Length of involved segment	< 3 cm	> 3 cm
2.	Sites of ulcers	Circumferential	At mesenteric attachment
3.	Axis of ulcers	Perpendicular to long axis	Parallel
4.	Cobblestone mucosa	⊖	⊕
5.	Fistula	⊕	⊕++
6.	Perforation	⊕	++
7.	Anorectal disease	⊕	⊕++
8.	Mesenteric granuloma	⊕	⊖
9.	Bowel granuloma	⊕	⊕
10.	Caseation in granuloma	⊕	⊖
11.	Caseation in nodes	⊕	⊖
12.	Periadenitis	⊕	⊖
13.	Asymmetry	⊖	⊕
14.	Transmural inv (Target App.)	⊕	⊕
15.	Fibrosis in muscle propria	⊕	⊖

5.4 THICKENED GASTRIC FOLDS

Gastric folds are said to be thickened when they measure >1cm in thickness.

1. *Thickened folds in fundus and body.*
   – Hypertrophic gastritis

- Zollinger-Ellison syndrome
  - Gastrin producing tumor
  - Postbulbar ulcer in 1 and 2 part of duodenum are suggestive.
  - Ulcers distal to 2nd part of duodenum are virtually diagnostic.
  - Excessive acid secretion cause mucosal edema and fold thickening.
  - 50% multiple and 50% malignant.
- Ménétrier's Disease
  - Marked glandular hypertrophy
  - Hypochlorhydria and hypoproteinemia is associated
  - Course of disease is chronic and unremitting in adults but resolution occurs in children.
- Varices—associated with esophageal varices.
- Lymphocytic gastritis
  - Large
  - Varioli form erosions.

2. *Thickened folds predominantly in antrum.* (The thickened rugal fold of more than 5 mm in antral area and of more than 1.5 cm along greater curvature. There are also prominent area gastrica of 4-5 mm which are polygonal or regular throughout stomach).
- Inflammatory/Infiltrative
  a. Crohn's disease
    - Aphthous ulceration, fold thickening, deep ulcers, skin lesion and scarring are observed.
  b. Amyloidosis, sarcoidosis, cystic fibrosis.
    - Associated lung changes suggests the diagnosis in sarcoidosis.
  c. *Tuberculosis*: Caseous lymphadenopathy is characteristic.

    d. Eosinophilic gastritis
- 50% have peripheral eosinophilia and 50% have allergic history.

    e. Caustic ingestion

    f. Drugs like 5-fluorouracil

    g. Radiotherapy

    h. Watermelon stomach
- Vascular ectasia involving submucosal vessels

    i. Acute pancreatitis

    j. Pseudolymphoma
- This is a benign reactive nodular hyperplasia.
- 70% have ulcer near the center of affected area.

3. *Thickening Involving any Part of Stomach*
   - *Carcinoma*
     - Thickened folds are irregular with signs of mucosal destruction.
     - Loss of pliability of gastric wall.
   - *Lymphoma*
     - Usually NHL
     - Multifocal, usually large masses with coarse mucosal folds which may extend along GE junction or pylorus with preservation of wall pliability.

5.5 THICKENED DUODENAL FOLDS

1. *Inflammatory*
   - Duodenitis
   - Pancreatitis
   - Crohn's disease
     - Precedes aphthous ulcer
     - Duodenal cap and D2 predominantly affected

- Infections
  - HIV, CMV, MAI, Cryptosporidium
2. *Neoplastic*
   - Zollinger-Ellison syndrome
     - Associated ulcers are seen.
   - Lymphoma
   - Metastases - Rare
     From melanoma, breast, ovary, etc.
3. *Infiltrative Disorders*
   - Amyloidosis
   - Whipple's disease
   - Mastocytosis
   - Eosinophilic enteritis
   - Peripheral eosinophilia
   - H/o allergy
   - Intestinal lymphangiectasia
4. *Vascular*
   - Varices
     - Invariably associated with esophageal varices
   - Intramural hemorrhage
     - Trauma, bleeding diathesis
     - "Stacked-coin" appearance
   - Ischemia—Seen in vasculitis, collagen disease
5. *Edema*
   - Hypoproteinemia—Nephrotic syndrome, cirrhosis, etc.
   - Lymphatic obstruction
   - Venus obstruction
     - Budd-Chiari syndrome
     - Constrictive pericarditis
   - Angioneurotic edema
6. *Infestations*
   - Giardiasis
     - Associated with hypermotility

- • Spasm producing narrowing
- • Associated with nodular lymphoid hyperplasia or hypogammaglobulinemia
- – Hookworm
  - • Ankylostoma duodenale
- – Strongyloidosis stercoralis
- – Tapeworm
  - • Taenia saginata/Taenia solium.

5.6 MASSIVELY DILATED STOMACH

Gas or food filled stomach can be identified, with the wall of greater curvature convex caudally with pyloric antrum pointing cranially. Mottled translucencies can be seen due to air trapped within food residues.

Causes

1. *Paralytic Ileus*
   - – Common in elderly
   - – Associated with fluid and electrolyte disturbance
   - – High mortality rate

a. Postoperative
b. Trauma
c. Peritonitis
d. Pancreatitis
e. Cholecystitis
f. Diabetic coma
g. Hepatic coma
h. Uremic coma
i. Hypokalemia
j. Drugs like anticholinergics

2. *Mechanical Gastric Outlet Obstruction*
   a. Fibrosis/scarring secondary to ulceration
   b. Malignancy in antrum
   c. Gastric volvulus
      - – Organo-axial type is usually associated with hiatus hernia
      - – Elevation of Lt hemidiaphragm

- No gas beyond stomach
- Collapsed small bowel loops
 d. Proximal small bowel obstruction
 e. Bezoars
 f. Infantile/adult hypertrophic pyloric stenoses
  US is diagnostic
3. Miscellaneous
 - Air swallowing
 - Intubation

5.7 TARGET LESIONS IN STOMACH ON BARIUM STUDIES

Appearance is due to umbilication or ulceration at the apex of nodule.

1. Benign lesions
 a. Leiomyoma—apical/central ulceration
 b. Ectopic pancreatic rests
  - Primitive ductal system fill with barium producing a central niche at the apex of the tumor.
 c. Neurofibroma
  - May be multiple and multifocal
  - Other stigmata of neurofibromatosis

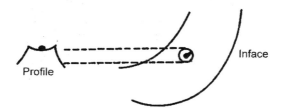

Fig. 5.7.1: "Bull's eye" (Target) lesions in the stomach

    d. Acute erosive gastritis
       – Ulcer surrounded by halo of edema.
2. Malignant lesions
    a. Leiomyosarcoma
       – Central ulceration but usually tumors are large
    b. Lymphoma
    c. Metastases from melanoma, carcinoid, breast, bronchus and pancreas.

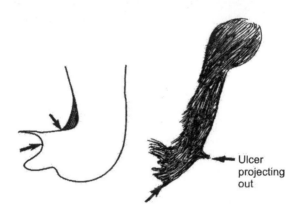

Ulcer projecting out

Fig. 5.7.2

Gastric adenocarcinoma polypoid type—shows abrupt narrowing of the pyloric canal due to mural infiltration of adenocarcinoma— polypoidal intraluminal component

Gastric lymphoma UGI – marked thickening of gastric ruge giving "Cobble-Stone" appearance and shrunken stomach

Table 5.7.1: CT-differentiation of gastric adenocarcinoma
from gastric lymphoma

CT	Lymphoma	Adenocarcinoma
Wall thickness	4.0 cm	1.8 cm
Mean	1.1 - 7.7 cm	1.1 - 3.2 cm
Range	Regular 42%	Regular 27%
Contour	Irregular 58%	Irregular 73%
Extent	Diffuse 80%	Focal 87%
Direct spread to adjacent organs	42%	73%
Lymph node above/ below renal hilum	42%	0%

5.8 GAS IN GASTRIC WALL

1. *Interstitial Gastric Emphysema*
   - Appear as linear or curvilinear lucent shadows along the gastric wall.
   Causes include
   - Raised intragastric pressure
   - Postendoscopy
   - Peptic ulceration
   - Necrotizing enterocolitis
2. *Emphysematous Gastritis*
   - Due to gas forming organisms in wall
   - Common in elderly, diabetes mellitus, alcohol abuse and following corrosive ingestion
3. *Cystic Pneumatosis*
   - Seen in elderly
   - Associated with COPD

5.9 COBBLE-STONE DUODENAL CAP ON BARIUM STUDY

1. *Small Size Cap*
   – Erosive duodenitis
     • Central fleck of barium with halo of edema
     • Duodenal cap is irritable
   – Benign nodular lymphoid hyperplasia
     • 1-3 mm nodules involving entire duodenal loop.
   – Heterotopic gastric mucosa
     • 1-6 mm nodules extending from pylorus towards apex of cap.
   – Food residue/effervescent granules
     • Move to most nondependent part
2. *Big Polypoidal Cap*
   – Large ulcer with surrounding edema
   – Hypertrophied Brunner's gland
     • Uniform size
     • Extend from pylorus to ampulla of Vater
     • Associated with end-stage renal failure in 25%
3. *Crohn's Disease*
   – Aphthoid ulcers are seen

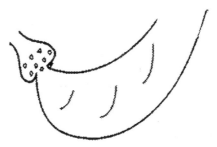

Fig. 5.9.1: "Cobble-stone" duodenal cap

4. *Varices*
   - Base of cap is usually affected
   - Decrease in erect position
   - Invariably associated with esophageal varices
5. Lymphoma
6. Carcinoma.

5.10 DILATED DUODENUM/OBSTRUCTION OF DUODENUM

1. *Congenital Causes*
   - Annular pancreas
   - Peritoneal bands = Ladd band
     - Commonest cause in neonates
     - Associated with malrotation and midgut volvulus
   - Aberrant vessel
   - Atresia, webs and stenosis
2. *Inflammatory Narrowing*
   - Chronic duodenal ulcer scar
   - Acute pancreatitis : Phlegmon, abscess, pseudocyst
   - Acute cholecystitis : Perforated gallstone
3. *Intramural Hematoma*
   - Blunt trauma (Accident, child abuse)
   - Anticoagulant therapy
   - Blood dyscrasia
4. *Tumoral Narrowing*
   - Primary duodenal tumors
   - Tumor invasion from pancreas, right kidney, lymph node enlargement
5. *Extrinsic Compression*
   - Aortic aneurysm
   - Pseudoaneurysm

6. *Miscellaneous*
   - Superior mesenteric artery syndrome from extensive burns, rapid weight loss, prolonged bedrest
     • Hold-up of barium in third part of duodenum
     • Delay of 4-6 hrs in gastroduodenal transit
     • Proximal dilatation and vigorous peristalsis with sharp cut off sign
     • Barium passes easily in making the patient prone
     • Postprandial pain relieved by lying on left side
     • Decrease aortomesenteric angle of 6-25° as opposed to normal of 45° as on U.S. and decreased aortomesenteric distance of 2-8 mm as opposed and normal 8-10 mm by CT.
     • 20% associated with duodenal ulcer
     • Very very rare in obese people.
   - Bezoar
   - Scleroderma
   - Paralytic ileus.

5.11 DILATED SMALL BOWEL/JEJUNAL AND ILEAL OBSTRUCTION

Criteria

Jejunal diameter shouldn't exceed 4 cm.
Ileal diameter shouldn't exceed 3 cm on small bowel enema.
The criteria limits are 0.5 cm less on barium meal follow through studies.

A. *Congenital*
   1. Ileal atresia/stenosis
   2. Enteric duplication cyst—commonest ileum
      - Location—antimesenteric border
   3. Midgut volvulus

    4. Mesenteric cyst—commonest ileum
        − Location mesenteric side
    5. Meckel's diverticulum.

B. *Extrinsic Bowel Lesions*
    1. Fibrous adhesions from previous surgery/peritonitis
        − Commonest cause in adults
    2. Hernias (inguinal, femoral, umbilical)
    3. Volvulus
    4. Masses—Neoplasms, abscess.

C. *Luminal Occlusion*
    1. Swallowed foreign body, bezoar, gallstone, etc.
    2. Meconium ileus
    3. Intussusception
    4. Tumor, e.g.: Lipoma.

D. *Intrinsic Bowel Wall Lesion*
    1. Strictures from neoplasm, Crohn's disease, tuberculosis enteritis, parasitic disease, radiotherapy, amyloidosis
    2. Intramural hemorrhage—blunt trauma, Henoch-Schönlein purpura
    3. Vascular insufficiency—Arterial/venous occlusion
    4. Celiac disease, tropical sprue, dermatitis herpetiformis
    5. Scleroderma
    6. Lymphoma.

E. *Miscellaneous*
    1. Postvagotomy and postgastrectomy
    2. Rapid emptying of stomach produce small bowel dilatation
    3. Extensive small bowel resection
    4. Zollinger-Ellison syndrome.

5.12 STRICTURES IN SMALL BOWEL

1. *Neoplasms*
   - Lymphoma
     - Usually secondary to lymph node involvement
     - Primary is usually NHL
     - Associated with thick folds
   - *Carcinoid*
     - Commonest site distal ileum
     - Produces intense fibroblastic response
   - *Carcinoma*
     - Commonest site is duodenum
     - Produce short segment stricture with mucosal destruction and ulceration
   - *Sarcoma*
     - Lympho - or leiomyosarcoma
     - Thick folds with eccentric lumen
   - *Metastases*
     - Flattened mucosal folds
2. *Crohn's Disease*
   - Aphthous ulcers
   - Skin lesions
3. *Tuberculous/Parasitic Infestation*
   - Long segment smooth strictures
   - Multifocal
4. *Ischemic*
   - Ulcers rare
   - Evolution more rapid ± strictures
5. *Radiation Enteritis*
   - Produce end arteritis and fibrosis
   - Doses >4500 rads

6. Enteric coated potassium chloride tablets
7. Surgical anastomosis
8. Amyloidosis.

5.13   SMALL INTESTINAL STRICTURE

Differential Diagnosis

1. Tuberculosis
2. Crohn's disease
3. Metastatic carcinoma
4. End-stage radiation enteritis
5. Endometriosis
6. Eosinophilic gastroenteritis
7. Post-traumatic
8. Drug induced
9. Primary malignancy

Tuberculosis

- Usually presents in a patient with a past or current history of pulmonary tuberculosis, either from swallowing of sputum or due to hematogenous spread.
- Sometimes primary, as from ingestion of infected cow's milk.
- Patient presents with loss of appetite, low-grade fever or sometimes subacute intestinal obstruction. Mantoux test may be positive and ESR is usually raised.
- Ulcerative form is most frequent, with ulcers presenting in an axis perpendicular to the long axis of intestines.
- Hypertrophic form present with gross thickening of bowel wall.
- Most common in the region of terminal ileum and caecum,

but may involve any part of the GI tract. In the ileocaecal area it usually presents with stricture and shortening of caecal pole. Multiple strictures may be seen in the small intestines or the whole of GI tract.

- Intestinal loops may be matted as seen on fluoroscopy, USG or CT.
- Mesenteric, peripancreatic or retroperitoneal adenopathy is seen with lymph nodes having caseous necrotic centers and peripheral enhancement on CECT.
- Ascites is usually present and is exudative with internal echoes and thick shaggy septations/adhesions seen on USG. On CT the ascitic fluid is of high attenuation value (20-45 HU).
- Omentum may be rolled up or may have irregular masses of soft tissue density. Similar masses may also be seen in mesentery.

Crohn's Disease

- A kind of regional enteritis is a disease of unknown etiology.
- Presents with discontinuous (skip areas) and asymmetric involvement of entire GI tract but most commonly involve the small intestines.
- There is transmural inflammation, ulceration and formation of non-caseating granulomas and enlargement of abdominal lymph nodes.
- Patients presents with colicky abdominal pains, diarrhea, low-grade fever, weight loss and malabsorption.
- There is cobblestone mucosae due to presence of abnormal edematous, ulcerated and fissured mucosa separated by normal uninvolved mucosa.
- Perianal abscess and fistula formation is very common.
- Terminal ileum alone or in combination with jejunum and ileum are most commonly involved.

- There is intense fibrosis of involved loops with formation of "string sign" due to stricture formation leading to marked narrowing of bowel loops.
- There is ulceration (aphthous ulcers) and fissuring of mucosa leading to appearances of thorns (rose thorns or raspberry thorns) on barium studies.
- Thickening of bowel loops lead to the "pseudokidney sign" seen on USG.
- "Creeping fat" appearances on CT is due to massive proliferation of intestinal fat leading to separation of bowel loops.
- Multiple intra-abdominal abscesses may also be seen.
- Multiple fistulous tracts (enterocolic, perianal, colovesical, colovaginal, enterocutaneous) etc. may also be seen either on barium studies or on CT.
- Extra intestinal manifestations like fatty infiltration of liver, sclerosing cholangitis, urolithiasis, digital clubbing, sero-negative arthropathy, erythema nodosum, may also be the presenting features.

Metastatic Carcinoma

- There is usually a history of primary carcinoma elsewhere.
- Intraperitoneal spread occurs from primary mucinous cancers of ovary, appendix, colon and breast.

Eosinophilic Enteritis

- Patients presents with relapsing attacks of gastroenteritis, there is peripheral blood eosinophilia in 50% of cases and positive history of atopy can be elicited.
- There is formation of eosinophilic granulomas and fibrosis.
- Fibrosis leads to stricture formation.

- There is separation of bowel loops and sometimes ascites may also be seen.

Post-traumatic

- The interval between trauma and onset of symptoms is usually 1 to 18 weeks.
- The stenotic segment may vary in length and outline.
- History may be suggestive and diagnosis is one of exclusion.

Drug Induced

- Usually due to non-enteric coated tablets of KCl and rarely NSAIDs.
- The drugs induce small bowel ischemia leading to ulceration, than fibrosis and subsequently stricture formation.
- The strictures are very short segment and diaphragm like and may be multiple.

Primary Malignancy

- Very rare
- May produce appearances like colonic carcinoma.
- There is evidence of mucosal destruction with overhanging edges.
- Hematogenous dissemination is seen in malignant melanoma, breast carcinoma, lung carcinoma, and Kaposi sarcoma.
- Direct extension may be seen in carcinoma ovary, uterus, prostate, pancreas, colon and kidney.
- There may be a single mass protruding into the lumen of

the bowel or encircling the bowel like an annular carcinoma leading to stricture formation.

- Stricture may also form due to direct compression either by the primary carcinoma itself or by involved nodes.
- On CT there is presence of soft tissue nodules or masses, sheets of tissue causing thickening of bowel wall, fixation and angulation of bowel loops and ascites.

Radiation Enteritis

- There is a history of radiotherapy done for a primary intra-abdominal or pelvic carcinoma usually seen in women with carcinoma ovary, cervix, endometrium or in patients with carcinoma bladder or colon.
- There is a latent period of usually 1-2 years before a full-blown picture emerges.
- There is irregular nodular thickening of folds with straight or transverse ulcers.
- Bowel wall is thickened with luminal narrowing and stricture formation.
- Strictures may be multiple and can be partial or complete.
- There may be shortening of small bowel.
- Bowel loops may be matted together due to intense desmoplastic reaction induced by radiation.

Endometriosis

- Rare but usually involves the rectum and colon, rarely small intestines are involved.
- There may be a history of endometriosis or colicky abdominal pain during menstruation.
- May presents as an intraluminal mass or stricture of bowel wall due to intense desmoplastic reaction invoked by periodic loss of blood by the endometriotic deposits.

(Flow Chart See Next Page)

Flow Chart 5.13.1

D/D-Small Intestinal Stricture

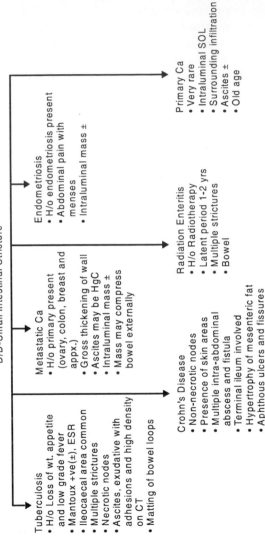

Tuberculosis
- H/o Loss of wt. appetite and low grade fever
- Mantoux +ve(±), ESR
- Ileocaecal area common
- Multiple strictures
- Necrotic nodes
- Ascites, exudative with adhesions and high density on CT
- Matting of bowel loops

Crohn's Disease
- Non-necrotic nodes
- Presence of skin areas
- Multiple intra-abdominal abscess and fistula
- Terminal ileum involved
- Hypertrophy of mesenteric fat
- Aphthous ulcers and fissures

Metastatic Ca
- H/o primary present (ovary, colon, breast and appx.)
- Gross thickening of wall
- Ascites may be HgC
- Intraluminal mass ±
- Mass may compress bowel externally

Radiation Enteritis
- H/o Radiotherapy
- Latent period 1-2 yrs
- Multiple strictures
- Bowel

Endometriosis
- H/o endometriosis present
- Abdominal pain with menses
- Intraluminal mass ±

Primary Ca
- Very rare
- Intraluminal SOL
- Surrounding infiltration ±
- Ascites ±
- Old age

5.14 THICKENED FOLDS IN SMALL BOWEL

Normal fold thickness—1.5-2 mm

Abnormal fold thickness— Jejunum > 2.5 mm

Ileum > 2.0 mm

Calibre—

Proximal jejunum— > 3.5 cm

(4.5 cm, of small bowel enema)

Mid small bowel— > 3.0 cm

(4.0 cm, of small bowel enema)

Ileum— > 2.5 cm

(3.0 cm, if small bowel enema)

Divided in to two Categories:

1. With dilated small bowel—common causes
   - Vascular insufficiency
   - Lesions of bowel and mesentery
   - Z-E syndrome
   - Amyloidosis
   - Lymphoma
   - Abetalipoproteinemia
   - Extensive small bowel resection

2. With nondilated small bowel

A. Localized (<50% of small bowel)

Smooth and Regular

a. Vascular
   Intramural hematoma
   - Trauma
   - Bleeding diathesis

Ischemia
- Acute—embolus, Henoch-Schönlein purpura
- Chronic—vasculitis, RT, atheroma, fibromuscular dysplasia

b. Edema
- Adjacent inflammation or mass

c. Infiltrative disease
- Early amyloidosis
- Early eosinophilic enteritis

Irregular and Distorted

a. Inflammatory
- Crohn's disease
- Z-E syndrome

b. Infective
- Tuberculosis

c. Neoplastic
- Lymphoma
- Carcinoid
- Melanoma or other metastases.

B. Generalized (> 50% small bowel involved)

Smooth and Regular

a. Vascular
- Bleeding diathesis
- Vasculitis, RT, etc.

b. Edema
- Hypoproteinemia
- Venous congestion
- Lymphatic obstruction
- Angioneurotic edema

c. Infiltrative
   - Late amyloidosis
   - Eosinophilic enteritis
d. Abetalipoproteinemia

Irregular and Distorted

a. Inflammatory
   - Crohn's disease
b. Infiltrative
   - Late amyloidosis
   - Eosinophilic enteritis
     - Whipple's disease
     - Mastocytosis
c. Infestation
   - Giardiasis
   - Strongyloidosis
d. Neoplastic
   - Lymphoma
e. Primary lymphangiectasia

5.15 THICKENED SMALL BOWEL FOLDS WITH GASTRIC ABNORMALITY

1. Lymphoma/metastases
2. Z-E syndrome
3. Ménétrier's disease
4. Amyloidosis
5. Eosinophilic gastroenteritis
6. Whipple's disease
7. Crohn's disease

5.16 NODULAR APPEARANCE OF SMALL BOWEL

1. Sandlike nodules (1 mm)
   - Seen in following infiltrative disorders as
     a. Waldenström's macroglobulinemia
        - Associated with normal fold.
     b. Mastocytosis—Associated with thick folds.
     c. Whipple's disease—Associated with thick folds.
2. Small nodules (> 2 mm)
   a. Thickened Folds
      1. Inflammatory – Crohn's disease
         - Cobblestone mucosa
         - With skip areas
      2. Neoplastic – Lymphoma

Normal Folds

1. Inflammatory
   - Nodular lymphoid hyperplasia
     - Associated with hypogammaglobulinemia
     - Associated malabsorption and giardiasis
2. Polyposis
   - Peutz-Jeghers syndrome
   - Autosomal dominant
   - Multiple hamartomas
   - May be associated with intussusception
   Gardner's and Canada-Cronkhite syndrome may occasionally involve small bowel
3. Lymphoma
4. Metastases – on antimesenteric border esp. melanoma, breast, GIT and ovary.
5. Infections as typhoid, yersinia, histoplasmosis.

5.17 MALABSORPTION

Defined as deficient absorption of any essential food materials within small bowel.

1. *Primary*
   - The digestive abnormality is the only abnormality
   - Celiac/–or tropical sprue
   - Disaccharidase deficiency.

2. *Secondary*
   - The abnormality occurs during the course of some disease.
   - Enteric
   - Gastric – fistula, gastrectomy, pyloroplasty
   - Pancreatic – cystic fibrosis, pancreatitis, carcinoma.
   - Hepatobiliary
   - Intra or extrahepatic biliary obstruction.
   - Acute and chronic liver disease.

5.18 MALABSORPTION

Clinical Features

- Diarrhea
- Steatorrhea
- Flatulence, abdominal distension
- Weight loss.
- Other—Paresthesia, bone pain, tetany, glossitis, cheliosis, anemia, lassitude.

Blood tests: Anemia, LFT, serum iron, folic acid, albumin, vit. K, D, B$_{12}$.

Fecal fat: 72 hour quantitative fecal fat analysis -estimation of 14c in breath after ingestion of radioactive triglyceride.

Small bowel N folds With			Dilated bowel		Thick straight folds		Thick nodular irregular folds	
	Fluid	Wet bowel	Dry	Wet	Dry	Wet	Dry	Wet
Disease								
1. Celiac disease commonest cause- Jejunal dilatation is hallmark		+		−				
2. Tropical sprue		+	+	+				
3. Whipple's disease							+	+ (rare)
4. Infestations as giardiasis, hookworm, tapeworm							+	
5. Mechanical defects as fistulas blind loop, volvulus anastomosis	+			+				
6. Neurologic-DM						+	+	
7. Inflammatory enteritis								

Contd...

Contd...

Small bowel N folds With	Fluid	Wet bowel	Dilated bowel		Thick straight folds		Thick nodular irregular folds	
			Dry	Wet	Dry	Wet	Dry	Wet
8. Endocrine-ZE syndrome						+		
9. Collagen disease scleroderma, lupus		+	+					
10. Neoplastic as lymphoma							+	
11. Vascular disease ischemic					+			
12. Abetalipoproteinemia-CNS damage, retinal abnormalities, steatorrhea, acanthocytosis						+		
13. Lymphangiectasia								
14. Pancreatic causes	+							+
15. Gastric causes	+							

D-14[c]-xylose Breath Test: Test of choice for detecting bacterial overgrowth.

- Gram-negative bacteria metabolize D-xylose to 14 CO_2 hydrogen test for lactase deficiency.
- A rise of more than 20 ppm in exhaled hydrogen above basal level after ingestion of lactose at 1g/kg body weight.

Barium

- Dilution of barium, because of hypersecretion of fluid by bowel.
- Flocculation
- Segmentation of the column of barium
- Moulage sign the appearance of barium in a feature less tube due to effacement of mucosal folds.

Malabsorption describes impaired absorption of normal dietary constituents, namely protein, carbohydrates, fats, minerals and proteins.

Causes

- Mucosal
  1. Coeliac disease
  2. Inflammation—Tropical sprue
     - Crohn's disease
     - Radiotherapy
  3. Infiltrative disorder:
     - Whipple's disease
     - Mastocytosis
     - Amyloidosis
     - Eosinophilic enteritis
  4. Lymphangiectasis
  5. Parasites
     - Giardiasis
     - Strongyloidosis
  6. Ischemia

- Inadequate digestion
  - Postgastrectomy
  - Deficiency or inactivation of pancreatic lipase
  - Gastrinoma
  - Disaccharidase deficiency (lactose intolerance)
- Reduced intestinal bile salt concentration
  - Liver disease
  - Blind loop syndrome
  - Pseudo-obstruction
  - Ileal resection
  - Ileal inflammatory disease (Crohn's, TB)
  - Drugs-by sequestration of bile salts
- Inadequate absorptive surface
- Intestinal resection or bypass
  (short bowel syndrome)
- Major resection
  - Severe ischemia/infarction
  - Volvulus
  - Trauma
- Repeated resections
  - Crohn's disease
  - Peutz-Jeghers syndrome
- With or without colon-150 cm
- With colon- 50-70 cm
- Normal ileum can assume the function of jejunum by adaptation
- Lost ileum is metabolically irreplacable.
- Resection of >100 cm of terminal ileum -interrupts extrahepatic circulation of bile salt.

Barium

- Show indication of the length of residual small bowel
- Features of adaptation—increased lumen diameter, thickened folds, more numerous krinkled folds.

Cystic fibrosis: Exocrine pancreatic secretion are low in bicarbonate and viscid.

Acid with pH—Maldigestion

- *Duodenum*—thickened or flattened folds, nodular filling defects, and lumen dilatation with sacculation along it's lateral border.
- In small bowel, particularly terminal ileum—Normal fold pattern is replaced by an irregular network of curving lines.

Celiac Disease

- Antibodies to gliadin fraction of gluten HLA-DR3.
- Gold standard in diagnosis–characteristic changes shown by mucosal biopsy.
- Favorable clinical response to gluten-free diet.
- Reversal to near normalcy on follow-up mucosal biopsies.

Radiological/Features

Lumen dilatation >3 cm in follow through—

- Increased separation or even absence of jejunal folds
- Reversal of normal fold character between the ileum and the jejunum
- Increase in number and thickness of folds
- Mosaic mucosal pattern—network of barium containing grooves separating areas 1-3 mm in size
- In duodenum—fewer and irregular folds
- On gluten-free diet—Number of folds in jejunum returns to normal
- Less improvement in number of ileal folds
- If bowel calibre increases while on gluten-free diet, suspect a complication, i.e. lymphoma, carcinoma or intersusception (rare and nonobstructive).

Tropical Sprue

- Post-infective malabsorption with subtotal villous atrophy.

- In tropical countries.
- Extends throughout the small bowel.
- Megaloblastic anemia, vitamin B_{12} and folate deficiency.
- Dramatic response to broad-spectrum antibiotics and folate.

Barium: Lumen dilatation, thickened folds, and flocculation.

Zollinger-Ellison Syndrome

- Gastric acid hypersecretion—maldigestion of fat
- Severe peptic ulcer disease—steatorrhea
- Gastrinoma—damage of jejunal mucosa.

R/F- dilated duodenum with coarse nodular folds with erosions.

- Thickened folds increased fluid, particularly in the proximal jejunum.
- 75-80% of gastrinomas pancreas
- 15%- duodenum
- Endoscopic USG- >50% of adjacent pancreatic gastrinomas
- CT/MR/ somatostatin receptor scintigraphy.

Eosinophilic Gastroenteritis

- H/o allergic disorders
- Diagnostic criteria
  - Symptoms related to GIT
  - Eosinophilic infiltration of mucosa on biopsy or a characteristic barium appearance with peripheral eosinophilia
  - Exclusion of parasitic or certain extraintestinal disease like polynodosa arteritis.
- Remissions and recurrences—typical
- Predominantly mucosal
  - Nausea, vomiting, diarrhoea
  - Fold thickening—antral
  - Straight thickened folds in small bowel

- Patchy distribution
- Predominant involvement of muscularis-thickening of muscularis with lumen narrowing -Antral
- Small bowel- segmental narrowing, not associated with fold thickening
- Serosal-rare, ascites, pleural effusion.

Whipple's Disease

Tropheryma whippelli.
- GIT, (small bowel) heart valves, CNS, joint capsule involvement.
- Lamina propria filled with macrophages containing PAS positive residue.
- Enteroclysis—Best radiological test for diagnosis of Whipple's disease.
- Diffuse or patchy micronodules, predominantly in the jejunum and at the duodenojejunal junction.
  CT—Abdominal lymphadenopathy with fatty material.

Pseudo-obstruction

Sign/symptom of obstruction without a mechanical cause.
- Primary familial *de novo*
  - Visceral neuropathy
  - Myopathy
- Dilated aperistaltic bowel loops.
- Antegrade barium study to exclude mechanical obstruction should be avoided.
- To be evaluated by CT.
- Secondary collagen vascular disease
  - Scleroderma
  - Dermatomyositis/Polymyositis
  - SLE

- Amyloidosis
- Endocrine disorder (a) Hypothyroidism (b) Diabetes.
- Neurological disease—Chaga's disease.
- Paraneoplastic visceral neuropathy—small cell lung carcinoma.
- Jejunal diverticulosis
- Drugs—Narcotics, tricyclic antidepressions.

Systemic Sclerosis

- Most common cause of chronic intestinal pseudo-obstruction.
- Esophagus—most common involved side, small bowel-60%.
- 35% patients present with malabsorption.

R/F—aperistalsis in distal two-third of esophagus with patulous lower esophageal sphincter and reflux esophagitis.

- Involvement of 2nd and 3rd parts of duodenum and jejunum
- Hidebound appearance
- Sacculation.

Amyloidosis

- Deposition of insoluble glycoprotein
- GIT involvement—more common in primary amyloidosis.
- Small bowel—non-specific dilatation, fold thickening, impaired motility, suspected of pseudo-obstruction.
- Localized deposition—filling defects either macro or micronodular.

Bacterial Overgrowth Syndromes

Normal 10^4 organisms /ml, aerobic-in jejunal aspirate
– >10^6/ml abnormal

Protective Mechanisms

1. Gastric acid
2. Peristalsis
3. Mucus and rapid turn over of enterocytes
4. Humoral and cellular immunity.

Causes

Stasis

- Strictures
- Diverticulosis
- Blind loop
- By passed bowel
- Pseudo-obstruction

Increased Bacterial Entry

- Impaired gastric acid output—Achlorhydria, hypochlor-hydria
- Gastrectomy
- Atrophic gastritis
- Omeprazole

Immunodeficiency

- Advanced age
- Hypogammaglobulinemia
- Malignancies
- AIDS

Affects

- Deconjugation of bile salts
- Reduced absorption of amino acids and carbohydrates
- Bind and utilize B_{12}

Jejunal Diverticulosis

Most common site of small bowel diverticula.
- Along mesenteric border
- Erect X-ray abdomen- numerous air-fluid levels in the upper abdomen
- Supine film- rounded air filled space without volvulae conniventes.
- Barium meal follow through/enteroclysis /CT
- Active bleeding—Tc 99m sulphur colloid scanning.

Parasitic Infestations

- *Giardiasis*: Villous atrophy, disruption of microvilli, bile salt decomposition -cytotoxic T cell.
- Acute self limiting diarrhea/chronic diarrhea, malabsorption, weight loss.
- *Diagnosis*: Stool examination/duodenal mucosal biopsy or duodenal aspirate
- Strongyloidosis: Increased or decreased motility, narrowing, ulceration, thickened folds, dilatation of lumen.
- Pipestem appearance of jejunum—chronic cases
- Megaduodenum
- Intestinal tuberculosis and extensive small bowel involvement by Crohn's disease may also lead to malabsorption syndrome.
- Radiation enteropathy-damage to mucosa malabsorption.

Lactose Intolerance

Primary
Acquired
- Celiac and tropical sprue, regional enteritis, viral and bacterial infections of GIT, giardiasis, cystic fibrosis, VC.

- Bloating, cramps, flatulence following milk ingestion.
- Measurement of breath hydrogen after 50 g lactose ingestion.

Lymphangiectasia

- Congenital malformation
- Blockage of lymph drainage in the mesentery or retroperitoneum extensive abdominal or retroperitoneal carcinoma/lymphoma, carcinoid, cirrhosis, chronic pancreatitis, congestive heart failure.
- Enteroclysis may reveal diffuse or patchy micronodules similar to Whipple's with thickened, edematous folds, with increased intraluminal fluid.
- Younger patients are affected.
- Mesenteric nodes are not enlarged except in patients with secondary cause, where primary pathology may be obvious.

Mastocytosis

- Mast cell infiltration.
- Urticaria
- Mucosal and submucosal infiltration with histamine release pain, nausea, vomiting, diarrhea.
  - Thicked irregular folds, diffuse mucosal nodularity, large urticaria like lesions.

Flow Chart 5.18.1
Malabsorption

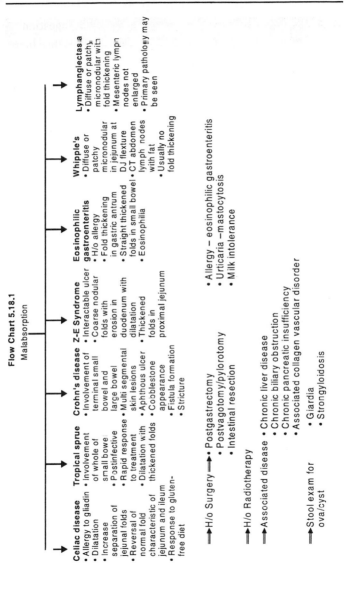

Celiac disease
• Allergy to gliadin
• Increase separation of jejunal folds
• Reversal of normal fold characteristic of jejunum and ileum
• Response to gluten-free diet

Tropical sprue
• Involvement of whole of small bowel
• Postinfective
• Rapid response to treatment
• Dilatation with thickened folds

Crohn's disease
• Involvement of terminal small bowel and large bowel
• Multi segmental skin lesions
• Aphthous ulcer
• Cobblestone appearance
• Fistula formation
• Stricture

Z-E Syndrome
• Interactable ulcer
• Coarse nodular folds with erosion in duodenum with dilatation
• Thickened folds in proximal jejunum

Eosinophilic gastroenteritis
• H/o allergy
• Fold thickening in gastric antrum
• Straight thickened folds in small bowel
• Eosinophilia

Whipple's
• Diffuse or patchy micronodular in jejunum at DJ flexure
• CT abdomen lymph nodes with fat
• Usually no fold thickening

Lymphangiectasia
• Diffuse or patchy micronodular with fold thickening
• Mesenteric lymph nodes not enlarged
• Primary pathology may be seen

⇒ H/o Surgery ⟶ • Postgastrectomy
• Postvagotomy/pylorotomy
• Intestinal resection

⇒ H/o Radiotherapy

⇒ Associated disease • Chronic liver disease
• Chronic biliary obstruction
• Chronic pancreatic insufficiency
• Associated collagen vascular disorder

• Allergy – eosinophilic gastroenteritis
• Urticaria –mastocytosis
• Milk intolerance

⇒ Stool exam for ova/cyst
• Giardia
• Strongyloidosis

5.19 PROTEIN LOSING ENTEROPATHY

1. *Disease with Mucosal Ulceration*
   - Carcinoma
   - Lymphoma
   - Villous adenoma
   - Inflammatory bowel disease
   - Peptic ulcer disease
2. *Nonulcerative Mucosal Disease*
   - Celiac disease
   - Tropical sprue
   - Whipple's disease
   - Allergic gastroenteropathy
   - Gastrocolic fistula
   - Villous adenoma of colon
3. *Associated with Hypertrophic Gastric Rugae*
   - Ménétrier's disease
4. *Lymphatic Obstruction*
   - Intestinal lymphangiectasia
   - Lymphoma
   - Retroperitoneal fibrosis
5. *Venous Obstruction*
   - Cirrhosis
   - IVC thrombosis
   - Constrictive Pericarditis
6. *Chronic Arterial Obstruction*
   - Atherosclerosis
7. *Heart Disease*
   Tricuspid insufficiency

5.20 PATHOLOGIC LESIONS IN TERMINAL ILEUM

1. *Inflammatory Lesions*
   - *Crohn's Disease*
     - Asymmetric involvement with skip lesions.
     - Predominates on the mesenteric border
     - Aphthoid ulcer – earliest sign
     - Fissure ulcer
     - Cobblestone pattern
     - Separation of bowel loops
     - Strictures and pseudosacculation
   - *Ulcerative Colitis*
     - Involves ileum in 10% of total colitis cases known as backwash ileitis.
     - Dilated ileum with granular mucosa.
     - No ulcers
   - *Radiation Enteritis*
     - Mural thickening with symmetrical stenosis
     - No ulceration or cobblestoning.
2. *Infective*
   - *Tuberculosis*
     - Cecum is predominantly involved.
     - Contraction and retraction of cecum.
     - Straightening of ileocecal angle.
     - Ulcer are uncommon.
   - *Yersinia*
     - Cobblestone mucosa with aphthous ulcers (resemble Crohn's disease)
     - No Deep fissure ulcer.
     - Spontaneous resolution in 10 wks.

- *Actinomycosis*
  - Very rare
  - Predominantly cecum is involved
- Histoplasmosis
  - Very rare
3. *Neoplastic*
   - *Lymphoma*
     - Usually non-Hodgkin's lymphoma
     - Irregular, nodular, thickened mucosa
     - Irregular polypoidal mass
     - Long segment annular stricture
     - Multiple ulcer
     - May be difficult to differentiate.
       from Crohn's disease radiologically.
   - *Carcinoid*
     - Invariably malignant if > 2 cm
     - Annular fibrotic stricture
     - Intraluminal filling defect
     - Mesenteric mass (produces stretching, rigidity and fixation of loops).
     - Intense desmoplastic response produces stellate arrangement of loops.
   - *Metastases*
   - Ischemia
     - Rare
     - Thickened
     - Folds, with 'cobblestoning' and 'thumb printing'.
     - Rapidly progressive, changes differentiate it from Crohn's disease.

5.21 COLONIC POLYPS

1. *Polyp* is a mass projecting into the lumen of hollow viscus above the level of mucosa. Arises from mucosa but may be derived from submucosa/muscularis propria.
   a. Neoplastic   – Adenomatous
   b. Nonneoplastic   – Hamartomatous/Inflammatory
2. *Pseudopolyp* refers to island of inflamed mucosa on a background of denuded mucosa.
   a. Pseudopolyposis of ulcerative colitis.
   b. Cobblestoning of Crohn's disease.
3. Postinflammatory/filiform polyps are finger like projections of submucosa covered by mucosa on all sides following healing and regeneration.
   1. *Adenomatous Polyps*
      A. *Single*: 1. Tubular, tubulovillous, villous
         – These form a spectrum both in size and degree of dysplasia.
         – Villous adenoma is the largest with severest dysplasia with highest premalignant potential.
         – Size: < 5 mm- 0% malignant
           5 mm - 1 cm - 1% malignant
           1 cm - 2 cm - 10% malignant
           > 2 cm - 50% malignant.
         – Puckering of bowel wall occurs at the base of polyp.
         – Villous adenomas are poorly coated because of mucous secretion; hence are associated with protein - losing enteropathy or hypokalemia.
      2. *Turcot's Syndrome*
         – Autosomal recessive
         – Increased risk of CNS malignancy.

B. *Multiple* : Familial adenomatosis coli, adeno-
matosis of GIT, Gardner's syndrome.
- May form a part of spectrum of same disease.
- Adenomas more numerous in distal colon and
rectum.
- Colon carcinoma develop in
  - 30% by 10 yrs after diagnosis.
  - 100% by 20 yrs after diagnosis.
- Carcinoma is multifocal in 50%
- Extra colonic abnormalities include
  - Hamartomas and adenomas in stomach
  - Adenoma of duodenum
  - Periampullary carcinoma
  - Jejunal and ileal polyps
  - Mesenteric fibromatosis
  - Multiple osteomas in skull and mandible
  - Dental abnormalitis – hypercementomas,
    odontomas, dentigerous cyst, etc.
  - Epidermoid cysts in leg, face, scalp, etc.
  - Pigmented lesion in fundi oculi.
  - Rarely thyroid carcinoma.
2. *Nonadenomatous Single Polyps*
   - Carcinoid
     - Commonest in appendix
     - Leiomyoma
     - Lipoma
     - Hemangioma, lymphangioma
     - Fibroma, neurofibroma
3. *Hamartomous Polyp*
   A. Single Juvenile Polyp
      - Commonest in rectum

B. Multiple
- Juvenile Polyposis—Nonhereditary
- Peutz-Jeghers syndrome - Hereditary
- Canada-Cronkhite syndrome-Nonhereditary
- Juvenile Polyposis
  - Seen in children < 10 yrs of age.
- Peutz-Jeghers syndrome
  - Autosomal dominant
  - 'Carpets' small bowel
  - Also affects colon and stomach in 30%
  - Pigmentation of mucosa and skin
  - Increased incidence of gastric, duodenal and ovarian carcinoma.
- Canada-Cronkhite syndrome
  - Predominantly affects stomach and colon.
  - Increased incidence of carcinoma of colon.
  - Skin pigmentation, nail atrophy and alopecia are associated features.

4. Hyperplastic Polyp
   A. Single/multiple—Commonest in rectum
   C. Nodular lymphoid hyperplasia
   - Seen usually in children
5. Inflammatory/postinflammatory polyp
   A. Single - Benign lymphoid polyp
   - Fibroid granulation polyp
   B. Multiple
   1. Ulcerative colitis - Polyps at all stages
   2. Crohn's disease - Less common than ulcerative colitis
   3. Schistosomiasis - Predominantly, involve rectum
   4. Amebiasis

5.22 COLONIC POLYPS

A. Adenomatous
B. Hyperplastic
C. Hamartomatous
D. Inflammatory
E. Infective
F. Others

ADENOMATOUS

1. Simple tubular adenoma, tubulovillous adenoma, villous adenoma - these three form a spectrum both in size and degree of dysplasia. Villous adenoma is the largest, shows most severe dysplasia and has highest malignancy incidence.

Signs suggestive of malignancy are:
a. Size
   - < 5 mm   -   0% malignant
   - 5 mm   -   1cm-1% malignant
   - 1 to 2 cm   -   10% malignant
   - >2 cm   -   50% malignant
b. Sessile - base is greater than height
c. 'Puckering' of colonic wall at base of polyp
d. Irregular surface.

Villous adenomas are typically fronded, sessile and are poorly coated by barium because of their mucous secretion. May cause a protein losing enteropathy or hypokalemia.

2. Familial polyposis coli and Gardner's syndrome—AD.
   Both conditions may represent a spectrum of the same disease. Multiple adenomas of colon which are more numerous in distal colon and rectum. Colonic carcinomas

develop in early adulthood (in 30% by ten years after diagnosis and in 100% by 20 years). Sixty percent of those who present with colonic symptoms already have colonic carcinomas. The carcinoma is multifocal in—
*50% extracolonic abnormalities may occur:-

a. *Hamartomas* of stomach (40%).
b. *Gastric adenomas* (more common in the Japanese).
c. *Adenomas* of duodenum (25%).
d. *Periampullary carcinoma* (12%).
e. *Jejunal and ileal* polyps (in 60%) of patients in Japanese literature).
f. *Mesenteric fibromatosis*—a noncalcified soft tissue mass which may displace bowel loops and produce mucosal irregularity from local invasion. USG reveals a hypo or hyperechoic mass and CT a homogenous mass of muscle density.
g. *Multiple osteomas*—most frequently in the outer table of the skull, the angle of mandible and frontal sinuses.
h. *Dental abnormalities*—hypercementomas, odontomas, dentigerous cyst, supernumerary teeth and multiple caries.
i. *Multiple epidermoid cyst*—usually on legs, face, scalp and arms.
j. *Pigmented lesions of the ocular fundus*: in 90% of patients with Gardner's syndrome and other extracolonic manifestations.
k. *Thyroid carcinoma* in 0.6%.

HYPERPLASTIC

1. *Solitary/multiple*- most frequently found in rectum.
2. *Nodular lymphoid hyperplasia*- usually children. Filling defects are smaller than familial polyposis coli.

HAMARTOMATOUS

1. *Juvenile polyposis*— ± Familial children under 10 yrs. Commonly solitary in rectum.
2. *Peutz-Jeghers syndrome*—Autosomal dominant. 'Carpets' small bowel, but also affects colon and stomach in 30%. Increased incidence of carcinoma of stomach, duodenum and ovary.

INFLAMMATORY

1. *Ulcerative Colitis*: Polyps can be seen at all stages of activity of the colitis (no malignant potential): *acute*: pseudo polyps (i.e. mucosal hyperplasia); chronic: sessile polyp (resembles villous adenoma); *quiescent*- tubular, filiform (wormlike) and can show branching pattern.

   Dysplasias in colitic colon is usually not radiologically visible. When visible it appears as solitary nodule, several separate nodules (both nonspecific) or as a close grouping of multiple adjacent nodules with apposed, flattened edges (the latter appearances being associated with dysplasia in 50% of cases).
2. *Crohn's disease*—polyps less common than in ulcerative colitis.

INFECTIVE

1. *Schistosomiasis*—predominantly involves rectum.± strictures.
2. Amebiasis.

OTHERS

1. *Canada-Cronkhite syndrome*—Not hereditary. Predominantly affect stomach and colon; but can occur anywhere in bowel. Increase incidence of carcinoma of colon.

Other features are alopecia, nail atrophy and skin pigmentation.

2. *Turcot's Syndrome*: Autosomal recessive.
   Increased incidence of CNS malignancy.

Polyposis Syndrome

Type	Trait	Gastric	SB	Colon	Histology	GI-Malignancy	Extra Intestinal
Familial polyposis	AD	< 5%	< 5%	100%	Adenoma	100%	–
Gardner's syndrome	AD	5%	5%	100%	Adenoma	100%	Osteoma
Peutz-Jeghers	AD	25%	95%	30%	Hamartoma	Rare	Perioral pigmentation
Juvenile polyposis	AD	–	–	100%	Hamartoma	?	–
Turcot's	AR	–	–	100%	Adenoma	100%	Glioma
Canada-Cronkhite	NH	100%	50%	100%	Inflammatory	None	Ectodermal
Cowden	AD	–	–	–	Hamartoma	None	Oral Papilloma

5.23 COLONIC STRICTURES/NARROWING

I. *Neoplastic*
  1. *Carcinoma*
     - Annular/scirrhous
     - Associated with mucosal distinction.
     - Short segment < 6 cm.
  2. *Lymphoma*
     - Cecum and rectum more frequently involved.
     - Radiologically, polypoid mass, diffusely infiltrative mass or annular lesion.
  3. *Metastatic*
     - From prostate, cervix, uterus, kidney, stomach, pancreas, etc.
II. *Chronic Stage of any Ulcerating Colitis*
  1. Inflammatory—are symmetrical, smooth and tapering.
     - Ulcerative Colitis
       - Common in sigmoid colon.
       - Require >5 yrs.
       - Malignant risk starts after 10 yrs and increase by 10% per decade.
       - Crohn's disease - Seen in 25% cases.
       - 50% are multiple.
       - Solitary rectal ulcer syndrome.
  2. Infective
     - Tuberculosis
       - Commonest in ileocecal region.
       - Short 'hourglass' stricture
     - Amebiasis
       - Common in descending colon.
       - Occurs in 2-8% cases.

- Multiple in 50%
- Improvement with metronidazole
- LGV
  - Sexually transmitted disease caused by Chlamydia.
  - Long and tubular stricture
  - Commonest in rectosigmoid region.
- Schistosomiasis
  - Commonest in rectosigmoid region.
- Other
  - H. zoster, CMV, strongyloidosis, etc.

3. *Ischemic*
   - Infarction heals rapidly by stricture formation.
   - Commonest site is splenic flexure.
   - Have tapering ends.

4. *Traumatic*
   - Radiotherapy
     - Latent period—Several years.
     - Commonest site—rectosigmoid.
   - Cathartic colon
     - Pseudostricture – Changes during exam.
     - Initially, ascending colon is involved.
   - Caustic colitis.

III. *Extrinsic Masses*

1. *Inflammation as in*
   - Retractile mesenteritis
   - Diverticulitis
   - Pericolic abscess

2. *Deposits*
   - Amyloidosis
   - Endometriosis
   - Pelvic lipomatosis

IV. *Postsurgical*
- Adhesive bands
- Surgical anastomosis

V. *Normal*
- Cannon point.

5.24 PNEUMATOSIS INTESTINALIS

Also known by the name of
- Pneumatosis cystoides intestinalis
- Bullous emphysema of intestine
- Intestinal gas cysts
- Peritoneal lymphopneumatosis

Causes

A. *Bowel Necrosis / Gangrene*
- Commonest cause
- There is damage and disruption of mucosa with entry of gas forming bacteria.
  a. Necrotizing enterocolitis—in neonate
  b. Ischemia and infarction as in mesenteric thrombosis.
  c. Neutropenic colitis.
  d. Sepsis.
  e. Volvulus.
  f. Caustic ingestion.

B. *Mucosal Disruption*
- Increased intraluminal gas pressure leads to overdistension and dissection of gas in bowel wall.
  a. Intestinal obstruction as pyloric stenosis, annular pancreas, imperforate anus, Hirschsprung's disease, meconium plug syndrome, etc.

    b. Intestinal trauma as in endoscopy, rent, perforation, bowel surgery, barium enema, penetrating and blunt abdominal trauma, etc.

    c. Infection and inflammation as peptic ulcer disease, tuberculosis, peritonitis, Crohn's disease, ulcerative colitis, Whipple's disease, etc.

C. *Increased Mucosal Permeability*
- Defects in lymphoid tissue allows bacterial gas to enter bowel wall.
  a. Immunotherapy
     - Graft versus host disease
     - Organ / bone marrow transplantation.
  b. Miscellaneous
     - AIDS enterocolitides, steroid therapy, chemo– and radiation therapy, collagen vascular disease, diabetes mellitus.

D. *Pulmonary Disease*

Alveolar rupture with air dissection into interstitium and mediastinum, followed by retroperitoneal dissection and then along vascular bundles into bowel wall.
- Chronic obstructive pulmonary disease.
- Chest trauma.
- Positive pressure ventilation.

5.25 MEGACOLON IN ADULT

Transverse colon diameter greater than 5.5 cm is known as megacolon.

Causes

I. *Nontoxic* (without mucosal abnormality)
   1. Distal obstruction as by carcinoma.

2. Ileus – Paralytic or secondary to hypokalemia
3. Pseudo-obstruction
   - No organic lesion evident
   - Few fluid levels and feces seen in rectum.
4. Purgative abuse.

II. *Toxic*
   - Acute transmural fulminant colitis produce neuro-muscular degeneration and loss of motor tone. Mortality is 20%.
   1. Inflammatory
      a. Ulcerative colitis
      b. Crohn's disease
      c. Pseudomembranous colitis
   2. Ischemic colitis
   3. Dysentery
      a. Amebiasis
      b. Salmonella

Radiological Findings

- Colonic ileus with marked dilatation of transverse colon and few air-fluid levels.
- Increasing caliber of colon on serial radiographs without redundancy.
- Loss of normal colonic haustra and interhaustral folds.
- Irregular mucosal surface with pneumatosis coli.
- Barium enema is contraindicated due to risk of perforation.

5.26 THUMB PRINTING IN COLON

This is due to thickened mucosal folds because of submucosal edema/hemorrhage.

Causes

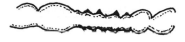

Fig. 5.26.1: Shows thumb printing in colon

I. *Colitides*
   a. Ischemic
      – Commonest site is splenic flexure
      – Peroral pneumocolon may obliterate it.
   b. Ulcerative colitis.
   c. Crohn's disease
   d. Amebic colitis
   e. Pseudomembranous colitis
   f. Schistosomiasis
II. *Neoplastic*
   a. Lymphoma
   b. Metastases

   Pseudo thumb printing is produced by mucosal indentation by mural air cysts. Careful examination will reveal intramural air.
III. *Miscellaneous*
   – Endometriosis
   – Amyloidosis
   – Diverticulitis / diverticulosis
   – Hereditary angioneurotic edema.

5.27 APHTHOUS ULCERS

These are fine erosions with a halo of edematous mucosa.

Causes

I. *In Colon*
   1. Crohn's disease - Earliest sign
   2. Amebic colitis
   3. Yersinia colitis

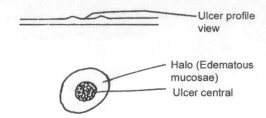

Fig. 5.27.1

- Produces thick mucosal folds with ulceration.
- Lymphoid nodular hyperplasia
4. Salmonella, shigella infection
5. Herpes virus infection
6. Behçet's disease
   - Usually simulates Crohn's disease
   - Occasionally resemble idiopathic ulcerative protocolitis
7. Ischemic colitis
8. Lymphoma.
II. *In Small Bowel*
   1. Crohn's disease
   2. Yersinia enteritis
   3. Polyarteritis nodosa.

5.28 ANTERIOR INDENTATION OF RECTO SIGMOID JUNCTION

1. Ascites
   - Commonest cause
   - especially in erect position
2. Abscess (pericolic)

3. Hematoma
4. Endometriosis
5. Surgery
   – Sling repair for rectal prolapse
6. Tumors
   – Peritoneal metastases – Common site for gastric, colonic, pancreatic and ovarian metastatic deposits.
   – Primary pelvic tumor esp. adnexal/Tubo-ovarian masses.
7. Hydatid Cyst
   – Metastatic from rupture of usually the hepatic cyst into peritoneal cavity with seedlings.

5.29 ° WIDENING/ENLARGEMENT OF PRESACRAL/RETRORECTAL SPACE

Normal width is < 5 mm in 95%
Width >1cm is considered abnormal.

I. *Normal Variation*
   – 40% cases and associated usually with obesity.

II. *Rectal Inflammation*
   1. Ulcerative colitis
      – Seen in 50% cases
      – Width increases as disease progresses.
   2. Crohn's colitis
   3. Idiopathic proctosigmoiditis
   4. Radiation therapy

III. *Rectal Infection*
   1. Proctitis (Tubercular, amebiasis, LGV, etc)
   2. Diverticulitis

IV. *Rectal Tumor*

A. *Benign*	B. *Malignant*
1. Developmental cyst – dermoid, enteric cyst	1. Adenocarcinoma, cloacogenic carcinoma
2. Lipoma, neurofibroma	2. Lymphoma, sarcoma, lymph node metastases
3. Epidermal cyst	3. Prostatic, uterine, vesical, ovarian causes
4. Rectal duplication	

V. *Body Fluids / Deposits*

1. Hematoma
   - Surgery, sacral fracture
2. Pus
   - Perforated appendix, presacral abscess.
3. Serum
   - Edema, venous thrombosis.
4. Fat
   - Cushing syndrome, pelvic lipomatosis.
5. Amyloidosis.

VI. *Sacral Tumors*

1. Metastases, plasmacytoma, chordoma in adults.
2. Sacrococcygeal teratoma, anterior sacral meningocele in children.

VII. *Miscellaneous*

1. Colitis cystic profunda.
2. Pelvic lipomatoses.

5.30 CYSTIC MESENTERIC MASSES

I. *Benign Cysts*

1. Pancreatic Pseudocyst
   - Sequelae of pancreatitis
   - Cyst contents reveal P. amylase.

2. Nonpancreatic Pseudocyst
   – Sequelae of mesenteric/omental hematoma/ abscess.
   – Thick-walled, usually septated with hemorrhagic/ purulent contents.
3. Enteric duplication Cyst.
4. Enteric cyst.
5. Mesothelial cyst.

II. *Masses*
   1. Cystic lymphangioma (Commonest).
   2. Pseudomyxoma peritonei.
   3. Cystic mesothelioma.
   4. Mesenteric cyst.
   5. Mesenteric hematoma.
   6. Benign cystic teratoma.
   7. Cystic spindle cell tumor.
      (leiomyoma / leiomyosarcoma).

5.31 NONVISUALIZATION OF GALLBLADDER ON ULTRASOUND

1. Contracted gallbladder.
2. Chronic cholecystitis.
3. Gallbladder carcinoma.
4. Perforation of gallbladder.
5. Congenital absence of gallbladder.

FILLING DEFECTS IN GALLBLADDER

1. *Fixed*
   A. *Single and Small*
      1. Calculus, wall adherent.

    2. Adenomyomatosis
- Usually fundal
- Stricture
- Rokitansky-Aschoff sinuses
- Visible after contraction

    4. Polyp
    5. Neurinoma

B. *Single and Large*
    1. Calculus
    2. Tumor – Primary / Secondary

C. *Multiple*
    1. Calculi
- 30% radiopaque

    2. Cholesterosis "strawberry" GB
- Characteristic multiple mural filling defects.

II. *Mobile*
    1. Tumefactive Sludge, biliary balls.
    2. Blood clot
    3. Calculus – usually nonshadowing.

III. *"Comet-Tail" Defect in GB*
    1. Rokitansky-Aschoff sinuses
    2. Intramural stone
    3. Cholesterolosis of GB.

5.32 GAS IN BILIARY TREE

These appear as irregularly branching gas shadows not reaching liver edge. Bile duct is outlined; GB may or may not be seen.

I. *Within the Bile Duct*
    1. Incompetence of sphincter of Oddi.
      (after sphincterotomy / passage of stone / patulous as in elderly)

2. Postoperative (cholecystoenterostomy / choledocho-enterostomy)
3. Spontaneous biliary fistula.
   - Gallstone ileus = Gallstone erodes the inflamed GB wall to enter duodenum (60%) and colon (20%)
   - Duodenal ulcer perforates into bile duct.
   - Malignancy
   - Trauma

II. *Within the Gallbladder*
1. All of the above
2. Emphysematous gallbladder
   - Seen in diabetes due to infection by gas forming organism.
   - Air bile level seen on erect films.
   - Intraluminal and intramural gas.

5.33 GAS IN PORTAL VENOUS

- Branching gas shadows within 2 cm of liver capsule.
- Gas may also be seen in portal and mesenteric venous and bowel wall.
- Considered a life-threatening event and sign of bowel infarction and gangrene unless proved otherwise.

I. *Children*
1. Necrotizing enterocolitis – 10% cases.
2. Umbilical vein catheterization
3. Erythroblastosis fetalis
4. Congenital GI obstruction : Duodenal atresia, esophageal atresia, imperforate anus.

II. *Adults*
   A. Intestinal necrosis (in 74% of adults)
      1. Bowel infarction

   2. Ulcerative colitis
   3. Necrotizing enterocolitis due to mesenteric arterial thrombosis
   4. Perforated ulcer (gastric / duodenal).
B. Miscellaneous
   1. Hemorrhagic pancreatitis
   2. Sigmoid diverticulitis
   3. Intra-abdominal abscess
   4. Pneumonia
   5. Inadvertant gas injection during endoscopy
   6. Dead fetus
   7. Diabetes, diarrhea
   8. During DCBE esp in severely ulcerated colon
   9. Acute gastric dilatation.

5.34   DIFFUSE HEPATOMEGALY

I. *Neoplastic*
   1. Diffuse metastases
   2. Diffuse HCC
   3. Lymphoma
   4. Angiosarcoma
II. *Metabolic/Storage*
   1. Fatty infiltration
   2. Amyloidosis
   3. Wilson's disease
   4. Hemochromatosis
   5. Glycogen storage disease
   6. Lipid storage disease
   7. Galactosemia
III. *Congenital*
   – Polycystic liver

IV. *Infective/Inflammatory*
1. Viral - infective and serum hepatitis, infectious mononucleosis
2. Bacterial – Tuberculous, brucellosis
3. Fungal – histoplasmosis
4. Protozoal – Malaria, ameba, kala-azar
5. Parasitic – Hydatid
6. Spirochetal – Syphilis
7. Other – Sarcoidosis

V. *Vascular*
Passive venous congestion as in
- CHF
- Constrictive pericarditis

VI. *Degenerative – Cirrhosis*

VII. *Myeloproliferative – Myelofibrosis*
Polycythemia rubra-vera

5.35 HEPATIC CALCIFICATION

I. *Multifocal and Small*
- Healed granulomas (Tuberculosis, histoplasmosis, brucellosis)
- Intrahepatic biliary calculi

II. *Curvilinear*
1. Hydatid seen in 20-30% cases
2. Congenital cyst
3. Abscess – esp amebic / old pyogenic
4. Porcelain gallbladder

III. *Localized in Mass*
1. Metastatic
   - Usually multifocal
   - Seen with mucinous carcinoma of colon, breast,

stomach, ovarian carcinoma, melanoma, pleural mesothelioma, osteosarcoma, carcinoid.
- Amorphous/flaky/stippled/granular
- May be seen following chemotherapy/RT

2. Hepatoma
   - Punctate, stippled or granular.
3. Hepatoblastoma
4. Cholangiocarcinoma

IV. *Sunray Spiculation*
1. Hemangioma/infantile hemangioendothelioma.
2. Metastatic as colloid carcinomas.
3. Rarely hepatoma.

V. *Irregular*
1. Hepatic artery aneurysm.
2. Portal vein thrombosis.
3. Capsule of regenerating nodules.
4. Chronic granulomatous disease of childhood.

VI. *Diffuse Increased Attenuation*
1. Iron accumulation
   - Primary/secondary hemosiderosis
2. Copper accumulation
   - Wilson's disease.
3. Iodine accumulation
   - Amiodarone therapy as an antiarrhythmic.
4. Gold
   - Gold therapy for rheumatoid arthritis.
5. Thallium
   - Ingestion of rodenticides.
6. Glycogen storage disease.
7. Thorotrast.

5.36 PRIMARY HEPATIC MASSES

I. *Primary Benign*
   A. *Epithelial*
      1. *Hepatocellular*
         - Regenerative nodules
         - Adenomatous hyperplastic nodules
         - FNH
         - Hepatocellular adenoma
      2. *Cholangiocellular*
         - Bile duct adenoma
         - Biliary cyst adenoma
   B. *Mesenchymal*
      1. *Tumor containing adipose*
         - Lipoma
         - Myolipoma
         - Angiomyolipoma
      2. *Tumor of muscle*
         - Leiomyoma
      3. *Tumor of vessels*
         - Infantile hemangioendothelioma
         - Hemangioma
         - Peliosis hepatis
      4. *Misc* - Mesothelioma
   C. *Mixed Tissue Tumor*
      - Mesenchymal hamartoma
      - Benign teratoma
   D. *Misc*
      - Adrenal rest tumor
      - Pancreatic rest tumor

II. *Malignant*
   A. *Epithelial*
      1. Hepatocellular
         − Hepatoblastoma
           (in pediatric age)
         − HCC
      2. Cholangiocellular
         − Cholangiocarcinoma
         − Biliary cystadenocarcinoma
   B. *Mesenchymal*
      1. Tumor of vessel
         − Angiosarcoma
         − Epithelioid hemangioendothelioma
         − Kaposi sarcoma
      2. Misc
         − Embryonal sarcoma
         − Fibrosarcoma
      3. Tumor of muscle
         − Leiomyosarcoma
         − Rhabdomyosarcoma
   C. *Miscellaneous*
      − Carcinosarcoma
      − Teratoma
      − Yolk sac tumor
      − Carcinoid
      − Squamous carcinoma
      − Lymphoma

5.37 NEONATAL OBSTRUCTIVE JAUNDICE

I. *Infections*
   a. Bacterial
      − *E.coli*, Syphilis

b. Viral
   - TORCH, HBV, Coxsackie

On USG—Liver echogenicity and size normal or increased
Tibida scan—May reveal delayed uptake by hepatocytes

II. *Metabolic*
   a. Inherited
      - α-1 antitrypsin deficiency, cystic fibrosis, galacto-semia, hereditary tyrosinemia
   b. Acquired
      - Inspissated bile syndrome (secondary to erythro-blastosis): Cholestasis due to total parenteral nutrition.

III. *Biliary Tract Abnormalities*
   a. Extrahepatic
      - Biliary obstruction/hypoplasia/atresia

Biliary atresia
   - Correctable type with patent intrahepatic ducts
   - Noncorrectable type with occluded intrahepatic ducts
   - Normal size, contractible GB rules out the diagnosis
   - Absence of small GB favors the diagnosis
   - Liver echogenicity on US may be normal or increased
   - Normal uptake by hepatocytes but no excretion into bowel on TBIDA scan favors the diagnosis but is not diagnostic.

Choledochal Cyst
   - May present in neonate or early childhood.

Todani's Type
   I. (Commonest) - Fusiform or focal dilatation of CBD
   II. – Diverticulum of CBD
   III. – Choledochocele – outpouching of CBD in wall of duodenum

IV. a. Dilated CBD with focal dilatation of intrahepatic ducts.
    b. Focal dilatation of CBD

V. Focal dilatation of intrahepatic ducts (Caroli's disease)
TBIDA scan - Photopenic areas with delayed uptake of tracer.
Complications: include calculi, pancreatitis, abscesses, cirrhosis, portal hypertension, malignancy.

- "Bile plug"syndrome
- Intrahepatic
  - Ductular hypoplasia/atresia
  - Alagille syndrome
    - Autosomal dominant
    - Dysmorphic facies with ocular abnormalities
    - CVS anomalies esp pulmonary stenosis
    - Hypoplasia of intrahepatic ducts
    - Butterfly vertebra
    - Radioulnar synostosis

5.38 FETAL/NEONATAL HEPATIC CALCIFICATION

I. *Peritoneal* - On hepatic surface
  1. Meconium peritonitis
     - Commonest cause of abdominal calcifications
     - Solid or cystic masses with calcified walls seen on USG.
  2. Ruptured hydrometrocolpos
     - Appearance similar to meconium peritonitis.
     - Dilated fluid filled uterus and vagina.

II. *Parenchymal*
  1. Congenital infections
     - TORCH complex

- Scattered nodular calcification
  Other stigmata of disease process
2. Hepatic tumors
   - Hemangioma, hamartoma, hepatoblastoma, teratoma, metastatic neuroblastoma
III. *Vascular*
1. Portal vein thromboemboli
   - Seen as subcapsular branching calcification
2. Ischemic infarcts
   - Calcification in branching pattern distributed throughout liver.

5.39 DIFFUSELY HYPOECHOIC LIVER

1. Acute hepatitis
   - Hepatomegaly with normal echopattern.
2. Diffuse malignant infiltration
   - Hepatomegaly with coarse or altered echopattern.

5.40 DIFFUSELY HYPERECHOIC LIVER (BRIGHT LIVER)

	Hepatomegaly	Echopattern
1. Fatty infiltration	+/−	Normal
2. Cirrhosis (fibrosis+fatty)	−	Coarse and nodular
	(Shrunken liver in late stage)	
3. Hepatitis (Chronic)	+/−	Coarse
4. Infiltration/deposition (Malignant, glycogen storage granuloma)	+	Coarse and may be nodular
5. Steatohepatitis	+	Coarse

5.41 FOCAL, HYPERECHOIC HEPATIC LESIONS

1. Metastases from GIT, ovary, pancreas, GUT.
   - Usually multiple and larger than 2cm
   - Hypoechoic halo around lesions
2. Capillary hemangioma
   - Usually single and <2cm
   - Central arteriole may be seen.
3. Adenoma·
   - Especially in case of associated hemorrhage
4. Focal nodular hyperplasia
5. Focal fatty infiltration
   - Esp. around ligamentum teres and GB fossa.
6. Debris within lesions
   - Abscesses and hematoma
7. Miscellaneous
   - Hepatoma, lipoma, hemochromatosis.

5.42 FOCAL, HYPOECHOIC, HEPATIC LESIONS

1. Hepatoma
2. Metastases esp. cystic from ovary/stomach
3. Lymphoma
4. Cavernous hemangioma
5. Cysts
   - Hydatid
6. Abscesses
   - Including complicated/infected cysts.
7. Hematoma is acute stage.

5.43 PERIPORTAL HYPERECHOGENICITY

1. Air in biliary tree
2. Recurrent pyogenic cholangitis
3. Cholecystitis
4. Schistosomiasis
5. Periportal fibrosis

5.44 THICKENED GALLBLADDER WALL

I. *Diffuse* (anterior wall>3mm except physiologically contracted)
   A. *Intrinsic*
      1. Ac. cholecystitis
      2. Chr. cholecystitis
      3. Xanthogranulomatous cholecystitis
      4. Hyperplastic cholecystosis
      5. Sepsis
      6. GB carcinoma
      7. AIDS cholangiopathy
      8. Sclerosing cholangitis
      9. GB varices
   B. *Extrinsic*
      1. Hepatitis
      2. Hypoalbuminemia
      3. Renal failure
      4. CHF
      5. Hepatic vein obstruction
      6. Benign ascites
      7. Cirrhosis
      8. GVH disease
      9. Lymphatic obstruction

II. *Focal*
  A. *Metabolic*
     – Hyperplastic cholecytosis
  B. *Benign tumor*
     – Adenoma
     – Neurinoma
     – Papilloma
     – Carcinoid
     – Fibroadenoma
  C. *Malignant*
     – Adenocarcinoma
     – Leiomyosarcoma
     – Metastases
  D. *Inflammation/Infection*
     – Polyp
     – Parasitic granuloma as in ascaris, filariasis, etc.
     – Retention cyst
     – Xanthogranulomatous cholecystitis
  E. *Miscellaneous*
     – Impacted gallstone
     – Heterotopic mucosa.

5.45 FOCAL HYPODENSE LESIONS ON NECT LIVER

Lesions	Enhancement on CECT
1. *Malignant*	
– Hepatoma, metastasis hemangiosarcoma, intrahepatic cholangio-carcinoma	– Heterogeneous pattern of enhancement esp in early arterial phase

2. *Benign*
   a. Hemangioma — Usually peripheral nodular enhancement advancing peripherally; persistent enhancement on delayed scans
   b. Adenomas—Seen in young females — Early arterial phase enhancement which fades rapidly
   c. Focal nodular hyperplasia
      – Seen in young females — Early arterial phase enhancement which fades rapidly
      – Asymptomatic unless large — Central stellate scar may be seen
3. *Cyst*—Benign, simple, hydatid, VHL, polycystic liver disease — No enhancement but margins clearly demarcated; imperceptible walls
4. Abscesses—Pyogenic, amebic, fungal — Peripheral enhancement with heterogeneous perilesional enhancement due to edema in adjacent hepatic parenchyma
5. *Focal fatty infiltration*
   – No mass effect — No change but increased Conspicuous
6. *Vascular*
   – Infarction, hematoma, laceration — No change but increased conspicuous
   – Hepatic artery aneurysm — Intense enhancement
7. Biliary Tree Dilatation — No change
   – Biloma, Caroli's disease choledochal cyst

5.46 HYPERPERFUSION ABNORMALITIES OF LIVER

There are areas of early enhancement on arterial-dominant phase due to decreased portal blood flow/formation of intrahepatic arterioportal shunts/increased aberrant drainage through hepatic veins.

1. Lobar/segmental
   – Portal v. thrombosis

- Obstruction by malignant neoplasm
- Ligation of arterioportal shunt
- Hypervascular GB disease
2. Subsegmental
   - Obstruction of peripheral portal branches.
   - Acute cholecystitis
   - FNAB
3. Generalized heterogeneous
   - Cirrhosis
4. Subcapsular
   - Idiopathic
5. Miscellaneous
   - Aberrant venous drainage as gastric or cystic veins.

5.47 HEPATIC TUMORS WITH VASCULAR "SCAR"

1. FNH
2. Hepatic adenoma
3. Giant cavernous—hemangioma
4. Fibrolamellar HCC
5. Intrahepatic cholangiocarcinoma
6. Hypervascular metastases.

5.48 DIFFUSELY HYPODENSE LIVER ON NECT

1. Fatty infiltration (obesity, early cirrhosis, Cushing's disease, late pregnancy, Ccl4 poisoning, etc
   - No change on postcontrast scans
   - No mass effect on vascular channels.
2. Malignant infiltration
   - Heterogeneous enhancement on CECT.

3. Amyloidosis
   - No change on CECT
4. Budd-Chiari syndrome
   - On CECT, non-visualized hepatic veins and/or IVC, multiple collaterals at porta
   - Hepatomegaly in acute cases
   - Shrunken liver with hypertrophied caudate lobe in chronic cases.

MRI in Important Hepatic Lesions

Lesions	T1W	T2W	Gadolinium
1. HCC	↓, Iso, ↑	↑	↑
2. Metastases except melanoma	↓	↑	±↑
3. Melanoma metastasis	↑	↓	±↑
4. Hemangioma	↓	↑	↑
5. Adenoma	↑	↓	–
6. FNH			
Central scar	↓	↑	↑
Margin	Isointense	↑	± ↑
7. Regenerating Nodules	↓, Isointense	↓ Hyperintense	–
8. Hemochromatosis	↓	↓++	–

5.49 SPLENOMEGALY

1. Massively
   - CML
     • Kala-azar
   - Myelofibrosis
     • Gaucher's disease

- Malaria
  - Lymphoma
2. Moderately
   - All the above
   - Storage disorders (Niemann-Pick disease, DM)
   - Hemolytic anemia (TTP, Spherocyctosis)
   - Portal hypertension
   - Leukemias
3. Mildly
   - All of the above
   - Infection
     a. *Viral*—Infectious mononucleosis
     b. *Bacterial*—Brucellosis, enteric fever
     c. *Fungal*—Histoplasmosis
     d. *Rickettsial*—Typhus
     e. Sarcoidosis
     f. Amyloidosis
     g. Rheumatoid arthritis
     h. SLE
     i. Splenic trauma

5.50 SPLENIC CALCIFICATION

I. *Diffusely Disseminated*
   1. Phleboliths
      - May have central lucencies
   2. Granulomas
      - Commonest; multiple, small nodular
      - Seen in tuberculosis, histoplasmosis, brucellosis.
II. *Vascular*
   1. Splenic artery calcification—Curvilinear

2. Splenic artery aneurysm.
III. *Calcified Cyst Wall* (Curvilinear)
    1. Congenital cyst
    2. Post-traumatic cyst
    3. Echinococcal cyst
    4. Cystic dermoid
    5. Epidermoid
IV. *Miscellaneous*
    1. Sickle cell anemia—fine granular
    2. *Pneumocystitis carinii*
    3. Healed abscess or infarct or hematoma.

5.51 HYPERECHOIC SPLENIC LESION

1. Granulomas
   - Miliary tuberculosis, histoplasmosis
2. Phleboliths
3. Myelofibrosis
4. Gamma Gandy nodules in portal hypertension.

5.52 FOCAL HYPOATTENUATING LESIONS IS SPLEEN

1. Lymphoma/leukemia
2. Metastases
3. Abscesses
4. Cystic lesions
   - Congenital cyst/epidermoid
   - Pseudocyst (Post-traumatic)
   - Cystic degeneration of infarct/hematoma
   - Cavernous hemangioma/lymphangioma

5.53 PANCREATIC CALCIFICATION

I. *Chronic Pancreatitis*
   - Numerous tiny stippled calcifications usually intraductal.
     a. Alcoholic
        • Calcification limited to head and tail.
     b. Biliary
     c. Idiopathic
     d. Hereditary
        • Autosomal dominant.
        • Calcification is typically rounded and large.
        • Diagnosis considered in young, non alcoholics.
     e. Pancreatic Pseudocyst
        • Curvilinear rim calcification is addiction.

II. *Neoplastic*
   a. Microcystic adenoma -"sunburst" appearance
   b. Macrocystic cystadenoma-amorphous and peripheral
   c. Adenocarcinoma (rare)
   d. Cavernous hemangioma—multiple phleboliths
   e. Metastases from colon, ovarian carcinomas.

III. *Hyperparathyroidism*
   - Similar to chronic pancreatitis
   - Concomitant nephrocalcinosis or urolithiasis.

IV. *Cystic Fibrosis*
   - Typically fine and grannular
   - Occurs late in disease and suggest advanced pancreatic fibrosis.

V. *Kwashiorkor*
   - Similar to chronic pancreatitis
     (Tropical pancreatitis) appears before adulthood.

VI. *Intraparenchymal hemorrhage*
   a. Old hematoma/abscess/infarct
VII. *Hemochromatosis.*

5.54 PANCREATIC MASSES

Focal pancreatitis
- H/o
- Usually in pancreatic head
- Calcification /cystic areas
- May be difficult

Serous cystadenoma (Microcystic)
- Benign
- F>M, 1.5:1, elderly female abdominal pain and /or mass.
- Hypervascular, multilocular cystic tumor with small cyst- with clear watery glycogen rich fluid.
- Central scar with sunburst pattern of calcification
- USG—homogenous hyperechoic solid looking encapsulated mass.

Mucinous Cystadenoma (Macrocystic)
- Malignant /premalignant
- Uni/multilocular
- F>M, body and tail of pancreas
- Large cystic areas may contain curvilinear calcification in cyst wall.
- Epigastric pain/abdominal mass.

May be difficult to differentiate from necrotic adenocarcinoma - but carcinoma has thick, irregular wall with calcification.
- *Intraductal papillary mucinous tumor*
   - Abdominal pain/recurrent pancreatitis
   - M>F
   - Ductal dilatation.

- *Islet cell tumors*
  - 80% functionally—small
  - 25% nonfunctioning—large
- *Most common Insulinoma*
  - 90% benign, 10% malignant, 90% solitary
  - Whipple triad-1 decrease blood glucose, (hypoglycemia) relief by glucose.
  CT- hypervascular-arterial phase
  - Post Gd. MR- Rim enhancement.
- Endoscopic-relatively hypoechoic with well-defined smooth margins.
  - *2nd MC Gastrinoma*- ZES-(Acid hypersecretion diarrhea, peptic ulcer)
    - 60% multiple, 60% malignant.
    - Hypervascular
  - Gastrinoma triangle-cystic and CD superior, 2nd and 3rd part of duodenum, pancreatic head and neck.

Adenocarcinoma

> 80% of all primary pancreatic neoplasms.
- M>F
- Risk factors
  - Cigarette smoking
  - Alcohol and coffee-not associated with increased adenocarcinoma.

C/F

- Pain
- Weight loss
- Jaundice—Ca head of pancreas
- Unexplained venous thrombosis
- 60% head, 13% body, 5% tail, 22% diffuse.

Imaging

- CT most popular means of determining the local tumor extent and assessing candidates for potential curative surgery.
- Should be the initial diagnostic procedure.

USG

Echopoor homogenous highly attenuating masses, becoming heterogenous as they enlarge, with irregular lobulated margin.

- Double duct sign, chain of Lakes appearance of main pancreatic duct.

Doppler

Involvement of PV, SV, hepatic and gastroduodenal arteries

NECT

Most adenocarcinoma have attenuation pattern similar to normal pancreas unless necrosis /cystic change present.

- Detected only as contour deformity.
- Calcification usually absent.

CECT

Hypovascular, with tumor pancreas contrast being maximum in pancreatic phase.

Other Features

- Focal contour change with or without descrete mass
- Focal lesion of soft tissue density in an otherwise fatty replaced gland
- Spherical enlargement of the head
- Convet rounded border of the uncinate process
- Abrupt termination of CBD
- Double duct sign

Criteria for Unresectability

- Tumor diameter 5cm or more
- Extra pancreatic invasion of adjacent tissues and organs, with the exception of the duodenum
- Distant metastasis > nodal hematogenous
- Occlusion, stenosis or encasement of vessels portal vein SMA, celiac trunk.

TMM staging

T	Tx-Primary tumor cannot be assessed
	TO-No e/o any primary tumor
	T1-Tumor limited to pancreas
	T1a-< 2.0cm
	T1b->2.0cm
	T2-extent into duodenum, bile duct or peripancreatic tissue
	T3-extent into stomach, spleen, colon or adjacent large vessels.
N	Nx-Could not be assessed
	N0- -ve
	N1- +ve
M	Mx- could not be assessed
	M0- -ve
	M1- +ve
MRI	Useful in tumor detection, staging, identification of level of obstruction and site of tumor.
	Gradient echo and T1W spin echo-used to evaluate vascular invasion
T1WI	To evaluate lymphadenopathy.
T2W	For hepatic mets.

T1WI	Hypointense relative to normal pancreatic parenchyma
T2WI	Variable signal intensity Post gadolinium-hypovascular
MRCP	heavily T2WI-level and degree of duct obstruction.
ERCP	1. When CT/MR findings unclear. 2. Ductal dilatation without identification of mass 3. To differentiate duodenal and ampullary tumors from periampullary tumors.

Endoscopic Ultrasound

• Currently under evaluation.

Advantages

• To visualize pancreas and surrounding structures with high resolution.
• To guide FNAC
• Vascular and LN invasion.

Disadvantages

• Invasive
• Operator dependence
• Inability to detect distant mets.

Solid and Papillary Epithelial Neoplasm

• Young female- 11-47yrs
  84% <35 yrs
• Large size tumor with solid and cystic areas with well-defined capsule in the body and /or tail of pancreas. Common intralesional hemorrhage and necrosis

- This unusual neoplasm is considered when characteristic CT findings are seen in young female patient.

Lymphoma

- Usually secondary to systemic disease
- Primary very rare
- Large homogenous solid mass, infrequently with central cystic areas
- Lymphadenopathy
- Displacement and stretching of peripancreatic vessels.

Metastasis

- Most common from melanoma-hyperintense on T1
- Also from-Breast, lung, kidney, prostate, GIT
- Multiple with H/o primary (Known primary)
- If solitary may be indistinguishable from primary.

Flow Chart 5.54.1

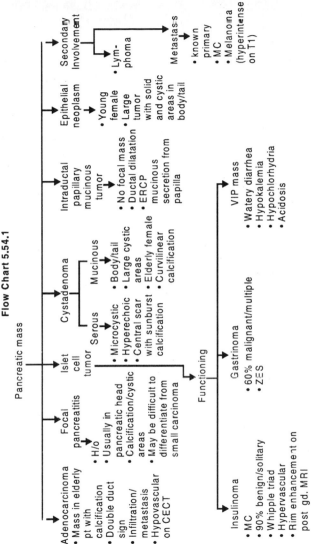

Pancreatic mass

Adenocarcinoma
- Mass in elderly pt with calcification
- Double duct sign
- Infiltration/ metastasis
- Hypovascular on CECT

Focal pancreatitis
- H/o
- Usually in pancreatic head
- Calcification/cystic areas
- May be difficult to differentiate from small carcinoma

Islet cell tumor

Functioning

Insulinoma
- MC
- 90% benign/solitary
- Whipple triad
- Hypervascular
- Rim enhancement on post gd. MRI

Gastrinoma
- 60% malignant/multiple
- ZES

VIP mass
- Watery diarrhea
- Hypokalemia
- Hypochlorhydria
- Acidosis

Cystadenoma

Serous
- Microcystic
- Hyperechoic
- Central scar with sunburst calcification

Mucinous
- Body/tail
- Large cystic areas
- Elderly female
- Curvilinear calcification

Intraductal papillary mucinous tumor
- No focal mass
- Ductal dilatation
- ERCP mucinous secretion from papilla

Epithelial neoplasm
- Young female
- Large tumor with solid and cystic areas in body/tail

Secondary Involvement
- Lymphoma
- Metastasis
  - known primary
  - MC
  - Melanoma (hyperintense on T1)

5.55 FOCAL PANCREATIC MASSES

Lesions	Features	Findings on CT
I. **Neoplastic**		
1. *Adenocarcinoma*	Commonest in head; followed by body and tail	Isodense of NECT; calcification very rare. Presence of metastasis invasion of vessel distinguish it from focal pancreatitis. Hyper attenuating in early arterial phase
2. *Islet cell tumor*	80% are functioning, except functioning Insulinomas all are Malignant : 75% of Nonfunctioning Tumor are benign, calcification common, diagnosis is usually by clinical symptomatology and hormonal markers	β-cell tumor – 90% benign and < 2cm. Usually isodense on NECT with marked contrast enhancement. Gastrinoma-60% malignant, marked contrast enhancement Associated with MEN-I Glucaganoma - > 4 cm
3. *Cystadenoma/ carcinoma Cystadenoma Cystadenocarci- noma*	Usually females > 60 yrs, Frequently calcified Calcification less common	Multiple small cysts in head (< 2cm). Multiple large cysts (>5cm) in body and tail.
4. *Lymphoma*	Usually secondary	Large homogenous solid mass with peri-pancreatic lymphade-nopathy causing dis-placement and stretch-ing of vascular structures

Contd...

Contd...

Lesions	Features	Findings on CT
5. *Solid and papillary epithelial neoplasm*	Rare	—
6. *Metastases*	Usually form RCC, HCC, bronchogenic, breast, ovarian cancer melanoma	Known primary at other site
II. **Inflammatory**		
1. *Focal pancreatitis*	Usually in head of pancreas. Calcification may be seen	Absence of associated metastases and adjacent invasion
2. *Pancreatic abscess*	Secondary to infected phlegmon/pseudocyst	Ring enhancing mass occurring as complication of pancreatitis
3. *Pseudocyst*	Complication of acute pancreatitis.	Thick wall cystic mass, may be multiple with a H/o acute pancreatitis

5.56 ADRENAL MASS

Width of normal limb is < 1cm

1. *Bilateral Large Adrenals*
   - Hodgkin's disease
   - Adrenal hyperplasia
   - Adrenal hemorrhage
   - Wilms' tumor
   - Infection as histoplasmosis/TB
   - Pheochromocytoma
   - Metastases

2. *Unilateral Adrenal Mass*
   – CT attenuation
     <OHU = benign mass
     0-15 HU = probably benign
     >15 HU = indeterminate
   – On 15 minute delayed contrast enhanced scan.
     <25 HU = benign lesion
     >25 HU = malignant lesion
   – Size of mass
     <3cm in diameter = likely benign (90%)
     >5cm in diameter = likely malignant

Small solid mass	*Large solid mass*	*Cystic masses*
– Cortical adenoma usually <10HU	– Cortical carcinoma – Pheochromocytoma	– Pseudocyst (old hemorrhage infarction)
– Metastases usually from lung, breast, RCC, etc.	– Neuroblastoma/ ganglioneuroma – Myelolipoma	– Lymphangioma/ hemangioma
– Pheochromocytoma – Granulomatous disease – Myelolipoma (Typically fat density)	– Metastases – Hemorrhage – Abscesses – Hemangioma	– True cyst – Hydatid cyst – Cystic degeneration of tumor/ hemorrhage – Cortical adenoma with low density

5.57 ADRENAL CALCIFICATION

Child
1. *Tumor*
   – Neuroblastoma (90%)
   – Ill-defined, nonhomogeneous, stippled calcification.

- Ganglioneuroma(20%)
  Inhomogeneous and stippled
- Dermoid (Tooth/calcified focus)

2. *Vascular*
   - Hemorrhage (secondary to sepsis, birth trauma)
     Partial or complete ring like calcification in cyst wall formed secondarily.

3. *Miscellaneous*
   - Wolman's disease - AR lipidosis
     Punctate cortical calcification.

Adults

1. *Tumors*
   - Pheochromocytoma(rare)but when present is usually in "eggshell pattern".
   - Carcinoma—irregular and punctate
   - Adenoma—punctate and small.
   - Ganglioneuroma—flocculant calcification.

2. *Vascular*
   - Hemorrhage (trauma)
     similar to that in child.

3. *Infection*
   - Tuberculosis, histoplasmosis, Waterhouse-Friderichsen syndrome.
   - Irregular and punctate.

4. *Endocrinal*
   - Addison disease
   - Commonly due to TB

5.58 EXTRALUMINAL INTRA-ABDOMINAL GAS

1. *Pneumoperitoneum*
   - Gas within the peritoneal cavity.
2. *Gas in Bowel Wall*
   - *Pneumatosis coli.*
   - *Pneumatosis intestinalis*—ischemia/infarction of bowel wall as in necrotizing enterocolitis.
3. *Gas in Biliary Tree*
   - Irregular branching gas shadows which don't reach the liver edge. Seen in conditions as patulous sphincter, following passage of gallstones and following postoperative procedures in biliary tree, enterobiliary fistulas, etc.
4. *Gas in Urinary Tract*
   - Fistula between urinary tract and intestine (Congenital, postoperative, trauma, etc.) emphysematous pyelonephritis and cystitis, etc.
5. *Gas in Portal Vein*
   - Branching gas shadows which extend to within 2 cm of the liver capsule.
   - Following bowel/mesenteric infarction, air embolus following DCBE.
6. *Abscess*
   - Mottled gas pattern. Lack of normal mucosal/haustral pattern help differentiate it from gas in fecal matter.
7. *Necrotic Tumor*
   - Usually in large tumors esp. following treatment.
8. *Retroperitoneal Gas*
   - Secondary to bowel perforation, postoperative procedures/diagnostic retroperitoneal air insufflation.

5.59 PNEUMOPERITONEUM

The collection of free air in the peritoneum because of a diverse group of diseases is known as pneumoperitoneum. An erect chest film is preferred to an erect abdominal film for this diagnosis. With careful radiographic techniques as little as 1ml of free gas in the peritoneum can be demonstrated, the views done usually to detect this little amount of gas are either an erect chest or left lateral decubitus abdominal film. A patient should be at least in position 10 min. before the radiograph is taken so that the gas collects in the desired highest point in the abdomen. A pneumoperitoneum can be detected in 76% of cases using an erect chest film, however if a left lateral decubitus suspected of having pneumo-peritoneum are critically ill, an erect film may not be obtained so it is important to identify the signs of pneumoperitoneum on a supine abdomen film.

Signs on a Supine Film

- Collection of gas in the right upper quadrant adjacent to liver lying mainly in the subhepatic space and the hepatorenal or Morrison's pouch (doge's sign), and is visible as an oval, linear or triangular collection of gas.
- Visualization of outer as well as inner wall of a bowel loop (Rigler's sign).
- Small triangular collection of gas in between three loops of bowel (stelltale triangle sign).
- Reflection of peritoneum like the falciform ligament, the medial and lateral umbilical ligaments and the urachus can occasionally be identified when very large amount of free gas is present.

- Very large amount of gas may accumulate beneath the diaphragm (cupola sign) or in the center of abdomen (football sign).
- Ligamentum teres sign is air outlining fissure of ligamentum teres hepatis seen as vertically oriented sharply defined slit like area of hyperlucency between 10th and 12th rib within 2.5-4.0 cm of vertebral border, 2-7 mm wide and 6-20 mm long.
- Gas bubbles may be seen lateral to right edge of liver.

Etiology

a. *Disruption of wall of a hollow viscus:*
    - Infectious bowel diseases like typhoid, tuberculosis. Typhoid being the commonest cause.
    - Perforated gastric/duodenal ulcer.
    - Blunt/penetrating trauma.
    - *Iatrogenic:* Laparoscopy, laparotomy, leaking surgical anastomosis, endoscope induced perforations, enema tip injury, diagnostic pneumoperitoneum.
    - Perforated appendix.
    - Ingested foreign body perforation.
    - Diverticulitis (ruptured Meckel's diverticulum).
    - Necrotizing enterocolitis with perforation.
    - Inflammatory bowel disease (Toxic megacolon)
    - Intestinal obstruction secondarily leading to perforation.
    - Ruptured pneumatosis cystoides intestinalis with 'balanced pneumoperitoneum' (free intraperitoneal air act as tamponade of pneumatosis cysts thus maintaining a balance between intracystic air and pneumoperitoneum.

- Idiopathic gastric perforation, i.e. spontaneous perforation in premature infants (congenital gastric wall defects).

b. *Through peritoneal surface*:
  - Transperitoneal manipulations like needle biopsy, catheter placements.
  - Mistaken thoracocentesis/chest tube placement.
  - Extension from chest as in dissection of pneumomediastinum, bronchopleural fistula.
  - Penetrating abdominal injury.

c. *Through female genital tract*:
  - Iatrogenic as in culdocentesis, Rubin test for tubal patency and pelvic examinations.
  - Spontaneous as during intercourse, douching, horse back riding and knee chest exercises.

d. *Intraperitoneal pathologies*:
  - Peritonitis by gas forming organisms
  - Ruptured abscess.

PSEUDOPNEUMOPERITONEUM

These are processes that mimic free gas in the peritoneum:
- Pseudo wall sign: This is seen when two gas distended bowel loops come in close apposition.
- Chilaiditi syndrome: is a specific radiological abnormality seen in very thin asthenic individuals due to interposition of colon between the liver and diaphragm leading to a false impression of free gas. The colon can however be recognized on careful inspection of presence of the haustral pattern.
- Subdiaphragmatic intraperitoneal fat or interposition of omental fat between liver and diaphragm.

- Curvilinear collapse: sometime a band of curvilinear collapse with a crescent of normal lung between it and diaphragm may simulate free gas.
- Subpulmonary pneumothorax
- Uneven diaphragm.
- Retroperitoneal air.
- Subdiaphragmatic abscess.

Flow Chart 5.59.1

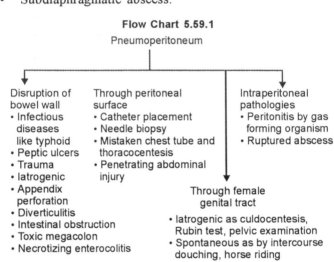

Pneumoperitoneum

Disruption of bowel wall
- Infectious diseases like typhoid
- Peptic ulcers
- Trauma
- Iatrogenic
- Appendix perforation
- Diverticulitis
- Intestinal obstruction
- Toxic megacolon
- Necrotizing enterocolitis

Through peritoneal surface
- Catheter placement
- Needle biopsy
- Mistaken chest tube and thoracocentesis
- Penetrating abdominal injury

Intraperitoneal pathologies
- Peritonitis by gas forming organism
- Ruptured abscess

Through female genital tract
- Iatrogenic as culdocentesis, Rubin test, pelvic examination
- Spontaneous as by intercourse douching, horse riding

5.60 PNEUMOPERITONEUM

- It indicates presence of gas within the peritoneal cavity.
- A little as 1 ml of free gas may be detected on erect chest or left lateral decubitus abdominal films, but gas may take upto 10 min to rise.
- On erect films, gas accumulate beneath the domes "cupola or moustache" sign.
- On supine films, gas may be seen in subhepatic space

(dolfin sign); outlining falciform ligament; outlining outer margin of bowel wall (Rigler's sign), and at times gas may collect in the center of the abdomen over a fluid collection (football sign).

Causes

1. *Perforation*
   a. Peptic ulcer-75-80% show pneumoperitoneum.
   b. Inflammation-toxic megacolon, diverticulitis.
   c. Infarction (bowel or mesentery)
   d. Obstruction (volvulus, neoplasms, etc)
   e. Pneumatosis coli/intestinalis.
2. *Iatrogenic*
   a. Postprocedure (following peritoneal dialysis, endoscopy, embolization) or postoperative. It may take 2-3 wks, for reabsorption of air, however, serial radiographs will show a definite decrease.
3. *Associated Chest Conditions*
   a. Pneumonia.
   b. Emphysema.
   c. Carcinoma of lung.
   d. Pneumomediastinum.
   e. Intermittent positive pressure ventilation.
   f. Pulmonary peritoneal fistula.
4. *Introduction per vaginum as following vaginal douches.*
5. *Idiopathic.*

5.61 GASLESS ABDOMEN

Characterized by Ground glass Haziness in abdominal radiograph with normal properitoneal fat lines or bulging of flank lines is some cases.

In children-

a. *High Obstruction*
   – Isolated esophageal atresia.
   – Duodenal atresia.
   – Annular pancreas.
   – Hypertrophic pyloric stenosis.
   – Choledochal cyst.
   – Volvulus.

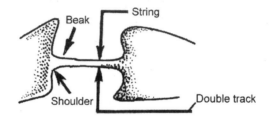

Fig. 5.61.1: Infantile hypertrophic pyloric stenosis

b. *Excessive vomiting.*
c. *Excessive nasogastric aspiration.*
d. *Fluid filled bowel loops as closed loop obstruction, bowel wash out.*
e. *Relative absence of bowel loops in abdomen as in congenital diaphragmatic hernia.*

In Adults

a. *High Obstruction*
   – Volvulus.
   – Benign and malignant strictures.

b. *Ascites*
c. *Pancreatitis* and other *acute* abdominal conditions producing excessive vomiting.
d. *Fluid filled bowel.*
   - Mesenteric/bowel infarction.
   - Active colitis.
e. *Large abdominal mass pushing* and collapsing the bowel loops laterally.
f. *Normal variant.*

5.62 ASCITES

It is defined as accumulation of fluid in the peritoneal cavity. Smaller amounts of fluid is first detected in pelvis.

Radiographic Signs

1. Obliteration of fat lines at the superior border of bladder.
2. Linear lucency of pelvic fat between the fluid density and bony pelvis.
3. Symmetric densities on both sides of bladder due to fluid in peritoneal recesses (dogs ears) appearance.
4. With larger amounts of fluid.
   a. Elevation of both domes of diaphragm.
   b. Homogeneous shadow of soft tissue density called "ground glass appearance."
   c. Poor visualization of psoas and renal outline.
   d. Obliteration of right lateral inferior margin of liver.
   e. Displacement of ascending and descending colon medially with obliteration of haustral markings and of the flank stripes.

    f. Visualization of lateral lucent band between the lateral abdominal wall and right lobe of liver.
- Hellmer's sign.

5. On barium study—Separation of small bowel loops is seen.

6. Ultrasonography is very sensitive is detecting ascites even the minute amounts esp. with a full bladder.

Technique

However, small, fluid collections in pelvis are more sensitively detected by transvaginal/transrectal ultrasound than trans-abdominal approach. Hyperechoic reflections are seen with complicated ascites.

7. On CT/MRI ascites appear as extravisceral collection and in addition may reveal the underlying cause is some instances.

Causes

1. *Neonatal Ascites*
    a. Urinary causes
- Bladder/renal rupture.
- Posterior urethral valves.

    b. Chylous ascites
- Perforation of GB/CBD.
- Intestinal lymphangiectasia.

    c. Hemoperitoneum
- Ruptured adrenal/spleen/liver.
- Ruptured congenital neuroblastoma.
- Ruptured hepatic tumor or hemangioma.

    d. Intestinal contents (Bowel perforation)
- Meconium ileus.

          – Atresia.
            Stress ulcer.
    e. Transudate
          – Fetal hydrops.
          – Cardiac failure.
          – Idiopathic.
2. *Adults*
    – Cirrhosis with portal hypertension.
    – Hypoalbuminemia.
    – Infectious peritonitis—particularly tubercular.
    – Perforation peritonitis.
    – Tumoral ascites.
          a. Malignancy
              – Mesothelioma, peritoneal metastases, carcinoma of GIT and ovary.
          b. Benign
              – Fibroma of ovary (Meig's syndrome)

Increased Pressure in the Vascular System

a. CHF
b. Constrictive pericarditis.
c. Thrombosis of IVC.

Lymphatic Obstruction

a. Obstruction of visceral lymphatic drainage or of the origin of lymphatic duct at the level of cisterna of Pecquet.
b. Lymphoma.
c. Postradiotherapy.
d. Trauma.
e. Filariasis.
    – Miscellaneous as myxedema, extrahepatic causes of portal hypertension.

5.63 ABDOMINAL MASS IN NEONATE

I. *Renal (55%)*
   1. *Hydronephrosis*: Dilated pelvicalyceal system. May be associated with hydroureter and bladder hypertrophy. It may be due to PUJ obstruction, posterior urethral valves, ectopic ureterocele, prune-belly syndrome and UVJ obstruction.
   2. Multicystic dysplastic kidney.
   3. Infantile polycystic kidneys.
   4. Mesoblastic nephroma.
   5. Renal vein thrombosis.
   6. Renal ectopia.
   7. Paranephric collection (urinoma).
   8. Wilms' tumor (rare).
II. *Genital (15%)*
   1. Hydrometrocolpos—Dilated fluid filled vagina and/or uterus.
   2. Adnexal cysts—Follicular cysts (commonest), corpus luteal cyst, theca lutein cyst, paraovarian cyst, teratoma, cystadenomas.
   3. Gastrointestinal (15%) commonly associated with obstruction.
      – Duplication cyst—Commonest bowel mass.
      – Mesenteric cyst.
      – Meconium pseudocyst.
      – Dilated bowel.
   4. Non-renal retroperitoneal (10%)
      – Adrenal hemorrhage—Commonly due to neonatal stress.
      – Neuroblastoma.
      – Teratoma.

5. Hepato/Spleno/Biliary (5%)
   - Hepatoblastoma.
   - Hepatic cyst.
   - Splenic cyst.
   - Splenic hematoma.
   - Choledochal cyst.
6. Miscellaneous.
   1. Urachal cyst.
   2. Meningocele in lower abdomen.
   3. Sacrococcygeal teratoma.

5.64 ABDOMINAL MASS IN CHILD

I. *Renal 55%*
   1. Wilms' tumor.
   2. Hydronephrosis—due to PUJ obstruction, PU valves, reflux disease, associated with UTI.
   3. Cyst—Multicystic dysplastic kidney, polycystic disease, simple cysts, cystic nephroma, calyceal cyst, etc.
II. *Non-renal Retroperitoneal 23%*
   1. Neuroblastoma.
III. Gastrointestinal 18%
   1. Appendicular abscess.
   2. Hepatoblastoma commonly in right lobe, 40% is bilateral lobes and 40% calcify.
   3. Hemangiomas—multiple, involving entire liver +/- CHF and may be associated with cutaneous hemangiomas.
   4. Choledochal cyst—10% present with a classical triad of mass, pain and jaundice. Dynamic radionuclide scintigraphy with 99Tc-TBIDA is diagnostic.
   5. Omental cyst (greater omentum/lesser sac, multi-locular).

   6. Mesenteric cyst (between leaves of small bowel mesentery).
   7. Duplication cyst.
   8. Pancreatic pseudocyst.
   9. Meckel diverticulum.
 10. Mesenteric lymphoma.

IV. *Genital*
   1. Ovarian cyst.
   2. Teratoma.

V. *Miscellaneous*
   Cystic lymphangioma.

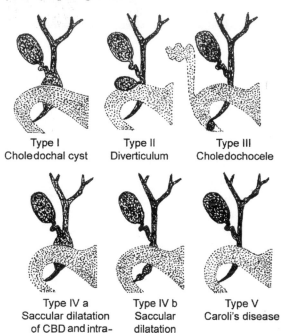

    Type I   Type II   Type III
Choledochal cyst   Diverticulum   Choledochocele

   Type IV a   Type IV b   Type V
Saccular dilatation   Saccular   Caroli's disease
of CBD and intra-   dilatation
hepatic ducts   of CBD

Fig. 5.64.1

DD of Wilms' Tumor and Neuroblastoma

	Wilms' Tumor	*Neuroblastoma*
1. Age	80%<3years	15-30% <1yr; 75% <5yrs
2. Site	Kidneys	Adrenal (40%), sympathetic chain in abdomen (25%), chest (15%), neck (5%), pelvis(5%)
3. Plain Film		
1. Calcification	10%	2/3 cases
2. Renal outline	Lost or enlarged	Maintained but displaced
3. Intervertebral formina	Normal	May be enlarged
4. Bone lesion	Uncommon	Common
4. On USG/CT/MRI		
1. Major vessels	Displaced	Encased
2. Hemorrhage/ necrosis	Common	Uncommon
3. IVC/renal vein thrombosis	Commoner	Uncommon
5. Radionuclide scanning	Not useful	MIBG scanning is useful for skeletal metastases
6. Associated syndrome	Beckwith synd. [macroglossia, organomegaly, exomphalos hemihypertrophy] Cryptorchidism, hypospadias, aniridia, hemihy-pertrophy may also be associated	Opsomyoclonus (cerebellar ataxia and jerky eye movement),hypertension and +/- diarrhea due to VIP secretion

5.65 INTESTINAL OBSTRUCTION IN NEONATE

I. *Duodenal—Commonest*
1. Stenosis/Atresia -"double-bubble" sign; may be associated with annular pancreas, mongolism or with other abnormalities of GIT.
2. Annular pancreas—May not present until adulthood.
3. Peritoneal bands—Congenital fibrous Band's of Ladd-connects cecum to posterior abdominal wall and commonly crosses duodenum.
4. Aberrant vessel as preduodenal portal vein.
5. Congenital web.
6. Choledochal cyst.

II. *Jejunal and Ileal Obstruction.*
CT is best modality for evaluation (95% accurate with 94% sensitivity and 96% specificity).
1. Atresia/stenosis.
2. Midgut volvulus results from arrest in rotation and fixation of small bowel in fetal life.
3. Meconium ileus—Mottled lucencies are seen due to gas entrapment in meconium. Peritoneal calcification secondary to perforation seen in 30% cases.
4. Inguinal hernia.
5. Inspissated milk—dense amorphous intraluminal masses surrounded by rim of air with or without mottled lucencies within them. Resolves spontaneously.
6. Paralytic ileus usually due to drugs administered during labor.
7. Enteric duplication cyst—Located on antimesenteric side, mostly in ileum.
8. Mesenteric cyst from meconium peritonitis located on mesenteric side.

3. *Colonic*
    1 Hirschsprung's disease.
    2. Small left colon syndrome.
    3. Meconium plug syndrome.
    4. Atresia.
    5. Anorectal malformation.
        – *High type*—With or without sacral agenesis and gas in bladder (due to rectovesical fistula)
        – *Low type*—perineal/urethral fistula may be associated.

5.66 ABNORMALITIES OF BOWEL ROTATION

1. *Exomphalos*
    – It refers to total failure of bowel to return to the abdomen from the umbilical cord which are contained within a sac. This is a midline lesion.
    DD: Gastrochisis—paramidline abdominal wall defect through which the bowel protrudes.
2. *Non-rotation*
    – Asymptomatic.
    – Small bowel located on right side of abdomen.
    – Colon located on left side of abdomen.
    – Small and large bowel lie on either side of SMA with a common mesentery.
    – SMV is situated to the left of SMA.
3. *Malrotation*—DJ flexure lies to the right of midline and caudal to its usual position.
    – The cecum is more cephalad than normal.
       Invariably complicates left sided diaphragmatic hernia.
    – SMV is anterior to SMA.

4. *Reverse Rotation*
   - Colon is dorsal to SMA with jejunal and duodenum anterior to it.
5. *Paraduodenal hernias (Rare)*
   1. Through fossa of Landzert on left side (3/4)
      - Lateral to 4th part of duodenum and behind descending and transverse mesocolon.
   2. Through fossa of Waldeyer on right side (1/4)
      - Caudal to SMA and inferior to 3rd part of duodenum.
6. *Extroversion of Cloaca—Rare.*
   - No rotation of bowel.
   - Ileum and colon open separately onto the extroverted area in the midline below the umbilical cord.

5.67 INTRA-ABDOMINAL CALCIFICATION IN NEONATE

1. *Extraluminal*
   - Peritoneal calcification following fetal bowel perforation and meconium peritonitis.
2. *Intraluminal*
   - Intestinal obstruction following imperforate anus, small bowel atresia or Hirschsprung's disease.
   - Multifocal GI atretic sites.

5.68 HEMATEMESIS

It occurs due to upper GI bleed where the bleeding site is proximal to the ligament of Treitz. Mortality approx 10%. Barium exam should be avoided in acute cases.

Causes

I. *Esophageal Causes*
  1. Hiatus hernia
  2. Esophageal varices—mortality 50%
  3. Esophageal neoplasms
  4. Mallory-Weiss tears—very low mortality.

II. *Gastric Causes*—Mortality <10% if < 60 yrs and >35% if >60 yrs.
  1. Acute hemorrhagic gastritis—secondary to steroids, NSAIDs or alcohol intake.
  2. Gastric ulcers.
  3. Malignancy esp. leiomyosarcoma.

III. *Duodenal Causes*
  1. Blood dyscrasias.
  2. Hereditary telangiectasia—autosomal dominant.
  3. Connective tissue disorders as Ehlers-Danlos syndrome, pseudoxanthoma elasticum.

IV. *Visceral Artery Aneurysm*

V. *Vascular Malformation*

5.69 DYSPHAGIA IN ADULTS

Difficulty in swallowing can be due to:

I. *Intrinsic Causes*
  1. Benign strictures.
     – Peptic strictures due to reflux esophagitis.
     – Ingestion of corrosive acids and alkalis or foreign bodies.
     – Iatrogenic following prolonged nasogastric intubation or fibrosis secondary to radiotherapy.
     – Cutaneous diseases as epidermolysis bullosa and pemphigus.

- Syndromes as Plummer-Vinson syndrome which produces anterior indentation in the form of web. Common in females with iron deficiency anemia and in males with postgastrectomy status. Web can occur from C4 to D1 level. The condition is premalignant.
    - Tumors as leiomyomas.
2. Malignant strictures.
    - Carcinomas
    - Lymphomas

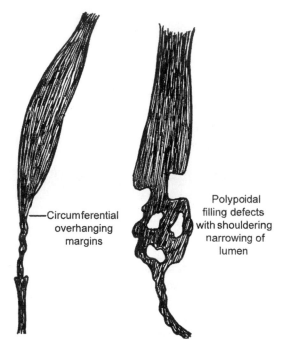

Fig. 5.69.1: Annular carcinoma in midportion esophagus (Left). Polypoidal carcinoma involving mid and lower esophagus (Right)

3. Miscellaneous.
   - Infections as moniliasis, HSV or CMV infections. They all produce shaggy ulcerated appearance and odynophagia (painful deglutition)
   - Schatzki ring may produce dysphagia if internal diameter is < 6 mm.

II. *Extrinsic Causes*
   1. *Tumors*
      - Mediastinal lymphomas and other tumors, mediastinal lymphadenopathy.
   2. *Vascular*
      - Aortic aneurysm.
      - Aberrant right subclavian artery produces posterior indentation (dysphagia lusoria).
      - Aberrant left pulmonary artery produces anterior indentation.
      - Right sided aortic arch produces right lateral and posterior indentation.
   3. *Pharyngeal Pouch* may indent the esophagus. May produce air-fluid level with signs of aspiration pneumonitis on chest radiograph.
   4. *Goiter*
   5. *Enterogenous Cyst*—lies adjacent to the esophagus. Evidence of associated hemivertebra and anterior meningocele may be there.
   6. *Prevertebral Abscess*/hematoma.

III. *Neuromuscular Disorders*
   1. Megaesophagus as in Chaga's disease, achalasia cardia.
   2. Systemic disease as scleroderma, myasthenia gravis.
   3. Bulbar/pseudobulbar palsy.

IV. *Psychiatric Disorders*
   1. Globus hystericus.

5.70 NEONATAL DYSPHAGIA

I. *Congenital Anomalies*
  1. Cleft palate.
  2. Macroglossia associated with syndromes as Pierre Robin or Beckwith-Wiedemann syndrome.
  3. Esophageal atresia.
  4. Brain malformation as Chiari malformation.
  5. Vascular anomalies.
     – Aberrant right subclavian artery compressing the esophagus from behind.
     – Aberrant left Pulmonary artery indenting the esophagus anteriorly.
     – Right side aortic arch producing a posterior and right lateral indentation over esophagus.
  6. Choanal atresia.

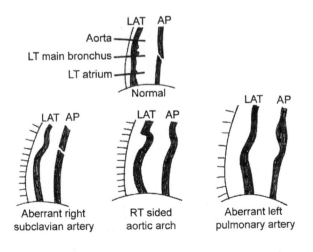

Fig. 5.70.1

II. *Miscellaneous*
1. Delayed/subnormal mental development.
2. Prematurity.

5.71 PHARYNGEAL/ESOPHAGEAL DIVERTICULA

Diverticulum is a blind sac or pouch arising from pharynx or esophagus.

I. *Upper Third*
1. *Zenker's/Pharyngoesophageal/ Hypopharyngeal Diverticulum.*
    - Present in middle aged and elderly esp >50yrs of age.
    - Arises through the posterior wall of hypopharynx usually on left side through Killian's triangle [weak area between the inferior constrictor and cricopharyngeus sphincter].
    - Causes oropharyngeal dysphagia, regurgitation, aspiration and hoarseness of voice.
    - May present as a mass in neck or superior mediastinal mass on chest X-ray with or without an air-fluid level.
    - It is a pulsion type of diverticulum.
2. *Lateral Pharyngocele*
    - Congenital—is remnant of 2nd branchial arch.
    - Acquired—Seen in trumpeters, glassblowers.

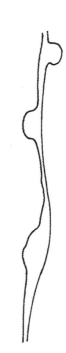

Fig. 5.71.1: Esophagogram showing multiple pulsion diverticula

II. *Middle Third*
1. Traction
    - Usually at the level of carina.
    - Secondary to mediastinal inflammation or adenopathy as in tuberculosis and histoplasmosis.
2. Developmental as in tracheo-esophageal fistulas.

III. *Lower Third*
1. *Epiphrenic*
    Causes include
    - Long standing peptic esophagitis and strictures.
    - Iatrogenic—postendoscopy or surgical injury.
    - Motility disorders as diffuse esophageal spasms, achalasia, hypertensive lower esophageal sphincter.
    - Collagen disorders—Ehlers-Danlos syndrome.

IV. *Miscellaneous*

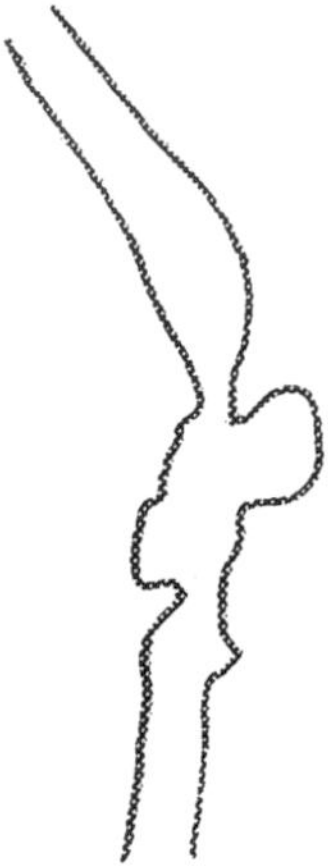

Esophageal

Intramural Pseudodiverticulosis

Fig. 5.71.2: "Cock screw" esophagus—Nonpropulsive segmental contractions producing multiple areas of pronounced luminal narrowing with areas of sacculations

- Very rare.
- There is dilatation of submucosal glands producing numerous tiny outpouching within the wall.
- Segmental/diffuse.
- Strictures/dysmotility of esophagus is usually associated.

5.72 ESOPHAGITIS/ESOPHAGEAL ULCERS

Signs of Esophagitis

- · Fine mucosa with nodularity in double contrast studies.
- Thickening of longitudinal folds (wider than 3mm).
- Thickening of transverse folds.
- Reduced or absent peristalsis.

1. *Disease*
   - Reflux esophagitis

Part of Esophagus Involved

   - Lower third esophagus.

Features

- Blurring of squamocolumnar junction.
- Fine, punctate ulcer which ultimately become punched out immediately above the esophagogastric junction.

Comments/Additional Features

- Hiatus hernia is commonly associated.

2. *Disease*
   - Barret's esophagitis.

Part of Esophagus Involved

- Lower third

Features

- Ulceration at junction of columnar and squamous esophageal mucosa.
- Fine reticular pattern of mucosa resembling area gastricae due to islands of columnar mucosa.

Comments/Additional Features

- Increased risk of carcinomatous change.
3. *Disease*
   - Moniliasis

Part of Esophagus Involved

- Any part but mainly upper third.

Features

- Early
  - Mucosal plaques
  - Folds become nodular.
- Late
  - Deep marginal ulceration, perforation, fistula and stricture may occur.

Comments/Additional Features

- Common in immunocompromised.
4. *Disease*
   - Herpetic esophagitis

Part of Esophagus Involved

- Mid esophagus

Features

- Sessile filling defects.
- Punched out ulcers on a background of normal mucosa.
- Ultimately, diffuse ulceration.

Comments/Additional Features

- Common in immunocompromised.
- Oral herpetic lip-lesions suggest the diagnosis.

5. *Disease*

 CMV esophagitis.

Part of Esophagus Involved

- Any part

Features

- Discrete, superficial ulcer.
- Giant ulcers on a normal mucosal background.

Comments/Additional Features

- Seen invariably in AIDS patient.
- Endoscopic biopsy differentiate them from similar looking HIV ulcers.

6. *Disease*
 – Tuberculous esophagitis.

Part of Esophagus Involved

- Any part

Features

- Deep ulcers and fistulas.
- Scarring and stricture formation.

Comments/Additional Features

- Caseating mediastinal nodes are associated.

7. *Disease*
 – Drug-induced esophagitis.

Part of Esophagus Involved

- Midesophagus

Features

- Ulceration

Comments/Additional Features

- Prolonged contact with certain drugs at sites of esophageal impression above the aortic arch or that produced by left main bronchus, above the impression caused by dilated left atrium and left ventricles. [Tetracycline, KCl, quinidine, aspirin, phenylbutazone.

8. *Disease*
   – Caustic esophagitis

Part of Esophagus Involved

- Sites of anatomical holdup.

Features

- Ulceration with mucosal sloughing.
- Fibrosis, long-segment smooth strictures.
- Perforation into pleural/pericardial cavity.
- Ultimately, esophagus may be atonic, especially if myenteric plexus is destroyed.

Comments/Additional Features

- Dyes include sodium hydroxide and carbonate, iodine and bleaches.
- Increased risk of squamous cell carcinoma latent period =20-40 years.

9. *Disease*
   – Radiation esophagitis.

Part of Esophagus Involved

- Part included in radiation field.

Features

- Doses >2500 and <4500 rads produce transient changes as—

- Mucosal granularity.
- Minute ulcers.
- Narrowing of lumen from mucosal edema.
  Doses >4500 rads.
- Severe esophagitis due to obliterative endarteritis.
- Long smooth tapered strictures.

Comments/Additional Features

- Drugs like adriamycin and actinomycin-D potentiate esophagitis.

10. *Disease*
   – Nasogastric tube esophagitis.

Part of Esophagus Involved

- Lower third.

Features

- Features of peptic esophagitis.

Comments/Additional Features

- Nasogastric intubation for as short as 3 days can make LES incompetent.

11. *Miscellaneous*
Cause include Crohn's disease – intramural diverticulosis.

5.73 ESOPHAGEAL STRICTURES

		Inflammatory	Neoplastic
1.	Type	– Smooth	– Irregular
2.	Length	– Usually long	– Usually short
3.	Shouldering	– Absent	– Present

Contd...

Contd...

	Inflammatory	Neoplastic
4. Mucosal fold destruction	– Usually absent	– Present
5. Age group	– Early childhood young adults upto middle age	Middle-age and above
6. Proximal dilatation	– More pronounced	Less pronounced
7. Causes	– Peptic, corrosives, achalasia, scleroderma, iatrogenic	Carcinoma, leiomyosarcoma postradiotherapy

Causes of Smooth Esophageal Strictures

I. *Inflammatory*
   1. *Peptic*—Usually lower esophagus.
   2. *Scleroderma*—Lower 2/3 esophagus; poor functioning LES, hypoperistalsis produces reflux esophagitis and stricture.
   3. *Corrosives*—Strictures at sites of potential hold-up as aortic arch, esophagogastric junction. Alkalis are more prone than acids.
   4. *Iatrogenic*—Prolonged nasogastric intubation produces prolonged dilated LES with reflux and stricture formation in lower third esophagus.
   5. *Infections* as tuberculosis.

II. *Neoplastic*
   1. *Carcinoma* with submucosal spread.
   2. *Benign tumors* as leiomyoma may produce smooth, eccentric, polypoid mass.
   3. *Extrinsic mass* as mediastinal lymphadenopathy and carcinoma bronchus, etc.

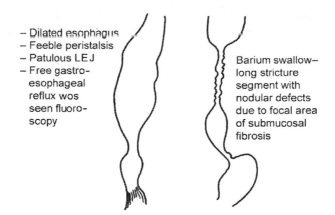

- Dilated esophagus
- Feeble peristalsis
- Patulous LEJ
- Free gastro-
  esophageal
  reflux wos
  seen fluoro-
  scopy

Barium swallow–
long stricture
segment with
nodular defects
due to focal area
of submucosal
fibrosis

Fig. 5.73.1: Scleroderma (Left), case of
caustic esophagitis (Right)

Irregular Esophageal Strictures

1. *Neoplastic*
   - Carcinoma.
   - Leiomyosarcoma.
   - Carcinosarcoma.
   - Lymphoma.
2. *Iatrogenic*
   - Radiotherapy.
   - Postoperative:-Fundoplication.

5.74 TERTIARY CONTRACTIONS IN ESOPHAGUS

These are noncoordinated, nonpropulsive contractions in
esophagus seen mainly in distal 2/3 esophagus 5-10% of
normal adult in 4th-6th decade show them.

Causes Include

1. Presbyesophagus
   - Elderly patients with severely disordered motility due to muscle atrophy.
   - May cause chest pain or dysphagia.
2. Diffuse esophageal spasm.
3. Hyperactive achalasia.
4. Neuromuscular disease.
   - Diabetes
   - Parkinsonism.
   - Multiple sclerosis.
   - Thyrotoxic myopathy.
   - Myotonic dystrophy.
5. Obstruction at the cardia.
   - Neoplasm.
   - Distal esophageal stricture.
   - Benign lesion.
   - Surgery (repair of hiatus hernia)

Findings

- Spontaneous repetitive nonpropulsive contraction. "yo-yo" motion
- Corkscrew appearance.
- Compartmentalization of barium ("Rosary bead", "Shish Kebab")

5.75 GASTRIC MASSES AND FILLING DEFECTS

1. *Primary Malignant Neoplasms*
   a. *Carcinoma*
      - Usually polypoidal with granular/lobulated surface.

- Sessile lesions are detected by alteration in pattern of area gastricae or rugal folds.
- Usual site is pyloric region.

b. *Lymphoma*
- Most are NHL.
- May be polypoidal, ulcerating or infiltrative.
- Multiple polypoidal, tumor esp. with central ulceration giving "bulls-eye" appearance is characteristic.
- Giant cavitating lesions with pronounced thickening of folds is suggestive of diagnosis.

c. *Leiomyosarcoma*
- Large exophytic tumors with central necrosis.
- Usual site is fundus and body.
- Association with functional extra-adrenal paragangliomas and pulmonary chondromas.

d. *Kaposi Sarcoma*
- Frequently seen in AIDS.
- Multifocal, submucosal and occasionally polypoidal tumors.
- Associated duodenal and small bowel involvement may be present.

e. *Carcinoid*
- Arise in distal antrum and along lesser curvature.
- Submucosal nodule which may be sessile or pedunculated.
- Highly vascular tumor with hypervascular metastases.

2. *Metastases (Secondary Malignancies)*
- Frequently ulcerate producing bull's eye lesion.
- Common primaries include melanoma, bronchus, breast, etc.

3. *Benign Lesions*
- Polyps.

A. Type
- Hyperplastic [local glandular hyperplasia]

Features

- Usually <1cm
- Multiple

Location

- Fundus and body.

Comments

- Commonest.
- Associated with familial polyposis coli
- Associated with atrophic gastritis.
- No premalignant potential.

B. Type
- Adenomatous polyps [dysplastic]

Features

- Usually >1cm.
- Often solitary with nodular surface.

Location

- Antrum.

Comments

- Associated with atrophic gastritis.
- Premalignant.
- May prolapse into pyloric canal to produce gastric outflow obstruction.

C. Type
i. Villous [Hamartomas]

Features

- Usually >3cm
- Reticular appearance.

Location

- Antrum is spared.

Comments

- Associated with Peutz-Jeghers syndrome and Cowden's disease.
  ii. Submucosal lesion.
  Produces smooth bulge into lumen with obtuse angle with the normal wall.
- Leiomyoma
  - Commonest, difficult to separate from leiomyosarcoma.
- Lipoma
  - Soft; change shape with gastric peristalsis.
- Others
  - Neurofibromas, hemangiomas, lymphangiomas, ectopic pancreatic rests, duplication cyst, etc.
4. *Extrinsic Indentation*
  - Pancreatic tumors.
  - Splenic enlargement.
  - Hepatic enlargement.
  - Other retroperitoneal tumors.
  - Subdiaphragmatic masses/collection.
5. *Miscellaneous*
  Bezoars
  - Mobile mass in lumen with no attachment to wall.
  - Trichobezoar are commonly seen in psychiatric patients.

– Phytobezoars are commonest.
– When large take the shape of stomach with contrast/
barium entering into the interstices of the bezoar.

5.76 LINITIS PLASTICA

Linitis plastica or *"leather bottle" stomach* is a result of
submucosal spread of pathological process, leaving in most
cases an intact mucosa resulting in a negative endoscopy.
There is intense desmoplastic reaction which leads to a rigid
stomach wall and narrow lumen. There is loss of normal
mucosal pattern and reduced capacity. The stomach wall is
thickened and there is loss of normal peristalsis.

DIFFERENTIAL DIAGNOSIS

1. *Malignancy*
   – Scirrhous gastric carcinoma.
   – Lymphomas both Hodgkin's and NHL (Non-Hodgkin's
     lymphoma).
   – Metastatic involvement.
2. *Inflammation*
   – Chronic gastric ulcer disease with intense spasm.
   – Crohn's disease.
   – Sarcoidosis.
   – Eosinophilic gastroenteritis.
   – PAN (Polyarthritis nodosa)
   – Stenosing antral gastritis.
3. *Infection*
   – Tertiary stage of syphilis.
   – Tuberculosis.
   – Histoplasmosis.

- Actinomycosis.
- Strongyloidiasis.

4. *Trauma*
   - Corrosive gastritis
   - Radiation injury.
   - Gastric freezing.

5. *Others*
   - Amyloidosis
   - Pseudolymphoma
   - Cystic fibrosis.

RADIOLOGICAL APPEARANCE

Barium Meal: There is generalized narrowing of gastric lumen (tubular shape of stomach), with reduced capacity, the mucosa is often nodular and fold pattern is lost. There is loss of peristalsis appreciated on fluoroscopy.

Ultrasound: There is evidence of wall thickening, usually more than 6 mm. No evidence of active peristalsis is seen.

CT Scan: Water distension with gas effervescence is used to demonstrate the true thickness of gastric wall which is usually more than 1 cm, the nodular mucosal pattern can be appreciated, and surrounding organs and areas can be examined for associated changes like infiltration and lymphadenopathy in cases of malignancy. One peculiar property of linitis plastica associated with malignancy is contrast enhancement on CECT, this helps identify infiltrative tumors less than 1 cm in thickness.

COMMON ETIOLOGIES

Scirrhous gastric carcinoma: There is intense desmoplastic reaction associated with this carcinoma. It usually involves the antrum of stomach, but may extend to involve the entire stomach. There is firmness, rigidity, reduced capacity and aperistalsis of involved areas. On double contrast barium studies and CECT there is loss of normal mucosal fold features, with sometimes granular or polypoid folds, and encircling growth. There is intense enhancement on CECT and surrounding infiltration may be present.

Lymphoma: Both Hodgkin's and NHL may involve the stomach either partially or diffusely. Stomach is the most common site of GI tract lymphoma especially NHL or extranodal Hodgkin's. The flexibility of gastric wall is preserved and mucosal folds and wall may be grossly thickened (4-5 cm). On CT there is homogenous overall attenuation and minimal enhancement after contrast administration. There may be diffuse retroperitoneal and mesenteric adenopathy.

Metastatic involvement: There is usually a history of primary malignancy elsewhere like malignant melanoma, breast, lung, colon, prostate, leukemia, secondary lymphoma. Breast Ca. is the most common malignancy producing linitis plastica like appearance.

Radiation injury: There is a positive history of radiotherapy received for primary malignancy in near by organs. There is intense desmoplastic reaction produced by radiotherapy leading to effacement of gastric folds. There is a latent period of 1 month to 2 years.

Acids: A positive history of acid ingestion can usually be elicited and is usually found in female patients. There are associated changes in esophagus.

Granulomatous disease: (*Tuberculosis, Sarcoidosis*): These may cause changes like linitis plastica. Usually associated changes are seen in the lungs. In cases of TB changes may

Flow Chart 5.76.1

Linitis plastica

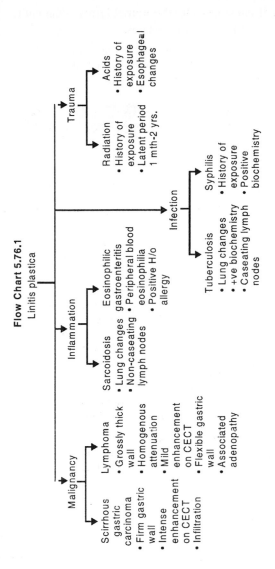

- **Malignancy**
  - Scirrhous gastric carcinoma
    - Firm gastric wall
    - Intense enhancement on CECT
    - Infiltration
  - Lymphoma
    - Grossly thick wall
    - Homogenous attenuation
    - Mild enhancement on CECT
    - Flexible gastric wall
    - Associated adenopathy

- **Inflammation**
  - Sarcoidosis
    - Lung changes
    - Non-caseating lymph nodes
  - Eosinophilic gastroenteritis
    - Peripheral blood eosinophilia
    - Positive H/o allergy
  - **Infection**
    - Tuberculosis
      - Lung changes
      - +ve biochemistry
      - Caseating lymph nodes
    - Syphilis
      - History of exposure
      - Positive biochemistry

- **Trauma**
  - Radiation
    - History of exposure
    - Latent period 1 mth-2 yrs.
  - Acids
    - History of exposure
    - Esophageal changes

be seen in small intestines and abdominal lymphadenopathy may be present with or without ascites.

Eosinophilic gastroenteritis: The patients may have a positive history of atopy and peripheral blood eosinophilia may be seen in 50% of the cases. Ascites may or may not be present.

5.77 LINITIS PLASTICA

Disease	Features	Additional Points
1. *Gastric carcinoma*	Loss of wall pliability	– Irregular mucosal folds with destruction. – Commonest cause
2. *Lymphoma*	Wall pliability preserved, multifocal submucosal nodules. Disease extend cross the GE junction and/or pylorus	Folds architecture preserved. Massive associated lymphadenopathy
3. *Metastases esp breast*	Wall pliability preserved	Fold architecture preserved. Known primary
4. *Local invasion as pancreatic carcinoma*	Localized mucosal destruction	Pancreatic mass with evidence of invasion into stomach
5. *Corrosives*	Associated with strictures. Nonspecific findings.	H/o ingestion
6. *Radiation therapy*	Mucosal fold effacement. Large antral ulcers may be associated	H/o radiation exposure
7. *Granulomatous disease as Crohn's disease syphilis, TB.*	Nonspecific findings. Wall pliability preserved	Other stigmata elsewhere
8. *Eosinophilic gastritis*	Evidence of peripheral eosinophilia. History of allergy. Nonspecific features	Diagnosis by biopsy

5.78 GASTROCOLIC FISTULA

1. *Inflammatory*
   - Peptic disease with ulcer and perforation.
   - Crohn's disease with multiple fistulas and mucosal involvement and skip areas.
   - Chronic pancreatitis with enzyme leakage or duct rupture.
   - Granulomatous infections as tuberculosis, actinomycosis.

2. *Neoplastic*
   - Carcinomas of stomach, pancreas or colon.
   - Metastases with perforation and fistulation.

5.79 RETROPERITONEAL FIBROSIS

Also known *as ormonds disease* or *chronic periaortitis*.

It is a rare fibrotic process frequently involving the caudal aspect of retroperitoneum without effects on ureter, great vessels, lymphatic and even CBD, caused by proliferation of fibroblasts, acute infective cells and capillaries, all of which are surrounded by collagen fibers.

In 15%- Associated with fibrotic process else where in body.

D/D-

Causes

A. *Primary-2/3rd*

Autoimmune with antibodies to 'CEROID' (insoluble lipid) systemic vasculitis associated with fibrosis outside retroperitoneum in 8-15%.

Age—Middle-aged to elderly

Sex—M:F 2:1

Usually responsive to steroid.

B. *Secondary*

Benign

- Medication 12%—Most common is Methysurgide, but β blocker, methyldopa, hydralazine, antibiotics and other analgesics prolonged use- causes abdominal, pulmonary and endocardial fibrosis, early withdrawal often results in regression of disease.
- Retroperitoneal hemorrhage-because of trauma, ruptured aneurysm or retroperitoneal surgery like translumbar aortography and percutaneous renal biopsy.
  Aneurysm rupture- on CT-acute extra luminal blood is of soft tissue attenuation. Vermiform finger like extension in the retroperitoneum.
- Post-traumatic chronic hematoma- Decreased mass with a thick dense rim-peripheral calcification may also be seen.

INFECTION

Like TB, syphilis, actinomycosis, brucellosis and fungal infection, etc. can lead to retroperitoneal fibrosis.

MISCELLANEOUS

Variety of intra-abdominal inflammatory conditions (diverticulitis, appendicitis, Extravasation from the urinary tract, aneurysm of aorta and iliac artery.

MALIGNANT

8-10%.

Primary neoplasm or metastatic disease or lymphoma can provoke an extensive desmoplastic reaction.

Primary Retroperitoneal Tumor

Majority are malignant.

- Liposarcoma-Most common.
  On CT- is a attenuation of fat density.
- Leiomyosarcoma- large heterogenous masses.
  Low attenuation component- necrosis
  No fat or calcification.
- *MFH*- Heterogenous soft tissue, necrosis positive

Metastasis

Mets from colon and breast, soft tissue, lung, kidney, prostatic tumor incites a fibrotic reaction around itself.

Lymphoma

HL (Hodgkin lymphoma)>NHL (Non-Hodgkin lymphoma).
Enlarged lymph node may appear as discrete masses or confluent- soft tissue obliterating the retroperitoneal fat—Loss of definition of fat plane but not involving aorta and IVC.

- *Excretory urography*- ureteric obstruction.
- Bilateral in 75%
- Tapering lumen or complete obstruction- usually at L4-5
- Medial deviation of ureter which is obstructed and dilated other causes = Normal in 18%
  - Pelvic lipomatosis
  - Following abdominoperineal resection.
  - Retrocaval ureter—Right ureter passes behind the IVC at the level of L4
  - Hypertrophy of psoas muscle of L3.
- USG- Hypoechoic smoothly marginated mass that often appear as plaque around the distal aorta. Due to medial deviation of ureter.

CT: From minimal periureteral stranding to large lobulated masses obliterating the fat plane but not involving the aorta and IVC, indistinguishable from bulky lymphadenopathy.

D/D feature of retroperitoneal fibrosis from primary RPF Tumor.

RPF: Usually located at the level of L4 and plaque like and infiltrating rather then nodular RPF usually surrounds the ant. and lateral aspect of great vessels, whereas marked displacement of aorta or IVC is seen in primary retroperitoneal Tumor or in malignant LAP.

LAP in lymphoma is often-centered more cephalad in-RP and may be bulkier at the level of renal hila.

- Malignant or infective may invade and destroy adjacent bones or organ.

NCCT: RPF-similar to that of muscle/focal or uniform hyper-density -increase collagen.

CECT: Exuberant Enhancement.

MRI: Non-malignant RPF

- Homogenous decrease signal intensity (similar to psoas muscle) on both T1 and T2- reflects mature and quiscent phase.
- Acute benign RPF-Intermediate or increase on T2- increase cell ularity and fluid.

Malignant

Heterogeneous on T2 WI

Both malignant and non-malignant enhancement after IV Gadognium.

MRA and GRE are effective- to see the vascular involvement and collateral vessel formation.

- Radionuclide- Ga67 uptake during active infection.

Flow Chart 5.79.1
RPF (Retroperitoneal Fibrosis)

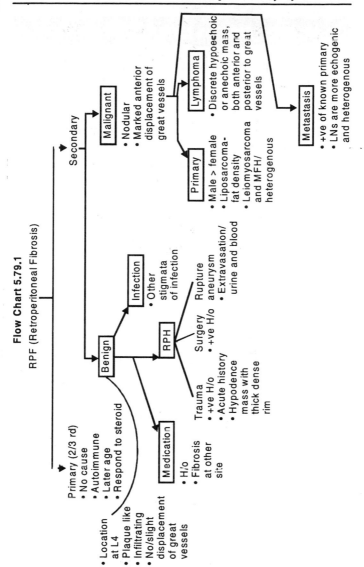

5.80 MASS OF ILIO-PSOAS COMPARTMENT

- Iliacus and psoas major muscles are chief flexors of lower limb.
- Due to their common *origin* and *insertion* both are considered together.
- Structuraly they are structures located in posterior abdominal wall.
- Psoas minor is a small muscle absent in upto 70%.
- CT- Isoattenuating; minimal/nil enhancement.
  MRI- Intermediate (T1, T2, PD)
  USG- Hypoechoic to liver/ISO - to renal medulla with linear echogenic fascial strips.
  Plain X-ray- soft tissue density
- Maximally thick at L3-4. A linear area within -fat about lumbar plexus

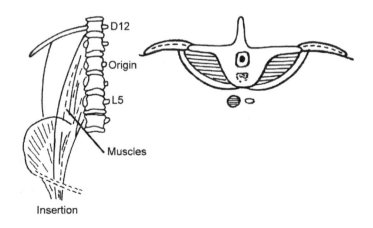

Fig. 5.80.1: Ilio-psoas compartment

Pathologies/Masses

Inflammatory

Neoplastic

Pseudoaneurysm of lumbar artery

Hemorrhage

Ilio-psoas bursitis

Imaging

1. Plain X-ray
2. Retroperitoneal air insufflation and tomography
3. CT
4. MRI
5. USG
6. Indirect-IVP, aortography, IVC graphy.

SALIENT FEATURES

1. *Inflammatory*- Most common
   - Pyogenic/tubercular.
   - Mostly secondaries- Surgery, spine, kidney, pancreas, bowel, sometimes primary also aortic bed.
   - On CT and MRI
     - Diffuse bulkiness.
     - Focal masses.
     - Iso to hypo on CT and with homogenous/rim enhancement.
     - T1- iso/hypo; T2-hyper; PD-hyper
     - Gas +−
     - Calcification⊥- TB.
     - Destruction and sclerosis of adjacent bone.
     - ± a phlegmon or an abscess
   - On USG

- Hypoechoic collection
- Bulky muscle.
- Plain X-ray-loss of psoas silhoutte.
- Apart from imaging radiologist helps in diagnostic and intervention. We should also try and find out the source of infection.

2. *Neoplastic*
   - 1/3-1/4 the causes of ileo psoas masses.
   - Sometimes primary soft tissue tumor or sometimes secondarily by invading lesion as lipoma, liposarcoma, rhabdomyoma and sarcomas, teratoma, dermoid, etc.
   - Presence of fat is a sign of fat containing mass
   - Difficult to differentiate from above.

3. *Hemorrhage*
   - Due to trauma, iatrogenic, graft, VWD, hemophilia.
   - Expansile mass of various appearances, dual phase of resolution is seen.
   - Bone destruction is not seen.
   - Slowly it resolves forming a level or low density area. Calcification, rim enhancement, confuse it to infection. Superinfection is rarely a problem.

4. *Bursitis*
   - Presents as a flocculant mass in inguinal area with invagination towards hip.
   - Communication to hip is seen early 15% by arthrography.
   - Due to rheumatoid arthritis, osteoarthritis. Seen as areas of fluid in all modalities.

5. *Pseudoaneurysm of lumbar arteries*
   - Due to trauma /surgery
   - Doppler USG/MRA give good demonstration.

Flow Chart 5.80.1
Masses in ilio-psoas compartment

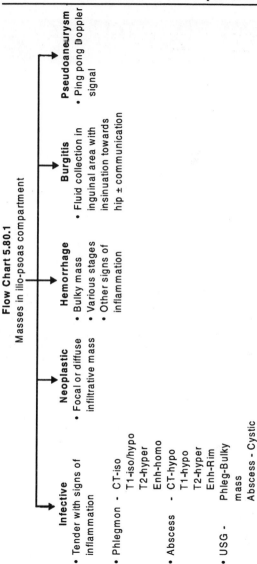

Infective
- Tender with signs of inflammation

- Phlegmon - CT-iso
  - T1-iso/hypo
  - T2-hyper
  - Enh-homo
- Abscess - CT-hypo
  - T1-hypo
  - T2-hyper
  - Enh-Rim
- USG - Phleg-Bulky mass
  - Abscess - Cystic

Neoplastic
- Focal or diffuse infiltrative mass

Hemorrhage
- Bulky mass
- Various stages
- Other signs of inflammation

Burgitis
- Fluid collection in inguinal area with insinuation towards hip ± communication

Pseudoaneurysm
- Ping pong Doppler signal

– From above it is evident that radiologists have a supportive, land marking and confirmatory role

5.81 ANATOMY OF LIVER, BILE DUCTS, AND PANCREAS

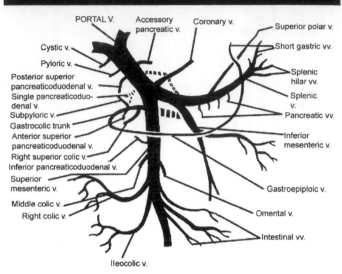

Fig. 5.81.1: Extrahepatic portal vein branches

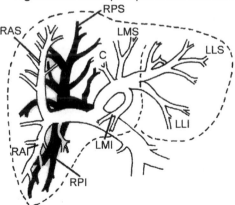

Fig. 5.81.2: Intrahepatic portal vein branches

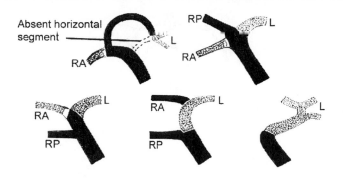

Fig. 5.81.3: Variations of intrahepatic portal venous system (20%)

A. Left portal vein
   1. Absence of horizontal segment (0.2%)
B. Right portal vein
   1. Trifurcation of main portal vein (11%)
   2. Origin of RP segment from main portal vein (5%)
   3. Origin of RA segment from left portal vein (4%)
   4. Absence of main right, RA and RP portal segments

RAS = right anterior segment	RPI = right posterior inferior	LMI = left median inferior
RAI = right anterior inferior	RPS = right posterior superior	LMS = left median superior
RAS = right anterior superior	C = caudate lobe	LLI = left lateral inferior
RP = right posterior segment	L = left portal vein	LLS = left lateral superior

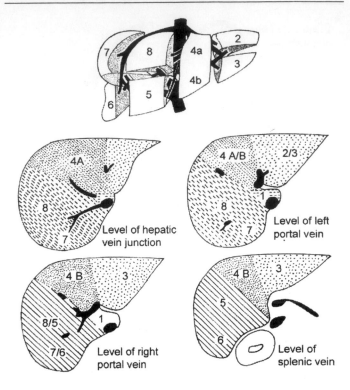

Fig. 5.81.4: Liver

Functional Segmental Liver Anatomy

(Goldsmith and Woodburne)	*(Couinaud and Bismuth)*
Caudate lobe	
Left lobe Left lateral segment	Left lateral superior subsegment
	Left lateral inferior subsegment
Left medial segment	Left medial superior subsegment
	Left medial inferior subsegment

Contd...

Contd...

(Goldsmith and Woodburne)		(Couinaud and Bismuth)
Right lobe	Right anterior segment	Right anterior inferior subsegment
		Right anterior superior subsegment
	Right posterior segment	Right posterior inferior subsegment
		Right posterior superior subsegment

Functional Segmental Liver Anatomy

Based on distribution of 3 major hepatic veins:

a. Middle hepatic vein

Divides liver into right and left lobe

Also separated by main portal vein scissura (Cantlie line) passing through IVC + long axis of gallbladder).

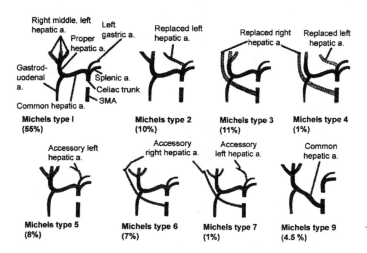

Fig. 5.81.5

b. Left hepatic vein
   Divides left lobe into medial + lateral sectors
c. Right hepatic vein
   Divides right lobe into medial + lateral sectors
   Each of the four sections is further divided by an imaginary transverse line drawn through the right + left portal vein into anterior + posterior segments; the segments are numbered counterclockwise from IVC.

Hepatic Arterial Anatomy (Michels classification)

Type I (55%):

- Celiac trunk trifurcates into LT gastric a. + splenic a. + common hep. a.
- Common hep. a. divides into gastroduodenal a. + proper hep. a.
- RT hep. a. + LT hep. a. arise from proper hep. a.
- Middle hep. a. (supplying caudate lobe) arises from
  a. LT/RT hep. a.
  b. Proper hep. a. (in 10%)

Type II (10%):

- Common hep. a. divides into gastroduodenal + RT hep. a.
- LT hep. a. replaced to LT gastric a.
- Middle hep. a. from RT hep. a.

Type III (11%):

- Common hep. a. divides into gastroduodenal + LT hep. a.
- RT hep. a. replaced to superior mesenteric a.
- Middle hep. a. from LT hep. a.

Type IV (1%):

- Common hep. a. divides into middle hep. a. + gastro-duodenal a.

- RT hep. a. + LT hep. a. are both replaced

Type V (8%):

- Accessory LT hep. a. arises from LT gastric a.

Type VI (7%):

- Accessory RT hep. a. arises from superior mesenteric a.

Type VII (1%):

- Accessory RT + LT hepatic a.

Type VIII (2%):

- Combinations of accessory + replaced hepatic aa.

Type IX (4.5%):

- Hepatic trunk replaced to superior mesenteric a.

Type X (0.5%):

- Hepatic trunk replaced to LT gastric a.

Hepatic Fissures

1. Fissure for ligamentum teres = umbilical fissure = invagination of ligamentum teres = embryologic remnant of obliterated umbilical vein connecting placental venous blood with left portal vein
   - Located at dorsal free margin of falciform ligament
   - Runs into liver with visceral peritoneum
   - Divides left hepatic lobe into medial + lateral segments (divides subsegment 3 from 4)

2. Fissure for ligamentum venosum
   = Invagination of obliterated ductus venosus
   = Embryologic connection of left portal vein with left hepatic vein
     - Separates caudate lobe from left lobe of liver
     - Lesser omentum within fissure separates the greater sac anteriorly from lesser sac posteriorly.

3. Fissure for gallbladder
   = shallow peritoneal invagination containing the gallbladder
     – Divides right from left lobe of liver.
4. Transverse fissure
   = Invagination of hepatic pedicle into liver
     – Contains horizontal portion of left + right portal veins.
5. Accessory fissures
   a. Right inferior accessory fissure
      = From gallbladder fossa/just inferior to it to lateroinferior margin of liver
   b. Others (rare)

Normal Size of Liver

Sonographic measurements along vertical (craniocaudal) axis:
a. Midclavicular line

< 13 cm	=	normal
13.0 – 15.5 cm	=	indeterminate (in 25% of patients)
> 15.5 cm	=	hepatomegaly (87% accuracy)

b. Preaortic line > 10 cm
c. Prerenal line > 14 cm

Normal Hemodynamics Parameter of Liver

Portal vein velocity: > 11 cm/sec
Congestion index (= cross-sectional area of portal vein divided by average velocity): 0.070 ± 0.09
Hepatic artery resistive index: $0.60–0.64 \pm 0.06$

Liver Function Tests

1. Alkaline phosphatase (AP)
   Formation: bone, liver, intestine, placenta

    high increase: cholestasis with extrahepatic biliary obs-
                      truction (confirmed by rise in GT drugs,
                      granulomatous disease. (sarcoidosis),
                      primary biliary cirrhoses primary +
                      secondary malignancy of liver.
    mild increase: all forms of liver disease, heart failure

2. γ-glutamyl transpeptidase (GGT)
   very sensitive in almost all forms of liver disease
      Utility: confirms hepatic source of elevated AP,
                     may indicate significant alcohol use.

3. Transaminases
   High increase: viral / toxin-induced acute hepatitis
   a. Aspartate transaminase (AST); formerly serum
      glutamic oxaloacetic transaminase (SGOT)
      Formation: liver, muscle, kidney, pancreas, RBCs
   b. Alanine aminotransferase (ALT); formerly serun
      glutamic pyruvic transaminase [SGPT]
      Formation: primarily in liver
      • rather specific elevation in liver disease.

4. Bilirubin
   Helps differentiate between various causes of jaundice
   a. Unconjugated / indirect bilirubin = insoluble in water
      Formation: breakdown of senescent RBCs
      Metabolism: tightly bound to albumin in vessels
                     actively taken up by liver, cannot be
                     excreted by kidneys
   b. Conjugated / direct bilirubin = water-soluble
      Formation: Conjugation in liver cells
      Metabolism: Excretion into bile; not reabsorbed by
                     intestinal mucosa + excreted in feces

Elevation:
- Overproduction: hemolytic anemia, resorption hematoma, multiple transfusions
- Decreased hepatic uptake: drugs, sepsis
- Decreased conjugation: Gilbert syndrome, neonatal jaundice, hepatitis, cirrhosis, sepsis
- Decreased excretion into bile: hepatitis cirrhosis, drug-induced cholestasis, sepsis, extrahepatic biliary obstruction.

5. Lactic dehydrogenase (LDH)
   Nonspecific and therefore not helpful
   high increase: primary or metastatic liver involvement

6. Alpha fetoprotein (AFP)
   > 400 ng/mL: strongly suggests that focal mass represents a hepatocellular carcinoma.

Normal Size of Bile Ducts

- CBD at point of maximum diameter:
  ≤ 5 mm = normal; 6-7 mm = equivocal; ≥ 8 mm = dilated
- CHD at porta hepatis + CBD in head of pancreas: 5 mm
- Right intrahepatic duct just proximal to CHD: 2-3 mm
- CHD at porta hepatis + CBD in head of pancreas: 5 mm
- Right intrahepatic duct just proximal to CHD: 2-3 mm
- Cystic duct diameter: 1.8 mm
  Average length of 1-2 cm
  Distal cystic duct posterior to CBD (in 95%), anterior to CBD (in 5%)

Bile Duct Variants

Incidence

2.4% of autopsies;
13% of operative cholangiograms

A. Aberrant Intrahepatic Duct

May join CHD, CBD, cystic duct, right hepatic duct, gallbladder

- anomalous right hepatic duct entering CHD/cystic duct (4-5%)

Cx: 1. postoperative bile leak if severed

2. segmental biliary obstruction if ligated

B. Cystic Duct Entering Right Hepatic Duct

C. Ducts of Luschka

= small ducts from hepatic bed draining directly into gallbladder

D. Duplication of Cystic Duct/CBD

E. Congenital Tracheobiliary Fistula.

= Fistulous communication between carina and left hepatic duct

• Infants with respiratory distress

• Productive cough with bilious sputum

√ Pneumobilia

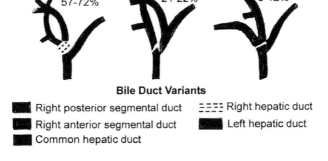

Bile Duct Variants

■ Right posterior segmental duct   ≡≡≡ Right hepatic duct

■ Right anterior segmental duct   ■ Left hepatic duct

■ Common hepatic duct

Fig. 5.81.6: Bile duct variants

Pancreaticobiliary Junction Variants

A. Angle between CBD + pancreatic duct:
   a. Usually acute at 5° – 30°
   b. Occasionally abnormal at up to 90°
B. Sphincter of Oddi
   = Muscle fibers encircling the CBD + pancreatic duct at choledochoduodenal junction.
   a. Choledochal sphincter = encircles distal CBD
   b. Pancreatic duct sphincter (in 33% separate)
C. Types of union between CBD + pancreatic duct:
   a. 2-10 (mean 5) mm short common channel (85%) with a diameter of 3-5 mm
   b. Separate entrances into duodenum
   c. 8-15 mm long common channel
   d. Pancreatic duct inserting into CBD > 15 mm from entrance into duodenum
   e. CBD inserting into pancreatic duct

CONGENITAL GALLBLADDER ANOMALIES

Agenesis of Gallbladder

Incidence

0.04 - 0.07% (autopsy)

Associated with:

Common: Rectovaginal fistula, imperforate anus, hypoplasia of scapula + radius, intracardiac shunt.

Rare: Absence of corpus callosum, microcephaly, atresia of external auditory canal, tricuspid atresia, TE fistula, dextroposition of pancreas + esophagus, absent spleen, high position of cecum, polycystic kidney.

Hypoplastic Gallbladder

a. Congenital
b. Associated with cystic fibrosis

Septations of Gallbladder

A. Longitudinal Septa
   1. Duplication of gallbladder
      = two separate lumens + two cystic ducts
      Incidence: 1:3,000 to 1:12,000
   2. Bifid gallbladder = double gallbladder
      = two separate lumens with one cystic duct
   3. Triple gallbladder (extremely rare)
B. Transverse Septa
   1. Isolated transverse septum
   2. Phrygian Cap (2-6% of population)
      = kinking/folding of fundus ± septum
   3. Multiseptated gallbladder (rare)
      = multiple cyst-like compartments connected by
        small pores
      Cx: Stasis + stone formation
C. Gallbladder Diverticulum
   = Persistence of cystohepatic duct

Gallbladder Ectopia

Most Frequent Locations

(1) beneath the left lobe of the liver > (2) intrahepatic > (3) retrohepatic

Rare Locations

(4) within falciform ligament (5) within interlobar fissure
(6) suprahepatic (lodged between superior surface of right

hepatic lobe + anterior chest wall) (7) within anterior abdominal wall (8) transverse mesocolon (9) retrorenal (10) near posterior spine + IVC (11) intrathoracic GB (Inversion of liver).

Associated with: eventration of diaphragm

"Floating GB"

= gallbladder with loose peritoneal reflections, may herniate through foramen of Winslow into lesser sac

"Torqued GB"

= results in hydrops

PANCREAS

Pancreatic Development and Anatomy

A. Dorsal anlage (in mesoduodenum)

   Origin: arises from dorsal wall of duodenum

   – Forms cranial portion of head + isthmus + body + tail of pancreas.
   – Prone to atrophy (poor in polypeptides)
   √ Drains to the minor papill through accessory duct of Santorini.

B. Ventral Anlage (below primordial liver bud)

   Origin: ventral bud arises from ventral wall of duodenum and is composed of right + left lobes (the left ventral bud regresses completely), migrates to opposite side of duodenum + fuses with dorsal anlage during 6th week GA

   – Forms caudal portion of the pancreatic head + uncinate process + CBD.
   – Not prone to atrophy (rich in polypeptides)

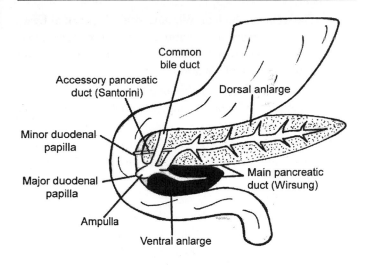

Fig. 5.81.7: Anatomy of pancreatic ducts

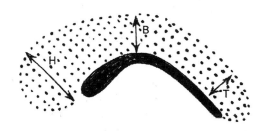

Fig. 5.81.8: Pancreatic diameters (on TRV image)

H	=	head	= 1.5 – 3.0 cm
B	=	body	= 1.2 – 2.5 cm
T	=	tail	= 1.0 – 2.5 cm

√ The ventral duct of Wirsung drains with the CBD through ampulla of Vater and becomes the major drainage pathway for the entire pancreas after fusion with the duct of Santorini.

C. Main pancreatic duct of Wirsung distal portion of dorsal duct connects with ventral duct; proximal portion of dorsal duct may disappear.

D. Accessory pancreatic duct of Santorini
= Proximal portion of dorsal duct which has not atrophied.

E. Ampulla of Vater
= Space within medial wall of second portion of duodenum below surface of papilla of Vater.

F. Major Duodenal Papilla = Papilla of Vater
– Drainage of common bile duct in 100%
– Drainage of main pancreatic duct of Wirsung in 90%

G. Minor Duodenal Papilla (Present in 60%)
– Drainage of accessory pancreatic duct of Santorini
– Drainage of main pancreatic duct in 10%
– Located a few cm orad to papilla of Vater.

SPLEEN

A. Normal Size
In adults : 12 cm length, 7-8 cm anteroposterior diameter, 3-4 cm thick; splenic index ($L \times W \times H$) of < 480
In children : Formula for length = $5.7 + 0.31 \times$ age (in years)

B. Normal weight 150 (100–265) g
estimated weight = Splenic index $\times$ 0.55

C. CT Attenuation
   a. Without enhancement:
      40-60 HU; 5-10 HU less than liver
   b. With enhancement:
      Normal heterogeneous enhancement during paren-
      chymal phase after bolus injection (due to varying
      blood flow rates through the cords of the red pulp).
D. MR Signal Intensity
   a. on T1WI: liver > spleen > muscle
   b. on T2WI: spleen > liver

IRON METABOLISM

Total body iron: 5 g
a. Functional iron: 4 g
   Location: Hemoglobin of RBCs, myoglobin of muscle,
                various enzymes
b. Stored iron: 1 g
   Location: Hepatocytes, reticuloendothelial cells of liver
                (Kupffer cells) + spleen + bone marrow
   Absorption: 1-2 mg/day through gut
   Transport: Bound to transferrin intravascularly

Deposition

a. Transferrin-transfer to:
   hepatocytes, RBC precursors in erythron, parenchymal
   tissues (e.g. muscle)
b. Phagocytosis by:
   Reticuloendothelial cells phagocytize senescent erythro-
   cytes (= extravascular hemolysis); RBC iron stored as
   ferritin/released and bound to transferrin.

5.82 INFLAMMATORY BOWEL DISEASE (IBD)

- The term IBD encompasses two forms of chronic, idiopathic, intestinal inflammation—Ulcerative colitis and Crohn's disease.
- *Unknown Etiology*
- *Ulcerative Colitis*
  - Diffuse inflammatory disease of unknown etiology.
  - Involves primarily the colorectal mucosa.

Epidemiology

- More common than Crohn's disease.
- Steady incidence (2-10/100000)
- Bimodal age distribution
  Peak– 15-25 yr
    – 50-80 yrs (smaller)
- Risk factors
  - White –2-5 *risk
  - Jewish –2-4 *risk
  - Developed country
  - Urban dweller
  - Family H/o –30-100 *risk
  - Sibling –(8.8% incidence)
  - Single
  - Non-smoker
  - Unknown

Etiology and Pathogenesis

- Speculations
- Genetic and familial factors:
  - Familial aggregation, increase frequency in mono-zygotic twins.

- ? Polygenes
- HLA- B5, BW- 52, DR2
- Association with autoimmune disorder—sacroiliitis, ankylosing spondylitis, enteropathic oligoarthritis, anterior uveitis.
- Anatomic and physiological factors: Abnormal mucin production.
- Infectious factors: Chlamydia, mycobacteria, gut anaerobes, CMV, Yersinia and bacterial cell wall components have all been proposed.
- Enteric nervous system and gut hormones: sub P and VIP = increased release.
- Psychologic and stress factors: personality (neurotic, introverts).
- Chemical mediators: Proinflammatory cytokines = IL-1 increased.
- Environmental factors:
  - Smoking: Protective
  - Oral contraceptives: Increased incidence

Diet

Cow's milk protein, lactose intolerance, chemical food additives - carrageenan.

Clinical Findings

Variable in clinical course, waxes and wanes.
- Acute exacerbations of bloody diarrhea.
- M/C clinical features—diarrhea, abdominal pain, rectal bleeding, weight loss, tenesmus.
- Vomiting, fever, constipation, arthralgias = less common.

Radiologic Findings

- Plain film
  - Colonic fecal residue: distal extent of fecal residue gives an indication of the proximal extent of the colitis.
  - Mucosa
    - Smooth
    - Granular irregular fuzzy, if ulceration = distrupted
    - Intramural gas/pneumatosis
  - Haustration
    - Widening of haustral cleft with loss of parallel line
  - Diameter
    - Upper limit of N- 5.5 cm
      = Other associated abnormalities like—Renal calculi, sacroiliitis, ankylosing spondylitis, AVN of femoral head.
  - Mural thickness
    - > 3 mm
    = Barium enema
    - To confirm clinical diagnosis
    - To assess the extent and severity of disease
    - To differentiate ulcerative colitis from Crohn's disease and other collitides.
    - To follow the course of disease
    - To detect complications.

Findings

Acute Changes

- Mucosal granularity
  - Hyperemia and accumulation of inflammatory cells in mucosa, gradual transition.
    Abnormality in quality and quantity of mucus.

- Mucosal stippling
  - Due to Crypt microabscesses which rupture into lumen, cause ulcers and barium flecks to adhere.
- Collar Botton ulcers = crypt abscess breach the lamina propria and muscularis mucosae and undermine submucosa.
- Haustral thickening or loss = edema
- Inflammatory polyps
- Contiguous, confluent, circumferential disease.

Chronic Changes

- Haustral loss:
  - Alteration in tone of the taeniae, which are relaxed
  - Colonic shortening due to massive hypertrophy and fixed shortening of muscularis mucosae (contraction) foreshortening of the colon.
- Luminal narrowing:
  - Benign strictures seen in 10% of pt's
  - Smooth tapering, rarely cause obstruction.
- Sometimes reversible, usually in distal colon.
- If irreversible, and located in proximal colon = suspicion of malignancy.
- Widening of presacral space
  - 1-1.5 cm moderate increase
    - mural thickening due to proliferation, inflammation and infiltration of perirectal fat.
  - > 1.5 cm definately abnormal
- Rectal value abnormality: N < 5mm, S3-S4 level

Proctitis

- Fold thickness > 6.5 mm with or without increase persacral space.

- Absent fold with increased presacral space = absent fold with normal presacral space = normal variant.
- *Backlash ilitis*:
  - Patulous and fixed ileocecal value that easily refluxes with persistent dilatation of terminal ileum.
  - Absent normal fold pattern with granular mucosa.
- Post-inflammatory pseudopolyps

Ultrasound

- Moderately thick hypoechoic wall
- Typical wall stratification maintained
- If extensive pseudopolyposis = wall stratification may be lost.
- Loss of haustra

Computed Tomography

- Mural thickening
- Target appearance of wall
  - Due to submucosal edema (acute)
  - Due to fat proliferation (chronic)
- Rectal narrowing and widening of presacral space. Hallmarks of chronic UC.
- When sufficiently large pseudopolyps can be identified on CT.
- Mural thickening, un-suspected perforations and pneumatosis can be identified on CT in patients with toxic megacolon.

MRI

- Can identify mural stratification
- Thickening and abnormal hypointensity of mucosa on T1 and T2 WI.

- Degree of mural enhancement correlates well with disease severity. (on fat suppressed gradient echo).

Scintigraphy

- Ga 67 citrate
- In labelled leukocytes
- Useful when there is danger of bowel perforation and extent and degree of disease activity must be assessed
- FDG-PET.

Prognosis

- Most patients = Mild to moderate disease
- 15 to 25% require colectomy
- Mortality
  - In first 2 yrs of disease in > 40 yrs old pt's
  - 1/3rd- colonic disease
  - 1/3rd- complication
  - 1/3rd- unrelated cause

CROHN'S DISEASE

- Chronic cicatrizing disorders of the alimentary tract, characterized by granulomatous inflammation of the mucosa, bowel wall and surrounding mesentery.
- Any part of alimentary tract
- Terminal ileum and proximal colon most common site

Epidemiology

- Uncommon disorder
- Increasing in incidence
- Bimodal age distribution- Peak- 15-25 yrs.
  Smaller peak - 50-80 yr.

Risk factors

- White race
- Jewish (8-fold increase)
- Urban
- Family history positive
- Sibling with disease (30 fold increase)
- Single
- Oral contraceptive use
- Smoking (4-fold increase)
- Season (highest relapse rate autumn and winter, lowest in summer).

Pathogenesis and Etiology

- Unknown etiology
- Genetic, environmental, infection, immunological, and psychological factors.
- Increase PAF, PG, LT
- Failure of suppressor T-cell generation, coupled with hyperactive state of helper T-cells.
- Defect in mucosal permeability = absorption of complex sugars and macromolecules.
- Increased deposition of type 5 collagen.

Clinical Features

Rectal bleeding, diarrhea, abdominal pain.
- Two type - colicky pain in lower abdomen relieved by defecation, severe pain in right lower quadrant simulating appendicitis.
- Abscess, fistula, perianal lesion.
  O/E - pallor, dehydration, anemia, weight loss, clubbing, abdominal distension tachycardia, fever.
- Abdominal, tenderness, profound wasting and emaciation.
- Palpable intra-abdominal mass.

Radiologic Findings

Plain Film

- When confined to colon- plain film features are similar to ulcerative colitis.
- An extended gas filled stricture is suggestive of granulomatous colitis.
- Small bowel obstruction.
- Evidence of - nephrolithiasis, gallstones, ankylosing spondylitis, sacroiliitis, avascular necrosis of femoral head.

Barium Examination

For evaluation of small bowel, enteroclysis should be the method of choice for the following indications.
- To demonstrate early changes.
- To demonstrate the full extent and possible presence of skip lesions, if surgery is contemplated.
- To determine the cause of any clinical deterioration in previously stable patient.
- To distinguish between spasm, active stenotic disease, and a fibrous stricture.
- To investigate postoperative complications of .Crohn's disease.
- To definitively rule out the presence of Crohn's disease in small bowel.
- A fluoroscopic small bowel barium meal follow through is adequate for.
- As a follow-up study in clinically stable patients with known small bowel Crohn's disease.
- To investigate patients with Crohn's disease know to involve predominantly terminal ileum (with pneumocolon)
- To investigate possible recurrence of Crohn's disease in the neo-terminal ileum after ileo-cecal resection.

- In patients with ileostomy - retrograde small bowel enema is recommended for the demonstration of more distal small bowel loops.
  Early disease:
  - – Smooth symmetric fold thickening (obstructive lymphedema of sub-mucosa)
  - – Coarse villous pattern (thickened adherent villi)
  - – Hyperplasia of lymphoid follicles with aphthoid ulcers.
  - – (Shallow mucosal erosions, 1-3 mm, surrounded by small halo of edema.

Intermediate disease

- Progressive submucosal edema with widening of base of fold with partial or complete obliteration.
- Variable submucosal infiltrate with patchy fibrosis = distortion and interruption of fold.
- Enlargement and deepening of aphthoid ulcers.
- Stellate or rose thorn appearance
- May fuse—crescenteric or linear
  Typical—Long linear ulcer on mesenteric border
- Thickening, sclerosis and retraction of mesentery = straightened mesenteric border, with redundant anti-mesenteric border.
- Localized mucosal thickening or inflammatory polyps Nodular pattern of Crohn's disease. (Inflammatory infiltrate with patchy profound edema and granulation tissue).

Advanced Disease

- Deep linear clefts of ulcers or fissures axial and transaxial fissuring
- Pseudopolyps ulceronodular or cobblestone pattern.
- Antimesenteric redundancy of bowel wall disappears with transaxial extension of ulceration.

- Bowel wall thickening with inflammation and fibrosis.
- Fat wrapping = hypertrophied subperitoneum is tethered towards the bowel wall by mesenteric perivascular fibrosis = spiral CT may show parallel thickened vessels traversing this (comb sign).

Barium enema	*Late findings*
Early findings	
Nodular lymphoid hyperplasia	• Fissures
• Aphthoid ulceration	• Fibrosis
• Deep ulceration/confluent	• Haustral loss
ulceration	• Sacculations
• Cobblestone appearance	• Postinflammatory
• Asymmetric, involvement	• Pseudopolyps
• Segmental distribution	• Intramural abscess
• Skip lesions	stricture
• Inflammatory pseudopolyps	

Anorectal Disease

Fissures ulcer, abscess, fistulae, hemorrhoids.

CT

- Bowel wall thickening
- During acute non-cicatrizing phase = stratification is maintained - with target or double halo appearance.
- With long-standing disease—transmural fibrosis—loss of stratification.
- CT may reveal - fibrofatty proliferation with creeping fat of mesentery. Stranding of fat, lymph node in mesentery, hypervascularity with perivascular fibrosis - comb sign (vascular jejunization of the ileum)
- Phlegmon, abscess

USG

TRUS - (Transrectal ultrasound)
- Mural thickening is >4mm - loss of stratification
- Perianal and perirectal abscesses, fistulas
- Heterogenity of the anal sphincter.

Transabdominal Ultrasound

- Thickening of colonic and small bowel wall (target or bull's eye appearance)
- Loss of haustration
- Absent peristalsis
- Increase blood flow in SMA with decreased RI
- Deminished compressibility.

MRI

- Can show extent and severity of inflammatory change
- Detection of perianal and perirectal fistula, sinus tracts and abscesses

Extraintestinal Complications of IBD

- Hepatobiliary
  - Steatosis
  - Cholelithiasis - impaired enterohepatic circulation of bile salts
1. Sclerosing cholangitis
  - Fibrous mural thickening of bile ducts
  - Focal clustering of IH ducts
  - Discontinuous areas of IH biliary dilatation without hepatic, porta hepatis or pancreatic masses.
    - Cholangiography - beading, pruning
    - Cholangiocarcinoma
    - Secondary biliary cirrhosis
    - Liver abscess
    - Pancreatitis

Urinary Tract Complications

- Nephrolithiasis - oxalate calculi
- Hydronephrosis
- Fistulas - enterovesical
- Musculoskeletal
  - Arthropathy
    - Ankylosing spondylitis
    - Sacroilitis
    - Avascular necrosis of femoral head
    - Osteomyelitis, septic arthritis
    - Osteoporosis
    - Psoas abscess
- Pulmonary complication
  - Serositis
  - ILD (interstitial lung disease)
  - Bronchiolitis/Bronchiectasis/chronic bronchitis
  - Necrobiotic nodules.

Skeletal System and Joints

6.1 ABNORMAL SKELETAL MATURATION

SKELETAL MATURATION DISORDERS

Retarded

1. *Chronic Ill Health*
   - Congenital cardiac disorders.
   - Chronic renal failure.
   - Inflammatory bowel disease.
   - Malnutrition including rickets.
   - Maternal deprivation.
2. *Chromosomal Disorders*
   - Down's syndrome.
   - Turner's syndrome.
   - Trisomy 18, etc.
   - Noonan syndrome.
   - Prader-Willi syndrome.

3. *Endocrinal Disorders*
   - Hypothyroidism
   - Hypogonadism
   - Hypopituitarism
   - Cushing's disease and steroid therapy.
4. *Congenital Syndromes*
   - Bone dysplasias.
   - Malformation syndromes.
5. *Miscellaneous*
   - Extreme emotional deprivation.

Accelerated

a. *Localized*
   1. Local hyperemia secondary to inflammation/infection.
   2. Trauma.
   3. Vascular malformations (hemangioma/AVM)
   4. Klippel-Trenaunay-Weber syndrome.
   5. Maffucci syndrome.
   6. Neurofibromatosis.
   7. Macrodystrophia lipomatosa.

b. *Generalized*
   i. *Endocrinal*
      - Idiopathic sexual precocity
      - Hypothalamic masses
      - Adrenal and gonadal tumors
      - Hyperthyroidism
   ii. *Congenital*
      - MeCune-Albright's syndrome
      - Cerebral gigantism
      - Lipodystrophy
      - Pseudohydroparathyroidism

- Weaver-Smith syndrome
- Marshall-Smith syndrome
iii. *Miscellaneous*
    - Obesity in children

Asymmetric

a. *Localized Gigantism*
   Causes similar to localized accelerated maturation.
b. *Localized Atrophy*
   1. Paralysis.
   2. Radiation treatment in childhood.

Premature Closure of Growth Plate

1. Localized hyperemia due to chronic inflammation as in arthritides or infection, hemophilia.
2. Vascular malformation—AVM.
3. Trauma.
4. Radiation treatment during childhood.
5. Thermal injury—Burns and frostbite.
6. Multiple exostoses and enchondromatosis.
   (Ollier's disease)

6.2 SHORT LIMB SKELETAL DYSPLASIA

RHIZOMELIC

(Proximal Limb Shortening)

1. *Achondroplasia*
   - Large skull with small base and sella and a small foramen magnum.
   - Short ribs with deep concavities to anterior ends.
   - Decreased interpedicular distance caudally in lumbar spine.
   - Short pedicles with narrow lumbar canal.

- Posterior scalloping with anterior vertebral body beaking.
- Square iliac wings with Champagne glass pelvic cavity.
- Rhizomelic micromelic with bowing of long bones.
- Trident hands.

2. *Hypochondroplasia*
   - Similar to achondroplasia except skull never affected.
   - Height normal or mildy reduced.

3. *Pseudochondroplasia*
   - Similar to achondroplasia.
   - Except that skull is normal.
   - No changes seen in 1st year of life.

4. *Chondrodysplasia punctata*
   - Stippling in long bone epiphysis, spine or larynx.

Mesomelic

(Middle Segment Shortening)

1. *Dyschondrosteosis*
   - Also known as Léri-Weill's disease.
   - Usually affects females.
   - Madelung's deformity.
   - Medial aspect of proximal/distal tibia defective with or without hypoplastic fibula.

2. *Mesomelic Dysplasia*
   - Type Langer.
   - Type Reinhardt-Pfeiffer.

Acromesomelic

(Middle and Distal Segment Shortening)

1. *Chondroectodermal Dysplasia*
   - Also known as Ellis-van Creveld syndrome.

- Paired long bones are short with dome-shaped metaphyses.
- Abnormal medial tibial plateau with defective epiphyses laterally.
- Postaxial polysyndactyly.
- Carpal fusions seen esp. capitate and hamate with delayed development of carpal bones.
- Partial/total absence of teeth.
- Abnormal hair and nails.
- Rib cage similar to asphyxiating thoracic dystrophy.

2. *Acromesomelic Dysplasia.*
3. *Mesomelic Dysplasia.*
   - Type Nievergelt.
   - Type Robinow.
   - Type Werner.

Acromelic

(Distal Segment Shortening)

1. *Asphyxiating Thoracic Dystrophy*
   - Also known as Jeune disease.
   - Thorax is stenotic.
   - Ribs are short and horizontal and clavicles are highly placed
   - Polydactyly.
2. *Peripheral Dysostoses*

6.3 SHORT SPINE SKELETAL DYSPLASIA

DISEASE

1. *Pseudoachondroplasia*
   Spinal abnormality besides short spine
   - Platyspondyly with exaggerated grooves for ring apophyses.
   - C_1 and C_2 dislocation.
   Other features
   - Short limbs.
     - Marked joints laxity.
2. *Spondylometaphyseal Dysplasia*
   Like type Kozowski.
   - Limb abnormalitis besides spine involvement.
3. *Spondyloepiphyseal Dysplasia*
   a. Dominant Variety.
      - Congenita.
      - Platyspondyly, maximal in thoracic spine.
   Other features
   - Severe tubular bone involvement.
     - Retinal detachment common.
   b. X-linked-tarda.
      Spinal abnormality besides short spine
      - Mounds of dense bone are found on superior and inferior surfaces of the posterior part of vertebral endplates.
   Other features
   - Tubular bones minimally affected.
     - Iliac wings are small.
     - Hip degeneration frequently occurs prematurely.
   c. Recessive.
      Spinal abnormality besides short limbs
      - Generalized platyspondyly of least severity.

Other features
Nil

4. **Diastrophic Dwarfism**
Spinal abnormality besides other limb abnormalities
   – Interpedicular narrowing in lumbar spine.
      – Progressive kyphoscoliosis.
   Other features
   – Delta-shaped epiphyses.
   – Hitch Hiker thumb.

5. **Metatrophic Dwarfism**
Spinal abnormality besides limb abnormalities
   – Hypoplastic odontoid.
      – Severe progressive scoliosis.
   Other features
   – Short limbs.
      – Dumb-bell-shaped long bones.

6. **Kniest Syndrome**
Spinal abnormality besides limb abnormalities
   – Platyspondyly.
   – Kyphoscoliosis.
   – Interpedicular narrowing of lumbar spine.
   Other features
   – Dumb-bell-shaped long bones.
   – Irregular epiphyses.
   – Limited and painful joint movements.

6.4   LETHAL NEONATAL DYSPLASIA

1. *Osteogenesis Imperfecta*

Type II
   – Lethal *in utero*/early infancy.
   – Sclera are dark blue.

- Bones are grossly demineralized with thin cortices.
- Numerous healed or healing rib fracture.
  - *Type IIA* – Long bones are short, broad and bowed.
    - Ribs are broad with continuous beading.
  - *Type IIB* – Long bones as in Type IIA.
    - Ribs show less or no beading.
  - *Type IIC* – Long bones are thinned and show multiple fractures
    - Ribs are too thin and beaded.
- Skull is enlarged with numerous wormian bones; Mineralization may be retarded.

2. *Thanatophoric Dwarfism*
   - Infants are stillborn or die immediately after birth.
   Rhizomelic Dwarfism with Bowing of Long Bones.
   - Metaphyses are irregular.
   - Epiphyses of knee absent.
   - Short, wide, metacarpals and phalanges.
   - Marked platyspondyly with 'H-shaped' vertebra on AP view of spine.
   - Poor mineralization of pelvic bones with small square iliac blades.
   - Clover leaf skull.
   - Ribs are short and flared anteriorly.

3. *Chondrodysplasia Punctata*
   - Rhizomelic type (recessive) is lethal.
     - Stippling or punctate calcification of tarsus and carpus, long bone epiphyses, vertebral transverse processes and pubic bones.
     - Long bones show gross asymmetric shortening and metaphyseal irregularity.

4. *Asphyxiating Thoracic Dystrophy*—Patients die in infancy from respiratory distress.
   - Thorax is stenotic.

- Ribs are short and horizontal.
- Clavicles are highly placed.

5. *Campomelic Dwarfism*
   - Long bones are bowed.

6. *Achondrogenesis Type I and II*

7. *Short rib syndromes with or without polydactyly (Type I,II,III)*

8. *Homozygos achondroplasia*

9. *Hypophosphatasia—Gross general failure of Ossification of skeleton.*

6.5   DUMB-BELL-SHAPED LONG BONES

1. *Metatropic Dwarfism*—Short spine and short limb dwarfism.

2. *Pseudochondroplasia*—Short limb (Rhizomelic dwarfism).

3. *Kneist syndrome*—Short spine and short limb dwarfism.

4. *Diastrophic dwarfism*—Short spine and short limb dwarfism.

5. *Osteogenesis Imperfecta*
   Type III– Sclera blue at birth but usually normal in adolescence.
   - Bones are demineralized.
   - Vertebral compression and kyphoscoliosis.
   - Long bones shows multiple fracture and bowing.
   - Sutures are wide with multiple wormian bones.
   - Dentinogenesis imperfecta.

6. *Chondroectodermal Dysplasia*—Acromesomelic dwarfism with ectodermal dysplasia.

6.6 MUCOPOLYSACCHARIDOSES AND MUCOLIPIDOSIS

- They are characterized by constellation of radiological signs related to skeletal system and share some common characteristics as:
  a. Abnormal bone texture
  b. Widening of diaphyses.
  c. Tilting of distal radius and ulna towards each other.
  d. Pointing of proximal ends of metacarpals.
  e. Large skull with calvarial thickening.
  f. Anterior beaking of upper lumbar vertebrae.
  g. J-shaped sella.
  h. Flared ilia.
  i. Fragmented femoral ossific nucleus.

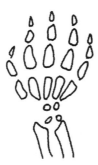

Fig. 6.6.1: Appendicular skeleton

6.7 MUCOLIPIDOSES

1. Type I (Neuraminidase deficiency)
2. Type II (I-cell disease)
3. Type III (Pseudopolydystrophy of Maroteaux)

CLASSIFICATION

Type	Eponym	Inheritance	Age of onset	Osseous abnormalities other than common characteristics	Other abnormalities
I-H	Hurler syndrome/ Gargoylism	Autosomal recessive	By 1-2 years	Nil	Corneal clouding. Severe neurological abnormalities
I-S (V)	Scheie syndrome	Autosomal recessive	Childhood	Nil	Carpal tunnel syndrome. Mild neurological abnormalities
II	Hunter syndrome	X-linked recessive	2-4 years	Nil	Nil, no corneal clouding Mild to moderate neurological changes
III	Sanfilippo syndrome	Autosomal recessive	Childhood	Nil	Nil. Severe neurological abnormalities
IV	Brailsford-Morquio syndrome	Autosomal recessive	1-3 years	Marked kyphosis due to short spine	Nil. No neurological changes
VI	Maroteaux-Lamy syndrome	Autosomal recessive	Childhood	Nil	Nil. No neurological abnormalities. Except meningeal involvement
VII	Sly syndrome	Autosomal recessive	—	Nil	Nil. Absent to severe neurological abnormality

6.8   GENERALIZED OSTEOSCLEROSIS

CHILDREN

i. *Dysplasias*
   - Osteopetrosis.
   - Pyknodysostosis.
   - Craniotubular dysplasia.
   - Craniotubular hyperostoses.
ii. *Metabolic*
   - Renal osteodystrophy.
iii. *Poisoning*
   - Lead   = Dense metaphyseal bands.
                 = Flask-shaped femora.
   - Fluorosis   = Thickened cortex with narrow medulla.
                 = Ossification of tendons, ligaments and interosseous membranes.
   - Hyper-   = Dense metaphyseal bands.
     vitaminoses D = Widened zone of provisional calcification.
                 = Soft tissue calcification.
   - Hyper-   = Subperiosteal new bone
     vitaminosis A formation.
                 = Reduced metaphyseal density.
iv. Idiopathic.
   - Caffey's disease.
   - Idiopathic hypercalcemia of infancy.

Adults

i. *Myeloproliferative.*
   = Myelosclerosis.

  =   Marrow cavity narrowed by endosteal reaction.
  –   Patchy lucencies due to fibrous tissue.

 ii. *Metabolic*
  –   Renal osteodystrophy.

 iii. *Poisoning*
  –   Fluorosis.
  •Similar as in children.

 iv. *Neoplastic*
  –   Osteoblastic metastases.
  –   Lymphoma.

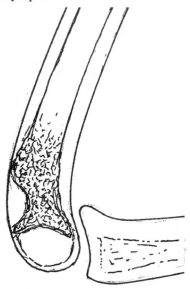

Fig. 6.8.1: Paget's disease: Early long-bone changes. Lateral view of the humerus in a middle-aged man shows an "advancing wedge" ("blade of grass" or "flame shadow") appearance at the end of the bone, characteristic of early Paget's disease. Since the disease process generally proceeds from one articular end of the long bone to the other, all three phases—early, intermediate and late—may be seen in the same bone

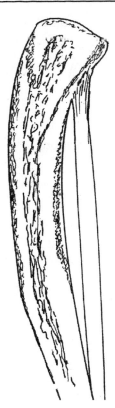

Fig. 6.8.2: Paget's disease: Late long-bone changes. Lateral view of the tibia shows anterior bowing secondary to late-phase

  – Mastocytosis.
  = Sclerosis of marrow with patchy areas of lucency.
  v. *Idiopathic*
    – Paget's disease.
    = Coarsened trabeculae.
    = Bone expansion.

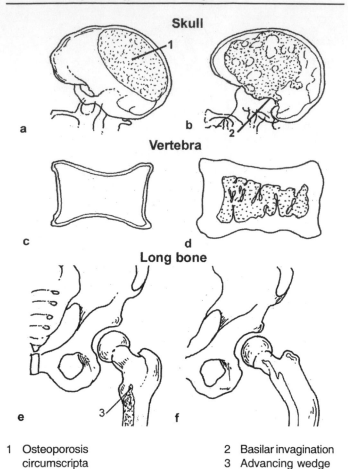

1 Osteoporosis circumscripta
2 Basilar invagination
3 Advancing wedge

Fig. 6.8.3: Progression of Paget's disease: a, c, and e Early (osteolytic) "hot" phase and b, d, f late (osteoblastic) "cold" phase manifestations of Paget's disease in (a, b) the skull, (c, d) vertebrae, and (e, f) long bones, a Osteoporosis circumscripta, b. "Cotton-wool" appearance. c. Biconcave vertebra. d. "Picture frame" ivory vertebra. e. "Flame," "blade of grass" deformities. f. Dense, larger diameter deformities

6.9 SCLEROTIC BONE LESIONS

DEVELOPMENTAL

i. *Single*

a. *Fibrous Dysplasia.*

b. *Bone Islands* (Enostosis)
   = Round/Oval dense lesion in medullary location with radiating thorn like spicules.
   = Usually <15 mm.
   = Grow upto skeletal maturity.

ii. *Multiple*

a. *Bone Islands.*

b. *Fibrous Dysplasia.*
   = Cyst like lesion in diaphysis or metaphysis with endosteal scalloping +/- bone expansion with thick sclerotic border (rind sign)
   = Age =3 to 15 years.

c. *Osteopoikilosis/Osteopathia Condensans Disseminata*
   = Dense round/Oval/Lancelete lesion arranged parallel to long axis of bone.
   = Seen usually at ends of long bones and around joints; in the carpus and tarsus.
   = No interval change.

d. *Osteopathia Striata/Voorhoeve's Disease*
   Sclerotic striations in long bones parallel to long axis affecting both diaphysis and metaphyses.

e.   *Tuberous Sclerosis*
    = Patchy, sclerotic lesions in skull, vertebrae, pelvis and long bones with irregular periosteal new bone formation.

Vascular

- Bone infarcts.
  (Single/Multiple)
- an in sickle cell anemia.
- = Sclerotic lesions in femoral or humeral head in medullary bone.
- = Sharply defined or ill-defined diffuse sclerosis.

Traumatic

- Callus (Single/multiple fracture sites)

Infective
- Sclerosing osteomyelitis of Garré.
- = Localized gross sclerosis in absence of apparent bone destruction.

Idiopathic
- Paget's disease.
  (Single/Multiple)
- = Coarsened trabeculae, cortical thickening and bone expansion.
- = Encroachment of medullary cavity with epiphyseal involvement as well.
- = "Cotton-Wool spots" in skull.

Neoplastic
  i. Single

a. Metastases.
b. Lymphoma. *De novo* or after RT of a lytic lesion)
c. Osteoma.
   = Usually skull, PNS and mandible.
d. = Ivory or dense type; spongy or trabeculated type. Broad based with smooth well-defined margins.
e. *Osteoid Osteoma*
   = Round/oval radiolucent lesion with dense surrounding sclerosis with a central nidus <1cm.
   = Lesion sited in relation to cortical bone with dense scleroses extending into medullary cavity as well.
f. *Osteoblastoma*
   = Similar to osteoid osteoma but central radiolucency is larger approx. 2-10 cm in diameter.

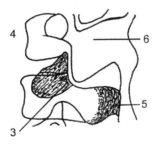

Fig. 6.9.1: Osteoid osteoma. The frontal projection shows an enlarged, dense right pedicle (3) and pars interarticularis (5), characteristic of osteoid osteoma (compare with normal pedicle on left (4 & 6).

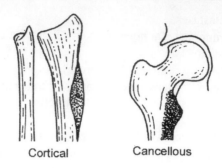

Cortical   Cancellous

Fig. 6.9.2: Osteoid osteoma

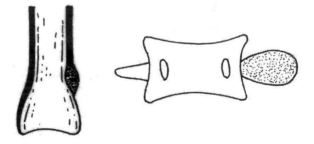

Fig. 6.9.3: Nonossifying fibroma (A) and osteoblastoma (B)

   g. *Primary Bone Sarcoma*
- = Commonest being osteosarcoma.
- ≃ Wide zone of transition with periosteal reaction and soft tissue extension.
- – Healed/Healing benign or malignant bone lesions as lytic areas following RT on CT, bone cyst, fibrous cortical defect, etc.

  ii. *Multiple*
- – Metastases.
- – Lymphoma.

–   Osteomas.
 (Gardner's syndrome).
=   Osteomas, soft-tissue tumors, polyposis coli)

d. *Mastocytosis*
  = Circumscribed areas of increased density due to thickening of medullary trabeculae.
  = Coarsened appearance of bone with indistinct endosteum.

e. *Multifocal Osteosarcomas*
  – Multiple myeloma.
  = in 2 to 3%

f. *Multiple healed/healing benign or malignant bone lesions.*

6.10 BONE SCLEROSIS ASSOCIATED WITH PERIOSTEAL REACTION

Traumatic

- Healing fractures with callus formation.

Neoplastic

- Metastases.
- Lymphoma.
- Osteoid osteoma/osteoblastoma.
- Osteosarcoma.
- Ewing's sarcoma.
- Chondrosarcoma.

Infective

- Osteomyelitis.
- Syphilis.

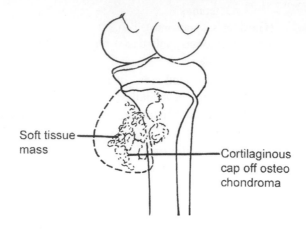

Fig. 6.10.1: Chondrosarcoma (peripheral)

Idiopathic

  i. *Infantile Cortical Hyperostoses (Caffey's disease)*
      = Age of onset is 9 weeks.
      – Marked periosteal proliferation and cortical thickening beneath soft tissue swellings.
      = Bones affected are mandible, ribs, scapula, ulna and any other bone except phalanges and spine.
      = In long bones, diaphyses is only involved.
 ii. *Melorheostosis/Leri's Disease*
      = Dense irregular bone running along cortex of long bone both externally and internally.
        (Dripping candle wax appearance).
      = Lower limbs are commonly involved.
      = Lesions are segmental and unilateral in distribution.

6.11 SOLITARY SCLEROTIC LESION WITH LUCENT CENTER

NEOPLASTIC

  i. *Osteoid Osteoma*
- Central lucent center <1 cm.

  ii. *Osteoblastoma*
- Central lucency
- 2-10 cm in diameter.

Infective

  i. *Brodie's Abscess*
- Metaphyseal lytic lesion with surrounding sclerosis.
- Tunnelling toward epiphyseal plate is pathognomonic.

  ii. *Granulomatous*
(Syphilis, Tuberculosis).

6.12 COARSE TRABECULAR PATTERN OF BONE

1. Paget's Disease:
   - Expansion of bone is associated.
2. Osteoporosis ⎤ — Resorption of secondary
3. Osteomalacia ⎦ trabeculae produces prominent and thickened primary trabeculae.
4. Hemoglobinopathies
   - Esp. thalassemia
   - Expansion of marrow cavity destroys medullary trabeculae.

5. Hemangioma
   - Of vertebral bodies produces vertical coarse trabecular pattern with slight expansion (caudry cloth appearance).
6. Renal osteodystrophy
   - Associated sclerosis and subperiosteal bone formation is evident.
7. Osteonecrosis
   - Cystic defects with coarse trabecular pattern; periostitis and increased bone density may be seen if infection is causative factor.
8. Fibrogenesis imperfecta ossium
   - Obliteration of trabecular architecture with coarsening of remaining trabeculae.
9. Gaucher's disease
   - Associated with hypoplasia of vertebral bodies, thining of cortices of tubular bones and subperiosteal new bone formation.
10. Neoplasms as chondromyxoid fibroma where new bone is laid in pattern of coarse trabeculae.

6.13 RELATIONSHIP OF METASTATIC LESIONS TO THE PRIMARY TUMORS

Location of primary tumor/ variety of primary tumor	Characteristic of metastatic lesions			
	Lytic	Blastic	Mixed	Expansile
1. Bronchogenic carcinoma	√			
2. Bronchogenic carcinoid		√		
3. Breast	√		√	

Contd...

Contd...

Location of primary tumor/ variety of primary tumor	Characteristic of metastatic lesions			
	Lytic	Plastic	Mixed	Expansile
4. Gastric carcinoma		√	√	
5. Colon	√	√ (occasionally)		
6. Rectum	√			
7. Renal cell carcinoma	√			
8. Wilms' tumor	√			√
9. Bladder		√	√	
10. Prostate		√		
11. Thyroid	√			
12. Pheochromocytoma				√
13. Adrenal carcinoma	√			
14. Neuroblastoma	√			√
15. Cervix	√			√ (rarely)
16. Uterus	√			√
17. Ovary	√			
18. Testes	√		√ (rarely)	
19. Squamous cell carcinoma of skin	√			
20. Melanoma	√			√

6.14 CHILDHOOD TUMORS METASTASIZING TO BONE

1. Neuroblastoma.
2. Leukemias and lymphoma.
3. Clear cell sarcoma (Variant of Wilms' Tumor)

4. Rhabdomyosarcoma.
5. Retinoblastoma.
6. Ewing's sarcoma.
7. Osteosarcoma.

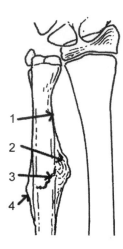

Fig. 6.14.1: Ewing's sarcoma. A permeative destructive lesion can be observed in the diaphysis of the distal ulna. Fracture callus merges with a "sunburst" periosteal reaction. The cortex on the radial aspect of the ulna is destroyed by a soft-tissue mass growing out into the soft tissue. A short, oblique pathologic fracture is also evident. Ewing's sarcoma cannot be differentiated radiologically from a nonHodgkin's lymphoma, the latter occurs in an older age group (third and fourth decades). Differentiation from osteomyelitis can be difficult, however, unlike Ewing's sarcoma, metaphyseal involvement is usually a prominent feature of childhood osteomyelitis (See labelling next page)

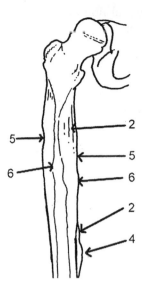

1 Destructive lesion
2 Soft-tissue mass
3 Pathologic fracture
4 Periosteal reaction
5 "Saucerization"
6 Well-organized periosteal reaction

Fig. 6.14.2: Ewing's tumor

6.15 BUBBLY BONE LESIONS

NEOPLASTIC

i. *Benign*
   1. GCT
   2. Angiomas

     3. Chondromyxoid fibroma
     4. Enchondroma
  ii. *Malignant*
     1. GCT
     2. Osteoblastoma
     3. Multiple myeloma
     4. Metastases (Kidney and Thyroid)

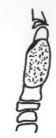

Infection

Fig. 6.15.1: Enchondroma

1. Brodie's abscess.
2. Coccidioidomycosis.
3. Echinococcus.

Endocrinal

1. Hyperparathyroidism.

Tumor Like Lesions
1. Nonossifying fibroma.
2. Aneurysmal bone cyst.
3. Simple cyst.

Idiopathic
1. Histiocytosis X.
2. Fibrous dysplasia.

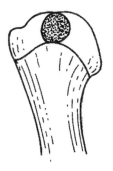 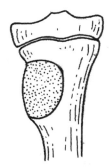

Fig. 6.15.2: Chondroblastoma   **Fig. 6.15.3:** Chondromyxoid fibroma

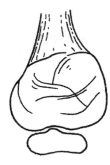

Fig. 6.15.4: Aneurysmal
bone cyst

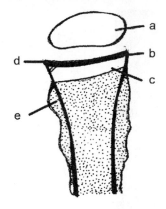

Fig. 6.15.5: Scurvy
a. Loss of epiphyseal density
with a pencil thin cortex
(Wimberger's sign)
b. Dense zone of provisional
calcification
c. Metaphyseal lucency
(Trummerfield zone)
d. Metaphyseal corner
fracture - Pelken Spur
e. Subperiosteal hematoma

6.16 PRIMARY BONE TUMORS: CLINICAL FEATURES, SITE OF PREDILECTION, RADIOLOGICAL PRESENTATION

Tumor	Age (Decades)	Sex ratio	Location	Radiologic presentation
1. Simple bone cyst	1st, 2nd	2:1	Proximal humerus, proximal femur	Expansile, well-defined medullary lucency with sclerotic margin
2. Aneurysmal bone cyst	1st, 2nd	1:1	Posterior vertebral arch, metaphysis of long bone	Medullary, expansile lucency abutting growth plate, marked attenuation of cortices, buttressing and lesion wider then growth plate are characteristic
3. Fibrous cortical defect	1st	1:1	Distal femur, proximal tibia	Oval lucency in cortex with fine sclerotic margins continuous with cortex
4. Nonossifying fibroma	1st, 2nd	1:1	Distal femur, proximal tibia	Cortical lucency with wavy sclerotic margin with penetration into medullary space

Contd...

Contd...

Tumor	Age (Decades)	Sex ratio	Location	Radiologic presentation
5. Enchondroma	3rd, 4th	1:1	Long tubular bone, tubular bones of hand	Lucent, expansile medullary lesion with characteristic punctate or 'pop-corn' calcification.
6. Chondroblastoma	2nd	2:1	Epiphyses (Usually before closure of growth plate)	Lucent epiphyseal lesion with areas of calcification.
7. Chondromyxoid fibroma	2nd, 3rd	Slight male preponderance	Lower extremities (Periarticular)	Eccentric, expansile lesion with thick sclerotic margin with or without foci of calcification
8. Polyostotic fibrous dysplasia	1st, 2nd	—	Proximal femur, innominate bones, skull facial bones	Multiple expansile lesions with variable amount of sclerosis with or without pathologic fractures
9. Monostotic fibrous dysplasia	2nd, 3rd	—	Ribs, proximal femur and tibia ,facial bones	Localized medullary expansile lesion with sclerotic margin and faint calcification

Contd...

Contd...

Tumor	Age (Decades)	Sex ratio	Location	Radiologic presentation
10. Osteochondroma	1st to 3rd	Slight male preponderance	End of long tubular bones, scapula, rib, innominate bone, spine	Sessile or pedunculated exostosis with cortices and medulla continuous with the parent bone
11. Osteoblastoma	2nd, 3rd	1:1	Spine, long tubular bone, small bones of hands and feet	Eccentric oval lucency (nidus) with surrounding sclerosis involving both cortical and medullary region with periosteal reaction and buttressing (Size of nidus >2 cm)
12. Osteoid osteoma	2nd	2:1	Proximal femur, tibia, posterior vertebral arch	Oval lucency with surrounding sclerosis (Size of lucency <1 cm)
13. Giant cell tumor	3rd, 4th	1:1	Articular ends of femur, tibia or tibia after epiphyseal closure	An expansile, subarticular, lucent lesion with no or minimal reactive sclerosis

Contd...

Contd...

Tumor	Age (Decades)	Sex ratio	Location	Radiologic presentation
14. Ewing's sarcoma	1st, 2nd	3:1	Long tubular bones, pelvis, vertebrae, ribs, scapula	Permeative destruction with extensive periosteal reaction with large soft tissue component producing saucerization in the diaphyseal region
15. Fibrosarcoma	3rd, 6th	1:1	Pelvis, facial bones, long tubular bones	Localized, expansile destructive and permeative lesion
16. Reticulum cell sarcoma	4th, 5th	—	Pelvis, femur	Permeative destructive lesion with no sclerosis
17. Malignant fibrous histiocytoma	Any age	Slight male preponderance	Femur, tibia, humerus, ribs, skull, facial bones	Well-defined destructing lesion with no sclerosis and often soft tissue extension
18. Eosinophilic granuloma	1st to 3rd	1:1	Any bone	Well-defined destructive lesion with no sclerosis in inactive or resolving stage

Contd...

Contd...

Tumor	Age (Decades)	Sex ratio	Location	Radiologic presentation
19. Multiple myeloma	7th, 8th	Slight male preponderance	Axial skeleton	Well-defined destructive lesion in medullary cavity with endosteal erosion; no sclerosis or soft tissue mass
20. Central chondrosarcoma	5th, 6th	-do-	Pelvis, femur, tibia, humerus	Destructive medullary lesion with cortical destruction; soft tissue component and soft tissue calcification
21. Osteosarcoma	2nd, 3rd	-do-	Distal femur, proximal tibia	Subcortical sclerotic lesion with cortical destruction periosteal reaction and soft tissue component
22. Juxtacortical osteosarcoma	3rd, 4th	1:1	Distal femur (Posterior Cortex)	Well-demarcated sclerotic lesion with periosteal reaction but no soft tissue component

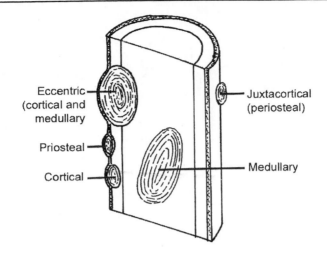

Fig. 6.16.1: Locations of tumors within bone

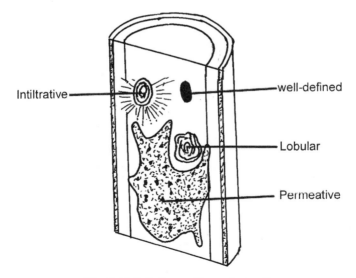

Fig. 6.16.2: Patterns of bone destruction

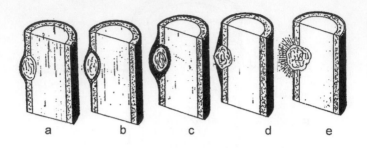

Fig. 6.16.3: Types of periosteal reaction (a) Well-organized (b) Buttress (c) Onion skin (d) Codman's triangle (e) Sunburst

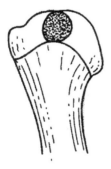

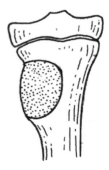

Fig. 6.16.4: Chondroblastoma   **Fig. 6.16.5:** Chondromyxoid fibroma

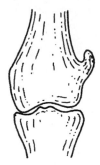

Fig. 6.16.6: Osteochondroma (Exostosis)

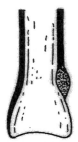

Fig. 6.16.7: Non-ossifying fibroma (Fibrous cortical defect)

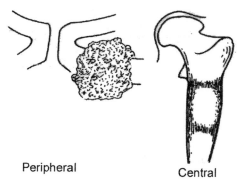

Peripheral

Central

Fig. 6.16.8: Chondrosarcoma

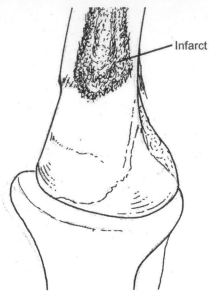

Fig. 6.16.9: Diaphyseal infarct. Lateral view of the distal femur in a 50-year-old man shows a typical diaphyseal infarct. This lesion, which is remote from the knee joint, was asymptomatic. The absence of punctate calcifications and lobular margins differentiates a bone infarct from an enchondroma

6.17 RADIOLOGIC CHARACTERISTICS OF BENIGN AND MALIGNANT BONE LESIONS

		Benign	*Malignant*
1.	Margination	Well-defined	Destructive, poorly defined
2.	Border	Sclerotic	Infiltrating
3.	Periosteal reaction	Less aggressive	More aggressive
4.	Zone of transition	Narrow	Wide
5.	Soft tissue mass	Absent	Present

6.18   SUBARTICULAR LYTIC BONE LESION

ARTHRITIDES

1. *Osteoarthritis*
   - Marginal osteophytes.
   - Subchondral sclerosis.
   - Reduced joint space.
   - Multiple cyst in load bearing regions.
2. *Rheumatoid Arthritis*
   - Cysts at/near the regions of capsular insertion.
   - Joint space narrowing.
   - Juxta-articular osteoporosis.
   - No sclerosis.
3. *Calcium Pyrophosphate Arthropathy*
   - More collapsed and fragmented articular surface.

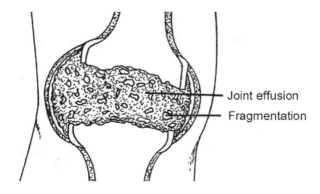

Fig. 6.18.1: Diarthrodial joint with neuropathic arthritis

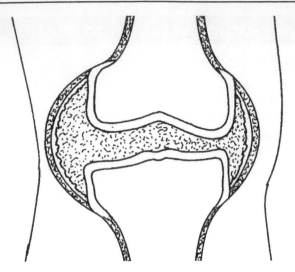

Fig. 6.18.2: Diarthrodial joint in lupus erythematosus

- Cysts larger than osteoarthritis
- Rest similar changes as in osteoarthritis
4. *Gout*
   - Punched out erosions with overhanging edge with adjacent soft tissue masses.
5. *Hemophilia*
   - Erosions and subchondral cyst with periarticular osteoporosis with Preserved joint space until late in disease.

Neoplastic

1. Metastases/multiple myeloma.
2. Aneurysmal bone cyst.
3. GCT.
4. Chondroblastoma.

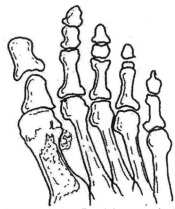

Fig. 6.18.3: Reiter's syndrome. Dorsiplantar projection of the foot shows marked resorption of the proximal side of the interphalangeal joint of the great toe resulting in a "mortar-in-pestile" or "pencil-in-cup" deformity. Note also resorption at the distal interphalangeal joint of the fourth toe, fusion of the distal interphalangeal joint of the fifth toe, and marginal erosion at the proximal interphalangeal joint of the fifth toe. Involvement of the distal interphalangeal joints is not uncommon in the arthritis of Reiter's syndrome

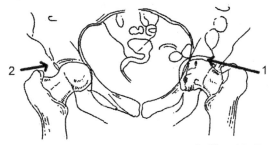

1. Medial wall of acetabulum   2. Iliopubic line

Fig. 6.18.4: Rheumatoid arthritis. Anteroposterior projection of the hips shows concentric narrowing of both hip joints with axial migration of the femoral heads resulting in protrusioacetabulum (i.e. the medial wall of the acetabulum is medial to the iliopubic line). The intense sclerosis of the left femoral head and left acetabulum indicates secondary osteoarthritis; however, osteophytes are absent

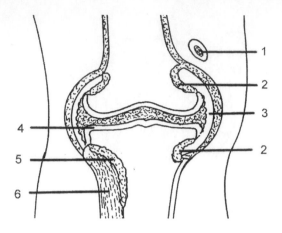

1 Subcutaneous nodule   2 Marginal erosion
3 Synovial hypertrophy   4 Diffuse articular loss
5 Enthesopathy   6 Tendon insertion

Fig. 6.18.5: Diarthrodial joint with rheumatoid arthritis

5. Pigmented Villonodular Synovitis.
   – Mainly lower limbs esp. knee.
   – Soft tissue mass.
   – Cyst like defects with sharp sclerotic margins.
   – Joint space destruction.

Miscellaneous

1. *Post-traumatic*
   Esp. in carpal bones.

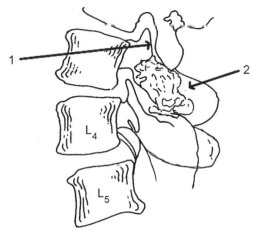

1 Posterior apophyseal joint   2 Hypertrophic bone

Fig. 6.18.6: Osteoarthritis of spine. Lateral tomogram of an old woman shows advanced degenerative change in the posterior apophyseal (facet) joints of the lumbar spine. Hypertrophic bone encroaches on the central spinal canal. Note also spondylolisthesis at L4-L5, with calcification in the outer fibers of the annulus fibrosus at this level. The intervertebral discs are relatively well-maintained. Note that the spinal apophyseal (facet) joints are synovial joints which may undergo degenerative change. The resulting sclerosis and hypertrophic bone may encroach upon the central spinal canal and produce a secondary form of spinal stenosis, as in this patient

2. *Osteonecrosis*
   - Associated sclerosis, collapse and fragmentation of trabeculae.
   - Preserved joint space.
3. *Tuberculosis*
   - Completely or partially epiphyseal or partly metaphyseal.
   - No sclerosis.

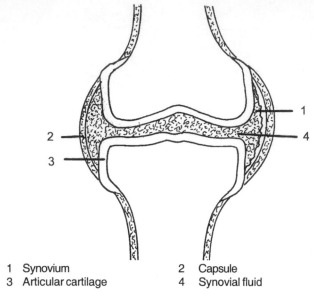

1 Synovium
2 Capsule
3 Articular cartilage
4 Synovial fluid

Fig. 6.18.7: Normal diarthrodial joint

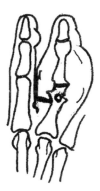

Fig. 6.18.8: Chronic tophaceous gout

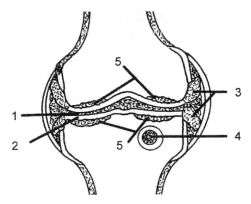

1 Joint-space narrowing 2 Diffuse articular loss
3 Osteophytes 4 Subchondral cyst
5 Subchondral sclerosis

Fig. 6.18.9: Osteoarthritis of diarthrodial joint

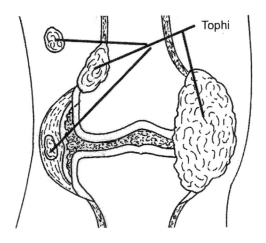

Fig. 6.18.10: Diarthrodial joint with chronic tophaceous gout

6.19   OSTEOLYTIC DEFECT IN THE MEDULLA

WELL-DEFINED

i. *Nonexpansile*
   a. *Marginal Sclerosis*
      • *Unilocular*
         – Geode (associated with arthritis).
         – Healing benign/malignant osseous lesion.
         – Brodie's abscess.
         – Simple bone cyst.
         – Enchondroma.
         – Chondroblastoma.
         – Fibrous dysplasia.
      • *Multilocular*
         – Fibrous dysplasia.
         – Simple bone cyst.
   b. *No marginal Sclerosis*
      – Metastases.
      – Multiple myeloma.

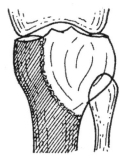 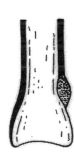 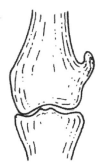

Fig. 6.19.1: Giant cell tumor   **Fig. 6.19.2:** Non-ossifying fibroma   **Fig. 6.19.3:** Osteochondroma (Exostosis)

      – Eosinophilic granuloma.
      – Brown tumor of hyperparathyroidism.
      – Enchondroma.
      – Chondroblastoma.

ii. *Expansile*
- *Eccentric expansile*
  - Giant cell tumor.
  - Aneurysmal bone cyst.
  - Enchondroma.
  - Nonossifying fibroma.
  - Chondromyxoid fibroma.
- *Grossly Expansile*
  - Malignant lesions.
  - Metastases.
  - Plasmacytoma.
  - Central chondrosarcoma.
  - Telangiectatic osteosarcoma.
- *Benign lesions*
  - Aneurysmal bone cyst.
  - GCT.
  - Enchondroma.
- *Nonneoplastic*
  - Fibrous dysplasia.
  - Hemophilic pseudotumor.
  - Brown tumor of hyperparathyroidism.
  - Hydatid disease.

Ill-defined

i. *Without Periosteal Reaction*
- *Nonexpansile*
  - Metastases.
  - Multiple myeloma.

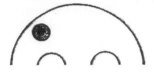

Fig. 6.19.4: Hemangioma of bone

- Hemangioma.
- Lymphoma.
- Malignant fibrous histiocytoma.
- *Expansile*
  - Chondrosarcoma.
  - Giant cell tumor.
  - Metastases from kidney/thyroid.
  - Fibrosarcoma.
ii. *With Periosteal Reaction*
  - Osteomyelitis.
  - Ewing's sarcoma.
  - Osteosarcoma.

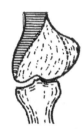

Fig. 6.19.5: Osteosarcoma

6.20 LUCENT BONE LESION CONTAINING BONE/CALCIUM

NEOPLASTIC

1. Metastases esp. breast.
2. Chondroid lesions.
   - Benign
     - Enchondroma.

- Chondroblastoma.
  Chondromyxoid fibroma
- Malignant
  - Chondrosarcoma.
3. *Osteoid Lesions*
  - Benign
    - Osteoid osteoma.
    - Osteoblastoma.
  - Malignant
    - Osteosarcoma.
4. *Fibrous Tissue Lesions*
  - Malignant
    - Fibrosarcoma.
    - Malignant fibrous histiocytoma.

Miscellaneous

- Fibrous dysplasia.
- Osteoporosis circumscripta
  (Paget's disease).
- Avascular necrosis/infarction of bone.
- Osteomyelitis with sequestrum.
- Eosinophilic granuloma.
- Intraosseous lipoma.

6.21 COMMON LYTIC BONE LESIONS

WITH MARKED SCLEROSIS

- Brodie's abscess.
- Osteoblastoma.
- Osteoid osteoma.
- Stress fracture.
- Tuberculosis.

Multiple

- Fibrous dysplasia.
- Enchondroma.
- Eosinophilic granuloma.
- Metastases.
- Multiple myeloma.
- Brown tumors in hyperparathyroidism.

Seen <30 years of age

- Chondroblastoma.
- Aneurysmal bone cyst.
- Infection.
- Nonossifying fibroma.
- Eosinophilic granuloma.
- Solitary bone cyst.

Seen on both sides of joint
- Synovioma.
- Angioma.
- Chondroid lesion.

6.22 LOCATION OF SOME COMMON NEOPLASM/LESIONS

EPIPHYSIS

- Chondroblastoma.
- Giant cell tumor.
- Intraosseous ganglion.

Metaphysis

- Nonossifying fibroma.
- Chondromyxoid fibroma.

- Simple bone cyst.
  Osteochondroma
- Brodie's abscess.
- Giant cell tumor.
- Osteosarcoma.
- Chondrosarcoma.

Diaphysis

- Ewing's sarcoma.
- Nonossifying fibroma.
- Simple bone cyst.
- Enchondroma.
- Fibrous dysplasia.
- Osteochondroma.

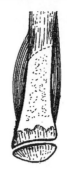

Fig. 6.22.1: Ewing's sarcoma

6.23 SEPTATED BONE LESIONS

Lesions	Type of septations
1. Aneurysmal bone cysts	Delicate, horizontally oriented
2. Chondromyxoid fibroma	Coarse, thick
3. Giant cell tumor	Delicate, thin
4. Hemangioma	Striated, radiating
5. Nonossifying fibroma	Lobulated

6.24 MOTH-EATEN BONE

Characterized by multiple, scattered lytic lesions of varying sizes with no major central lesion, less well-defined/demarcated lesional margin with larger zones of transition.

1. Neoplastic
   1. Metastasis/multiple myeloma-including neuroblastoma in child.
   2. Leukemias/lymphomas.
   3. Ewing's sarcoma.
   4. Osteosarcoma/chondrosarcoma.
   5. Fibrosarcoma and malignant fibrous histiocytoma.
   6. Histiocytosis X/ Langerhans' cell histiocytosis.
2. Infective.
   - Osteomyelitis.

6.25   OSTEOPENIA

GENERALIZED

1. Osteoporosis (diminished osteoid production)
   - In axial skeleton and appendicular skeleton.
     - Decreased number and thickness of trabeculae.
     - Cortical thinning.
     - Juxta-articular osteopenia with trabecular bone predominance.
     - Delayed fracture healing with poor callus formation.
   - In spine only.
     - Diminished radiographic density.
     - Increased vertical striations.
     - Prominence of endplates.
     - Picture framing and compression deformities with protrusion of disks.
   a. *Congenital*
     - Osteogenesis imperfecta.
     - Turner's syndrome.
     - Homocystinuria.
     - Neuromuscular disease.

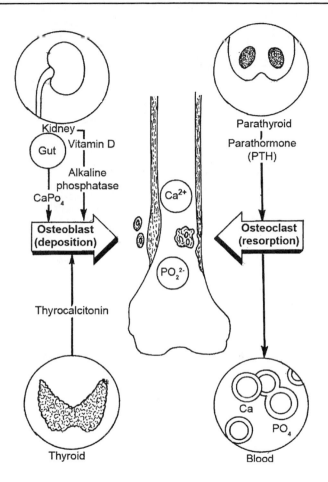

Fig. 6.25.1: Factors affecting resorption (Osteoclastic activity) and deposition (Osteoblastic activity) of calcium and phosphorus

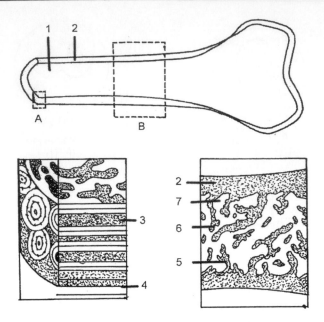

1 Medulla	5 Spongiosa
2 Cortex	6 Osteocytes
3 Haversian canal	7 Marrow
4 Lacunae with osteocytes	

Fig. 6.25.2: Normal bone. Cross-sectional anatomy of normal adult bone indicating osteocytes and their effect on bone metabolism. Inset A: Location of osteocytes within bone cortex. Inset B: Location of osteocytes within bone spongiosa. Note the conduits of metabolite transport within each area: Haversian canals in the cortex, vascular marrow in the medulla

- Mucopolysaccharidosis
- Trisomy 13 and 18.
- Pseudo- and pseudohypoparathyroidism.

   – Glycogen storage disease.

   – Progeria.

b. *Idiopathic*
- Juvenile   : < 20 yrs.
- Adult   : 20-40 yrs.
- Postmenopausal : > 50 yrs.
- Senile   : > 60 yrs.

c. *Miscellaneous*
- Renal osteodystrophy.
- Disuse: immobilization.
- Collagen disease and rheumatoid arthritis.
- Bone marrow replacement by leukemia/lymphoma, multiple myeloma/metastases.
- Drugs
  (Heparin, steroids, methotrexate, vit A)
- Radiation therapy.

d. *Nutritional Deficiency*
- Scurvy.
- PEM.
- Calcium deficiency.

e. *Endocrinopathy*
- Hypogonadism.
- Cushing's syndrome.
- Hyperthyroidism.
- Hyperparathyroidism.
- Acromegaly.
- Addison's disease.
- Diabetes mellitus.
- Pregnancy.
- Mastocytosis.

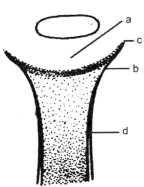

Fig. 6.25.3: Rickets
a. Widened growth plate
b. Fraying, splaying and cupping of metaphysis
c. Thinbony spur
d. Indistinct cortex

2. *Osteomalacia*—accumulation of excessive amounts of uncalcified osteoid with bone softening.
   - Uniform osteopenia.
   - Fuzzy indistinct trabecular detail of endosteal surface.
   - Thin cortices of long bone
   - Coarsened, frayed trabeculae decreased in number and size
   - Bone deformity from softening
     - Hourglass thorax
     - Bowing of long bones
     - Buckled/compressed pelvis
   - Increased incidence of fractures, biconcave vertical bodies
   - Mottled skull and pseudofracture

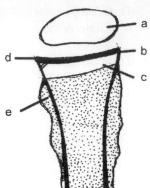

Fig. 6.25.4: Scurvy
a. Loss of epiphyseal density with pencil thin cortex
b. Dense zone of provisional calcification
c. Metaphyseal lucency
d. Pelken spur
e. Subperiosteal hematoma

Causes of Osteomalacia

- Dietary deficiency of vitamin D_3 and lack of solar irradiation
- Deficiency of metabolism of vitamin D
  - Chronic renal tubular disease
  - Chronic administration of phenobarbitone
  - Diphenylhydantoin
- Decreased absorption of vitamin D
  - Malabsorption syndrome
  - Partial gastrectomy

- Decreased deposition of calcium in bone
  - Diphosphonatos
  - (Used for treatment of Paget's disease)
3. *Hyperparathyroidism*—Increase bone resorption by osteoblasts.
   Causes: Adenoma (commonest), hyperplasia, carcinoma, ectopi hormone production, etc.)
   - Loss of fine trabeculae with ground glass appearance
   - Subperiosteal bone resorption affecting radial side of middle phalanx of middle finger, medial proximal tibia, lateral end of clavicle, symphysis pubis, ischial tuberosity, medial femoral neck, dorsum sellae, superior surface of ribs and proximal humerus
   - Cortical tunnelling producing 'basketwork' appearance and 'pepperpot' skull
   - Brown tumors in mandible, ribs, pelvis and femora
   - Bone softening leading to basilar invagination, wedged or codfish vertebra, triradiate pelvis, pathological fracture
   - Soft tissue calcification
   - Marginal erosion at DIP, ulnar side of base of little finger metacarpal and hamate with normal joint space
   - Chondrocalcinosis and periarticular calcification (Capsular and tendenous)
4. *Diffusely infiltrating bone disease*
   - For example: Multiplc mycloma, lcukcmia, metastases.

Localized/Regional

1. *Disuse* due to local immobilization secondary to fractures, neuromuscular paralysis.
   Pattern of bone loss:
   - Uniform (Commonest)
   - Spotty (Periarticular)
   - Bandlike (metaphyseal or subchondral)

- Endosteal cortical scalloping.
- Linear cortical lucencies.

2. *Sudeck's atrophy*
   (Reflex sympathetic dystrophy)
   - associated with post-traumatic/postinfective states, myocardial infarction, calcific tendinitis, cervical spondylosis.
   - Affects shoulder and hands.
   - Disuse osteoporosis.
   - Subperiosteal bone erosion.
   - Small periarticular erosions.

3. *Transient osteoporosis of hip*
   - Severe, progressive, osteoporosis of femoral head, neck, acetabulum.
   - Full recovery in 6 months.

4. *Regional migratory osteoporosis*
   - Swelling and osteoporosis of joints of lower limbs.
   - Migratory nature differentiates it from other cause.

5. Osteolytic tumor.

6. Lytic phase of Paget's disease.

7. Inflammation—rheumatoid arthritis, osteomyelites, tuberculosis.

8. Early phase of bone infarct and hemorrhage.

9. Burns and frostbite.

6.26A PERIOSTEAL REACTIONS— TYPES AND CONDITIONS

A. CONTINUOUS

a. Cortex Destroyed

1. Simple shell-like or expanded cortex.

2. Lobulated shell like.

3. Ridged shell—trabeculated or soap bubble like.

Causes
- Giant cell tumor.
- Aneurysmal bone cyst.
- Enchondroma.
- Nonossifying fibroma.
- Chondromyxoid fibroma.
- Expansile metastases.
- Plasmacytoma.
- Central chondrosarcoma.
- Telangiectatic osteosarcoma.
- Fibrous dysplasia.
- Hemophilic pseudotumor.
- Brown tumor of hyperparathyroidism.
- Hydatid.

b. **Intact Cortex**

1. Solid—even, uniform thickness >1 mm, persistent and unchanged for week.

Patterns
- Thin—Eosinophilic granuloma, osteoid osteoma.
- Dense undulating—Vascular disease.
- Thin undulating—Pulmonary osteoarthropathy.
- Dense elliptical—Osteoid osteoma, long-standing malignant disease.
- Cloaking—Storage disease, chronic infection.

2. *Unilamellar*

- Osteomyelitis.
- Histiocytosis.
- Benign tumors.
- Healing fractures.

3. *Multilamellar*

- Osteomyelitis.
- Histiocytosis.
- Aneurysmal bone cyst.
- Ewing's sarcoma.
- Osteosarcoma.

4. *Parallel spiculated—Hair on end*

- Ewing's sarcoma.
- Osteosarcoma.
- Metastases.
- Thalassemia.
- Syphilis.
- Infantile cortical hyperostoses.

B. INTERRUPTED

1. Buttressing

- Solid periosteal bone is formed at lateral extraosseous margin of growing bone lesion, e.g.: Ewing's sarcoma.

2. Codman's triangle—angular periosteal configuration with underlying cortex.

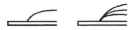

E.g.: – Hemorrhage.
   – Malignancy (osteosarcoma, Ewing's sarcoma).
   – Acute osteomyelitis.
   – Fracture.
   – Hemangioma.
3. Parallel or spiculated.

– Osteosarcoma.
– Ewing's sarcoma.
– Chondrosarcoma.
– Fibrosarcoma.
– Leukemia.
– Metastases.
– Acute osteomyelitis.

C. COMPLEX

1. Divergent spiculated.
   "Sunray" appearance.

– Osteosarcoma.
– Metastases (Colorectal).
– Ewing's sarcoma.
– Hemangioma.
– Meningioma.
– Tuberculosis.
– Tropical ulcer.

2. *Combination types*
   – Ewing's sarcoma.
   – Osteosarcoma.

6.26B PERIOSTEAL REACTION

SOLITARY AND LOCALIZED

1. Traumatic.
2. Inflammatory/infective.
3. Neoplastic
   – Benign.
   – Malignant.

Bilateral Involvement

a. *Symmetrical*
   1. *Vascular Insufficiency*
      (Venous, lymphatic, arterial)
      – Usually confined to lower limbs.
      – Soft tissue swelling is seen.
      – Solid, undulating periosteal reaction.
      – Phleboliths seen in venous causes.
   2. *Hypertrophic Osteoarthropathy*
      – Periosteal reaction seen in metaphysis and diaphysis of radius, ulna, tibia, fibula, less commonly femur and humerus and bones of hands and feet.
      – Thickness of periosteal reaction corresponds to duration of disease.
      – Periarticular osteoporosis, soft tissue swelling and joint effusions seen.
   3. *Pachydermoperiostoses*
      – Self-limited, familial condition, affecting boys at puberty with predilection for blacks.

- Bone affected are radius and ulna, tibia, fibula mainly followed by bones of hands and feet.
- Periosteal reaction is solid and spiculated and also involves the epiphysis in addition metaphysis and diaphysis.

4. *Thyroid Acropachy*
   - Solid, spiculated, lace-like periosteal reaction affecting diaphysis of metacarpals and phalanges of hands and less commonly of feet.

5. *Fluorosis*

   Solid undulating periosteal reaction in long bones, flat bone with osteosclerosis, ligamentous and interosseous membranous-calcification.

b. *Asymmetrical*
   1. Arthritides
      - Rheumatoid arthritis
      - Psoriatic arthropathy
   2. Metastases
   3. Disseminated osteomyelitis
   4. Osteoporosis/osteomalacia
      - Multiple fractures
   5. Nonaccidental injuries
   6. Bleeding diathesis
   7. Hand foot syndrome (Sickle cell dactylitis)
   8. Idiopathic
      - Degenerative

6.27 PERIOSTEAL REACTION IN CHILDHOOD

BENIGN

1. Physiological
   - Symmetrical involvement of diaphysis during 1st 6 months of life.
2. Battered child syndrome.
3. Infantile cortical hyperostoses (<6 months of age)
   - Mandible, clavicles and ribs usually affected.
4. Hypervitaminosis A.
5. Scurvy/rickets.
6. Osteogenesis imperfecta.
7. Congenital syphilis
   - Usually diaphyseal.
8. Drugs like Prostaglandins E1 to treat ductus dependent CHD.
9. Eosinophilic granuloma.
10. Osteomyelitis/trauma.
11. Sickle cell disease.
12. Kinky hair syndrome.

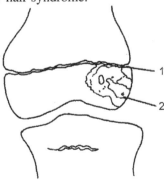

1 Destructive lesion   2 Involucrum

Fig. 6.27.1: Epiphyseal abscess. Anteroposterior views shows a well-demarcated destructive lesion in the epiphysis. The joint is normal

13. Juvenile chronic arthritis.
    – Bilaterally symmetrical in periarticular regions of phalanges, metacarpals and metatarsals.

Malignant

1. Multicentric osteosarcoma.
2. Metastases from neuroblastoma and retinoblastoma.
3. Acute leukemia.
4. Ewing's sarcoma.

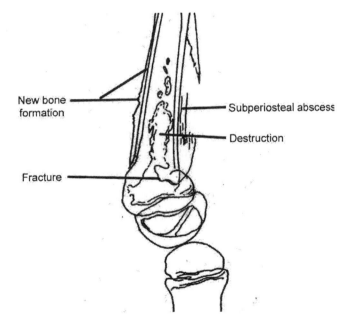

Fig. 6.27.2: Acute osteomyelitis: Anteroposterior views shows a mottled, destructive pattern along the entire metaphysis. There is extensive periosteal new bone formation. Periosteal elevation by a subperiosteal abscess is evident only on the lateral projection

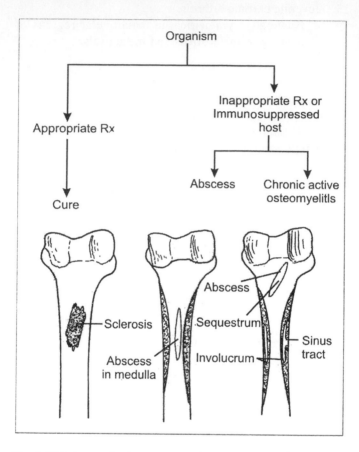

Fig. 6.27.3: Interaction between organism and host. Whether a bone infection will progress or be cured is determined by host factors and the efficacy of the therapy

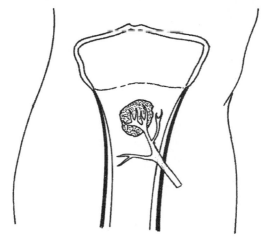

Fig. 6.27.4a: Routes of bone invasion: In hematogenous osteomyelitis, organisms gain access to bone via the nutrient arteries, which are most numerous in the metaphysis of a growing bone

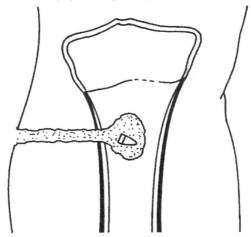

Fig. 6.27.4b: Contiguous spread from a soft-tissue infection allows organisms to penetrate the periosteal lining and the underlying cortex, gaining access to the medullary cavity. Pus elevates the periosteum, stimulating formation of new bone (periosteal reaction)

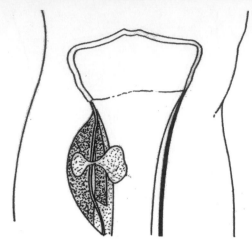

Fig. 6.27.4c: A missile wound enables organisms and debris to gain entry via a traumatic break in the skin and bone

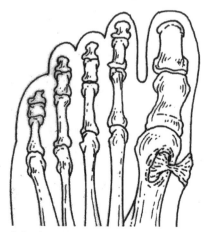

Fig. 6.27.4d: In diabetic osteomyelitis, fissures and ulcers form in the overlying skin secondary to diabetic vascular disease and organisms enter via these openings. As a consequence of vascular obstruction, leukocytes, antibodies, and antibiotics fail to reach the infected focus in the bone

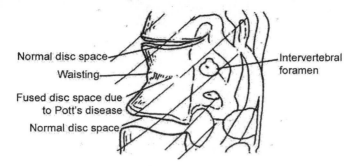

Fig. 6.27.5: Vertebral deformity following childhood Pott's disease

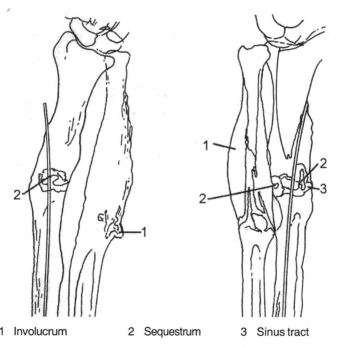

1 Involucrum	2 Sequestrum	3 Sinus tract

Fig. 6.27.6: Chronic active osteomyelitis

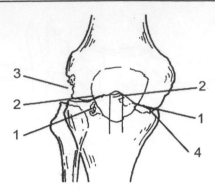

1	Destruction	2	Joint space loss
3	Marginal erosion	4	Joint effusion

Fig. 6.27.7: Joint tuberculosis

6.28   HYPERTROPHIC OSTEOARTHROPATHY

PULMONARY

– Carcinoma bronchus esp.oat cell carcinoma.
– Lymphoma.
– Abscess.
– Bronchiectasis.
– Metastases.

Pleural

– Pleural fibroma
– Mesothelioma.

Cardiovascular

– Cyanotic CHD.

Gastrointestinal

- Ulcerative colitis/Crohn's disease.
- Dysentery.
- Lymphoma.
- Whipple's disease.
- Celiac disease.
- Cirrhosis.
- Nasopharyngeal carcinomas.
- Juvenile polyposis.

6.29 DIFFERENTIAL DIAGNOSIS OF SKELETAL LESION IN NONACCIDENTAL INJURY

Disease	Shaft fractures	Abnormal metaphyses	Osteopenia	Periosteal reaction	Comments
1. Birth trauma	+	+/-	–	+/-	Clavicle, humerus and femur most commonly involved
2. Copper deficiency	+	+	+	+/-	Seen with prematurity, TPN, malabsorption, etc.
3. Congenital insensitivity to pain	+	+	–	+	—
4. Congenital syphilis	–	+	–	+	—
5. Menke's syndrome	–	+	+	+	Only males are affected, Wormian bones may be seen
6. Nonaccidental injury	+	+	–	+	—
7. Osteogenesis imperfecta	+	+/-	+	–	Wormian bones, associated dentinogenesis imperfecta
8. Osteomyelitis	–	+	Localized	+	—
9. Paraplegia	+	+	+	+	Lower limbs are only involved
10. Prost. E therapy	–	–	–	+	—
11. Rickets	+	+	+	+	Increased alkaline phosphatase
12. Scurvy	–	+	+	+	After 6 months of age
13. Caffey's disease	+	–	–	+	—

6.30 BONE DYSPLASIAS-ASSOCIATED WITH MULTIPLE FRACTURES

REDUCED DENSITY

1. Osteogenesis imperfecta.
2. Achondrogenesis.
3. Hypophosphatasia.
4. Mucolipidosis II.
5. Cushing's syndrome.

Normal Osseous Density

1. Cleidocranial dysplasia.
2. Enchondromatosis.
3. Fibrous dysplasia

Increased Density

1. Osteopetrosis.
2. Pyknodysostosis.

6.31 EXCESSIVE CALLUS FORMATION

CAUSES

1. Steroid therapy and Cushing's syndrome.
2. Neuropathic arthropathy.
3. Osteogenesis imperfecta.
4. Nonaccidental injury.
5. Paralytic states.
6. Renal osteodystrophy.
7. Multiple myeloma.

6.32 BONE WITHIN BONE APPEARANCE

It results from endosteal new bone formation.

CAUSES

1. Normal
   - In thoracic and lumbar spine (in infants)
   - Growth recovery lines (after infancy)
2. Infantile cortical hyperostosis (Caffey's disease)
3. Sickle cell disease/thalassemia.
4. Congenital syphilis.
5. Osteopetrosis/oxalosis.
6. Radiation.
7. Acromegaly.
8. Paget's disease.
9. Heavy metal poisoning (Bi,Pb,Th)
10. Prostaglandin E therapy.
11. Leukemia.
12. Tuberculosis.
13. Rickets.   *Rare*
14. Scurvy.
15. Vit D toxicity.
16. Reflex sympathetic dystrophy.

6.33 FATIGUE FRACTURES

Normal bone subjected to repetitive stresses (none of which is alone capable of producing a fracture) leads to mechanical failure over a period of time.

Radiographic Signs

1. *Cancellous Bone*
   - Subtle blurring of trabecular margins.
   - Faint sclerotic area due to peritrabecular callus.
   - Sclerotic band (due to trabecular compression and peritrabecular callus) perpendicular to cortex.
2. *Compact Bone*
   - Subtle ill-defined cortex.
   - Intracortical lucent striations.
   - Solid thick lamellar periosteal new bone formation.
   - Endosteal thickening.

Fracture	*Related activity*
1. Clay Shovelers fracture (fracture spinous process of lower cervical/upper thoracic spine)	Clay shovelling
2. Coracoid process of scapula	Trap shooting
3. Ribs	Carrying heavy pack, golf, coughing
4. Distal shaft of humerus	Throwing ball
5. Coronoid process of ulna	Pitching ball, throwing javelin, propelling wheelchair
6. Hook of hamate	Swinging golf club/tennis racquet/ baseball bat
7. Spondylolysis (pars interarticularis fracture)	Ballet, lifting heavy weights, scrubbing floor
8. Femoral neck	Ballet, long distance running
9. Femoral shaft	Ballet, long distance running, gymnastics, marching
10. Obturator ring of pelvis	Stooping, bowling, gymnastics
11. Patella	Hurdling

Contd...

Contd...

Fracture	Related activity
12. Tibial shaft	Ballet, jogging
13. Fibula	Long distance running, jumping, parachutting
14. Calcaneus	Jumping, parachutting, prolonged standing, etc.
15. Navicular	Stooping on ground, marching, prolonged standing, ballet.
16. Metatarsal (commonly 2nd)	Marching, prolonged standing, stamping on ground.
17. Sesamoids of metatarsals	Prolonged standing.

6.34 PSEUDOARTHROSIS

CAUSES

1. Nonunited fracture.
2. Congenital in tibia and fibula—usually in neurofibromatosis.
3. Fibrous dysplasia.
4. Idiopathic juvenile osteoporosis.
5. Osteogenesis imperfecta.
6. Cleidocranial dysplasia—in femur.
7. Ankylosing spondylitis.

6.35 IRREGULAR/STIPPLED EPIPHYSIS

CAUSES

1. Normal variant
   – In distal femur.

2. Avascular necrosis
   - Single in Perthes' disease.
   - Multiple in sickle cell anemia.
3. Hypothyroidism
   - Delayed appearance and growth of ossification centers.
   - Femoral capital epiphysis divided into inner and outer half.
4. Chondrodysplasia punctata
   - Stippling in long bones epiphyses, spine, larynx which disappears by 2 yrs of age.
   - Asymmetrical shortening of limbs.
5. Multiple epiphyseal dysplasia
   - Delayed appearance and growth of epiphysis.
   - With or without metaphyseal irregularity.
6. Spondyloepiphyseal dysplasia.
7. Hypoparathyroidism.
8. Down's syndrome.
9. Trisomy 18.
10. Fetal warfarin syndrome
    - Stippling of uncalcified epiphysis particularly axial skeleton, proximal femora and calcanei.
    - Disappears after 1st year.
11. Homocystinuria
    - Distal ulnar and radial epiphysis—pathognomonic.
12. Zellweger cerebrohepatorenal syndrome.
13. Fetal alcohol syndrome
    - Mostly calcaneus and lower extremities.
14. Meyer dysplasia
    - Confined to femoral heads.
15. Morquio's syndrome
    - Irregular ossification of femoral capital epiphysis.

6.36 AVASCULAR NECROSIS/OSTEONECROSIS/ ASEPTIC NECROSIS

This is the consequence of interrupted blood supply to bone with death of cellular elements.

CAUSES

a. *Toxic*
   - Steroids (>2 yrs of treatment)
   - NSAID-Indomethacin.
   - Alcohol.
   - Immunosuppressives.
b. *Traumatic*
   - Idiopathic—Perthes' disease.
   - Fractures—Femoral neck, talus, scaphoid.
   - Radiotherapy.
   - Heat-burns, electrical.
   - Fat embolism.
   - Frostbite.
c. *Inflammatory*
   - Rheumatoid arthritis.
   - Psoriasis.
   - SLE.
   - Scleroderma.
   - Neuropathic arthropathy.
   - Osteoarthrosis.
   - Infection.
   - Pancreatitis.
d. *Metabolic/Endocrinal*
   - Pregnancy.
   - Diabetes.
   - Cushing's syndrome.

- Hyperlipidemia.
- Gout.
- Hypercholesterolemia.
- Hyperuricemia.

e. *Hematopoietic Disorders*
   Hemoglobinopathies as sickle cell anemia.
   - Hemophilia.
   - Gaucher's disease
   - Histiocytosis.
   - Polycythemia.

f. *Thrombotic/Embolic*
   - Dysbaric osteonecrosis.
   - Giant cell arteritis.
   - Endocarditis.
   - Polyarteritis nodosa.
   - Peripheral vascular disease.

Steinberg Classification for AVN of Hip

Stage 0	– Normal.
Stage 1	– Normal-barely abnormal trabecular pattern, abnormal bone scan/MRI.
Stage 2A	– Focal sclerosis and osteopenia.
2B	– Distinct sclerosis with osteoporosis and early crescent sign.
Stage 3A	– Subchondral undermining (Crescent sign) and cyst formation.
3B	– Mild alteration in femoral head contour and subchondral fracture with normal joint space.
Stage 4	– Marked collapse of femoral head with significant acetabular involvement.
Stage 5	– Joint space narrowing with acetabular degenerative changes.

MR Changes in AVN (Mitchell-staging)

Stage	T1WI	T2WI	Comments
A	Increase	Intermediate	Fat
B	Increase	Increase	Subacute blood
C	Decrease	Increase	Fluid/edema
D	Decrease	Decrease	Fibrosis

6.37   SOLITARY RADIOLUCENT METAPHYSEAL BANDS

It represents a periods of poor endochondral bone formation.

CAUSES

1. Normal variant.
2. Any severe systemic illness.
3. Healing rickets.
4. Scurvy.
5. Leukemia, lymphoma.
6. Metastatic neuroblastoma.
7. Congenital infection as syphilis.
8. Growth lines.
9. Metaphyseal fracture esp. in nonaccidental injuries.

6.38   SOLITARY DENSE METAPHYSEAL BAND

1. Normal variant.
2. Heavy metal poisoning (lead, bismuth, phosphorus, etc)
3. Systemic illness.
4. Rickets (healed)
5. Scurvy.
6. Sickle cell disease.

7. Vit. D intoxication.
8. Crotinism.
9. Congenital syphilis.
10. Estrogen to mother during pregnancy.
11. Leukemia.
12. TORCH infection.
13. Idiopathic hypercalcemia.
14. Radiation.
15. Osteopetrosis.

6.39   ALTERNATING RADIOLUCENT/DENSE METAPHYSEAL BANDS

1. Growth arrest or Park's lines.
2. Rickets esp. Vit D resistant.
3. Osteopetrosis.
4. Chemotherapy.
5. Chronic anemias
   – Sickle cell/thalassemias.
6. Treated leukemia.

6.40   DENSE VERTICAL METAPHYSEAL LINES

1. Congenital rubella
   – Produces a characteristic "celery stalk" appearance.
2. Congenital CMV infection.
3. Hypophosphatasia.
4. Localized metaphyseal injury.
5. Osteopathia striata
   – Bony exostosis may be associated.

6.41   FRAYED METAPHYSIS

1. Achondroplasia.
2. Congenital infections (Rubella, Syphilis)
3. Copper deficiency.
4. Chronic stress, e.g. wrist of gymnasts.
5. Hypophosphatasia.
6. Metaphyseal dysostosis.
7. Rickets.
8. Scurvy.

6.42   CUPPING OF METAPHYSIS

1. Normal variant esp. distal end of ulna and proximal end of fibula.
2. Bone dysplasias as achondroplasia, pseudoachondroplasia, etc.
3. Rickets
   – Associated with metaphyseal blurring and fraying.
4. Scurvy
   – Usually follows fracture.
5. Trauma
   – To growth plate; the changes will be asymmetrical.

6.43   ERLENMEYER FLASK DEFORMITY

This deformity is characterized by expansion of distal ends of long bones esp. femora.

CAUSES

It include:

1. Storage disorders as Gaucher's disease, Niemann-Pick disease.

2. Rickets.
3. Anemias, e.g. thalassemia with coarse trabecular pattern.
4. Fibrous dysplasia.
5. Osteopetrosis.
6. Heavy metal poisoning, e.g. lead with thick transverse dense metaphyseal bands.
7. Metaphyseal dysplasia (Pyle's disease)
   - Rare autosomal recessive disease. Characterized by sclerosis of skull vault and base, widening of medial ends of clavicle and expansion of pubic and ischial bones.
8. Down's syndrome.
9. Achondroplasia.
10. Rheumatoid arthritis.
11. Hypophosphatasia.
12. Diaphyseal aclasia.
13. Ollier's disease.
14. Craniometaphyseal dysplasia
    - Common, autosomal dominant condition.
15. Osteodysplasty (Melnick-Needles syndrome)
    - Seen in females. Characterized by distorted irregular ribs and sigmoid shaped clavicles; cortical irregularity, patchy sclerosis and bowing of bones are also seen.

6.44 EROSION OF MEDIAL METAPHYSES OF PROXIMAL HUMERUS

- Normal variant
- Neoplastic
  - Leukemia.
  - Metastatic neuroblastoma.
- Storage disorders
  - Gaucher's disease.

- – Hurler's syndrome.
- – Niemann-Pick disease.
- Endocrinal
  - – Hyperparathyroidism.
- Arthropathies
  - – Rheumatoid arthritis.

6.45 ABNORMALITY RELATED TO CLAVICLES

EROSION OR ABSENCE OF OUTER END OF CLAVICLE

- Rheumatoid arthritis.
- Hyperparathyroidism.
- Post-traumatic osteolysis.
- Metastasis.
- Multiple myeloma.
- Cleidocranial dysplasia.
- Pyknodysostosis.

PENCILED DISTAL END OF CLAVICLE

- Scleroderma.
- Hyperparathyroidism.
- Infection.
- Rheumatoid arthritis.
- Trauma.
- Progeria.

DESTRUCTION OF MEDIAL END OF CLAVICLE

- Metastasis.
- Infection.
- Lymphoma.

- Eosinophilic granuloma.
- Rheumatoid arthritis.
- Sarcoma.
- Rarely cleidocranial dysplasia.

6.46 RIB LESIONS

NEOPLASTIC

i. *Benign*
- Fibrous dysplasia (Commonest)
- Eosinophilic granuloma.
- Benign cortical defect.
- Hemangioma.
- Enchondroma (at costochondral/costovertebral junction)
- Osteochondroma.
- Giant cell tumor.
- Aneurysmal bone cyst.
- Langerhans' cell histiocytosis.
ii. *Malignant*
   a. Primary
   - Chondrosarcoma.
   - Osteosarcoma.
   - Fibrosarcoma.
   - Ewing's sarcoma.
   - Multiple myeloma/plasmacytoma.
   b. Secondary
   - Adults.
     - Metastases.
     - Desmoid tumor.
   - Child
     - Metastatic neuroblastoma.

Nonneoplastic

- Healing fractures.
- Radiation osteitis.
- Paget's disease.
- Brown tumor of hyperparathyroidism.
- Osteomyelitis.

6.47 RIB NOTCHING

SUPERIOR MARGIN

  i. *Connective Tissue Disorders*
  - Rheumatoid arthritis.
  - Scleroderma.
  - SLE.
  - Sjögren's syndrome.

  ii. Metabolic
  - Hyperparathyroidism.

  iii. Miscellaneous
  - Marfan's syndrome.
  - Restrictive lung disease.
  - Neurofibromatosis.
  - Poliomyelitis.
  - Osteogenesis imperfecta.
  - Progeria.

Inferior Margin

  i. *Arterial*
  - Coarctation of aorta (CoA) (4-8th ribs bilaterally)
    - U/L and Rt.sided if coarctation is proximal to Lt. Subclavian artery

- U/L and Lt side if associated with anomalous
  Rt. subclavian artery distal to coarctation.
- Aortic thrombosis.
- Pulmonary stenosis, Fallot's tetralogy or absent
  pulmonary artery (all causes of pulmonary oligemia)
- Subclavian obstruction.
  (Post Blalock-Taussig shunt)
- Upper 3 or 4 ribs ipsilateral to operation side.

ii. *Venous*
- AV chest wall malformation
- SVC obstruction
- Pulmonary AV malformation

iii. *Neurogenic*
- Neurofibromatosis
- Intercostal neuroma
- Poliomyelitis/quadriplegia

iv. *Osseous*
- Hyperparathyroidism
- Thalassemia
- Mclnick needles syndrome

6.48 ABNORMAL SHAPE, SIZE AND DENSITY OF RIBS

a. *Ribbon Ribs*
- Osteogenesis imperfecta.
- Neurofibromatosis.

b. *Wide/Thick Ribs*
- Chronic anemias.
- Fibrous dysplasia.
- Paget's disease.

- Achondroplasia.
- Mucopolysaccharidosis.
- Healed fracture with callus.

c. *Bullous Costochondral Ends*
- Rachitic Rosary.
- Scurvy.
- Achondroplasia.

d. *Short Ribs*
- Achondroplasia.
- Achondrogenesis.
- Thanatophoric dysplasia.
- Asphyxiating thoracic dysplasia.
- Mesomelic dwarfism.
- Short rib polydactyly syndrome.
- Spondyloepiphyseal dysplasia.
- Enchondromatosis.
- Chondroectodermal dysplasia.

e. *Dense Ribs*
- Osteopetrosis.
- Fluorosis.
- Mastocytosis.

f. *Hyperlucent Ribs*
- Osteopetrosis.
- Cushing's disease.
- Acromegaly.
- Scurvy.

6.49 MADELUNG DEFORMITY

Characterized by shortening of distal radius with posterior subluxation of distal ulna.

CAUSES

- Isolated congenital
    - Usually bilateral and commoner in females.
- Leri Weill syndrome (dyschondrosteosis)
- Turner's syndrome.
- Post-traumatic.
- Postinfectious.

6.50 CARPAL FUSION

ISOLATED

i. *Congenital*
    - Triquetral lunate.
      (Commonest)
    - Capitate-Hamate.
    - Trapezuim Trapezoid.
ii. *Acquired*
    - Inflammatory arthritides as rheumatoid arthritis.
    - Pyogenic arthritis.
    - Post-traumatic.
    - Postsurgical.

Syndrome Related

- Acrocephalosyndactyly
  (Apert's syndrome).
- Arthrogryposis multiplex congenita.
- Ellis-van Creveld syndrome.
- Holt-Oram syndrome.
- Turner's syndrome.
- Symphalangism.

6.51 ABNORMAL DIGITS

a. *Brachydactyly*
   (Shortening/Broadening of metacarpal +/- phalanges)
   - Idiopathic.
   - Post-traumatic.
   - Osteomyelitis.
   - Postinfarction as sickle cell disease.
   - Turner's syndrome.
     (4th +/- 3rd and 5th)
   - Arthritis.
   - Osteochondrodysplasia.
   - Pseudo and pseudopseudohypoparathyroidism.
     (4th and 5th)
   - Mucopolysaccharidosis.
   - Hereditary multiple exostoses.
   - Basal cell nevus syndrome.

b. *Arachnodactyly*
   (elongated/slender)
   - Marfan's syndrome
     (Metacarpal index = 8.4-10.4)
   - Homocystinuria.

c. *Syndactyly*
   (osseous +/- cutaneous fusion of digits)
   - Apert's syndrome.
   - Carpenter syndrome.
   - Down's syndrome.
   - Neurofibromatosis.
   - Poland syndrome.

d. *Polydactyly*
   - Carpenter syndrome.

  - Ellis-van Creveld syndrome.
  - Meckel-Gruber syndrome.
  - Polysyndactyly syndrome.
  - Short rib-polydactyly syndrome.
  - Trisomy 13.
e. *Clinodactyly* (Curvative of fingers in mediolateral plane)
  - Normal variant.
  - Clinodactyly
  - Multiple dysplasia.
  - Trauma.
  - Arthritis.
  - Contractures.

6.52 ABNORMAL THUMB

a. *Broad*
  - Acrocephalopolysyndactyly.
  - Acrocephalosyndactyly.
    (mitten hand and sock foot deformity)
  - Rubinstein-Taybi syndrome.
  - Oropalatodigital syndrome.
    (Large cone epiphysis of distal phalanx)
b. *Large*
  - Klippel-Trenaunay-Weber syndrome.
  - Maffucci syndrome.
  - Neurofibromatosis.
  - Macrodystrophia lipomatosa.
c. *Short/small*
  - Fanconi's anemia.
  - Holt-Oram syndrome.
  - Brachydactyly.
  - Cornelia de Lange syndrome.
  - Fetal hydantoin.

d. *Absent*
   - Fanconi's anemia.
   - Poland syndrome.
   - Thalidomide.
   - Trisomy 18.
e. *Triphalangeal*
   - Fanconi's anemia.
   - Holt-Oram syndrome.
   - Blackfan-Diamond syndrome.
   - Poland syndrome.
   - Trisomy 13 and 21.
   - Thalidomide.
f. *Abnormal position*
   - Proximal placed.
     (Cornelia de Lange syndrome)
   - Diastrophic dysplasia and Rubinstein-Taybi syndrome.

6.53   LYTIC LESION IN DIGITS

WELL-DEFINED

i. *Neoplastic*
   a. *Benign*
      - Implantation dermoid.
      - Enchondroma.
      - Glomus tumor.
      - Osteoid osteoma.

Malignant

- Osteoblastoma.
ii. *Nonneoplastic*

- Sarcoid.
- Solitary bone cyst.
- Fibrous dysplasia.

Poorly Defined

i. Neoplastic.
   a. *Benign*
     - Aneurysmal bone cyst.
     - Giant cell tumor.
   b. *Malignant*
     - Metastases.
     - Multiple myeloma.
     - Osteosarcoma.
     - Fibrosarcoma.
ii. Nonneoplastic.
   - Osteomyelitis.
   - Brown tumors of hyperparathyroidism.
   - Hemophilic pseudotumor.
   - Leprosy.

6.54 ACRO-OSTEAL CHANGES

ACRO-OSTEOLYSIS

- Familial
- Massive osteolysis.
- Essential osteolysis.
- Ainhum disease.
- Acquired.
  - Psoriasis.
  - Porphyria.
  - Ehlers-Danlos syndrome.
  - Thromboangiitis obliterans.
  - Ergot therapy.

- Raynaud disease.
- Diabetes.
- Arteriosclerosis.
- Dermatomyositis.
- PVC workers.
- Rheumatoid arthritis.
- Scleroderma.
- Leprosy.
- Syringomyelia.
- Hyperparathyroidism.

Acro-osteosclerosis

- Patchy in nature
  - Incidental (Middle-aged and females)
  - Rheumatoid arthritis
  - Sarcoidosis
  - Scleroderma
  - SLE
  - Hodgkin's disorders
  - Hematological disorders.

RESORPTION OF DISTAL PHALANGES

a. *Congenital*
b. *Dysplasia*
  - Cleidocranial.
  - Pyknodysostosis.
  - Acro-osteolysis of Hajdu and Cheney syndrome.
  - Pachydermoperiostosis.
c. *Infective*
  - Osteomyelitis.
  - Leprosy.
  - Sarcoid.

d. *Trauma*
   - Frostbite.
   - Thermal injuries.
   - Electrical injury.
   - Amputation.
e. *Poisons*
   - Ergot.
   - PVC.
   - Phenytoin.
   - Snake/scorpion venom.
f. *Metabolic*
   - Hyperparathyroidism and porphyria.
g. *Vascular*
   - Scleroderma.
   - Pseudoxanthoma elasticum.
   - Occlusive vascular disease.
h. *Neurotrophic*
   - Tabes dorsalis.
   - Diabetes.
   - Congenital in difference to pain.
   - Myelomeningocele.
i. *Neoplastic*
   - Kaposi sarcoma.
j. *Miscellaneous*
   - Psoriasis.
   - Pityriasis rubra.
   - Epidermolysis bullosa.
   - Reticulohistiocytosis.
   - Ainhum.
   - Progeria.
   - Neurofibromatosis.

6.55 MONOARTHRITIS

a. *Traumatic*
   - Associated fracture.
   - Joint effusion esp. lipohemarthrosis include.
   - Secondary osteoarthritis.
   - Neurotrophic arthritis.
   - Pigmented villonodular synovitis.
b. *Septic Arthritis*
   (Tuberculous, pyogenic, lyme, fungal).
   - Periarticular erosions.
   - Joint space narrowing.
   - Periosteal reaction.
   - Bony/fibrous ankylosis.
c. *Collagen-like Disease*
   - Rheumatoid arthritis esp. chronic juvenile arthritis.
   - Rheumatic fever.
d. *Sarcoidosis*
   - Psoriatic arthritis.
   - Ankylosing arthritis.
e. *Biochemical Arthritis*
   - Gout.
   - CPPD disease.
   - Chondrocalcinosis.
   - Ochronosis.
   - Hemophilic arthritis.
f. *Degenerative*
   - Osteoarthritis.
g. *Sympathetic*
   - In response to, e.g. tumor.
h. *Neuropathic arthropathy.*

6.56 ARTHRITIS WITH PERIOSTITIS

CAUSES

1. Juvenile rheumatoid arthritis.
2. Psoriatic arthritis.
3. Reiter's syndrome.
4. Infectious arthritis.
5. Hypertrophic osteoarthropathy.
6. Hemophilia.
7. Uncommonly, rheumatoid arthritis.

6.57 ARTHRITIS WITH DEMINERALIZATION

CAUSES

1. Hemophilia.
2. Osteomyelitis.
3. Rheumatoid arthritis, juvenile chronic arthritis.
4. Reiter's syndrome.
5. Scleroderma.
6. SLE.

6.58 ARTHRITIS WITHOUT DEMINERALIZATION

CAUSES

1. Psoriatic arthritis.
2. Osteoarthritis.
3. Neuropathic arthropathy.
4. Gout.
5. Sarcoidosis.
6. Reiter's disease.

7. Pigmented villonodular synovitis.
8. Ankylosing spondylitis.
9. Calcium pyrophosphate arthropathy.

6.59 ARTHRITIS WITH PRESERVED/ WIDENED JOINT SPACE

CAUSES

1. Infective/inflammatory arthritis
   - early stage due to joint effusion.
2. Psoriatic arthropathy
   - Due to fibrous tissue deposition.
3. Gout.
4. Pigmented villonodular synovitis.
5. Acromegaly
   - Due to cartilage overgrowth.

ARTHRITIS WITH

SOFT TISSUE NODULES

- Gout.
- Rheumatoid arthritis.
- Pigmented villonodular synovitis.
- Reticulohistiocytosis.
- Sarcoidoses.
- Amyloidosis.

LOOSE INTRA-ARTICULAR BODIES

- Osteochondrosis dessicans.
- Synovial osteochondromatosis.

- Chip fracture from trauma (Osteochondral fracture).
- Severe degenerative joint disease (detached osteophyte).
- Neuropathic arthropathy.

Arthritis Mutilans

Characterized by telescoping joints due to resorption of bone ends secondary to destructive arthritis.

Causes:

1. Leprosy
2. Diabetes.
3. Neuropathic arthropathy.
4. Rheumatoid arthritis.
5. Juvenile chronic arthritis.
6. Psoriatic arthropathy.
7. Reiter's syndrome.

6.60 ENLARGED FEMORAL INTER-CONDYLAR NOTCH

CAUSES

1. Hemophilia.
2. Juvenile chronic arthritis.
3. Psoriatic arthropathy.
4. Rheumatoid arthropathy.
5. Tuberculous arthritis.

6.61 PLANTAR CALCANEAL SPUR

CAUSES

1. Idiopathic.
2. Diffuse idiopathic skeletal hyperostosis.
3. Ankylosing spondylitis.
4. Psoriatic arthropathy.
5. Reiter's syndrome.
6. Rheumatoid arthritis.

6.62 CHONDROCALCINOSIS

Characterized by calcification of articular or hyaline cartilage.

a. *Idiopathic*
b. *Crystal deposition disease*
   - CPPD.
   - Gout.
c. *Metabolic*
   - Wilson's disease.
   - Hemochromatosis.
   - Familial hypomagnesemia.
   - Ochronosis.
   - Diabetes.
   - Hypophosphatasia.
d. *Endocrinal*
   - Hypothyroidism.
   - Primary hyperparathyroidism.
   - Acromegaly.

e. *Arthropathy associated*
  – Rheumatoid arthritis.
  – Postinfectious arthritis.
  – Post-traumatic arthritis.
  – Degenerative arthritis.
f. *Miscellaneous*
  – Hemophilia.
  – Amyloidosis.

6.63 ANKYLOSIS OF INTERPHALANGEAL JOINTS

CAUSES

1. Psoriatic arthritis.
2. Ankylosing spondylitis.
3. Still's disease.
4. Erosive osteoarthritis.

6.64 ENTHESIOPATHY

Characterized by osseous attachment of tendon.

CAUSES

1. Degenerative disorder.
2. Seronegative arthropathies as ankylosing spondylitis, Reiter's disease, psoriatic arthritis.
3. DISH.
4. Acromegaly.
5. Occasionally, rheumatoid arthritis.

6.65 SACROILIITIS

UNILATERAL

i. *Infective*
   - Pyogenic.
   - Tubercular.
ii. *Degenerative*
   - Osteoarthrosis secondary to abnormal mechanical stress
     - Narrowing of joint space with subchondral sclerosis.
     - Osteophytosis.

BILATERAL

i. Symmetrical
   - Ankylosing spondylitis.
     - Ankylosis of joint.
     - Ossification of ligaments.
   - Enteropathic arthropathy as in CD, UC, etc.
   - Osteitis Condensans illi.
     - Seen in young multiparous women.
     - Bone sclerosis with normal joint space.
   - Rheumatoid arthritis (in late stages)
     - Joint space narrowing.
     - Osteoporosis.
   - Deposition arthropathy (gout, CPPD, ochronosis)
     - Slow loss of cartilage.
     - Subchondral sclerosis + osteophytosis.
   - Hyperparathyroidism
     - Subchondral bone resorption.
     - Widening of joint space.

- Paraplegia
  - Joint space narrowing.
  - Osteoporosis.
ii. *Asymmetrical*
  - Psoriatic arthropathy.
    - Extensive erosion.
    - Ankylosis less common.
  - Reiter's syndrome.
  - Juvenile chronic arthritis.
  - Gouty arthritis.
    - Large well-defined erosion with adjacent sclerosis.
    - Osteoarthrosis.

6.66 PROTRUSIO ACETABULI

Characterized by acetabular floor bulging into pelvis. Criteria is acetabular line projecting medially to ilioischial line by >3 mm in males and >6 mm is females.

CAUSES

Unilateral

- Tubercular arthritis.
- Trauma.
- Fibrous dysplasia.
- Marfan's syndrome.

Bilateral

- Rheumatoid arthritis and juvenile chronic arthritis.
- Paget's disease.

- Osteomalacia/osteoporosis.
- Ankylosing spondylitis.
- Idiopathic/familial.
- Marfan's syndrome.

6.67 WIDENING OF SYMPHYSIS PUBIS (DIASTASIS)

Normal Measurements:

≤ 10 mm in newborn.

≤ 9 mm at 3yrs of age.

≤ 8 mm at 7yrs of age and over.

CONGENITAL

i. *With Normal Ossification*
   - Exstrophy of bladder.
   - Epispadias.
   - Hypospadias.
   - Imperforate anus with rectovaginal fistula.
   - Urethral duplication.
   - Prune belly syndrome.
   - Sjögren-Larson syndrome.
   - Goltz syndrome.

ii. *With Poorly Ossified Cartilage*
   - Achondrogenesis/hypochondrogenesis.
   - Campomelic dysplasia.
   - Chondrodysplasia punctate.
   - Wolf's syndrome.
   - Trisomy 9.

- Cleidocranial dysplasia.
- Hypophosphatasia.
- Hypothyroidism.
- Pyknodysostosis.
- Spondyloepiphyseal dysplasia.
- Osteogenesis imperfecta.
- Larson's syndrome.
- Spondylometaphyseal dysplasia.

Acquired

- Pregnancy (resolves spontaneously by 3rd month postpartum)
- Trauma.
- Osteitis pubis(Symmetrical bony irregularity with resorption and sclerosis).
- Osteolytic metastases.
- Osteomyelitis.
- Ankylosing spondylitis.
- Rheumatoid arthritis.
- Hyperparathyroidism (subperiosteal bone resorption).

6.68 FUSION OF SYMPHYSIS PUBIS

CAUSES

1. Postinfective.
2. Post-traumatic.
3. Osteitis pubis.
4. Osteoarthrosis.
5. Ankylosing spondylitis.

6. Alkaptonuria.
7. Fluorosis.

6.69 RADIOGRAPHIC FINDING IN DEGENERATIVE, INFLAMMATORY AND NEUROPATHIC ARTHRITIS

	Degene-rative	Inflam-matory	Neuro-pathic
1. Soft tissue swelling/nodules	−	++	+
2. Soft tissue calcification	−	++	−
3. Joint effusion	+	+	++
4. Enthesopathies	−	++	−
5. Alignment deformities	+	++	++
6. Osteoporosis	−	++	−
7. Diffuse joint loss	+	++	+
8. Central/marginal erosions	−	++	−
9. Articular destruction	+/−	+	++
10. Subchondral cysts	++	+/−	−
11. Osteophytes	++	−	+
12. Subchondral sclerosis	++	−	+/−
13. Vacuum phenomena	++	−	+/−

++, occurs very commonly

+/−, may or may not occur

+, occurs commonly

−, does not occur.

| 6.70 | COMPARATIVE FEATURES OF SERONEGATIVE SPONDYLOARTHRITIDES | | | |

	Ankylosing spondylitis	Psoriatic arthropathy	Reiter's arthritis	Enteropathic arthropathy
1. Onset	Gradual	Variable	Sudden	Peripheral-sudden axial-gradual
2. HLA-B27 positivity	90%	20%	90%	5%
3. Peripheral joint involvement	Uncommon	Upper extremities	Lower extremities	Uncommon
4. SI joint involvement	Symmetric bilateral	Asymmetric	Asymmetric	Symmetric bilateral
5. Spinal involvement	100%	20%	30-40%	5%
6. Syndesmophytes	Symmetric, marginal, contiguous, fine, delicate, anterior/ anterolateral	Asymmetric, non-marginal, skip areas, coarse, lateral/ posterolateral	Asymmetric, non-marginal, skip areas, coarse, lateral/ posterolateral	Asymmetric, marginal, contiguous, fine, delicate anterior/ anterolateral
7. Paravertebral ossification	Not seen	Seen	Seen	Not seen
8. Bone density	Decreased	Preserved	May be decreased	May be decreased

6.71   D/D OF DWARFISM

A. Osteochondrodysplasias—Short Limb Dysplasias
1. *Rhizomelic*
   (Proximal limb shortening)
   a. Achondroplasia.
   b. Hypochondroplasia.
   c. Pseudoachondroplasia.
   d. Chondrodysplasia punctata.
   e. Thanatotropic dwarfism.
2. *Mesomelic*
   (Middle segment limb shortening)
   a. Dyschondrosteosis.
   b. Mesomelic dysplasia.
3. *Acromesomelic*
   (Middle and distal limb shortening)
   a. Chondroectodermal dysplasia.
4. *Acromelic*
   (Distal limb shortening)
   a. Asphyxiating thoracic dystrophy.

B. Short Spine Type
1. Pseudoachondroplasia.
2. Spondyloepiphyseal dysplasia.
3. Diastropic dwarfism.
4. Metatropic dwarfism.
5. Kniest syndrome.

C. Dysostosis Multiplex (Short limb) + Short Trunk
- Hurler's syndrome.
- Morquio's syndrome.

D. Chromosomal Aberration
- Turner's syndrome.

E. Primordial Dwarfism

F. Endocrine Disease
Hypopituitarism, cretinism.
Hypergonadism.

G. Metabolic Disorder
Hypophosphatasia, rickets.

A. Primordial Dwarfism

– Congenital growth disturbance, genetically transmitted.
– Appearance and fusion of ossification centers is normal.
– Bones are radiologically normal except that they are unusually small.
– These patients are dwarfs at birth and never attain normal stature.
– They are sexually normal and transmit dwarfism to their children.

B. Endocrine Disorders

Hypopituitarism

• Due to partial or complete-lack of growth hormone.
• Typical hypopituitary dwarfism is k/as Lorain-Lévi dwarfism.
• Patient presents with short stature usually after 18 months of age, and are usually slender and well-proportioned.
• Mentality is unaffected, delayed skeletal age and are sexually immature.
• MRI shows small sella and hypoplastic pituitary gland.

Cretinism

• Delayed skeletal maturation, i.e. delayed appearance and fusion of ossification centers.

- Dwarfism with delayed dentition, delayed closure of font anelle, wormian bones. Fragmented epiphysis.
- Kyphosis with bullet-shaped vertebrae usually L1 and L2.

Hypergonadism

- Ovarian granulosa cell tumor in females, pineal tumors in males, hyperfunction of adrenal cortex.
- Sexual precocity with early appearance and rapid closure of epiphysis resulting in dwarfism.

Turner's Syndrome

- XO chromosome pattern.
- Ovarian dysgenesis.
- Short stature with retarded epiphyseal development.
- Webbed neck, broad chest, pectus excavatum, cubitus valgus, short fourth metacarpal.

Metabolic Disorders

Hypophosphatasia

- Severe forms result in dwarfism.
- Lack of calcification of metaphyseal ends of long bones.
- Decrease alkaline phosphatase activity.

Rickets

Causes delayed skeletal maturation, bowed legs and other deformities and may result in short stature.

DYSPLASIAS

1. Rhizomelic

Achondroplasia

- Long bones are short and broad.

- Small square iliac blades, horizontal acetabula.
- Lumbar canal stenosis due to decreased interpedicular distance.
- Large calvarium.
- Short stubby fingers.

Hypochondroplasia

- Short and broad femoral neck.
- Small iliac blades.
- Lumbar canal stenosis.
- Skull never affected.

Pseudoachondroplasia

- Long bones are short with broad metaphysis and irregular epiphysis.
  - Ilia are large, platyspondyly with central anterior tongue.
- Skull normal.
- Short stubby fingers.

THANATOTROPIC DWARFISM

- Rhizomelic dwarfism with bowing of long bones k/as Telephone handle long bones.
- Severe platyspondyly, vertebrae resemble letter H.
- Short ribs, short wide metacarpals and phalanges.
- Skull shows lateral temporal bulging k/as clover leaf skull.

Chondrodysplasia Punctata

a. Rhizomelic
b. Nonrhizomelic.
  - Asymmetric shortening of long bones with metaphyseal irregularity.
  - Stippling of carpus, tarsus and long bone epiphyses, around joints.

MESOMELIC DWARFISM

Dyschondrosteosis (Léri-Weill disease)

- Bilateral madelung deformity.
- Shortening of radius with triangular distal epiphysis.
- Carpal bones wedged between radius and protruding ulna with lunate at apex.

ACROMESOMELIC DWARFISM

1. Chondroectodermal dysplasia (Ellis-van Creveld syndrome)
   - Short stature with short limbs.
   - Shortening of paired long bones and hypoplasia of fingers and nails.
   - Hypoplastic lateral tibial plateau.
   - Polydactyly is most characteristic.

ACROMELIC DWARFISM

Asphyxiating Thoracic Dystrophy

- Narrow thorax and short ribs causing respiratory distress.
- Polydactyly, clavicles are highly placed.

Short Spine Dysplasias

Spondyloepiphyseal dysplasia.
- Ovoid or pear-shaped vertebral bodies in infancy with severe platyspondyly in later life.
- Normal metaphysis.
- Retarted development of symphysis pubis and femoral heads, coxa vara.

Diastrophic Dwarfism

- Progressive kyphoscoliosis.
- Hypermobile and abducted thumbs k/as Hitch Hiker's thumb.
- Delta-shaped epiphysis.
- 1st metacarpal is oval and hypoplastic—most distinctive feature.

Metatrophic Dwarfism

- Progressive kyphoscoliosis.
- Dumbell shaped long bones.
- Tail like appendage at distal end of gluteal cleft.

Short Limb + Short Trunk Dwarfs

Dysostosis Multiplex

1. *Hurler's Syndrome*
   - Macrocephaly, J-shaped sella, hook-shaped vertebral bodies.
   - Flaring of ilia, tapering of proximal ends of metacarpals.

Hunter's Syndrome

- Similar to Hurler's but less severe.

Brailsford-Morquio Syndrome

- Severe platyspondyly with central protrusion.
- Short and wide tubular bones.
- Narrow pelvis.

Maroteaux Lamy Syndrome

Dwarfism without mental impairment similar to Hurler's syndrome.

Flow Chart 6.71.1: Dwarfism

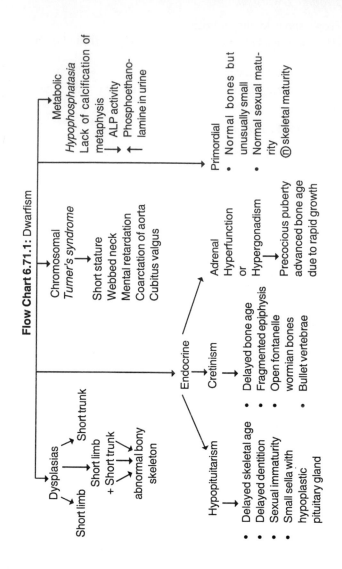

6.72 SCLEROTIC LESIONS OF BONE

- Bone reaction can be:
  a. Offence.
  b. Defence.

It can also be classified as:

1. Focal
2. Multifocal.
3. Generalized.

- Basically it is the role of osteoblasts.

  $\downarrow \rightarrow$ Central Reactive
      tumorogenic.

  Periosteal Reactive
      tumorogenic.

- Generic D/D of sclerotic lesion: "Vindicate"

Vascular	=	E.g. Hemangioma; infarcts.
Infections	=	E.g. Chronic osteomyelitis.
Neoplasm	=	E.g. Osteoma; osteoblastoma; secondaries
Drugs/poisons	=	E.g. Vitamin A and D; fluorosis; oxalosis.
Idiopathic	=	E.g. Caffey's; idiopathic hypercalcemia of infancy; Paget's.
Congenital	=	E.g. Bone island; osteopoikilosis; osteopetrosis; pyknodystosis.
Autoimmune	–	E.g. Mastocytosis.
Trauma	–	E.g. Stress fracture.
Endocrine/metabolic	=	E.g. Hyperparathyroidism; Paget's disease; hypoparathyroidism, pseudohypoparathyroidism and pseudopseudohypoparathyroidism.

IMAGING

a. Plain X-ray and tomography.
b. CT scan.
c. MRI.
d. Dexa (i.e. Densitometry).
e. Bone scintigraphy.

Role of Radiologist

Preop

1. Soft tissue extent.
2. Description.

3. Pathological fracture may be seen.
4. Aggressiveness.

5. Specific diagnosis if Possible.
6. Site of biopsy study.

7. Follows up the cases.

Postop

1. Record site of operation.
2. Excision Biopsy specimen.

3. Examination of adjacent normal bone.
4. Correlation of Microradiographic. Details to HPE.

5. X-ray diffraction to matrix.
6. Decide whether bone seaking.

SALIENT FEATURES

Osteopetrosis

• Primary fetal spongiosa—Not replaced properly by adult bone.

↓

—Grows in layers
(high in calcium   Prone to secondary
and Brittle)   infection.

Encroaches Marrow

↓

Extra Medullary
Hematoposis-
Anemia.

- **4 Types**

1. AR; severe; fatal; diagnosed early.
2. AD; Mild; Late diagnosed-   A. Skull vault.
3. AR; intermediate   B. Skull base +
4. Carbonic anhydrase   Rugger Jersy spine.
   deficiency with RTA
   and basal ganglia calcification.
- **Skull:** Thick, sclerotic bones (especially of base) with poorly pneumatized sinuses and encroached foramina. Dental abnormality.

Spine

Rugger Jersy spine with listhesis.

Extremities

Bone within Bone+Erlenmeyer Flask + Cigar lucencies.

Pyknodysostosis

- Autosomal recessive; short stature; multiple fracture with dense bones.

Skull

Brachycephaly; Persistent fontanelle and sutures wormian bones; sclerotic skull (esp base) with facial hypoplasia; obtuse mandible angle.

Spine

'Standing spool' vertebrae; listhesis, unfused neural arches) and ribs, etc. clavicle defect-lateral ends.

Extremities

Normal modelling with patent medulla.

Fibrous Dysplasia

- Woman 10-30 yrs monostotic and is mostly asymmetrical, U/L>>B/L.
- Usually the lesion stop growing with age.
- Radiological appearance of a cyst; cotton wool; ground glass depends upon the degree and distribution of calcium over the fibroid matrix. Basically it is a disease of medulla.
- Spinal involvement is rare while lesion is mainly metadiaphyseal. Longitudinal with a thinned but preserved cortex.
- Deformities like Shephard Crook, Mask Facies, proptosis.
- Fractures, Endocrinopathies, Fibrosarcomas (1%).

Renal Osteodystrophy and Hyperparathyroidism

- 9-34% patients of ROD and rarely patients of primary and tertiary HP show e/o sclerosis: occur because of poor renal function (global).
- Predilection for axial skeleton and metaphysis of long bones.
- Other features are that of osteoporosis, osteomalacia.
- Osteitis cystica fibrosa, soft tissue changes.

Hypopseudohypo and Pseudopseudohypoparathyroidism

- Pelvis, inner skull table, proximal femur, vertebral body.

associated with abnormal dentition and basal ganglion calcification.
- Associated features in PHP is short 4th and 5th metacarpal, coxa vara valga, cone-epiphysis, bowing of bones and soft tissue calcification.
- PPHP shows no radiological difference but has a normal blood chemistry.

Osteosclerotic Metastasis

- Prostate; Pheochromocytoma; Pancreas, Carcinoid; Cervix; Colon;. Breast; Stomach; TCC; Testis; Medulloblastoma; NP; Neuroblastoma.
- Tumor new bone—Osteosarcoma TCC; Mucinous Adenocarcinoma;

Carcinoma Prostate

- Cortical-Lung.

Caffey's Disease

- Idiopathic 9 wks-5 months; Sibling/cousin; presenting with fever-increase ESR-pleural effusion.
- Triad of hyperirritability, soft tissue swelling and bony cortical thickening.
- Patchy distribution; Remission and relapses.
- Soft tissue swellings—Painful; deep; proceed bony change and unrelated to it.
- A/E fibula and spine purelydiaphyseal
  - Rickets
  - Scurvy
  - Congenital syphilis.
- Periosteal reaction is associated.

Idiopathic Hypercalcemia of Infancy

- Elfin facies, failure to thrive.
- Generalized bone density increased; sclerotic bands at metaphysis.
- ? vit. A excess

Hypervitaminosis—A, D

- Basically periosteal reaction (Painful), Reversible; >1 yrs, bands.
- Soft tissue calcification (in vit- D), normal mandible.

Fluorosis

- Usually due to excess fluorine in drinking water.
- Due to increased osteoclastic activity to fluorine.
- Adults>>, Encroachment on medulla/foramina/spinal canal, etc.
- Membranes/Ligament ossification.

Lead

- Again due to lead in water.
- Due to lead deposition + reactive changes.
- Increased density +metaphyseal bands+modelling deformity.

Paget's Disease

- Elderly; Men; Polyostotic (80%); fibula (rare)
- 3 phases—Lytic, mixed; sclerotic; mosaic bone with lost corticomedullary differentiation
- Bones are large, thick, deformed, coarsened; joint deformities.

- Picture frame vertebra with collapse; lost lamina dura; hypercementosis.
- Skull has a cotton wool appearance with the lytic lesions starting in outer while sclerosis in inner table.

Myeloma

- i.e. Poems—seen in young men; spine, pelvis mostly involved.

Lymphoma

- Seen in low grade NHL and in HL (Hodgkin's lymphoma).
- Sclerotic lesion may occur as a result of healing.

Myelosclerosis

A part of myeloid metaplasia
- A group of conditions ranging from myeloid metaplasia, myelofibrosis to polycythemia rubra vera and CML.
- Marrow-fibrous tissue-bone formation.
- Has to be differentiated from osteopetrosis. Fluorosis, mastocytosis.

Mastocytosis

- 1/3 cases, presenting with urticaria pigmentosa, show bone changes.
- Coarsened trabecular pattern with focal lumpy/confluent areas of sclerosis. May terminate as leukemia.

Bone Island and Osteopoikilosis

- Island is just a lump of bone (hamartoma). In osteopoikilosis multiple islands are seen especially in periarticular areas. Well-defined, lanceolate, along the trabecular.

- Familial and has to be differentiated from secondaries and tuberous sclerosis which shows ill-defined patchy, cotton wool, flame-shaped opacities with islands.

OSTEOMA

Ivory spongy osteoid   Differentiation from Neuroblastoma, Osteomyelitis, Granuloma; Bleed; Stress fracture

- Small, well-defined tumor consisting primarily of well-differentiated bone; skull, PNS, Mandible, Pressure symptoms.
- *Osteoid osteoma:* Diaphysis of long bone; neural arch; central nidus with surrounding sclerosis; periosteal reaction, if tumor is near surface. Bone scintigraphy has an important role to play.

OSTEOBLASTOMA

- < 30 yrs; flat bones and vertebral appendages; some call it a large irregular and aggressive osteoid osteoma.
- Large, irregular, well-defined, expansile tumor with internal punctate calcification d/d GCT, ABC, osteoid osteoma, osteosarcoma.

OSTEOSARCOMA

- Most common primary malignant bone tumor; may be osteoblastic, chondroblastic, fibroblastic or telangiectatic.
- Most common about the knee; 10-25 yrs; metadiaphyseal; medulla is site of origin.
- Metastasis especially to lungs causing pneumatocele; Codman's triangle.

- A sclerotic destructive eccentrically growing mass showing good vascularity, differentiated other sarcomas, osteomyelitis; secondaries.

Rare Variants

Multifocal; diaphyseal; central; soft tissue osteosarcoma.
- Due to radiotherapy [3000 rad for 7-10 yrs]-Lytic aggressive: Radium ingestion known as secondary osteosarcoma.
- Other variants are parosteal and periosteal osteosarcoma.

OSTEOMYELITIS

- Especially pyogenic, syphilitic, fungal, sarcoidosis, Garre's and Brodie's osteomyelitis.

BONE INFARCTS

- Whether septic or aseptic, an infarct leads to an irregular sclerotic serpantine area in the medulla.

Flow Chart 6.72.1: Sclerotic Bone Lesions

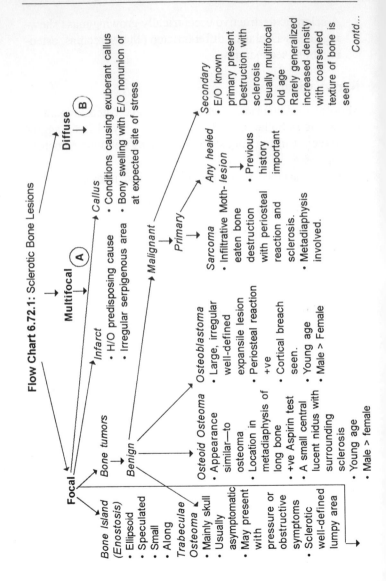

Focal

Bone Island (Enostosis)
- Ellipsoid
- Speculated
- Small
- Along

Trabeculae

Osteoma
- Mainly skull
- Usually asymptomatic
- May present with pressure or obstructive symptoms
- Sclerotic well-defined lumpy area

Bone tumors

Benign

Osteoid Osteoma
- Appearance similar—to osteoma
- Location in metadiaphysis of long bone
- +ve Aspirin test
- A small central lucent nidus with surrounding sclerosis
- Young age
- Male > female

Osteoblastoma
- Large, irregular well-defined expansile lesion
- Periosteal reaction +ve
- Cortical breach seen.
- Young age
- Male > Female

Infarct
- H/O predisposing cause
- Irregular serpigenous area

Malignant

Primary

Sarcoma
- Infiltrative Moth-eaten bone destruction with periosteal reaction and sclerosis.
- Metadiaphysis involved.

Any healed lesion
- Previous history important

Multifocal (A)

Callus
- Conditions causing exuberant callus
- Bony swelling with E/O nonunion or at expected site of stress

Diffuse (B)

Secondary
- E/O known primary present
- Destruction with sclerosis
- Usually multifocal
- Old age
- Rarely generalized increased density with coarsened texture of bone is seen

Contd...

Contd...

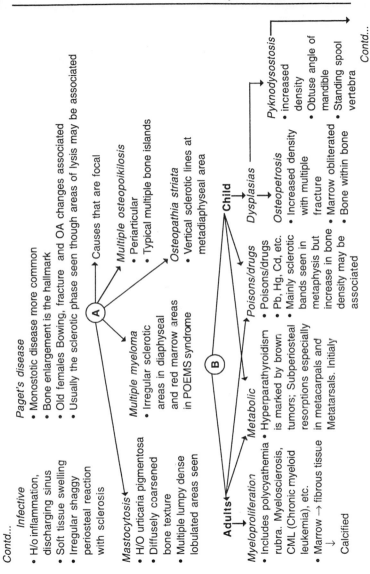

Contd...

Infective
- H/o inflammation, discharging sinus
- Soft tissue swelling
- Irregular shaggy periosteal reaction with sclerosis

Paget's disease
- Monostotic disease more common
- Bone enlargement is the hallmark
- Old females Bowing, fracture and OA changes associated
- Usually the sclerotic phase seen though areas of lysis may be associated

→ Causes that are focal

Multiple osteopoikilosis
- Periarticular
- Typical multiple bone islands

Osteopathia striata
- Vertical sclerotic lines at metadiaphyseal area

A

Mastocytosis
- H/O urticaria pigmentosa
- Diffusely coarsened bone texture
- Multiple lumpy dense lobulated areas seen

Multiple myeloma
- Irregular sclerotic areas in diaphyseal and red marrow areas in POEMS syndrome

B

Child

Dysplasias

Pyknodysostosis
- increased density
- Obtuse angle of mandible
- Standing spool vertebra

Osteopetrosis
- Increased density with multiple fracture
- Marrow obliterated
- Bone within bone

Poisons/drugs
- Poisons/drugs
- Pb, Hg, Cd, etc.
- Mainly sclerotic bands seen in metaphysis but increase in bone density may be associated

Metabolic
- Hyperparathyroidism is marked by brown tumors; Subperiosteal resorptions especially in metacarpals and Metatarsals. Initially

Adults

Myeloproliferation
- Includes polycythemia rubra. Myelosclerosis, CML (Chronic myeloid leukemia), etc.
- Marrow → fibrous tissue → Calcified

Contd...
- Diffusely increased density with coarse echotexture
- Marrow-hard to see
- Signs of extramedullary hematopoisis clinch the diagnosis

density decrease then increase with a coarse trabecular pattern. Blood profile is confirmatory
- Hypoparathyroidism and associated. Conditions may show sclerosis with short 4th/5th Metacarpal/tarsal. Blood profile is important. Cone epiphysis with soft tissue calcification seen.

- Stunted Growth and modelling abnormality is present
- Fluorine in adults causes extensive. Soft tissue calcification with increased bone density vitamin A and D poisoning show definite history.

- Cigar lucencies
- Erlenmeyer flask

- Normal modelling
- Clavicle defect
- Short stature

Idiopathic Hypercalcemia of infancy
- Elfin facies if with failure to thrive
- Increased density with metaphyseal bands

Caffey's disease
- 9 weeks-5 months
- Triad of hyperirritability, soft tissue swelling. Bony cortical thickening.
- Patchy distribution;
- Remission and relapses.
- Soft tissue swelling painful but not related to bone swellings.
- Purely diaphyseal.

- Cortex preserved but thinned

Fibrous dysplasia
- Female: 10-30 years
- Longitudinally growing medulary lesions.
- Cyst, cotton wool, Ground glass appearances depending on type of calcification.
- Metadiaphyseal.
- Fracture, endocrinopathy fibrosarcoma may be seen.
- Bone deformed.
- Dense sclerotic rim seen.

6.73   LYTIC LESION IN BONE

Single

With Marginal Sclerosis
- Geode/subarticular lucent cysts
- Brodie's abscess.
- Fibrous dysplasia
- Implantation dermoid
- Neoplasm-Benign-osteoid osteoma
- Simple bone cyst
- Chondroblastoma
- Enchondroma
- Adamantinoma

Malignant
Healing benign or malignant

Without marginal sclerosis
- Eosinophilic granuloma (EG)
- Brown tumor
- Multiple myeloma (MM)
- Metastasis
- Enchondroma
- Chondroblastoma
- Metastatic neuroblastoma

Multiple

- Metastasis

- Multiple myeloma
- FD (Polyostotic)
- Brown tumour
- Eosinophilic granuloma
- Metastatic neuroblastoma.
- Geode (Multiple)

EXPANSILE BONE LESION

- Giant cell tumor (GCT)
- Aneurysmal bone cyst (ABC)
- Enchondroma

- NOF (Non-ossifying fibroma)
- Chondromyxoid fibroma

GEODE

- Subarticular lucent bone lesion.
- Seen in osteoarthritis, rheumatoid arthritis. Calcium pyrophosphate deposition disease (CAPD).
- OA and CPPD = Multiple cysts in the load bearing areas of multiple joints with surrounding sclerotic margin.
- RA = No sclerosis.

BRODIE'S ABSCESS

- Localized bone infection presenting as subacute on chronic-infection.
- Clinical presentation.
- Site-metaphysis-diaphysis
- Radiological features—Circumscribed area of bone destruction with a variable degree of surrounding bone reaction.

Tunneling

- CT and MR-ovoid lesion with long axis parallel to bone.
- Scintigraphy-Enhances on the delayed isotope scan.
- Fibrous dysplasia (FD)-Unknown etiology, M>F, 10-30 years

Radiological Features

Monostotic or polyostotic (multiple bones)
Location—Diametaphyseal, pelvis, femur and rib, smooth, dense margin of varying width-'RIND OF an orange'.
Cortex—scalloped and thinned but intact

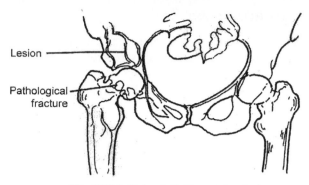

Fig. 6.73.1: Polyostotic fibrous dysplasia

MRI—Fluid filled cyst.
mineralization/fibrous tissue

IMPLANTATION DERMOID

Cyst lined by epidermis.
Previous history
R/F—Well-defined round lytic lesion
Minimal sclerosis is seen surrounding the lesion

Age

2nd and 3rd decade,   M:F = 2.5:1

Clinical Presentation

Site	—Diaphysis or metaphysis of tubular bone
R/F	NIDUS-Characteristic feature 10 mm or less surrounding the nidus is a region of reactive sclerosis and periosteal new bone formation
CT	—Thin section 2 mm. Scintigraphy-an intense focal abnormality and intense activity persistent on delayed image.

SOLITARY BONE CYST

Unilocular: Site-proximal humerus and femur – before epiphyseal closure calcaneum = mature skeleton

M > F

In metaphysis may extend into diaphysis

Radiological Features

Area of lucency in metadiaphysis.

Overlying cortex is thinned out, sclerotic reaction around the margin, No calcification.

Scintigraphy — No abnormality in blood pool phase as in aneurysm bone cyst (ABC).

Delayed image—Increase activity around the margin.

CHONDROBLASTOMA

Second decade of age, epiphysis or apophysis

Frequently extend into metaphysis

Well-defined, radiolucent, oval lesion with thin rim of sclerosis and cortical expansion.

Stippled calcification	—25%
Adjacent periosteal reaction	
CT and MR	—Extension into soft tissue
Bone scan	—Increase activity in blood pool phase.

ENCHONDROMA

50%	—Hands, 20% = Femur, Humerus and Tibia, 10% small bones feet
20%	—Flat bones
Age	—2nd and 3rd decade, flecks of calcification within the tumor—popcorn appearance

Scintigraphy   — Unremarkable
MRI   — Hyperintense on T2(hyaline cartilage)

ADAMENTINOMA OF LONG BONES

Midhalf of tibia(femur)
Age   — 10-50 (Avg-35 years)
Sex   — M : F = 5:4

Radiological Features

Multilocular appearance and satellite lesion are diagnostic.

Eosinophilic Granuloma

Age   — 3-12 years
Site   — Skull, pelvis, femur and spine. Diaphysis in long bones 2/3rd solitary
R/F   — Lucent lesion with sharply defined margins active phase, No sclerosis
Healing phase   — Peripheral sclerosis
Vertebrae plana   — Associated with paravertebral soft tissue mass.

BROWN TUMOR OF HYPERPARATHYROIDISM

Site   — Metaphysis and diaphysis unusually responsive to PTH solitary or multiple other associated feature resorption of bones.
- Chondrocalcinosis
- Pepper pot skull.
- Renal lithiasis

MULTIPLE MYELOMA (PLASMACYTOMA)

Solitary or multiple
> 40 years, M:F =2:1

- Persistent-bone pain or pathalogical fracture
- Radiological features-Diffuse osteoporosis
- Rounded or oval defects with sharp margin
- No marginal sclerosis
- Long bones, spine, clavicle, scapula and skull.
- Laboratory investigation- increase total serum protein, Bence Jones proteinuria (abnormal urinary protein/ hypercalcemia increase).

METASTASES

Elderly age group	:	Spine, pelvis and ribs, proximal end of humerus and femur
Females	:	Most common breast
Males	:	Prostate, lung and kidney. Majority are osteolytic

- Soft tissue extension is uncommon without much periosteal reaction, lung, Breast = lytic
- Renal cell carcinoma=Solitary lesion in pelvis and lumbar spine, if multiple <6 in number.
- Thyroid—Expansile and lytic and often solitary.
- Lab- alkaline phosphatase increased
  serum carcinoma increased

GCT (OSTEOCLASTOMA) OR GIANT CELL TUMOR

Age	—	20-40 years, M>F
Site	—	Subarticular, bones adjacent to knee joint and wrist, eccentric. No calcification/ossification, No periosteal reaction.
40%	—	Soap bubble pattern or trabeculation. May produce well-defined extension into soft tissue.

Blood pool phase of bone scan show increased activity

ABC (Aneurysmal bone cyst)

Age — Before epiphyseal fusion and usually central
Site — Long bones and lumbar spine. Neural arch increase
RIF — An area of bone resorption with expansion of overlying cortex thinned out and expanded.
CT and MR — Fluid level in the vascular space.

Chondromyxoid Fibroma

Peak - 20-30 years
Site - Metaphysis, around the knee joint

Radiological Features

Eccentric space occupying lesion in metaphysis
margins are well-defined with surrounding sclerosis, no calcification.

Bone Scan

Increased activity localized to reactive sclerosis.

Metastatic Neuroblastoma

< 5 years Already known to have abdominal mass
R/F — Multiple often symmetric, lytic bone lesion
    — skull lesions are common
    • Cranial sutural margin may be infiltrated with widening of suture lines.

- Long bones and shaft may be penetrated.
- Diagnosis identification of primary tumor and raised blood level and urinary catecholamine.

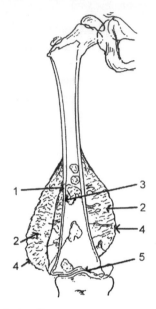

1. Areas of bone destruction
2. "Sunburst" periosteal reaction
3. "Codman triangle"
4. Circumferential soft-tissue mass
5. Pathologic fracture through growth plate

Fig. 6.73.2: Metastatic neuroblastoma. The permeative destructive lesion throughout the entire femoral shaft in a child with metastatic neuro-blastoma. The tumor has penetrated into the soft tissues along the distal half of the shaft, resulting in a large, circumferential soft tissue mass. The presence of a "sun-burst" periosteal reaction and Codman's triangles indicates the rapidity with which the tumor has broken through the periosteum. There is a pathologic fracture through the distal femoral growth plate

Table 6.73.1: Lytic lesion in bone

	Geode	FD	SBC	C blast	En.ChO	EG	BT	MM	Mets	GCT	ABC
Age	Mid/Late	10-30	2nd decade D	2nd decade	2-3 D	3-12	Mid	Elderly	Elderly	20-40	3-12
Sex	—	♀>♂	♂>♀	—	—	—	—	—	—	♀>♂	♀>♂
Site	S/A	DM	M/D	E/apo	Shaft	D	M/D	—	—	S/A	M
Location	At knee/Jt	P/F/R	Phox H&F Cal.	Long B	Small B of hand	SK, P.F and Sp.	Long B mandible R, P	Rare below elbow & knee scap ribs	Lt knee/chest	Long B and L spine	—
Surr. sclerosis	+	++	+	+	-/+	—	—	—	—	—	—
Multiplicity	+/-	+/-	—	—	+/-	+/-	+/-	⊕/—	+/-	—	—
Ca++	—	—	—	25% stippled corn	Pop-corn	—	—	—	—	—	Thin end strand
Other ch. feature	Arthritis	Stephabrook Albright	—	—	Maffucic syndrome olilier	Chest	Sub per bone	—	Known primary	Soap bubble	—
Exp. of bone	—	—	—	⊕	⊕	—	—	—	—	⊕	⊕
Lab. test	—	±	—	—	—	—	↑PTH	↑total Spot. Ca++↑ BJP in urine	Al.Phosp↑ serum Ca++↑	—	—

D—Decade

NON-OSSIFYING FIBROMA

10-20 years, around the knee joint.

Radiological Features

Increase radiolucency with well-defined margin in meta-diaphysis thin zone of reactive sclerosis.

Cortex is expanded but remains intact and thinned.

6.74 D/D OF GENERALIZED OSTEOPOROSIS

OSTEOPENIA

Generalized or regional rarefaction of the skeleton is decrease in bone density.

Causes of Diffuse Osteopenia

1. *Osteoporosis*—Diminished quantity of bone matrix but normal mineralization of remaining bone.
2. *Osteomalacia*—Normal quantity of bone but defective mineralization of osteoid.
3. *Hyperparathyroidism*—Increased bone resorption by osteoclasts.
4. Diffuse infiltrative bone diseases, e.g.
   • Multiple myeloma-leukemia
   • Gaucher's disease.

Generalized Osteoporosis

1. *Disorders of multiple/uncertain cause*
   a. Senile osteoporosis
   b. Juvenile osteoporosis
   c. Postmenopausal osteoporosis

2. *Endocrine*
   a. Cushing's disease
   b. Hypothyroidism
   c. Hyperthyroidism
   d. Hypogonadism
   e. Hypopituitarism
   f. Acromegaly
   g. Diabetes mellitus
3. *Congenital*
   a. Osteogenesis imperfecta
   b. Homocystinuria
4. *Nutritional disturbances*
   a. Scurvy
   b. Protein deficiency
   c. Calcium deficiency
5. *Drugs*
   a. Heparin
   b. Steroids
   c. Vitamin A
6. *Chronic diseases*
   a. Chronic renal disease—Renal osteodystrophy
   b. Hepatic insufficiency
   c. Chronic inflammatory polyarthropathies
   d. GI malabsorption syndromes
   e. Chronic debility or immobilization.

Osteoporosis

- No evidence of hyperparathyroidism or osteomalacia
- Evidence of condition such as senility, immobilization. Postmenopausal state, or other causes to explain it.

Roentgenological Changes

Most prominent in axial skeleton, proximal humerus, femur, wrist and ribs.

1. *Long Bones*
   - Cortical thinning with irregularity of endosteal surface.
   - The thin cortex maintains normal mineral content and appears dense.
   - Deossification of spongy bone.
   - Prominence of trabeculae in lines of stress.
   - Delayed fracture healing with poor callus.

2. *Spine*
   - Diminished radiographic density.
   - Vertebral end plates are thin and dense with "Pencilling in" of vertebrae.
   - Irregular endosteal surface of vertebral end plates.
   - Vertical striations because of loss of horizontal trabeculae and accentuation of vertical trabeculae along lines of stress.
   - Compression deformities with biconcave vertebral bodies—cod fish vertebrae
   - Absence of osteophyte formation.

Senile Osteoporosis

Etiology

- Reduced intestinal absorption
- Decreased adrenal function
- Secondary hyperparathyroidism
  - There is proportionate loss of cortical and trabecular bone.
  - Fractures most commonly in femoral neck, proximal humerus, tibia and pelvis.
  - F:M=2:1

Juvenile Osteoporosis

- Idiopathic self limiting disorder.
- Affects both sexes typically before puberty.
- Clinically bone pain, backache, limp
- Blood chemistry is normal.
- Fracture of metaphysis of long bones with minimal trauma
- Vertebral collapse, wedging, kyphosis

Postmenopausal Osteoporosis

- Affects women in 50-65 years age group.

Etiology

- Reduced estrogen levels.
- Nutritional status, level of activity and genetic causes also influence.
- There is disproportionate loss of trabecular bone with rapid bone loss.
- Fractures commonly affect vertebrae with wedging fracture of distal radius.

Cushing's Syndrome

- Due to excess of adrenocortical steroids.
- Negative calcium balance and hypercalciuria
- Decreased bone formation and increased resorption

Imaging

1. Osteoporosis
2. Exuberant callus formation causing increased density of endplates of compressed vertebral bodies.
3. Multiple painless rib fractures
4. Osteonecrosis.

Hypothyroidism

- Cretinism in children, myxedema in adults.
- Retarded skeletal maturation, fragmented epiphysis.
- Bullet shaped vertebrae
- Osteoporosis

Hyperthyroidism

- Increased metabolic activity with increase in bone formation and resorption.
- Bone resorption causes generalized osteopenia in skull, pelvis, spine and long bones.
- Vertebral wedging, cod fish vertebrae, kyphosis
- Pretibial myxedema.

Hypogonadism

- Due to decrease production of gonadal hormones or LH and FSH by pituitary.
  - *In boys*—Delayed closure of epiphysis with long limbs and short trunk.
  - *In females*—Turner's syndrome-short stature, cubitus valgus, osteoporosis, short 4th metacarpal, webbed neck. Cardiovascular anomalies.

Hypopituitarism

- Deficiency of growth hormone results in cessation of endochondral ossification.
- Retarded skeletal maturation, delayed skeletal growth
- Overall reduced bone density due to reduced bone formation.

Acromegaly

- Rarely causes osteoporosis
- Enlarged paranasal sinuses, prognathism, frontal bossing
- Enlargement and scalloping of vertebral bodies
- Arrow head terminal phalanges, increase heel pad thickness.

Osteogenesis Imperfecta

- Inherited disorder of connective tissue with abnormal maturation of collagen.
- *Classical clinical triad:* Fragile long bones, blue sclerae and deafness.
- Diffuse osteopenia with thin fragile long bones, multiple fractures and bowed bones.
- Exuberant callus

Scurvy

- Long-term deficiency of vitamin C (> 6 months)
- Children present with limb pain and irritability.

Imaging

1. Epiphysis is small and sharply marginated by a sclerotic rim.
2. Increase density of zone of provisional calcification
3. Transverse band of lucency in metaphysis known as Trümmerfeld zone.
4. Metaphyseal Spurs-Pelkan's spurs

Protein Deficiency

Protein deficiency produces osteoporosis due to deficiency of matrix production, e.g. in malnutrition nephrosis, diabetes mellitus, Cushing's syndrome and hyperthyroidism.

Heparin Toxicity

- Heparin has a direct local stimulating effect on bone resorption.
- Large doses of heparin >15000 units/day
- Hyperheparin states occur in Marfan's and Hurler's syndrome and mast cell disease.

Renal Osteodystrophy

- Bony changes in patients suffering from chronic uremia due to long standing renal disease.

Imaging Features

a. Secondary hyperparathyroidism-bone resorption
b. Osteoporosis
c. Osteosclerosis-Rugger Jersey spine
e. Soft tissue calcifications.

Arthropathies (Rheumatoid Arthritis)

- May cause osteoporosis due to steroids or limitation of movement due to pain or muscle wasting.
- Erosive changes, alignment deformities and soft tissue swelling may be found.

Disuse Osteoporosis

- Results from lack of stress and strain on bone.
- Frequently caused by paralysis or body cast.
- Osteoblasts remain inactive and older bone is not replaced.
- Relieved when affected part is mobilized.

Osteomalacia

- Due to vitamin-D deficiency in adults.

- Defective mineralization of osteoid in mature cortical and cancellous bone.
- Pseudofractures or looser's zones-B/L symmetrical focal accumulations of osteoid at right angles to long axis of bones.
- Intracortical resorption, osteopenia with coarse trabecular pattern.

Hyperparathyroidism

- Affects mainly middle aged women.
- Increase parathyroid hormone causes increase osteoclastic bone resorption.
- *X-Ray*—Subperiosteal, intracortical, subchondral, trabecular and subligamentous bone resorption.
  - Brown tumors, Pepper pot skull.
  - Osteopenia.

Diffuse Infiltrative Disorders

For example: Multiple myeloma, leukemia and Gaucher's disease may cause extensive deossification because of proliferation of plasma cells, leukemic cells or histiocytic cells in bone marrow.

Table 6.74.1: Generalized osteopenia

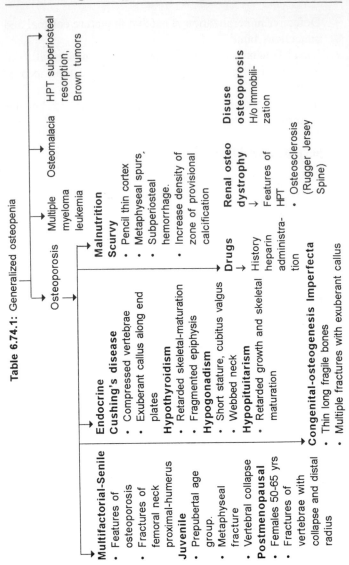

Generalized osteopenia

→ Osteoporosis

→ Multiple myeloma leukemia

→ Osteomalacia

→ HPT subperiosteal resorption, Brown tumors

Multifactorial-Senile
- Features of osteoporosis
- Fractures of femoral neck proximal-humerus

Juvenile
- Prepubertal age group.
- Metaphyseal fracture
- Vertebral collapse

Postmenopausal
- Females 50-65 yrs
- Fractures of vertebrae with collapse and distal radius

Endocrine
Cushing's disease
- Compressed vertebrae
- Exuberant callus along end plates

Hypothyroidism
- Retarded skeletal-maturation
- Fragmented epiphysis

Hypogonadism
- Short stature, cubitus valgus
- Webbed neck

Hypopituitarism
- Retarded growth and skeletal maturation

Malnutrition
Scurvy
- Pencil thin cortex
- Metaphyseal spurs,
- Subperiosteal hemorrhage
- Increase density of zone of provisional calcification

Drugs
→ History heparin administration

Congenital-osteogenesis Imperfecta
- Thin long fragile bones
- Multiple fractures with exuberant callus

Renal osteo dystrophy
→ Features of HPT
- Osteosclerosis (Rugger Jersey Spine)

Disuse osteoporosis
H/o Immobilization

6.75 SOLITARY DENSE VERTEBRA

LYMPH

- Lymphoma
- Low-grade infection
- Metastasis
- Paget's disease
- Hemangioma

Metastasis

1. Sclerotic metastasis
   - Medulloblastoma
   - Bronchus
   - Breast
   - Bladder
   - Bowel (Especially carcinoids)
   - Lymphoma
   - Prostate
2. Lytic metastasis-after T/F
3. No alteration in vertebral body size
4. Disc spaces preserved
5. Multiple
6. Lower thoracic and lumbar spine—Most common site
7. Sclerotic lesions are hypointense on both T1-and T2WI.

PAGET'S DISEASE

- Usually a single vertebral body is affected-lumbar spine and sacrum.
- Expanded body with thickened cortex and coarsened trabeculation. Picture frame vertebra.

- Disc space involvement is uncommon.
  - Fish vertebra-due to structural weakness (biconcave)
  - Involvement of posterior elements helps to differentiate from hemangioma.

Lymphoma

- HL>NHL—40-60 years.
- Normal sized vertebral body.
- Disc spaces intact.
- MR—focal or diffuse hypointensity than normal marrow on T1 WI and iso or hyperintensity than normal marrow on T2 WI.
- Low grade infection—
  - End plate destruction.
  - Disc space narrowing
  - Paraspinal soft tissue mass.

Hemangioma

Prominance of the secondary bony trabeculae of the vertebral body causing a striate or honeycomb pattern.
- Expansion +/−
- Lower thoracic and lumbar spine
- Multiple lesion in 25-30% cases
- *NECT:*—Lucent lesion with typical 'polka dot' densities in medullary spaces.
- Hyperintense on both T1 and T2 WI.
- Disc space-preserved.

Table 6.75.1: Solitary dense vertebrae

Feature	Metastasis	Paget	Lymphoma	Infection	Hemangioma
• Size	N	Ex	N	N or ↓	N or Ex
• Disc space	N	N	N	↓	N
• End plate destruction	–	–	–	+	–
• Paravertebral soft tissue	–	–	±	±	–
• Prominent vertical trabeculae	–	+	–	–	+
• Cortical thickening	–	+	–	–	–
• Post element involvement	+	+	–	–	–
• MR	↓ T1 and T2	Variable	↓ T1, iso or ↑ T1	↓ T1 and ↑ T2	↑ T1 and T2

6.76 ACRO-OSTEOLYSIS

- Loss of terminal tufts of digits
- Scleroderma/Connective tissue disease
- Psoriatic arthritis
- Reiter's disease
- Frostbite (thumbs spared) /burns
- Leprosy
- Polyvinyl chloride exposure
- Hyperparathyroidism
- Cleido cranial dysostosis
- Progeria
- Pycnodysostosis
- Sarcoidosis.

Cleidocranial Dysostosis

Autosomal dominant, 33% sporadic
- Skull
- Cranial dysplasia
- Wormian bones
- Basilar invagination.

Clavicles

- Aplasia/hypoplasia usually lateral portion.

Other Skeletal Abnormalities

- Small, high scapula
- Wide symphysis pubis
- Acro-osteolysis.

Hajdu-Cheney Syndrome

An osteolytic syndrome with skull deformities, characteristic facies, osteoporosis, premature loss of teeth, joint laxity, short stature, dissolution of the terminal phalanges, hearing loss and a hoarse voice.

- The changes in the terminal phalanges in this condition as well as in pycnodysostosis are 'pseudo-osteolysis, that is the disorder of defective development rather than bone destruction of bone already formed.
- The patients show bathrocephaly (projection of the occipital area and a deep groove at the lambdoid sutures both in the occipital and parietal bones)

PROGERIA

An abnormal congenital condition, associated with defect in the LAMIN Type A gene, which is characterized by premature aging in children, where all changes of cell structure occur.

- Normal at birth
- *"Wisened old man":* Alopecia, atrophy of muscles and skin
- Atherosclerosis = coronary artery disease
- Dwarfism
- Abnormal facies: Receding chin, beaked nose, exophthalmos.

Findings

- Acro-osteolysis
- Hypoplastic facial bones + sinuses
- Open cranial sutures + fontanelles, Wormian bone
- Coxa valga.

Pycnodysostosis

- Autosomal recessive
- Dense, sclerotic bones

Features

- Open cranial sutures + fontanelles
- Wormian bones
- Dolichocephaly
- Sclerotic vertebrae
- Fractured long bones
- Short, stubby bones
- Partial agenesis/aplasia of terminal phalanges.

Psoriatic Arthritis

Types

1. True psoriatic arthritis (1/3)
2. Resembling rheumatoid arthritis (1/3)
3. Combination of psoriatic and rheumatoid arthritis (RA) (1/3).

Findings

- No juxta-articular osteoporosis (unlike RA)
- Periosteal reaction-frequent
- Asymmetrical destruction of distal interphalangeal joints with ankylosis
- Resorption of terminal tufts with "pencil in cup" deformity.
- Ivory phalanges
- Destruction of 1st toe interphalangel joint with periosteal reaction and bony proliferation at distal phalangeal bone (Pathognomic)
- Asymmetrical syndesmophytes (lower cervical-to upper lumbar-spine)
- Squaring of vertebrae in lumbar-spine
- Paravertebral soft tissue calcification
- Bilateral asymmetrical sacroiliitis

Sarcoidosis

Non-caseating granulomatous disease
- Unknown etiology
- Young adults, blacks more than whites
- Prognosis usually good
- May affect any organ
- Chest most often involved
- Diffuse pulmonary infiltrate, may resolve or progress to fibrosis.
  - HRCT
    - Mediastinal adenopathy
    - Early = septal thickening, peribronchovascular nodules, alveolar ground glass opacity.
    - Late = Traction bronchiectasis, fibrosis, honey combing.
    - Skeleton involved in 10%
    - Differential diagnosis: Bronchial/transbronchial biopsy (60-95% diagnostic), liver or scalene biopsy.

Scleroderma/Progressive Systemic Sclerosis (PSS)

- Hypertrophy than atrophy of collagen fibers
- 4-6th decade, M:F = 1:3
- Bones
  - Punctate soft tissue calcification (finger tips, shoulder, hips)
  - Acro-osteolysis (63%).
- Intercarpal joint space narrowing (late).
- Chest
  - Evident in 10-25%
  - Pulmonary fibrosis with diffuse reticulate infilterate
  - Predominantly in lower lungs.

- GI
  - Esophageal dilatation and aperistalasis (>50%)
  - Hiatus hernia + GE reflux + Esophagitis +.

Distal Esophageal Stricture

- Gastroparesis
- Dilation and dysmotility of small bowel
- Pseudosacculation and dysmotility of colon.

Reiter's Syndrome

- Males
- Polyarthritis
  - Feet
  - SI joints
  - Knee/Ankles (Joint effusion)
- Urethritis
- Uveitis/Conjuctivitis.

Polyvinyl chloride may cause or feature the following:-

Miscellanous syndromes

  - Acro-osteolysis
  - Carcinogenosis

Symptoms and Signs

  - Raynaud's phenomenon.

Cranio-mandibular Dysostosis

- Acro-osteolysis
- Arthropathy
- GI bleeding
- Micrognathia
- Short stature

Flow Chart 6.76.1: Acro-osteolysis

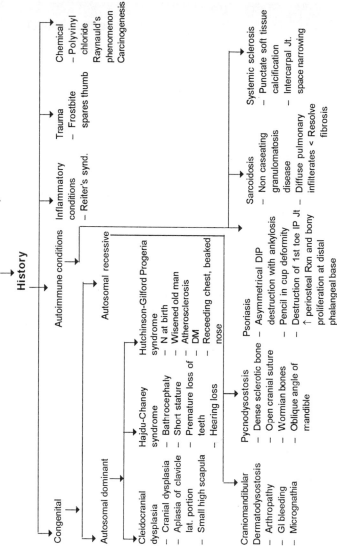

History

Congenital

Autosomal dominant

Cleidocranial dysplasia
– Cranial dysplasia
– Aplasia of clavicle lat. portion
– Small high scapula

Hajdu-Chaney syndrome
– Bathrocephaly
– Short stature
– Premature loss of teeth
– Hearing loss

Craniomandibular Dermatodysostosis
– Arthropathy
– GI bleeding
– Micrognathia

Pycnodysostosis
– Dense sclerotic bone
– Open cranial suture
– Wormian bones
– Oblique angle of mandible

Autosomal recessive

Hutchinson-Gilford Progeria syndrome
– N at birth
– Wisened old man
– Atherosclerosis
– DM
– Receeding chest, beaked nose

Psoriasis
– Asymmetrical DIP destruction with ankylosis
– Pencil in cup deformity
– Destruction of 1st toe IP Jt
– ↑ periosteal Rxn and bony proliferation at distal phalangeal base

Autoimmune conditions

Sarcoidosis
– Non caseating granulomatosis disease
– Diffuse pulmonary infiltrates < Resolve fibrosis

Systemic sclerosis
– Punctate soft tissue calcification
– Intercarpal Jt. space narrowing

Inflammatory conditions
– Reiter's synd.

Trauma
– Frostbite spares thumb

Chemical
– Polyvinyl chloride
Raynauld's phenomenon
Carcinogenesis

6.77 SACROILIITIS

Only anteroinferior aspects of SI joint is covered with cartilage (1mm hyaline cartilage on iliac side, 3-5 mm fibrous cartilage on sacral side, with normal joint width of 2-5 mm.
* Erosions—widening of joint space
* Subchondral bone sclerosis—bony ankylosis
* Periarticular osteoporosis—Eventual return of normal bone density.

D/D of Sacroiliitis

A. *B/L symmetrical:*
 – Ankylosing spondylitis
 – Psoriatic arthritis
 – Intrabowel disease: Crohn's, Whipple's
 – Rheumatoid arthritis
 – Deposition arthopathy,gout, CPPD.
 – Osteitis condensans ilei-More common in females, young, normal joint space
 – Hyperparathyroidism, subcondral—bone resorption and increase joint space
 – Paraplegia—Decrease joint space and osteoporosis.

B. *B/L Asymmetrical*
 Psoriatic arthropathy—40% of cases.

Reiter's Syndrome

Juvenile rheumatoid arthritis (JRA)
Osteoarthritis (OA): Smooth articular margins and well define, decrease joint space, subchondral bone sclerosis, anterior osteophytes.

C. *Unilateral (U/L)*

Infection
OA-abnormal mechanical stress.

ARTHRITIS INVOLVING SPINAL COLUMN

- Ankylosing spondylitis
- Rheumatoid arthritis
- Psoriatic arthritis
- Reiter's syndrome
- Osteoarthritis
- DISH
- JRA (juvenile rheumatoid arthritis).

ANKYLOSING SPONDYLITIS

Seronegative
97% of patient for HLA B27

Age	Late teens and 20's sex-equal in both sexes, osteopenia
SI joint	Symmetrical, erosions (more on iliac side) joint widening heals by sclerosis—joint narrowing (whiskering), fusion.

Spinal Column

After the SI joint, begins at dorsolumbar or L-S region and then progress to other areas.

Vertebral body squaring—

A. Osteitis and erosions adjacent to vertebral-endplate margins-shiny or ivory corner.

B. *All mineralization*

Syndesmophytes—hallmark (Annulus fibrosus calcification)

= maturation leading to "Bamboo spine" similar well defined ossification seen in interspinous ligament and around minor and major joints.

Enthesitis

Shaggy or whiskered pattern at IT and GT.

Spinal Fusion

After the calcification of IV disc.

Psoriatic Arthropathy

- 10% pt develop arthritis before skin lesions appear.
- In 25%—Develop simultaneously
- 65% = psoriasis precedies arthritis.

Clinical Feature

Normal bone, mineralization.

- *SI joint*—Seen in 50% of pt those have polyarthritis
- B/L symmetrical in 60%, asymmetrical is 40%
- *Erosion*—Joint widening-sclerosis. Fusion is less common than in ankylosing spondylitis.
- *Enthesitis*—IT and calcaneum.
- *Spine*—Segmental, asymmetrical, can involve any region. Paravertebral ossification-common and characteristically symmetric, squaring of vertebral body. Atlanto-axial subluxation in some cases.

Other Feature

- Frequently affection of hands.
- Sausage digit
- Erosion at DIP and IP of great toe, cup and pencil appearance (because of osseous fusion of IP joint)
- Arthritis mutilans.

Reiter's Syndrome

Young female, STD, characteristic triad of arthritis, urethritis and conjunctivitis associated with HLA B27 skeletal involvement seen eventually in 80%.

- *SI joint*—sacroiliitis-late in Reiter's, seen in 50% bilateral and asymmetrical

Fusion is less frequent than ankylosing spondylitis.

- *Spine*—Similar to psoriatic arthritis, except paravertebral ossification which is asymmetrical segmental around the dorsolumbar junction. Other feature-affects the feet rather than hand, MTP and IP of great toe. Normal mineralization.
- Irregular erosion and enthesis.
- Painful erosion and reactive spur very common around the calcaneum.

RHEUMATOID ARTHRITIS (RA)

- 20-55 yr, female more than M<G, mainly affects the small joints.
- *SI joint*—sacroiliitis-seen in few patients, erosive process is not as agressive as in other joints. Bone mineralization decreased.
- *Spine*—Most common site = upper cervical spine
- Subluxation-because of rupture of transverse ligament and
- Erosion of odontoid-finally leading to fracture of odontoid leading to basilar invagination.
- Apophyseal joint and disc space-rare-eroded-fused.
- Malalignment.

OA (DEGENERATIVE CHANGES)

- Degenerative arthritis of synovium—elderly.
- *SI joint*—rarely involved-smooth anterior margins, joint space decreased, subchondral sclerosis, anterior osteophytes
- *Spine*—Space bilateral and opposing bones become narrowed with marginal new bone formation-osteophyte-+ve and horizontal
- Most common site are cervical and lumbar spine (Lower cervical-C5-C6) and C6-C7.
- Vertebrae (C3 to C7) joints-narrowing of this joints with osteophytic lipping.

DISH (FORESTIET'S DISEASE)

- Elderly female, M:F=3:1, HLA B 27 in some patients. Excessive ossification found at many sites.
- *SI*—involves, the ligamentous part of joint fusion less common
- *Spine*—Cervical and lower thoracic (on right side)
- Flowing ossification of spine involving 4 or more continuous vertebrae and hyperostosis of some ligamentous attachment and around the iliac crest, is chia and above the acetabulum
- Normal vertebral and normal I/V disc space- No erosion.

Enteropathic Spondyloarthropathies

- Uncommon, Crohn's, Whipple's disease-may associated. with joint, disease of secondary type.
  1. Peripheral-ST swelling and local periostitis patients are sero -ve and HLA B27-ve.
  2. Sacroiliitis and spondylitis-identical to ankylosing spondylitis. Do not correlate with gut disease activity! Patients are usually male and increase positivity for HLA B27 antigen (appr. 60%).

Juvenile Rheumatoid Arthritis (JRA)

- Less than 16 yrs, 10%-Rh +ve, 90%- Rh-ve, osteopenia.
- *SI joint*—B/L asymmetrical, similar to ankylosing spondylitis.
- *Spinal*—cervical spine under developed vertebral, increase IV disc space
- Atlanto-axial subluxation -in sero+ve patients. Other joint-metacarpo and intercarpal joint-usual site
- Chronic synovitis and effusion-increase of carpal bones and epiphysis.

Table 6.77.1: Sacroiliitis

	AS	PA	Reiter syn.	RA	OA	DISH	JRA
Age and Sex	Adult age ♂ ≥ ♀	Middle age	Young ♂	Middle age ♀ > ♂	Elderly ♂ = ♀	Eld. ♂:♀ = 3:1	Young < 16
Sacroilitis	B/L Sym	B/L Sym	B/L Asym	B/L Sym	B/LA Sym U/L	B/L Sym L Asym	B/L Sym
Site of SI	Synovial part	Synovial	Synovial	Synovial	Synovial	Ligamentous C & lower thoracic	Synovium C spine
Spondylitis-site	T&L & rare C spine in ♀	Any region	Any region	C spine (C₁ and C₂)	Lower C spine	Ossi. of ALL ant. flowing	—
Ossification	Syndesmo-phyte (vertical)	Paraverte-bral symm.	Paraverte-bral, Asym	—	Osteophyte (Horizontal)	—	Under developed
Changes in V. body	Squaring	Squaring	Squaring	±	N or ↓ HCl	—	—
Erosions	+	+	+	++	—	—	+
Enthesitis	+	+	+	—	—	+	+
I/V dis sp.	N	N	N	N	→	N	←
I/V disc Ca⁺⁺	+	—	—	—	+	+	+
Bone mineral	→	N	N	→	Localized ↑ in B	N	→
Atlanto-axial subluxation	2% cases	+ 45% of PA	—	+	—	—	—
OPLL	+	—	—	—	—	+	—
Lab finding autoimmune markers	HLA B₂₇ Ag	HLA B₂₇ Ag	HLA B₂₇ Ag	+ve Rh factor	—	HLA B₂₇ in few	+ in sero, +ve / 10% Rh +ve

6.78   BONE CYST

Cyst in a well defined lucent lesion presenting in the bone. It can either be solitary or multiple and may be present in the epiphysis, metaphysis or diaphysis. It can be expansile, nonexpansile, uniloculated or multiloculated.

It may or may not have a sclerotic margin. The features however are not diagnostic and there is considerable overlap.

NONEXPANSILE UNILOCULAR CYSTIC LESIONS

- Fibrous cortical defect.
- Nonossifying fibroma.
- Simple unicameral bone cyst.
- Brown tumor of HPT.
- Eosinophillic granuloma.
- Enchondroma.
- Epidermoid inclusion cyst.
- Posttraumatic/degenerative cyst.
- Pseudotumor of hemophilia.
- Interosseous ganglion.
- Histiocytoma.
- Arthritic lesion.
- Endosteal pigmented villonodular synovitis.
- Fibrous dysplasia.
- Infectious lesions (Brodie's abscess)
- Metastasis.

NONEXPANSILE MULTILOCULAR CYSTIC LESION

- Aneurysmal bone cyst.
- Giant cell tumor.
- Fibrous dysplasia.

EXPANSILE UNILOCULAR CYSTIC LESIONS

- Simple bone cyst.
- Enchondroma.
- Aneurysmal bone cyst.
- Juxtacortical chondroma.
- Nonossifying fibroma.
- Eosinophillic granuloma.
- Brown tumor of HPT.
- Chondromyxoid fibroma.
- Hydatid cyst.
- Lipoma.

Lesions Surrounded by Marked Sclerosis

- Osteoid osteoma.
- Brodie's abscess.
- Chondroblastoma.
- Plasmacytoma.

Multiple Cystic Lesions

- Fibrous dysplasia.
- Enchondroma.
- Eosinophillic granuloma.
- Metastasis.
- Multiple myeloma.
- Brown tumors.
- Cystic angiomatosis of bone.
- Gaucher's disease.

Fibrous Cortical Defect

- Peak age 7-8 yrs mostly before epiphyseal closure.
- Present at metaphyseal cortex of long bones, most commonly posterior medial aspect of distal femur.

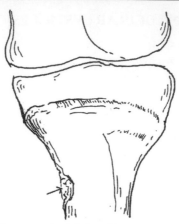

Fig. 6.78.1: Fibrous cortical defect. The most common benign bone tumor, it appears as a small oval lucency in the cortex of the posteromedial aspect of the proximal tibial shaft

- Round to oval, average diameter of 1-2 cm.
- Extends parallel to long axis of the bone.
- Cortical thinning and expansion may occur.
- Smooth well defined scalloped margins.
- Involutes over 2-4 years.

Nonossifying Fibroma

- Much larger than fibrous cortical defect and presents at an older age group 10-20 years.
- Majority are found near knee joint, distal end of femur being the most common site.
- Sharply defined radiolucent lesion at metadiaphysis and have a lobulated appearance with a thin zone of reactive sclerosis.
- May cause cortical expansion but the cortex remains intact.
- Lesions have a tendency to regress and multiple lesions may be associated with neurofibromatosis.

Simple Bone Cyst

- Also known as unicameral bone cyst.
- Always unilocular and well defined.
- Site of origin depends on the age of presentation, prior to epiphyseal fusion. They usually occur in the proximal humeri and femora, after epiphyseal fusion some lesions may occur in bones like calcaneum. By far the most common site is proximal humerus.
- During the stage of skeletal maturation the lesion is carried from its usual metaphyseal location to diaphysis. The usual location is thus metadiaphyseal.
- The overlying cortex is often thinned and slightly expanded with no periosteal reaction unless a fracture has occurred.
- The lesions may be surrounded by a discrete sclerotic margin.

Brown Tumor of HPT

- Alike osteoclastoma and pathologically is due to replacement of bone by vascularized fibrous tissue and collection of osteoclasts.
- Most common locations are jaw, pelvis, rib, metaphysis of long bones.
- Often eccentric and cortical in location and is most frequently solitary but may be multiple.
- They are expansile, well marginated and cyst like with endosteal scalloping.
- Other signs of hyperparathyroidism are present.

Eosinophilic Granuloma

- Most benign variety of histiocytosis X and in 60-80% cases is localized to bone with age incidence of 2-30 years.

Most common in 5-10 years of age. Solitary lesions are most common but it can be multiple.

- Lesions arise within medullary canal and skull is the site in 50% of cases and that too the diploic space of parietal bone being most frequent. The mono-ostotic involvement is most frequent.
- These are round or ovoid punched out lesions with beveled edges and with a sharply marginated sclerotic rim is present.
- Appearances may also be of hole within hole or that of button sequestrum.
- There may be an overlying soft tissue mass.

Enchondroma

- Benign cartilaginous growth in the medullary cavity. Bones with enchondral calcification are affected, the skull is thus not affected.
- Age of presentation is 10-30 years.
- An oval or round lucency is present near epiphysis with fine marginal line with scalloped well defined margins and ground glass appearance.
- Calcifications may be present in the lesion and there could be bulbous expansion of the bone with cortical thinning with no cortical breach or periosteal reaction.
- Multiple enchondromas may be seen in ollier's disease. In Maffuci syndrome multiple enchondroma are associated with soft-tissue cavernous hemangiomas.

Epidermoid Inclusion Cyst

- Alike implantation cyst and is most commonly seen in age group of 20-40 years.

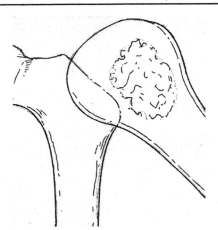

Fig. 6.78.2: Enchondroma

- Seen in superficially located bones as in the calvarium, phalanx, foot.
- These are well defiend lesions with a sclerotic margin and cortex is frequently expanded and thinned.
- No calcifications, soft tissue mass or periosteal reaction is noted.

Geodes

These are cystic lesion, usually subarticular in location and are secondary to arthritis and osteonecrosis. The etiology is similar to posttraumatic cysts and is due to bone necrosis leading to intrusion of synovial fluid and a connection with the joint may be demonstrated.

Intraosseous Ganglion

- These are benign subchondral lesions without degenerative arthritis.
- Usually presents in middle age with mild localized pain.

- Most common at the epiphysis of long bones.
- Well demarcated solitary lesions with a sclerotic margin and with no communication to the joint.

Histiocytoma

- Benign fibrous histiocytoma of bone may mimic a cystic lesions.
- Usually presents in 23-60 yrs age group with localized pain and soft tissue swelling.
- Long bone epiphysis are typically involved.
- Presents as a well defined lesion with or without a soap bubble appearance and may have a sclerotic rim with no evident periosteal reaction. May cause cortical expansion.

Fibrous Dysplasia

- Most common in the first two decades of life and the lesions are present in the medullary cavity.
- Mono-ostotic variety is commoner than polyostotic variety.
- Patient may present with limb length discrepancy, shepherd's crook deformity of femur, facial asymmetry, tibial bowing and rib deformity.
- Mc-cune Albright syndrome is the association of poly-ostotic fibrous dysplasia with cafe-au-lait spots and endocrine dysfunctions like precocious puberty and is usually seen in girls.
- Common locations are ribs, craniofacial bones, femoral neck, tibia and pelvis.
- Lesions have a smooth dense margins which may be as thick as to resemble a rind of an orange.
- The bone may be expanded and the cortex scalloped but intact.

- They may be multilocular and are usually diametaphyseal.
- In the skull the sclerosis may cause encroachment of neural foramina.
- There may be intra-lesional calcification so much so that some lesions may have increased density.

Brodie's Abscess

- This is a type of subacute pyogenic osteomyelitis usually occurring at the metaphysis of long bones.
- There is a central area of lucency surrounded by a dense rim of sclerosis.
- Lucent channel like tortuous configurations towards the growth plate are virtually pathognomic.
- There may be periosteal reaction and adjacent soft tissue swelling.

Aneurysmal Bone Cyst

- Expansile lesion of bone containing thin walled blood filled cystic cavities. Involving the vertebral neural arches and long bones more commonly.
- Age range is 10-30 years and female patients are affected more often.
- Purely lytic, expansile and eccentric radiolucency with soap bubble pattern of trabeculations is seen. There may be very slight sclerosis.
- There may be rapid progression and the tumor may present with a pathological fracture.
- The cortex may be thinned but is intact.
- Three quarter of these cysts present before epiphyseal fusion is complete.

Osteoclastoma

- Usually occur before epiphyseal fusion and most patients are less than 20 yrs of age.

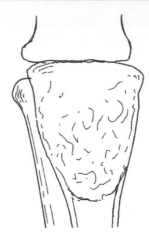

Fig. 6.78.3: Aneurysmal bone cyst. A large, medullary, expansile (blow out) lucency is seen in the proximal tibial diaphysis, abutting the growth plate (physis). The marked attenuation of the cortices, the well-organized triangular periosteal reaction along the distal margin of the lesion and the fact that the lesion is wider than the growth plate, are characteristic of an aneurysmal bone cyst

- May be associated with Paget's disease and usually present with pain swelling and tenderness at the affected site.
- It is an expansile solitary large lucent bone lesion causing exquisite cortical thinning near the epiphysis usually metaphyseal in location. The long bones are most frequently involved usually around the knee joint.
- There is a soap bubble appearance to the tumor with no evident sclerosis or periosteal reaction unless a fracture has occurred.
- There may be a soft tissue extension that characteristically has no calcification.
- When it involves vertebra it may lead to collapse and may involve the adjacent disks and may cross the joints.

Chondromyxoid Fibroma

- Peak age incidence 20-30 years and usually presents at the metaphysis of long bones.
- Expansile ovoid lesion with radiolucent center.
- Well defined sclerotic margin is present with no evident periosteal reaction.

Chondroblastoma

- Peak age incidence, 2nd decade and is usually epiphyseal in location involving the long bones more often.
- It's an oval to round eccentrically located lucent lesion with a well defined sclerotic margin and may contain punctate calcification.
- The cortex is intact, however a thick periosteal reaction may be seen.

Plasmacytoma

- Solitary bubbly grossly expansile lesion.
- Seen in 5th-7th decades of life, most commonly in thoracic or lumbar spine.

Multiple Myeloma

- Peak age is 5th-8th decades of life. There is an abnormal B-J protein in urine.
- Generalized osteoporosis with multiple widespread punched out lesions may be seen.
- There may be an associated soft tissue mass in the regions where bone destruction has occurred.
- May be associated with POEMS syndrome.

Metastasis

- Thyroid and kidney malignancies are the most common cause of metatastasis that resemble bone cysts however

lungs and breast carcinoma may also cause such appearance.
- Usually a history of primary can be elicited.

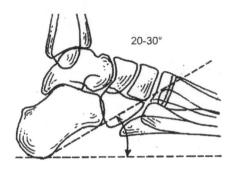

Fig. 6.78.4: Calcaneal pitch = Calcaneal inclination angle = determines longitudinal arch of foot; angle between line drawn along the inferior border of calcaneus connecting the anterior and posterior prominences + line representing the horizontal surface

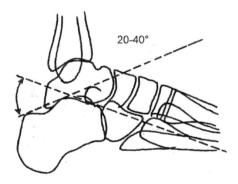

Fig. 6.78.5: Boehler angle = angle between first line drawn from posterosuperior prominence of calcaneus anteriorly to sustentaculum tali + second line drawn from anterosuperior prominence posteriorly to sustentaculum tail; measures integrity of calcaneus

Table 6.78.1: Bone cyst

Lesion	Age	Location	Uni or multi-loculated	Marginal sclerosis	Periosteal reaction	Cortical thickness expansion
Fibrous cortical defect	7-8 yrs	Metaphyseal cortex around knee	Uni	No	No	Normal
Nonossifying fibroma	10-20 yrs	Metadiaphyseal around knee	Uni	Thin rim	No	Expansile
Simple bone cyst	Bimodal	Metadiaphyseal	Uni	Present	No	Thinned and expanded
Brown tumor	No	Metaphysis and in jaw, pelvis, ribs	Uni	No	No	Expansile and thinned
Eosinophillic granuloma	5-10 yrs	Medullary canal	Uni	Present	No	Expansile
Enchondroma	10-30 yrs	Medullary canal	Uni	No	No	Expanded
Epidermoid inclusion cyst	20-40 yrs	Superficially located bones	Uni	Present	No	Expanded and thinned
Geodes	Later	Subarticular	Uni	No	No	Normal
Intra-osseous ganglion	Middle age	Epiphysis of long bones	Uni	Present	No	Expansion ±

Contd...

Contd...

Lesion	Age	Location	Uni or multi-loculated	Marginal sclerosis	Periosteal reaction	Cortical thickness expansion
Histiocytoma	23-60 yrs	Epiphysis of long bones	Multi	Present	No	Expansile
Fibrous dysplasia	10-20 yrs	Medullary canal	Uni	Thick	No	Thinned and expanded
Brodie's abscess	Children	Metaphysis	Uni	Present	Yes	Expansile
Aneurysmal bone cyst	10-30 yrs	Metadiaphyseal	Multi	Very mild	No	Thinned and expanded
Osteoclastoma	<20 yrs	Epiphysis around knee	Multi	No	No	Thinned and expanded
CMF	20-30 yrs	Metaphysis	Multi	Present	No	Expansile
Chondroblastoma	20-30 yrs	Epiphyseal	Uni	Present	Thick	Expansile
Plasmacytoma	50-70 yrs	Thoracic, lumbar spine	Multi	No	No	Expansile
Multiple myeloma	50-80 yrs	Wide spread	Uni	No	No	Normal
Metastasis	Later	Axial skeleton	Uni	No	No	Normal

BONE CYST
0-25 years

Epiphysis

Osteoclastoma
- Eccentric
- Multi-loculated
- Without sclerosis
- Without periosteal reaction
- Cortex usually intact, expansile

Chondroblastoma
- Eccentric
- Sclerotic margin
- Thick periosteal reaction
- Calcification +ve
- Expansile
- Cortex intact

Enchondroma
- Well defined
- Ground glass appearance
- Bulbous expansion
- Calcification +
- Expansile
- Cortex intact

Metaphysis

Fibrous Cortical defect
- Age 7-8 yr.
- Cortical in location
- Self regressing

Non-ossifying fibroma
- Larger at 10-20 yr
- Thin sclerotic margin
- Expansile
- Cortex intact
- Tendency to regress

Simple bone cyst
- Well defined
- Thin sclerotic rim
- Expansile
- Cortex intact
- No periosteal reaction

Brown Tumor
- Eccentric and Multiloculated
- Associated changes of hyper-parathyroidism

Fibrous Dysplasia
- Thick sclerosis
- No periosteal reaction
- Ground glass app.
- Expansile

Brodie's Abscess
- Thick sclerosis
- Periosteal reaction

CMF
- Periosteal reaction absent
- No calcification
- Sclerotic margin
- Expansile

Diaphysis

Eosinophillic Granuloma
- 5-10 yr age
- skull most common
- Punched out lesion
- Beveled edges
- Marginal sclerosis
- Expansile

Aneurysmal Bone Cyst
- Grossly Expansile
- Multiloculated
- Presents before epiphyseal closure
- Cortex intact

BONE CYST
25 yrs and above

Epiphysis

Geodes
– Subarticular
– Secondary to arthritis
  or trauma
– Changes of arthritis
  in nearby joints
– H/O trauma
– Secondary to arthritis
  may communicate to
  joint

Intraosseous Ganglion
– Subchondral
– Sclerotic margin
– No communication to
  joint

Histiocytoma
– Age 23-60 yr
– May be multiloculated
– Expansile.
– Marginal sclerosis
– No periosteal
  reaction

Metaphysis

Plasmacytoma
– 5th-7th decade
– Bubbly lesion
– Expansile
– Thoracic spine
  most common

Diaphysis

Simple bone
cyst

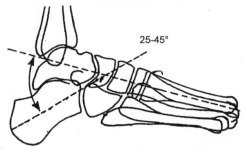

Fig. 6.78.6: Talocalcaneal angle on LAT view = angle between lines drawn through mid-transverse planes of talus + calcaneus; the midtalar line parallels the longitudinal axis of the first metatarsal

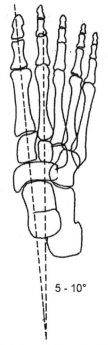

Fig. 6.78.7: Intermetatarsal angle amount that 1st + 2nd metatarsals diverge from each other

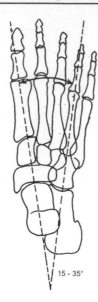

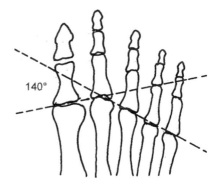

15 - 35°

Fig. 6.78.8: Talocalcaneal angle on AP view = Kite Angle = the midtalar and midcalcaneal lines parallel the 1st + 4th metatarsals; angle is greater in infants

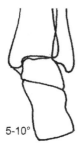

5-10°

Fig. 6.78.9: Heel valgus – cannot be measured directly on radiographs but inferred from the talocalcaneal angle and estimated on coronal CT sections

140°

Fig. 6.78.10: Angle of metatarsal heads = obtuse angle formed by lines tangential to metatarsal heads

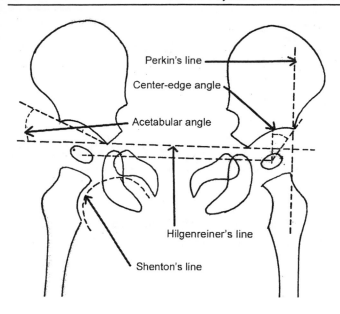

Fig. 6.78.11: AP pelvis view shows dislocation of hip
as evident by Broken Shenton line

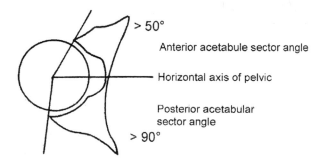

Fig. 6.78.12: Acetabular sector angles in normal Rt hip

7

Urogenital System

7.1 NEONATAL AND ADULT KIDNEY–DIFFERENCE

	Adult	*Neonatal*
Contour	Smooth	Lobed
Medullary	Reflectivity, −ve	−ve
Cortex	Reflectivity, +ve	++
Collecting	Echogenic	Echopoor
system	Inapparent	apparent

7.2 SMOOTH, SMALL KIDNEYS

Unilateral	*Bilateral*
• Ischemia due to focal arterial disease	Generalized arteriosclerosis
• Chronic infarction	Benign and malignant nephrosclerosis
• Radiation neoplasia	Atheroembolic renal disease
• Congenital hypoplasia	Chronic glomerulonephritis
• Postobstructive atrophy	Papillary necrosis
• Postinflammatory atrophy	Hereditary nephropathies
• Reflux atrophy	Hereditary chronic nephritis

Contd...

Contd...

Unilateral	Bilateral
	(Alpert's syndrome)
	Medullary cystic disease
	Arterial hypotension
	Amyloidosis (late)

SMALL, SMOOTH, UNILATERAL KIDNEY

With a small-volume collecting system.

A. Ischemia due to renal artery stenosis

Ureteric notching is due to enlarged collateral vessels and differentiates this from the other causes in this group.

Primary Uroradiologic Elements

Size–normal to decreased (left 1.5 cm less than right and right 2 cm shorter than left; may have less than normal increase in renal surface area in response to contrast material or diuretics).

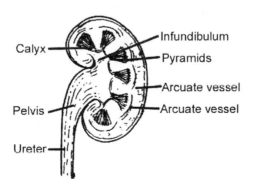

Fig. 7.2.1: Normal sectional anatomy of kidney

CONTOUR–SMOOTH (GLOBAL)

Secondary Uroradiologic Elements

- Pelvi-infundibulocalyceal system—attenuated (global)
- Notched proximal ureter (by ureteral arteries from lumbar branches of aorta), delayed opacification time
- Increased density of contrast material (decreased GFR allows increased salt and water absorption)
- Delayed washout of contrast material
- Parenchymal thickness—wasted (global)
- Calcification—linear (aneurysmal or atherosclerotic in renal hilus)
- Arteries—stenotic, aneurysmal, collateralized
- Angiography in atheromatous renal artery stenosis, there is an eccentric narrowing of the proximal third of the renal artery while in fibromuscular hyperplasia, there are segmental areas of stricturing and aneurysmal dilatation affecting the distal two-third of the renal arteries.
- Color Doppler shows the increase in peak systolic velocities to greater than 1.5 m/s, spectral broadening and increase in maximum diastolic flow velocities.

B. Chronic Renal Infarction

Primary Uroradiologic Elements

- Size—normal to small
- Contour—smooth (global)

Secondary Uroradiologic Elements

- Parenchymal thickness wasted (global, occasionally regional)
- Nephrogram—diminished to absent contrast material density
- Echogenicity—increased.

C. Radiation Nephritis

At least 23 Gy (2300 rad) over 5 weeks. The collecting system may be normal or small. Depending on the size of the radiation field both, one or just part of one kidney may be affected. There may be other sequelae of radiotherapy, e.g. scoliosis following radiotherapy in childhood.

Primary Uroradiologic Elements

- Size—normal to small
- Contour—smooth (global)
- Lesion distribution—consistent with radiation field material.

Secondary Uroradiologic Elements

- Parenchymal thickness—wasted (global, related to radiation field)
- Nephrogram—diminished density of contrast.

D. End Result of Renal Infarction

Due to previous severe trauma involving the renal artery or renal vein thrombosis.

The collecting system does not usually opacify during excretion urography.

E. With Five or Less Calyces

1. *Congenital Hypoplasia*

The pelvicalyceal system is otherwise normal.

Primary Uroradiologic Elements

- Size—decreased
- Contour—smooth (global)

Secondary Uroradiologic Elements

- Papillae—decreased number
- Calyces—decreased number
- Small renal artery and a normal ureter.

2. With a Dilated Collecting System

Post-obstructive atrophy

- There is thinning of the renal cortex and if there is impaired renal function, this will be revealed by poor contrast medium density in the collecting system.

Primary Uroradiologic Elements

- Size—small (normal or enlarged in minority of cases)
- Contour—smooth (global).

Secondary Uroradiologic Elements

- Papillae-effaced (global), may be normal in uncommon form
- Pelvi-infundibulocalyceal system—calyces dilated (global, may be normal in uncommon form)
  Parenchymal thickness—wasted (global).

3. Postinflammatory Atrophy

Primary Uroradiologic Elements

- Size—small
- Contour—smooth (global)

Secondary Uroradiologic Elements

- Papillae—disrupted
- Parenchymal thickness—wasted (global).

SMALL, SMOOTH, BILATERAL KIDNEYS

1. Generalized arteriosclerosis

Primary Uroradiologic Elements

- *Size*—normal to small
- *Contour*—smooth (global): May have random shallow scars

Secondary Uroradiological Elements

- Parenchymal thickness—wasted (global)
- Attenuation value—sinus fat increased

- Echogenicity- may be increased in sinus and renal parenchyma

2. *Medullary cystic disease*
   - Autosomal dominant disorder
   - Thin renal cortex
   - Variable number of small medullary cysts up to 2 cm on CT, US or MRI

3. *Amyloidosis, renal*
   - No specific radiological findings
   - Bilateral enlargement in presence of renal failure or nephrotic syndrome.
   - The nephrogram is normal or diminished
   - Renal thrombosis
   - Angiography is abnormal, but findings are nonspecific.
   - Gallium scans are extremely sensitive in the identification of renal amyloid.

4. *Papillary necrosis*
   - Thinning of the cortex
   - Partial sloughed papilla gives rise to density between papilla and pyramid. A fissure forms which communicate with central irregular cavity. In total sloughing, the sloughed papillary tissue may (a) fragment and passed in urine (b) cause ureteric obstruction (c) remain free in calyx (d) remain in pelvis and form a ball calculus.
   - With complete detachment, loss of normal cupping of the calyx with filling defect in the collecting system.
     A Analgesics other causes are- Adipose
     D Diabetes
     I Infant at shock
     P Pyelonephritis
     O Obstruction
     S Sickle cell disease
     E Ethanol

Flow Chart 7.2.1: Small smooth kidneys

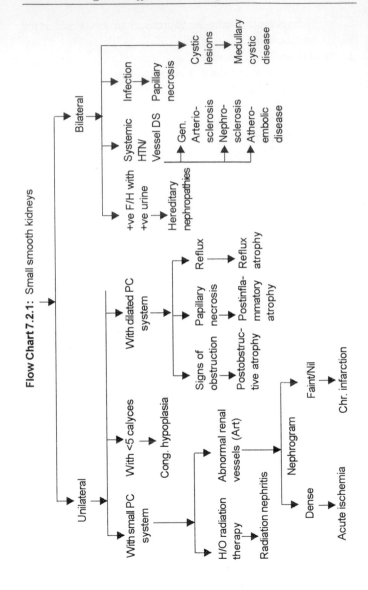

7.3 SMALL SMOOTH KIDNEYS

Smooth

- Uniform/undulating outline.
- No focal indentation (Esp against A calyx)
- Uniform cortical parenchymal thickness [1.5-2 cm]
- Uniform CMD [1:1/1:8]
- No focal variation in PT
- Vascularity adequate / mildly decreased
- Perirenal fascial planes uniform.

Small

- Anatomically
- Radiography   – 9-11 cm Rt
- USG   – 11-13 cm Lt
- CT /MRI
- Age variation   – Young
                                  – Old
- Body surface area variation.

U/L	B/L
1. Congenital	1. Generalized arteriosclerosis
2. Postobstructive	2. CGN (Chronic Glomerulonephritis)
3. Renal artery stenosis	3. Chronic papillary necrosis
4. Radiation nephritis	4. Arterial hypotension
5. Renal infarction.	5. U/L causes presenting B/L.

1. Congenital

- Quantitative decrease in renal tissue : Quality N.
- Pelvis calyceal system   :   Normal
- Ureter   :   Normal

- Opposite kidney : Enlarged
- Renal artery : Small /Normal
- Calyces <5

2. Postobstructive

- Early on the PCS +/- dilated but later it is normal.
- Parenchyma is thinned.
- Obstruction   Acute → Increased pressure in PCS
                       ↓   ↓
                   Chronic   decreased blood flow
                                            ↓
                                  decreased urine
                                     production
      Slow irreversible   ↓   ↓
Parenchymal damage.   ← Not relieved   Relieved
                       Return to normal function
- Calculus, PUJ obstruction, retroperitoneal fibrosis, ureterocele, clot, FB, bladder mass, fungus ball, stricture.
- On imaging, PCSU dilated /N :Size N /decreased;
- Cortex—N/decreased; nephrogram present/faint; poor
- Pyelogram—All depend upon level, severity duration.

3. Radiation Nephritis

- 2300 RAD (23 GY) for ≥ 5 wk.
- Due to small vessel disease.
- PCS—N/small.
- Global cortical thinning.
- Delayed but dense pyelogram with delayed washout.

4. End Result of Infarction

- Global decreased in size occurs when there is injury/ avulsion to main renal artery/segmental arteries.

- Non-visualization of kidney /PCS
- Kidney decreased in size and altered appearance on CT, MR, US.

5. Renal Artery Stenosis

- USE of IVP is nearly obsolete.
- Doppler examination
  - AT > .07 sec
  - AT < 2 cm/sec^2
  - PSV > 180 cm/sec
  - AO:RA <1/2 5-3
- Captopril scintigraphy — Proposed use for screening
- MRA/CTA — Useful corroborative
- Contrast invasive angiography — Conventional
  ↓
  DSA → I/A
  → I/V.

6. Generalized Arteriosclerosis and Arterial Hypotension

- Are systemic conditions presenting with multisystem involvement.
- Renal outline and PCS are normally seen.
- Delayed appearing and increasingly dense pyelogram is seen.
- Condition caused by AS is known as benign nephro-sclerosis.

7. Chronic Glomerulonephritis

- Hallmark is immediate faint and persistent nephrogram.
- On USG, CMD is lost with increased echogenicity.
- Diagnosis by HPE.

8. Chronic Papillary Necrosis

- Usually bilateral with multiple papillae affected.
- Different types of appearances depending upon stage and degree of papillary necrosis is seen.

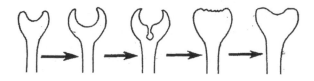

Fig. 7.3.1

- Main causes are analgesics and diabetes.

SMALL SMOOTH KIDNEY

U/L

Dilated PCS

- Postobstructive.
  - N /decreased function.
  - Thinned cortex.

Hypovolemic PCS

- RAS   – Increase BP.
- Radiation   – H/O
- Infarction   – H/O

Hypoplastic PCS

- Congenital.
  - Pt. Asympto.

B/L

Systemic

- Hypotension
- Arteriosclerosis
  These are systemic conditions with multisystem involvement.

Renal

- CGN   – Normal calyx.
- CPN   – Abnormal calyx.
- U/L causes

7.4 SMALL, IRREGULAR, KIDNEYS

- Reflux nephropathy (chronic atrophic pyelonephritis)
- Lobar infarction.
- Tuberculous.
- Renal dysplasia.

Chronic Pyelonephritis/Reflux Nephropathy

A focal scar over a dilated calyx. Usually multifocal and may be bilateral. Scarring is most prominent at the upper and lower poles. Minimal scarring, especially at a pole, produces decreased cortical thickness with a normal papilla.

Primary Uroradiologic Elements

- Contour—normal (early, intermediate)
- Focal scar (late: may be multifocal)
- Lesion distribution—unilateral (may be bilateral)

NORMAL
Cortex parallel to
interpapillary line

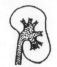
LOBAR INFARCTION
Broad depression over
a normal calyx

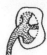
**REFLUX
NEPHROPATHY**
Focal scars over dilated
calyces. Most
prominent at upper
and lower poles. May be bilateral

SPLEEN IMPRESSION
Right kidney may
show hepatic
impression

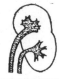
DUPLEX KIDNEY
Renal size usually
larger than normal

FETAL LOBULATION
Normal size.
Cortical depressions
between papillae

OVERLYING BOWEL
Spurious
loss of cortex

Fig. 7.4.1: Unilateral scarred kidney

Secondary Uroradiologic Elements

- Papillae—normal (early, intermediate)
- Retracted (late; focal)
- Calyces—normal (early, intermediate)
- Widened (late; focal)
- Parenchymal thickness—normal (early)
- Wasted (intermediate, late, focal)
- Focal compensatory hypertrophy.
- Nephrogram—deficient enhancement (lobar, sublobar; full-thickness; may be striated)

- Echogenicity—increased (focal)
- Increased central sinus complex.

Lobar Infarction

A broad contour depression over a normal calyx. Normal interpapillary line.

Primary Uroradiologic Elements

Early (within 4 weeks)	Late (after 4 weeks)
• Size—normal • Contour—normal	• Size—normal to small • Contour—focal scar (may be multifocal)
• Lesion distribution—unilateral (may be bilateral)	• Lesion distribution—unilateral (may be bilateral)

Secondary Uroradiologic Elements

Early (within 4 weeks)	Late (after 4 weeks)
• Pelvoinfundibulocalyceal system—attenuated (focal, occasional)	• Parenchymal thickness—wasted (focal) with normal interpapillary line.
• Nephrogram—absent (focal, occasional, global, rarely)	• Echogenicity –increased (focal)

Tuberculosis

- Calcification differentiates it from the other members.
- Usually hematogeneous from pulmonary disease, but

sometimes secondary to tuberculous infection of the gastrointestinal tract or bone.

- Initial lesion in renal tuberculosis—small tubercles in the glandular and cortical arterioles progress to necrotizing lesions.
- Tubercles enlarge and coalesce into necrotic irregular cavities.
- Ultimately, there is ulceration into the adjacent calyx, with formation of fistulae and strictures.
- The kidney becomes fibrotic and scarred.
- Renal involvement is probably always bilateral, in 25% of cases are unilateral.
- Imaging findings are typically asymmetrical.
- Renal calcification in up to 50% of cases, dense punctate calcification associated with healed tuberculomas or renal calculi.
- The classical urographic finding is multifocal caliectasis, due to irregular infundibular strictures. Parenchymal, scars in advanced cases.
- Ultimately, the kidney may become small, densely calcified, and nonfunctioning; the so-called autonephrectomy.

Renal Dysplasia

- Developmental parenchymal abnormalities resulting from abnormal development of the renal vasculature, renal tubules, collecting ducts, or drainage apparatus.
- Biopsy may be necessary for diagnosis.
- Multicystic dysplastic kidney is due to ureteric obstruction early in fetal life.
- Usually unilateral, bilateral disease is lethal.
- Antenatal diagnosis is possible in the third trimester.
- USG finding is of a multicystic mass without renal tissue.

- One-third have contralateral urological abnormalities as PUJ obstruction or VUR.
- Functional imaging with isotopes or IVU demonstrates lack of function.
- Arteriography outlines a small thread-like renal artery.

Table 7.4.1: Differential Diagnosis of Small, Irregular Kidneys

	Reflux nephropathy	Lobar infarction	TB	Renal dysplasia
1. Laterality	Unilateral	Unilateral	Bilateral	Unilateral
2. No. of foci	Multifocal	Unifocal	Multifocal	Multifocal
3. Involvement of papillae	+	–	+	NA
4. Status of calyces	Dilated	Attenuated	Dilated	NA
5. Parenchymal thickness	→	→	→	→
6. Nephrogram	Diminished	Absent	Diminished/Absent	Absent
7. Calcification	–	–	+	–
8. Cysts	–	–	–	+

7.5 LARGE SMOOTH KIDNEY

Unilateral

1. Renal vein thrombosis
2. Acute arterial infarction
3. Obstructive uropathy
4. Acute pyelonephritis
5. Xanthogranulomatous pyelonephritis
6. Misc— Compensatory hypertrophy.
          Duplicated pelvicalyceal system.

Renal Vein Thrombosis

Common Causes Children—Dehydration and shock, nephrotic syndrome, cyanotic heart disease.

Adults—
- Renal cell carcinoma
- Compression by tumor/lymph node or extension of thrombus from IVC, trauma.

Secondary to Renal Diseases—Chronic glomerulonephritis, amyloidosis.

Sudden Total Occlusion—Hemorrhagic infarct, permanant loss of function and eventual shrinkage of kidney.

Partial Obstruction—Collaterals develop and the renal function is undisturbed.

Primary Uroradiological Elements
- Size—Normal to large
- Contour—Smooth
- Unilateral.

Secondary Uroradiologic Elements

Collecting system—Attenuated, mucosal irregularity, nodularity, notching. Abnormalities disappear on retrograde pyelography.

Parenchymal thickness—Expanded.

Nephrogram—density varies from absent to normal, prolonged corticomedullary differentiation.

Echogenicity—variable (Initial 2 weeks—Hypoechoic-after-hyperechoic).

Renal vein—Dilated, intraluminal thrombus with diminished or absent flow.

Retroperitoneum—Dilated collaterals: Hemorrhage.

ACUTE ARTERIAL INFARCTION

Subtotal renal infarction is much common than infarction of the entire organ.

Most usual cause—embolus through thrombosis, super-imposed on underlying arterial disease, may also lead to infarction.

Primary Uroradiological Findings—Large, smooth, uni-lateral.

Secondary Uroradiological Findings:

Collecting system—attenuated

Nephrogram—absent/diminished density, cortical rim enhancement; focal nephrographic defect occurs in early subtotal infarction.

Echogenicity—normal/reduced.

Renal angiography defines the site of arterial block.

CT—well defined focal area of lower attenuation than that of adjacent normally enhancing parenchyma.

OBSTRUCTIVE UROPATHY

Dilatation of Pelvicalyceal System

Obstructive
- Cong-(E.g. PUJ, PUV)
- Acquired (stones, strictures, tumors)

Non-obstructive
- VUR
- Postobstructive dilatation
- Primary megaureter

IVU—Features of Acute Obstruction

- Increasingly dense nephrogram
- Modest kidney enlargement
- Delayed calyceal opacification
- Mild to moderate pelvicalectasis
- Spontaneous pyelosinus extravasation.

Features of Chronic Obstruction

Renal Size

Partial obstruction—increase complete obstruction—small nephrogram density—normal/decreased.

Parenchymal thickness—Reduced (Crescent, rim nephrogram).

Dilated Pelvicalyceal System—Ball pyelogram.

Ureters—Dilated/Tortuous

US—Excellent screening method.

Limitation
- Miss 1/3rd cases of acute obstruction
- Cannot differentiate extrarenal pelvis from PUJ obstruction.

- Unenhanced helical CT of KUB is the most sensitive technique for diagnosing acute obstructive uropathy.

ACUTE PYELONEPHRITIS

Clinically acute pyelonephritis refers to symptom complex of pyrexia, bacteriuria and flank pain.

IVU—Diffuse renal enlargement.
  — Delayed/poor pelvicalyceal system filling of reduced density.

Severe Acute Pyelonephritis—Nephrogram may be dense, persistent or striated.

US—Focal/generalized renal swelling, iso/hypoechoic.

CT—Patchy enhancement with bands and wedge-shaped areas of reduced enhancement extending from papillae to the edge of the kidney.

Delayed scans (3-6 hr)—increased enhancement in the prior areas.

Complication—abscess.

XANTHOGRANULOMATOUS PYELONEPHRITIS

- Chronic parenchymal inflammation caused by foamy histiocytes giving a yellowish appearance to the cut surface of the kidney.
- Usually associated with proteus infection in patients with calculus disease.

Radiological Features

- On IVU the pelvicalyceal system fails to fill in the presence of good thickness of renal substance.

- *US*—Dilated pelvicalyceal system with low level echoes, renal parenchyma is of low echogenicity, calculus is usually present.
- *CT*—Multiple rounded low attenuation areas of soft tissue density surrounded by thick parenchyma.
- Renal pelvis is contracted and contains calculus, associated perinephric and psoas collection may be present.

COMPENSATORY HYPERTROPHY

- Congenital absence of kidney.
- Postnephrectomy.
- Diseased, poorly functioning kidney.
- Maximum size of contralateral kidney is usually reached in approx 6 months.

Radiological Features

- Size of kidney increased
- Parenchymal thickness increased
- PCS and ureter appear prominent (as urine flow rate becomes the normal from the functioning kidney).

Flow Chart 7.5.1: Unilateral smooth enlarged kidney

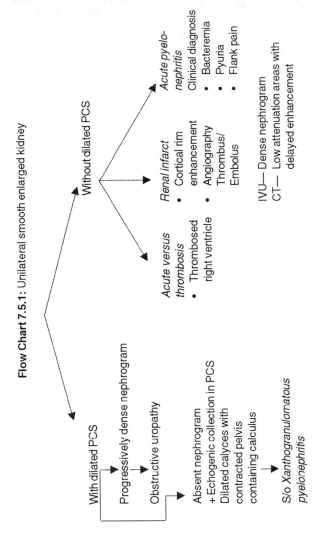

Unilateral smooth enlarged kidney

With dilated PCS
- Progressively dense nephrogram
- Obstructive uropathy

- Absent nephrogram + Echogenic collection in PCS
- Dilated calyces with contracted pelvis containing calculus

S/o *Xanthogranulomatous pyelonephritis*

Without dilated PCS

Acute versus thrombosis
- Thrombosed right ventricle

Renal infarct
- Cortical rim enhancement
- Angiography Thrombus/ Embolus

IVU— Dense nephrogram
CT— Low attenuation areas with delayed enhancement

Acute pyelo-nephritis
Clinical diagnosis
- Bacteremia
- Pyuria
- Flank pain

7.6 BILATERAL LARGE SMOOTH KIDNEYS

1. Proliferative /necrotizing disorders
2. Abnormal protein deposition
   - Amyloidosis
   - Multiple myeloma
3. Abnormal fluid accumulation
   - Acute tubular necrosis
   - Acute cortical necrosis
4. Neoplastic cell infiltration
   - Leukemia
5. Inflammatory cell infiltration
   - Acute interstitial nephritis
6. Miscellaneous
   - Autosomal recessive polycystic kidney disease
   - Acute urate nephropathy
   - Nephromegaly associated with diabetes mellitis Hyperalimentation and cirrhosis.
   - Renal vein thrombosis
   - Bilateral hydronephrosis.

PROLIFERATIVE/NECROTIZING DISORDERS

- Only kidneys involved

  - Acute (poststreptococcal)
- Glomerulonephritis
  - (RPGN)Rapidly progressive
- Glomerulonephritis (GN)
  - Idiopathic membranous GN

- Renal involvement is part of multisystem disorder
  - Wegener's granulomatosis

  - Goodpasture's syndrome

  - Diabetic glomerulosclerosis

- Membrano-
  proliferative GN
- IgA nephropathy
  glomerulosclerosis
- Glomerulosclerosis
  associated with
  heroin abuse
- Lobular GN
- PAN
- Allergic Anglis

- Hemolytic uremic
  syndrome

- Morphologic diagnosis of a specific disease within this group is dependent on integrating light, electron and immunofluorescent microscopic patterns of glomerulor involvement with other clinical or laboratory abnomalities.

R/F

Primary uroradiologic elements	:	Large, smooth, bilateral
Secondary uroradio-logical elements	:	Collecting system is attenuated.
	:	Parenchymal thickness is expanded. Echogenicity is increased.
	:	(HUS-selective hyperechogenicity of cortex relative to medulla)

Amyloidosis

Caused by accumulation of extracellular cosinophilic protein substance in various organs.

Primary—Renal involvement occurs is 35% cases.

Secondary—Secondary to chronic suppurative/inflammatory disease.

Renal involvement occurs in 80% cases.

- Tuberculosis
- Bronchiectasis
- Ulcerative colitis

- Osteomyelitis
- Rheumatoid arthritis

Radiological Features

Primary urological elements	: Large, smooth, bilateral
Secondary uroradio-logical elements	: Collecting system is attenuated
	: Parenchymal thickness expanded, becomes wasted with time.
	: Nephrogram—diminished density.
	: Echogenicity—Normal to increased.
	: Renal vein thrombosis (occasionally).

MULTIPLE MYELOMA

Multiple myeloma causes renal insult in 50% cases because of deposition—of abnormal proteins in the tubule lumina. Renal function is also compromised by:

- Increased blood viscosity.
- Nephrocalcinosis (Because of hypercalcemia)
- Bence Jones toxicity on tubules.

Amyloidosis

Radiological Features

Primary	B/L large smooth kidneys.
Secondary	Collecting system is attenuated.
	Parenchymal thickness is expanded.
	Nephrogram—diminished density.
	Echogenicity—increased.

Administration of contrast material in patients with multiple myeloma requires an awareness of potential hazards.

Dehydration should be avoided if the risk of complications is to be minimized.

Other Radiological Features

Osteopenia with well defined lucencies of uniform size in spine, pelvis, skull, ribs and shafts of long bones.
- Vertebral body collapse +/– paravertebral shadow +/–, intervertebral disc involvement.
- Expansile ribs lesions.
- Permeative mottled pattern of bone destruction present.

Extraskeletal Features

Hypercalcemia, hepatosplenomegaly, soft tissue tumors in sinuses, submucosa of pharynx, trachea, cervical lymph nodes and GIT.

ACUTE TUBULAR NECROSIS

State of reversible renal failure with or without oliguria that follows exposure of the kidney to certain toxic agents or to a period of prolonged, severe ischemia.

Toxic Agents

Bichloride of mercury, ethylene glycol, carbon tetrachloride, bismuth, arsenic, urographic contrast in particularly when administered to a patient of 2 pre-existing renal disease who has been dehydrated.

Ischemic Causes

Shock, crush injuries, burns, transfusion reaction, severe

dehydration, surgical procedure like renal transplantation or aortic resection.

R/F

Contrast material enhanced imaging studies should not be performed knowingly in patients with ATN.

Collecting System

Attenuated, opacification is diminished/absent.
* Nephrogram—75% patient's—immediate and persistently dense.
  25%—Increasingly dense and persistent.
* *Echogenicity:* Medulla—Normal to diminished.
  Cortex—Normal to increased.

ACUTE CORTICAL NECROSIS

Uncommon form of ARF in which there is death of the renal cortex and sparing of the medulla.
* A thin rim of subcapsular tissue on the external surface of the cortex and a thin rim of the juxtamedullary cortex are often preserved. This fine rim of viable cortex separate the necrotic cortex from the renal capsule externally and from the medulla internally.
* Calcification occurs at this inerface which is known as— *"Tram line calcification"*
* Calcification is detected microscopically at 6 days and radiologically—at approximately 24 days (Kidneys are still enlarged).

R/F

* B/L enlarged smooth kidney.

- Collecting system—Absent/faint opacification is effaced.
- Parenchymal thickness—Expanded.
- Nephrogram—Absent cortical nephrogram with selective enhancement of medulla.
- *Calcification*—Cortical-diffuse or tram line.
- *Echogenicity*—Center hypoechoic (early phase). Hyperechoic with acoustic shadow after calculm deposition.

Causes

Obstructive—Premature separation of placenta. Concealed hemorrhage, septic abortion, placenta previa.

Adults—Sepsis, dehydration, shock, burns, snakebite

Children—Dehydration, infection, transfusion reaction.

LEUKEMIA

Most common malignant cause of B/L global renal enlargement (Lymphoma occasionally produces such pattern but more commonly causes multifocal renal enlargement). Rarely, leukemia causes a unifocal renal mass due to chloroma, myeloblastoma or a myeloblastic sarcoma. Enlarged kidneys can occur in leukemic patients without leukemic infiltration because of:

- Acute urate nephropathy
- Amphotericin induced acute interstitial nephritis
- Renal candidiasis associated with intensive chemotherapy
- Lymphocytic rather than granulocytic tumors of leukemia are more frequently associated with renal enlargement
- Children with acute leukemia are more likely to develop nephromegaly as compared to adults
- Peripheral WBC count can be normal or depleted at the time of renal involvement.

R/F

Primary	B/L smooth enlarged kidneys
Secondary	Collecting system—attenuated.
	Parenchymal thickness—expanded.
	Nephrogram—diminished density.
	Echogenicity—Variable.

- Focal hemorrhage, subcapsular collections, obstructive clots in renal pelvis and other R/F in children.
- Metaphyseal lucencies—distal femur, proximal tibia and distal radius.
- Permeative destruction of bone.
- Osteolytic lesions—Diaphysis of long bone.
- Periosteal reaction—Proliferation of leukemic deposits deep to periosteum leading to subperiosteal hemorrhage. MR will show the marrow involvement clearly.

ACUTE INTERSTITIAL NEPHRITIS

Characterized histologically by infiltration of the interstitium by lymphocytes, plasma cells, eosinophils and a few polymorphonuclear leukocytes.

Usually results as a complication of exposure to certain drugs:

Antibiotics—Methicillin, ampicillin, penicillin, amphotericin, sulfonamides.

NSAIDs—Naproxen, ibuprofen.

Anticonvulsants—Phenytoin.

Antihistaminics—Cimetedine.

Cases usually evolve between 5 days to 5 weeks after exposure.

Clinical Features

Fever, rash, eosinophilia, hematuria, proteinuria and azotemia.

R/F

Primary	B/L smooth enlarged kidneys
Secondary	*Collecting system*—attenuated.
	Parenchymal thickness—expanded.
	Nephrogram—diminished density.
	Echogenicity—Increased.

AUTOSOMAL RECESSIVE (AR) (INFANTILE) PCKD (POLYCYSTIC KIDNEY DISEASE)

AR PCKD characterized by dilatation of renal collecting tubules, cystic dilatation of biliary radicles and periportal fibrosis.

AR PCKD Neonatal—Predominant renal and minimal hepatic involvement.

Juvenile—Predominant hepatic and minimal renal involvement.

R/F

Primary	B/L smooth enlarged kidney.
Secondary	Neonatal form: Collecting system is attenuated.

Parenchymal thickness is expanded.

Nephrogram—diminished density: Striated.

Attenuation value—Less than soft tissue (unenhanced CT)

Echogenicity—Diffusely increased, loss of corticomedullary differentiation.

Features of pulmonary hypoplasia—Small malformed thorax, pneumothorax and pneumomediastinum.

Juvenile Form

Nephrogram   :   Striated.

Calcification	:	Nephrocalcinosis (papillae)
Echogenicity	:	Increased.
Misc	:	Hepatosplenomegaly, varices, dilated bile ducts, increased hepatic echogenicity.

ACUTE URATE NEPHROPATHY

- Because of deposition of biurate crystals in the collecting tubules and interstitium leading to ARF.
- Seen most commonly during therapy for cancer particularly leukemia, malignant lymphoma.
- Myeloproliferative disorders and polycythemia vera.

R/F

- Bilateral smooth enlarged kidneys.
- Collecting system is normal.
- Nephrogram—Progressively dense.
- No opacification of pelvicalyceal system:
- Alkaline diuresis ⎫
- Large fluid intake ⎬ before administration of contrast medium
- Use of allopurinol ⎭

NEPHROMEGALY ASSOCIATED WITH CIRRHOSIS, HYPERALIMENTATION AND DIABETES MELLITIS

- Nephromegaly associated with cirrhosis.
- *Explanation*—Hyperplasia and hypertrophy of renal cells.
- *Hyperalimentation*—Because of hyperalimentation there is increase in fluid compartment of kidney related of hyperosmolality of the solution.
- Renal enlargement reverses following cessation of therapy.
- Diabetes mellitis—(in the absence of diabetic glomerulosclerosis).
- Renal enlargement is due to growth hormone effect nephron hypertrophy and glycosuric osmotic diuresis.

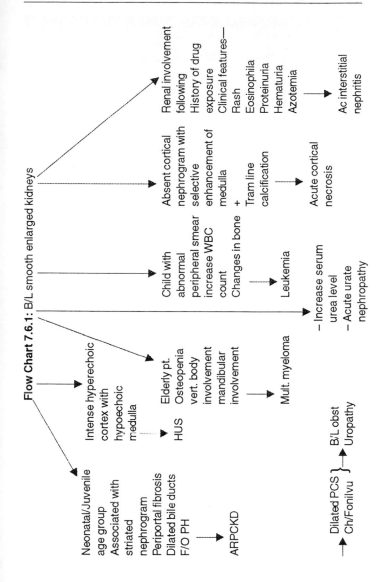

Flow Chart 7.6.1: B/L smooth enlarged kidneys

- Neonatal/Juvenile age group
- Associated with striated nephrogram
- Periportal fibrosis
- Dilated bile ducts
- F/O PH
→ ARPCKD

- Intense hyperechoic cortex with hypoechoic medulla
→ HUS

- Elderly pt.
- Osteopenia vert. body involvement mandibular involvement
→ Mult. myeloma

- Child with abnormal peripheral smear increase WBC count
- Changes in bone
→ Leukemia

- Increase serum urea level
- Acute urate nephropathy

- Absent cortical nephrogram with selective enhancement of medulla
+
- Tram line calcification
→ Acute cortical necrosis

- Renal involvement following
- History of drug exposure
- Clinical features—
  Rash
  Eosinophila
  Proteinuria
  Hematuria
  Azotemia
→ Ac interstitial nephritis

→ Dilated PCS Ch/Fonilvu } B/L obst Uropathy

7.7 NON-VISUALIZATION OF A KIDNEY DURING EXCRETION UROGRAPHY

1. Absent kidney—Congenital absence or postnephrectomy
2. Ectopic kidney
3. Chronic obstructive uropathy
4. Infection—Pyonephrosis
             —Xanthogranulomatous pyelonephritis
             —Tuberculosis
5. Tumor—An avascular tumor completely replacing the kidney or preventing normal functions of residual renal tissue by occluding the renal vein or pelvis, e.g. Renal cell carcinoma, Wilms' tumor
6. Renal artery occlusion-including trauma
7. Renal vein occlusion
8. Multicystic kidney

Salient Features

1. Absent kidney—Failure of the ureteric bud to reach the metanephron result in renal agenesis

Associated Anomalies

a. Failure of ipsilateral ureter and hemitrigone to develop
b. Adrenal agenesis
c. Absence of vas deferens, unicornuate uterus and absence or cyst of seminal vesicle
d. VATER syndrome—Vertebral and VSD
                —Anorectal atresia
                —Tracheal and esophageal lesions
                —Radial bone anomalies
e. Contralateral renal anomalies—Renal ectopia
                                —Malrotation
   Plain film—Absence of renal outline

Medial displacement of the splenic and hapatic flexure into renal bed.

Compensatory hypertrophy of contralateral kidney

CT or radionuclide imaging—Definitive showing absence of unilateral absence of renal tissue.

Other cause of atrophic kidney:
— Vesicoureteric reflux
— Infarct
— Bilateral renal agenesis associated with Pottar's syndrome characterized by oligohydramnios, characteristic facies and early death due to pulmonary hypoplasia.

Pyonephrosis

- Infeçtion of an obstructed kidney may lead to pus developing within the renal pelvis or calyx.
- Occurs in conjunction with the presence of calculi or undiagnosed PUJ obstruction.
- Imaging features—Obstructed system with particularly early or severe loss of renal outline.
- Cross-sectional imaging show evidence of pus and inflammatory debris within the dilated pelvicalyceal system (e.g. echogenic areas are USG or increased density on CT with possible layering).
- *Xanthogranulomatous pyelonephritis*
- Chronic inflammatory process in which lipid laden histiocytes invade and replace normal renal parenchyma.
- Seen in females, diabetics and infecting organism is usually E. coli and Proteus murabilis.
- IVU—Non-functioning kidney with calculi 80% Calculi is characterstically laminated or branched and fragmented.
- Initially the kidney is enlarged and this may have a focal

pattern simulating tumor but ultimately there is marked renal atrophy.

- *USG and CT*—Loss of normal corticomedullary differentiation and heterogenity which includes debris containing cystic areas and calculi.

Tuberculosis

IVU—Stricture affecting the calyceal neck, with the formation of hydrocalyces.

Strictures at the PUJ and at multiple level in the ureter.

Later the pelvis is affected and the entire kidney may become hydronephrotic and non-functioning (TB auto-nephrectomy).

—USG and CT demonstrates hydrocalyces and/or hydronephrosis which may contain a considerable amount of debris, areas of calcification and parenchymal loss.

In later stages there is inflamed and contracted bladder.

Renal Artery Stenosis

Reduction of the internal diameter by at least 60%
- Atheroma
- Fibromuscular dysplasia
- Polyarteritis nodosa
- Takayasu's arteritis
- Compression of the renal artery by retroperitoneal mass.

IVU—The affected kidney may be initially small and smooth. The reduced perfusion on the affected side produces a late nephrogram which is hyperdense.

Notching of the ureter due to compensatory hypertrophy of the ureteric artery.

USG—Excludes an obvious structural abnormality or coexistant condition that may relate to hypertension (renal scarring, hydronephrosis, calculus disease or tumors)

Doppler—Increase in the peak systolic velocity and renal: aortic velocity ratio of more than 3.5 or an absolute velocity of more than 180-200 cm/s.

Spectral Analysis of Intrarenal Arteries

- RAS of less than 75% is not detected by this technique
- More severe stenosis is characterized by reduction in the ascending slope of the systolic peak which can be measured as reduced acceleration (below 3m/s/s), lengthened time to systolic peak (above 0.0 75) and increased resistive index (above 5%) and pulsatility index (above 0.012) of the affected kidney compared with the other side.
- CT angiography
- MR angiography

Renal Vein Thrombous

- If thrombous is abrupt and complete the imaging features are similar to an arterial infarct.
- *Dopplar USG*—It demonstrates loss of venous rather than the arterial signal.

Subacute /partial thrombosis—Smooth renal enlargement. The IVU will show a delayed but subsequently hyperdense nephrogram and pyelogram with either normal calyces or some evidence of compression due to parenchymal swelling.

Notching of the ureter by dilated venous collaterals is occasionally seen.

USG—Loss of normal corticomedullary differentiation. Diffuse reduction in echogenicity. Thrombosis of the renal vein.

CT—Hypodense kidney

Multicystic Kidney

- Ureter fails to develop and is atretic while the kidney is non-functioning.
- *USG or CT*—The kidney is composed of non-communicating cyst of varying size.
- It is associated with an increased risk of contralateral pelviureteric junction obstruction.

Renal Tumors

Wilms' Tumor

- Present in first 3 years.
- Bilateral in 5%
- *Associated abnormalities*—Cryptorchidism, hypospadius hemihypertrophy, sporadic aniridia, Beckwith-Wiedemann syndrome.
- *Secondaries in*—Liver and lung.
                      —Tumor thrombus in IVC or Rt. atrium
- Plain film —Bulging flank.
                      —Loss of renal outline
                      —Enlargement of renal outline
                      —Displacement of bowel gas
                      —Loss of psoas outline

Calcification

USG—Large well defined mass, increased echogenicity than liver. Solid with haemorrhage/necrosis. Lack of IVC narrowing on inspection suggests occlusion.

CT—Large, well defined, low attenuating, heterogenous with foci of even lower attenuation due to necrosis. Minimal enhancement compared with the residual rim of functioning renal tissue.

MRI—Inhomogenous, Low signal (T_1W), high signal (T2W). Inhomogenous enhancement compared with residual renal tissue.

Renal Cell Carcinoma

- 90% of adult malignant tumors
- Bilateral in 10% and increased incidence of bilaterality in polycystic kidneys and von Hippel-Lindau disease. A mass lesion (showing irregular or amorphous calcification in 10% of cases). Calyces are obliterated, distorted and/or displaced. Half shadow filling defect in a calyx or pelvis. Arteriography shows a pathological circulation.

7.8 DILATED CALYX AND DILATED URETER

With a narrow infundibulum
1. Stricture
2. Extrinsic impression by an artery
3. Hydrocalycosis-congenital

With a wide infundibulum
1. Megacalyces
2. Postobstructive atrophy
3. Polycalycosis
4. PUJ obstruction

DILATED URETER AND CALYCES

Vesicoureteric Reflux

Obstruction   *No obstruction or reflux*
With in Lumen
1. Calculus   1. Postpartum
2. Blood clot   2. Following relief of
                                          obstruction

Flow Chart 7.8.1: Non-visualization of one kidney during excretion urography

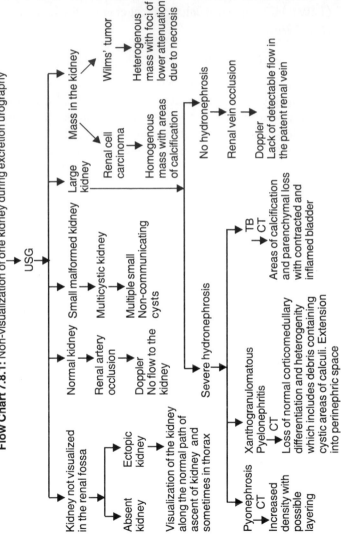

3. Sloughed papilla

In the Wall
1. Edema or stricture due to calculus
2. Tumor
3. Tubercular stricture
4. Schistosomiasis
5. Postsurgical trauma
6. Ureterocele
7. Megaureter

Outside the Wall
1. Retroperitoneal fibrosis
2. Ca. of cervix, bladder or prostate
3. Retrocaval ureter.

3. Urinary tract infection
4. Pri. non-obstructive ureter

DILATED CALYX

Stricture

- *Tumor*—usually a transitional cell carcinoma presenting as a mural growth. May be multiple
- Calculus
- *Tuberculosis*—Unilateral, collecting system—irregular margins, strictures, multifocal dilatation, distinctive feature communicating parenchymal cavities.
- Irregularity of papillary margin (Earliest)
- Calcifications, variable parenchymal thickness.

Extrinsic Impression by an Artery

- Rarely cause symptoms
- *Fraley syndrome*—Infundibular obstruction
- Nephralgia

- Right upper pole calyx
- IVP—Early opacification and delayed emptying
- Angiography—also useful.

Congenital Hydrocalycosis

- Congenital dilatation of calyx
- Diagnosis is safely made only in childhood.

Postobstructive Atrophy

- Kidney is usually small, smooth
- Effaced papillae, dilated PCS
- Parenchymal wasting
- Compensatory hypertrophy
- Megacalyces and polycalycosis
- Megacalyces—Dilated Calyces ± a slightly dilated pelvis
- Polycalycosis—Increased number of calyces—20-25
- Delayed visualization of calyceal system
- Cortical thickness—Normal
- Cause fetal obstruction, Boys > Girls

Calculus

- Can cause mechanical obstruction, edema or stricture
- Plain films, USG, CT—all help in diagnosis.

Blood Clot

- Volume of Blood loss is large enough
- Trauma, tumors, AVM, bleeding disorders- predispose
- Usually asymptomatic, dissolve in 2 weeks.
- IVP—Opaque urine, outlines the clot and may dissect.
- 'Hand in glove' appearance.
- USG—low level echoes that separate sinus echoes

- CT—appearance varies with time, does not enhance
- Persistent clot—may faintly calcify

Sloughed Papilla

- When papillary necrosis evolves to the stage of flank necrosis, separation occurs between viable and dead parts.
- Usually in analgesic nephropathy patients
- Obstruction at infundibulum, ureteropelvic junction or ureter.
- IVP—Triangle shaped filling defect
- One or more calyces will dilate reflecting loss of papillary tip.
- Calcium may deposit along periphery
- Occasionally very dense—Indistinguishable from calculus.

PUJ Obstruction

- More common left side, 20% b/l
- Cause neuromuscular incoordination, aberrant vessels
- *During acute episode-IVU*—delayed, increasing dense nephrogram and delayed appearence of PCS.
- calyces and dilated pelvis
- Contrast in collecting ducts-as crescents
- Ureters often not opacified
- Milder cases-difficult to diagnose

Tumors

- Tumors are very uncommon in ureter
- TCC—renal pelvis > ureter (3:1)
- Seen in lower 1/3rd of ureter, multicentricity and bilateral if TCC.
- Filling defects on IVU, never completely surrounded by opacified urine.

- Polypoid with smooth, irregular or lobular surface
- Squamous cell carcinoma—broad based and flat
- Bergman's sign—in ureteric carcinoma.
    —distinguishes from calculus
- USG—Similar to renal parenchyma in echogenicity
- CT—contrast enhancing mural mass projecting into lumen, circumferential or eccentric thickening.

Tuberculous Stricture

- Marked irregularity of part or all of the collecting system or ureter because of both submucosal granulomas and mucosal ulceration.
- Scars of healed TB produce sharply defined circumferential narrowings at one or several sites often with irregular margins.
- Fibrosis may progress during treatment of active TB.
- Pipe stem ureter, thimble bladder.

Schistosomiasis

- Ureteral abnormalities are found in half of patients with bladder schistosomiasis
- *Early*—minimal dilatation, slight mucosal irregularity and diminished peristalsis
- *Then with time*—calcification, mural thickening and straightening, beading, multiple narrowing
- Some cases-bilharzial polyps-seen as filling defects.
- No increase risk of TCC.

Ureterocele (Congenital)

- *Orthotopic ureterocele*—best seen by IVU
- The distal ureter is dilated, projects into the lumen of

bladder, opacified bladder urine surrounds the ureterocele separated by lucency, Cobra head deformity
- An ectopic ureterocele is seen on cystography as a smooth, non-opaque, intravesicular mass
- Ectopic ureter causes—UTI, bladder neck destruction.

Primary Megaureter

- Ureter has a normally tapered distal segment but is otherwise dilated over a varying length, from a few centimeters proximal to tapered end including PCS.
- Tapered segment is a peristaltic.

Retroperitoneal Fibrosis

- Ureteric destruction of variable severity (75% bilateral)
- Tapering lumen or complete obstruction—L4-L5
- Medial deviation of ureters
- Retroperitoneal, periaortic mass—CT or US.

Retrocaval Ureter

- Ureter passes posterior to IVC and partially encircles it at L3-L4 with proximal dilatation.
- Can cause flank pain, UTI.

Vesicoureteric Reflux

- Occurs when intrasegment of ureter in the UB is short and the angle of insertion is wide.
- VUR—decrease with age as lengthening of ureter occurs.
  Grading— 1. Ureter only
  2. Ureter, pelvis, calyces
  3. II + Mild dilatation of PCS, fornices normal
  4. Mod. dilatation of PCS

+ Unsharp fornices
5. Gross distention + Effaced papilla
- Small, scarred kidney.

Postpartum

- More common Rt. side
- Urinary tract obstruction
- Effect of P fimbriated E. coli on urothelium

Flow Chart 7.8.2: Dilated ureter

Obstruction
With in Lumen
- Calculus — Plain film and USG
- Blood clot — Filling defect on IVU
  — Disappears in 2 wks
- *Sloughed papilla*
  - Δ filling defect
  - Papillary necrosis—
    Analgesic Nephropathy

In the Wall
Tumor — Irregular, mural filling defect
  - Bergman sign
  - CT-enhancement
TB — Multifocal strictures,
    calcification, irregularity,
    Pipestem ureter,
    Associated findings
Schistosomiasis — Calcification, beading,
    multiple narrowings,
    polyps

VUR
- Mostly in children
- MCU—Diagnostic
- Small scarred kidneys

Uretrocele
- Terminally dilated ureter
- Cobra head deformity

Primary Megaureter
- A peristaltic distal tapered
  end with variable proximal
  dilation

No obstruction or Reflux
- Postpartum
- E.coli infection
- Postobstructive

Outside the wall
Retroperitoneal fibrosis
- 75% b/l
- Medial deviation of ureters
- Retroperitoneal mass

Retrocaval ureter
- On right side
- Ureter turns medially at L3-L4

Flow Chart 7.8.3: Dilated calyx

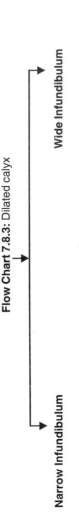

Wide Infundibulum

Megacalyx
– Dilated calyx ± pelvis
– Normal parenchymal thickness

Polycalycosis
– Associated with megacalyx
– Increase number of calyces 20-25
– Delayed visualization of calyces

Postobstructive Atrophy
– Small, smooth kidney
– Parenchymal wasting
– Compensatory hypertrophy

PUJ Obstruction
– Markedly dilated pelvis with
– Nonvisualization of ureter
– Crescents of contrast

Narrow Infundibulum

Stricture
– Calculus or tumor
– Tuberculosis-irregular calyces, dilatations multiple cavities, calcification

Extrinsic impression by an artery
– Upper right calyx
– Early opacification and delayed emptying
– Angiography

Congenital hydrocalycosis
– Seen in children

7.9 GAS IN URINARY TRACT

A. Gas inside the Bladder

1. Vesicointestinal fistula
2. Cystitis .
3. Following instrumentation
4. Penetrating wounds.

B. Gas in Bladder Wall

1. Emphysematous cystitis

C. Gas in Kidneys and Ureters

1. Any cause of gas in UB
2. Emphysematous pyelonephritis.
3. Ureteric diversion
4. Fistula with bowel.

A. Gas Inside the Bladder

1. Vesicointestinal fistula
   - Can be due to diverticular disease, carcinoma colon or rectum or Crohn's disease.
   - Pneumaturia is the presenting complaint.
   - Air visible in bladder lumen.
   - Fistulous communication can be demonstrated in 70% cases.
   - Focal thickening of bladder wall due to adjacent inflammation.
2. Cystitis
   - Due to gas forming organisms

- Esp. seen in diabetics and immunocompromised.
- Usually *E.coli* and rarely clostridium.

3. Following instrumentation
   - Cystoscopy and catheterization may lead to air in bladder lumen.
4. Penetrating wounds
   Trauma or any operative procedure may cause presence of gas in bladder lumen.

B. In Bladder Wall

Emphysematous Cystitis

- Uncommon complication of urinary tract infection by gas forming organisms.
- Almost pathognomonic of poorly controlled diabetes
- Plain film shows translucent streaks or rings of air bubbles in bladder wall

Intraluminal air fluid level may be +
U/S—shows echogenic foci with distal shadowing in area of bladder wall thickening.

C. Gas in Kidneys and Ureters

1. Any cause of gas in urinary bladder.
2. Emphysematous pyelonephritis
   - Rare fulminating form of acute pyelonephritis
   - Occurs usually in diabetics
   - Radiologically there is gas in renal parenchyma and in perirenal tissues and pelvicalyceal system.
   - Gas may have streaky/mottled/loculated pattern.
   - Crescent of subcapsular or perinephric gas may also be seen.
   - Absent-or decreased contrast excretion on IVP.

Ureteric Diversion into the Colon

- Ureterocolic anastomosis is performed after resection of bladder.
- Air is seen in pelvicalyceal system and ureters.

4. Fistula

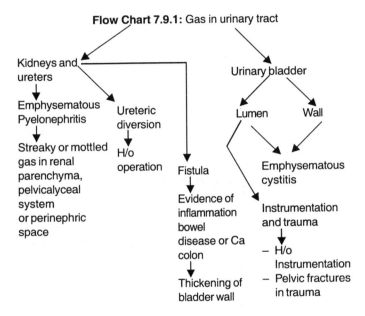

Flow Chart 7.9.1: Gas in urinary tract

7.10 LOSS OF RENAL OUTLINE ON PLAIN FILM

1. Technical factors
2. Absent kidney
   - Congenital
   - Postnephrectomy
3. Ectopic kidney
4. Perinephric hematoma
5. Perinephric abscess
6. Renal tumor

Technical Factors

- Poor radiographic technique
- Overlying fecal matter, gas filled bowel loops obscure renal shadows.

Congenital Absence of Kidney

- Can be unilateral or bilateral
- Unilateral renal agenesis—1:600 to 1:1000 live births
- M:F = 1.8:1
- Often associated with other anomalies of the vater anomalies, uterine anomalies
- Radiologically
  - Visualization of single kidney
  - Colon occupies renal fossa.
  - Compensatory hypertrophy of normal kidney.

Postnephrectomy

History of operation, scar in lumbar region. Surgical resection of 12th rib

Ectopic Kidney

– Kidney is normally located opposite 1st to 3rd lumbar vertebrae.
– Failure of ascent of kidney from pelvis may result in ectopic kidney.

There may be—

a. Longitudinal ectopia—pelvic, sacral or intrathoracic kidney.
b. Crossed ectopia

Pelvic kidney—on IVU malrotated kidney with short ureters.
• There may be associated contralateral renal agenesis, VUR and hypospadius.

Intrathoracic kidney—is more common on left.

Perinephric Hematoma

• Will fill the entire perinephric space and displaces the kidney.
• Plain film shows loss of renal and psoas outline. Kidney is displaced anteromedially on IVU.
• Ultrasound and CT show a perirenal collection.
• Signs of trauma, e.g. fractured transverse process.

Perirenal Abscess

• Extension of acute pyelonephritis or renal Abscess through the capsule.
• Loss of psoas margin and obscuration of renal contour.
• Scoliosis concave to involved side.
• Gas in perirenal tissue.

IVU—shows unilateral impaired excertion. Displacement of kidney

U/S and CT—Shows a complex, predominantly solid and hypoechoic mass with thick irregular wall. Perinephic collection and stranding gas within the lesion.

Renal Tumor

Tumor masses obliterate the perinephric fat planes and therefore cause loss of renal outlines on plain film.

Plain film—may show soft tissue mass with calcification

IVU—shows displacement and attenuation of pelvicalyceal system.

U/S—shows heterogenous mass displacing the collecting system and extending into perinephric fat planes.

CT—shows mass of heterogenous attenuation with perinephric extension.

Flow Chart 7.10.1: Loss of renal outline

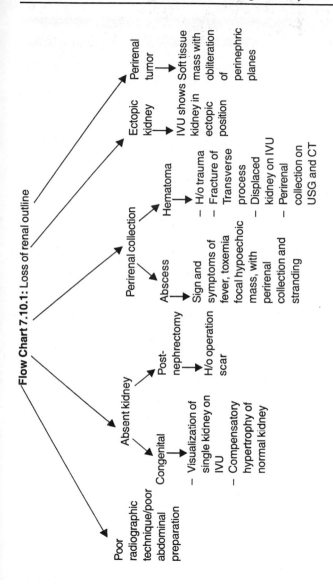

7.11 RENOVASCULAR HYPERTENSION

Renovascular hypertension is defined as hypertension that improves or resolves after correction of renal artery stenosis (RAS).

Signs of Unilateral RAS on IVU

1. Unilateral delay of 1 minute or more in the appearance of opacified calyces.
2. Small, smooth kidney
   – Left more than 1.5 cm shorter than the right
   – Right more than 2 cm shorter than the left.
3. Increased density of opacified calyces
4. Ureteric notching by collateral vessels.

Signs of RAS on ACE Inhibitor Renal Scintigraphy

1. Low probability suggested by a normal study
2. Intermediate probability when:-
   a. Small kidney contributing < 30% of total renal function.
   b. Time to maximum activity (Tmax) < 2 minutes and shows no change following administration of ACE inhibitor
   c. B/L symmetrical cortical retention of tracer
3. High probability when unilateral parenchymal retention indicated by:
   a. A change in the 20 minute/peak uptake ratio > 0.15, delayed excretion of tracer into the renal pelvis >2 minuts or increase in the time to maximal activity Tmax of > 2 minuts or 40% after administration of ACE inhibitor

4. Decreased sensitivity when B/L renal artery stenosis, impaired renal function, urinary obstruction or long-term ACE therapy

Signs of Renal Artery Stenosis on Doppler Sonography

1. Peak velocity in the renal artery >100 cm/s
2. Renal artery velocity >3.5 × aortic velocity
3. Tardus paresis waveform-slope of the systolic upstroke $< 3m/s^2$ and acceleration time (time from onset of systole to peak systole) > 0.075
4. Turbulent flow in the poststenotic renal artery.

Sign on Arteriography

- Reduction in luminal diameter > 75%
- Systolic pressure gradient across the stenosis > 15-25 mm kg or > 20% of aortic systolic pressure.
- Evidence of collateral circulation into distal vessels.
- Pharmacologic manipulation of collateral vessel flow (epinephrine restricts flow to the kidney and makes collaterals more apparent).

CT Angiography

- Demonstrates both wall and lumen of the vessel
- Extent of plaque projecting into the vessel lumen
- Can demonstrate ostial stenosis
- Can be used to examine the patency of vessel that have been dilated by intervascular stents.
- MRA—TOF MRA—Produced by unsaturated blood flowing into the plane of imaging

PC MRA

Causes

1. Atherosclerosis
2. Fibromuscular dysplasia
3. Thrombosis/Embolism
4. Arteritis
   - PAN
   - TAO
   - Takayasu's disease
   - Syphilis
   - Congenital rubella
5. Neurofibromatosis
6. Trauma
7. Aneurysm
8. AV-fistula
9. Extrinsic compression

Atherosclerosis

- 66% of renovascular causes.
- Stenosis of the proximal 2 cm of the renal artery
- Less frequently the distal artery or early branches at bifurcations
- More common in males.

Fibromuscular Dysplasia

- 33% of renovascular causes.
- stenosis +- dilatation which may give the characteristic 'string of beads' appearance.
- Mainly females less than 40 years.
- B/L in 60% of cases.

Takayasu's Arteritis

- Mainly young females less than 35 years of age
- Associated with fever and increased ESR
- Mainly involves the aorta or its major branches
- Luminal narrowing, occlusion, dilatation or formation of aneurysms
- Causes stenosis of aorta or main renal artery.

Polyarteritis Nodosa

- Usually affect medium or small sized vessels.
- Characterized by multiple aneurysms which are sharply defined and 2 to 3 mm wide.

Neurofibromatosis

- Coarctation of aorta
- +/- stenosis of other arteries
- +/- Intrarenal arterial abnormalities+

Flow Chart 7.11.1: Renal artery stenosis (RAS)

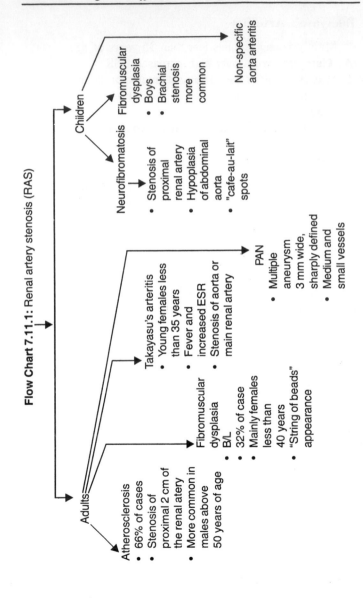

Adults

Atherosclerosis
- 66% of cases
- Stenosis of proximal 2 cm of the renal atery
- More common in males above 50 years of age

Fibromuscular dysplasia
- B/L
- 32% of case
- Mainly females less than 40 years
- "String of beads" appearance

Takayasu's arteritis
- Young females less than 35 years
- Fever and increased ESR
- Stenosis of aorta or main renal artery

PAN
- Multiple aneurysm 3 mm wide, sharply defined
- Medium and small vessels

Children

Neurofibromatosis
- Stenosis of proximal renal artery
- Hypoplasia of abdominal aorta
- "cafe-au-lait" spots

Fibromuscular dysplasia
- Boys
- Brachial stenosis more common

Non-specific aorta arteritis

7.12 RENAL CALCIFICATION

A. Calculi
B. Dystrophic Calcification due to localised disease:
1. Infections
2. Carcinomas
3. Vascular
4. Cysts
C. Nephrocalcinosis
1. Medullary
2. Cortical

A. Calculi:
- Stones with in the collecting system
- Usually sharp in outline
- Variable in size and number
- IVP—Shows hydronephrosis if obstructing
- USG—Echogenic with acoustic shadow

B. Dystrophic Calcification (Usually one kidney or part of one kidney)

1. *Infections*
   a. *Tuberculosis*
      - Irregular, indefinite and not dense as calculi.
      - Usually nodular, curvilinear or amorphous mottled calcification.
      - More common in cortex, in various segments.
      - Multifocal—Ureteric, UB, vas, seminal vesicles.
   b. *Hydatid*
      - Renal involvement in 3%
      - 50% of echinococcal cysts calcify.
      - Usually polar.
      - Curvilinear calcification.

    c. *Xanthogranulomatous pyelonephritis*
- Usually associated staghorn calculus in renal pelvis
- IVP—Non-functioning /poorly functioning kidney.
  - Ill-defined renal outline.
- U/S—Nephrolithiasis.
  - Decreased echogenicity.
  - Hydronephrosis.
- CT
  - Calculus with poorly functioning kidney.
  - Multiple non-enhancing masses (Some with fat density)
  - Perinephric extension.

    d. *Abscess*
- Calcification in wall.
- Or nodular calcification after resolution.

2. *Tumors*

    a. Renal cell carcinoma.
- 8-15% cases.
- Generally non-peripheral, amorphous and irregular.

    b. *Wilms' tumor*
- Amorphous, irregular calcification in soft tissue mass.

3. *Cysts*
- Due to hemorrhage or infection.
- May occur in
  - simple cyst
  - Multicystic dysplastic kidney
  - Adult polycystic kidney disease.

4. *Vascular*

    a. Subcapsular/perirenal hematoma.

    b. Aneurysm of renal artery.
- Curvilinear calcification or eggshell appearance.

    c. Nephrocalcinosis.

Parenchymal Calcification

Medullary Nephrocalcinosis (Pyramidal)

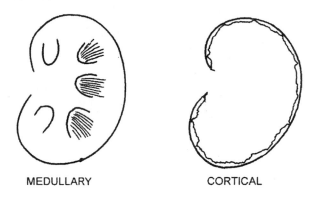

MEDULLARY   CORTICAL

Fig. 7.12.1

1. *Hyperparathyroidism*
   – Primary >> secondary.
   – Commonest cause (16%)
   – Other signs of HPT such as bone erosions, brown tumors, soft tissue calcifications.
2. *Renal Tubular Acidosis*
   – Commonest cause in children
   – May be associated with rickets/osteomalacia
   – Calcification often dense than other causes.
3. *Medullary Sponge Kidney*
   – Not a true cause of nephrocalcinosis as calcification is within ectatic ducts rather than in parenchyma.
   – Numerous medullary cysts communicating with tubules which opacify during IVU.
   – Cysts contain small calculi giving bunch of grapes appearance.

4. *Renal Papillary Necrosis*
   Calcification of shrunken necrotic papillae.

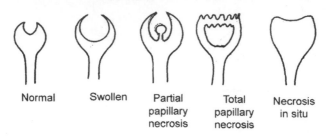

Normal   Swollen   Partial papillary necrosis   Total papillary necrosis   Necrosis in situ

Fig. 7.12.2

5. *Causes of Hypercalcemia or Hypercalcuria*
   a. Milk alkali syndrome
      – Due to long standing calcium and alkali ingestion.
      – Severe hypercalecmia, irreversible renal failure and ectopic calcification.
   b. Sarcoidosis.
      – Renal involvement in .2-5% cases.
      – Associated lung involvement—hilar LN, fibro-nodular infiltrate.
      – Bone lytic lesions.
   c. *Hypervitaminosis D*
      – In excess of 50,000 U/day
      – Deossification.
      – Widening of provisional zone of calcification.
      – Dense calvarium.
      – Metastatic calcification in arterial walls.
6. *Primary Hyperoxaluria*
   – 65% < 5 years
   – Generally diffuse and homogenous.
   – Recurrent nephrolithiasis.
   – Dense vascular calcification.

Cortical Nephrocalcinosis

    < 5% of cases.

1. *Acute cortical necrosis*
   - Small kidney
   - tramline/punctate calcification along margin of necrotic tissue.
   - USG shows hyperechoic cortex with shadowing.
2. *Chronic glomerulonephritis*
   - Small smooth kidneys with wasted parenchyma.
   - Normal papillae and calices.
   - Decrease density of contrast on IVU.
   - USG—increased echogenicity with prominent sinus fat.
3. *Hemolytic uremic syndrome*
   - Common cause in children
   - Cortical necrosis ?fibrosis? calcification
   - Clinically thrombocytopenia.
4. *Alport's syndrome*
   - Autosomal dominant.
   - Polyuria, anemia, nerve deafness, congenital cataract, Nystagmus.
   - Small smooth kidneys.
5. *Rejected renal transplant*
   - Small kidney.
   - Cortical calcifications

Flow Chart 7.12.1: Renal calcification

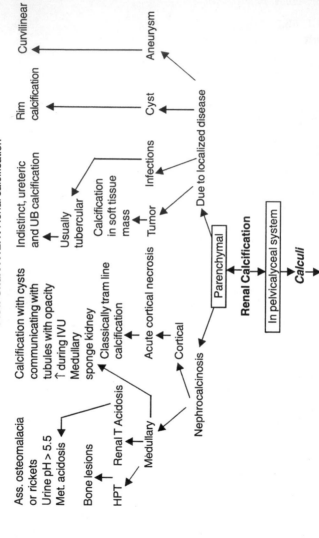

7.13 RENAL MASS

Adult

Unilateral	*Bilateral*
SOLID	

A. *Tumors:*
  a. *Malignant:*
    Adenocarcinoma
    (RCC)
    – Lymphoma
    – TCC
    – Metastasis
    – Adult
      neuroblastoma
  b. *Benign:*
    – AML
      (Angiomyolipoma)
    – Oncocytoma
    – Adenoma
    – Mesenchymal
      tumors
      (Lipoma, fibroma
      myoma, hemangioma

A. Tumors
  Lymphoma

Metastasis
B/L malignant or benign
Renal tumors

B. *Cysts:*

— Adult polycystic kidney
  disease

— Acquired cystic kidney
  disease.

B. *Inflammatory masses:*
  – Acute focal pyelonephritis.
  – Renal abscess.
  – Xanthogranulomatous pyelonephritis.
  – Malakoplakia.
  – Tuberculoma.

CYSTIC
a. Simple renal cysts

b. Inherited cystic disease
   - Multilocular cystic nephroma
   - Multicystic dysplastic kidney
c. Focal hydronephrosis.

CHILDREN (PEDIATRIC)

Single
- Wilms' tumor
- Multilocular cystic nephroma
- Mesoblastic nephroma.
- Focal hydronephrosis.
- Traumatic cyst, abscess.
- RCC

- Intrarenal neuroblastoma
- Malignant rhabdoid tumor

Multiple
- Multiple Wilms' tumors
- Angiomyolipoma.

- Lymphoma.
- Leukemia.
- Nephroblastomatosis.
- Adult polycystic kidney disease
- Abscesses

Renal Cell Carcinoma

- Most common urological malignant lesion in adults
- M:F=2:1, 6th and 7th decade.
- U/L, 2%-B/L, 9% multicentric (VHL, familial, dialysis).
- Diagnostic triad—flank pain, gross hematuria and palpable renal mass—4-9% of patients.
- Usually solid.
- < 3 cm-homogenous, smooth.
- Larger—necrosis and/or hemorrhage, dystrophic calcification.
- Plain X-ray—normal, soft tissue mass overlying/bulging renal outline, or loss of psoas outline.

- Calcification—in 20% of RCC.
  (Non-peripheral or central)—87%—carcinomas.
- IVP—67% sensitive in detecting solid mass lesion of the kidney.
- However cannot determine the nature of a renal mass.

Primary Uroradiologic Elements

Size	–	Large
Contour	–	Unifocal mass
Lesion distribution	–	U/L

Secondary Collecting System

Focal—dilatation, displacement, attenuation.

Nephrogram	:	Focal replaced, irregular margin.
Attenuation	:	Diminished,enhances less than normal parenchyma, unsharp parenchymal interface with ill-defined margin, a thick or irregular wall, enlargement of renal vein or IVC with or without filling defect.
Echogenicity	:	Variable
MR	:	SI similar to parenchyma on unenhanced T1-T2 WI, enhances with gd.
Angio	:	Most RCC-hypervascular, -presence of tumor vessels
	:	Irregular tortous, without normal tapering, randomly distributed, variable in caliber with unpredictable branching.
Lymphoma-	:	Primary lymphoma—rare
		Usually
		– Secondary hematogenous

- Direct extension.
- N.H.L. > H.L.
- B/L > U/L,
- Multiple nodular, diffuse infiltration, bulky single tumor, solitary nodule, invasion from perirenal disease, microscopic infiltration.

Earliest change metastatic nodules detected as nephrographic defects on contrast material enhanced imaging studies, at a time when kidneys may be (Normal) in size and contour.

Primary Uroradiological Elements

Size	:	Large
Contour	:	Normal to multifocal masses.
Lesion distribution	:	Bilateral.

Secondary Uroradiological Elements

Collecting system	:	Displaced, caliectasis without pelviectasis (from sinus spread)
Parenchymal thickness	:	Expanded (focal)
Nephrogram	:	Multifocal masses/attenuation value less than that of (Normal) tissue: minimal enhancement with contrast material.
Echogenicity	:	Multifocal hypoechoic solid masses.

Transitional Cell Carcinoma

Primary involvement of PCS and ureter.
- Focal, multifocal or diffuse, transform the normally smooth mucosa into a surface with is irregular or nodular.

- Twice as common in renal pelvis than in the ureter.
- B/L -10% multifocal 20-44%
- M>F, 7th decade
  - Gross or microscopic hematuria flank pain.

IVP

- Primary investigative modality
- Filling defect in renal pelvis, or calyx, calyceal cut off, infundibular narrowing, poor or non-visualization of one group of calyces, non-functioning kidney, due to or HDN.
    i. HDN
    ii. Extensive destruction and replacement of renal parenchyma.
    iii. Renal vein invasion.

USG

- Iso or hypoechoic solid mass separating the central sinus echoes.
- Focal enlargement of renal cortex if seen suggests infiltration of renal perenchyma.

CT

Pelvis or calyceal filling defect or a solid mass in renal sinus.
- Parapelvic fat line is initially compressed by the growing mass and if disrupted indicates invasion.
- In large masses a diagnosis of TCC is more likely if the mass is centrally located, with centrifugal extension, and preservation of renal shape.
- RCC tends to be eccenteric, distort renal outline and shows relatively more enhancement.

Metastasis

Relatively common at autopsy-seen in 20% patients

- M.C. sites of primary—Lung, breast, colon, malignant melanoma.
- Multiple and B/L
- If single large—impossible to differentiate from primary (Renal tumor—Biopsy indicated)
- USG—hypoechoic
- CT—small multiple solid renal lesion, < 2 cm, subcapsular in renal cortex.

Angiomyolipoma (AML)

- Radiologically most common, diagnosed benign renal neoplasm.
- Hamartoma—represents excessive growth of mature fat, smooth muscle and arteries normally present in the kidney.
- F > M—Most asymptomatic.
- Larger lesions—Mass, flank pain, hematuria, hypotension.
- Association with tuberous sclerosis (TS)—80% of patients with TS have AML.
- X-ray—in 10% of patients shows large soft tissue mass with fat radioleucency.

Typical Findings

Primary

Size	:	Large
Contour	:	Unifocal mass.
Distribution	:	U/L
Secondary	:	Collecting system—attenuated (focal); displaced (focal)
Nephrogram	:	Replaced (focal)
Attenuation value		mixed (negative and +ve values) (fat)

Echogenicity : Heterogenous, often hyperechoic.

MR : Signal intensity follows fat on T1 and T2 WI and fat suppressed images.

Oncocytoma
- Uncommon benign tumor arise from PCT
- 4-7% of all renal tumor.
- Average size—7cm
- Often detected incidently as they rarely bleed or cause pain unless extremely large.

USG : Solid homogenous mass with central stellate scar.

CT : Well defined solid mass with homogenous central echo with central scar.

MR : Homogenous signal intensity. low to moderate on T1 and relatively high on T2 WI. Central stallate scar with well defined capsule.

Angio : Well defined vascular renal tumor with a 'spoke-wheel' pattern of vessels penetrating into the center of the tumor and homogenous tumor blush.

Adenoma : Seen in =15% kidneys at autopsy.
: Usually as cortical subcapsular tumor
: Arise from tubular epithelium.
: Difficult to distinguish from RCC. Natural H/O—unknown.

Wilms' Tumor : Most common abdominal and renal malignancy in children.
: 7-8/10 children/years
: 80% in first three years
: Association with cryptorchidism, hypospadias, hemihypertrophy.

Sporadic Oniridia
- 10-15% B/L
- Plain film—abdominal mass displacing adjacent structures.
- Calcification - in 5%
- USG—Large well defined mass, greater echogenicity than liver.
  Solid with hemorrhage and necrosis.
  CT—well defined, low attenuation with hemorrhage and necrosis.
  MR—inhomogenous low signal on T1 and high on T2.
- Differentiation from neuroblastoma—2nd most common retroperitoneal tumor in children.

Wilms' Tumor	*Neuroblastoma*
• Intrarenal mass with distorted PCS anatomy.	• Intraspinal extension
• Vascular structures (IVC, aorta) displaced	• Encased
• Heterogenous with areas of necrosis.	• Solid homogenous
• Ipsilateral IVC./renal	• Extend into chest thoracoabdominal sign
• Vein tumor thrombus (+)	• (−)
• Lung metastasis	• Bone mets.
• Usually does not cross midline	• Crosses midline
	• Calcification more common.

Congenital Mesoblastic Nephroma

- Most common solid renal tumor in newborn—can be diagnosed in utero on ultrasound.
- Mean age at diagnosis—3 and half months, associated polyhydramnios.

US/CT—predominatly solid mass but even cystic and calcified component can be seen.

- Does not extend into IVC.

Primary

Size	:	Large
Contour	:	Infiltrative bean-shaped mass
Lesion distribution	:	U/L
Secondary collecting system	:	Attenuated, caliectasis with pelviectasis nephrogram-replaced.
Attenuation value	:	Soft tissue homogenous (common)
Echogenicity	:	Soft tissue homogenous (common)
others	:	Polyhydramnios (in utero)

Multilocular Cystic Nephroma

- Uncommon neoplasm composed of multiple variable sized cysts with prominent septa.
- Arises as U/L unifocal mass with the remaining portion of one kidney uninvolved or compressed by the tumors.
- Surrounded by dense fibrous capsule.
- Calcification of cyst wall uncommon.
- Characteristically one or more of the cysts herniate into the renal pelvis to form filling defects.

Nephroblastomatosis

- Remnant of primitive blastoma as sheets or more discrete nodules in cortex.
- Commonly associated with Wilms' tumor.
- IVP—multifocal distortion of PCS.
- CT—Multiple nodules of varying sizes, situated in the peripheral portion of the kidney, with enlargement.
- Surface—usually smooth
- Minimal—contrast enhancement

Simple Cysts/Localized Cystic Disease

Most common focal mass of the kidney.

- Pathogenesis—not conclusively established.
- Obstruction of renal tubule /blockage and expansion of calyceal diverticulum.
- Cyst fluid is serous, not urine, LDH level—lower than serum.
- Usually U/L and single, most common site—polar, (lower pole).
- Rarely numerous simple cysts completely replace the parenchyma of either the entire kidney or only a portion of one kidney—Localized cystic disease Composed of cluster of simple cysts that lacks a capsule and preserves the reniform shape of the enlarged kidney.

Cystic diseases to be distinguished from usually benign but sometimes malignant—multiloculated cystic neoplasms (grow by expansion and appears as ball shaped encapsulated mass).

SIMPLE CYST TYPICAL FINDINGS

Primary

Size	:	Variable
Contour	:	Unifocal mass
Lesion distribution	:	Variable
Secondary collecting system	:	Attenuated (focal), displace (focal)
Nephrogram	:	Displace (focal), replaced (focal), smooth margin, 'thin rim sign' when peripheral, 'beak sign' when peripheral.
Calcification	:	Uncommon, curvilinear, peripheral.
Attenuation value	:	Water, no contrast enhancement

Echogenicity	:	Anechoic, well defined far walls, enhanced through sound transmission.
MR	:	Signal intensity parellel's water.
Polycystic kidney disease	:	Multiple cysts in B/L kidneys

Primary

Size	:	Large
Contour	:	Multifocal masses.
Lesion distribution	:	B/L (may be asymmetric)

Secondary

Collecting system	:	Displaced, attenuated.
Nephrogram	:	Replaced (multiple masses with smooth margin, varying sizes, radiolucent with urography or angiography; water density/intensity, non-enhancing with CT/MRI
Echogenicity	:	Multiple fluid filled masses.
Cyst content	:	Serous with urea content equal to urine.

Acquired Cystic Kidney Disease

- Multiple renal cysts formation in patients with end stage renal disease.
- Seen in 40-50% of patients on long-term hemodialysis.
- Multiple small B/L cysts involving both renal cortex and medulla.
- Increased incidence of renal neoplasms.
- US—B/L small kidneys with increase echogenicity with multiple cysts.
- Solid or complex renal tumor may be present.

- CT—B/L small kidney, with multiple cysts.
- Cyst wall calcification—common.

Acute Focal Bacterial Pyelonephritis and Renal Abscess

- Usually secondary to ascending inferior gram -ve organism
- Most bacterial abscesses are associated with calculus in pelvis or ureter.
- IVP—reveals presence of focal renal mass.
- USG—hypoechoic poorly defined mass with internal echos.
- CT—Low density area with patchy enhancement.
- Lack of well-defined wall and central low density differentiates it from renal abscess.

ABSCESS TYPICAL IMAGING FEATURES

Primary

Size	:	Large
Contour	:	Unifocal mass
Lesion distribution	:	U/L

Secondary

Collecting system	:	Attenuated (focal), displaced (focal)
Nephrogram	:	Normal (early), replaced (focal), irregular, thick wall(late)
Attenuation value	:	Normal to slightly diminished before contrast administration.
	:	Enhances less than normal paren-chyma (early) decreased and non-enhancing (late)
Echogenicity	:	Variable (hypoechoic (early) to ane-choic (late).

Contd...

Flow Chart 7.13.1: Renal mass

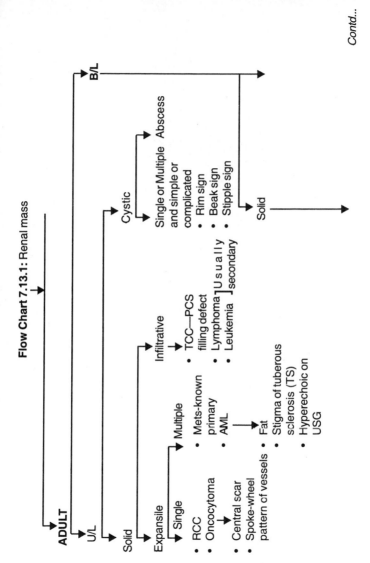

Contd...

Contd...

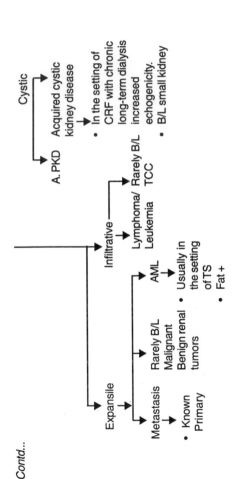

Cystic

A. PKD → Acquired cystic kidney disease
• In the setting of CRF with chronic long-term dialysis increased echogenicity.
• B/L small kidney

Infiltrative → Lymphoma/ Leukemia → Rarely B/L TCC

Expansile

Metastasis → • Known Primary

Rarely B/L Malignant Benign renal tumors

AML → • Usually in the setting of TS
• Fat +

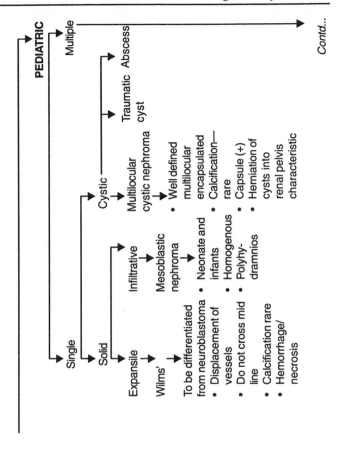

Contd...

Contd...

Contd...

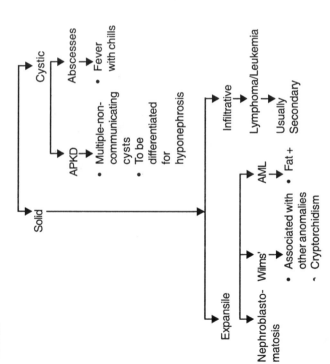

7.14 CYSTIC DISEASE OF KIDNEYS

Renal Cysts : Represent dilated nephrons or collecting ducts

Cystic Kidney : Is a kidney with 3 to 5 or more cysts

Renal Cystic Disease : Refers to any disorder that results from the presence of multiple renal cysts

- Simple Cysts
- Atypical Cysts

Cystic Neoplasams

Nongenetic Conditions	*Imaging Features*
• Cystic dysplasia or dysplasia	• U/L or B/L
• Multicystic dysplastic kidney	• Diffuse or Localised
• Multilocular cyst	• Size of kidneys
• Localized cystic disease of the kidney	• Extrarenal manifestations
• Parapelvic cyst	
• Simple cysts	
• Calyceal cysts	
• Medullary sponge kidney	
• Acquired cystic disease of kidney (in CRF)	

GENETIC CONDITIONS

Autosomal Dominant

- Autosomal dominant, polycystic kidney disease (ADPKD)
- Tuberous sclerosis, VHL

DILATATION OF
A SINGLE CALYX
Most commonly due
to extrinsic compression
by an intrarenal artery
(Fraley syndrome)

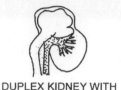

DUPLEX KIDNEY WITH
HYDRONEPHROTIC
UPPER MOIETY
drooping flower
appearance

PSEUDOTUMOR IN
REFLUX
NEPHROPATHY
Hypertrophy of
unscarred renal
parenchyma

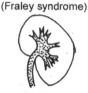

HILAR LIP
Hyperlasia of parenchyma
adjacent to the
renal hilum

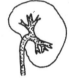

PROMINENT SEPTUM
OF BERTIN
Increased activity on
Tc-DMSA scanning

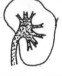

RENAL CYST
US confirms typical
echo-free cyst

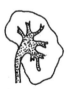

MULTIPLE RENAL CYSTS
e.g. adult type
polycystic disease
spider leg deformity
of calyces

TUMOR
Replacement of much
or all normal renal
tissue

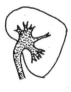

DROMEDARY HUMP
Left sided variant

Fig. 7.14.1: Localized bulge of the renal outline

- Medullary cystic disease
- Glomerulocystic disease

Autosomal Recessive

Autosomal recessive polycystic kidney disease (ARPKD)
Juvenile Nephronophthisis.

Cysts Associated with Syndromes

- Chromosomal disorders
- Autosomal recessive syndromes
- X-linked syndromes

CLASSIFICATION OF RENAL CYSTS

Renal Dysplasia

- Multicystic dysplastic kidney
- Focal segmental cystic dysplasia
- Multiple cysts associated with lower UT obstruction.

Polycystic Disease

- Childhood (AR)
- Adult (AD)

Cortical Cysts

- Simple cyst
- Multilocular cystic nephroma
- Syndromes associated with cysts
- Zellweger's
- Tuberous sclerosis
- Turner's syndrome.

- VHL
- Trisomy 13.
- Trisomy 18.
- Hemodialysis

Medullary Cysts

- Calyceal cyst (diverticulum)
- Medullary sponge kidney
- Papillary necrosis
- Juvenile nephronophthisis (medullary cystic disease MCD)

Miscellaneous

- Inflammatory
- TB
- Hydatid

Neoplastic

- Cystic degeneration of carcinoma.

Traumatic

- Intrarenal hematoma.

Extraparenchymal Renal Cysts

- Parapelvic
- Perinephric

Simple Cysts

USG Criteria: A renal fluid collection with the following features:
- No internal echoes
- Sharply defined distal wall

- Posterior acoustic enhancement
- Round or oval shape.

Atypical Findings in a Cyst

- Internal echoes
- Septa
- Discernible wall
- Solid components within cyst
- Calcification.

DDx

- Hydrocalyx
- Calyceal cyst
- Cavity
- Obstructed moiety of duplex system (upper pole)
- Hematoma
- Aneurysm or AVM.

CT Criteria

1. Sharp margination and demarcation
2. Smooth thin wall
3. Homogeneous attenuation (0-20 HU)
4. No enhancement
   If CT findings are atypical or if patient has hematuria, non-enhanced scan should be obtained.

MRI Criteria

1. Sharp margination and demarcation
2. Smooth thin wall
3. Homogeneous water like signal intensity decrease T1-WI, increase T2-WI.

4. No enhancement
   SS FSE sequences best suited.

ATYPICAL CYSTS

BOSNIAK categorization of cystic renal masses according to CT criteria:

Category 1: Classic simple cysts.

Category 2: Minimally complicated cysts, do not require surgery.

- Smooth, Thin (< 1mm) septa.
- Small smooth plaques of fine linear calcification in cyst wall or septa.
- High density cysts (40-100 HU)
- Can be followed with serial imaging, provided the following criteria are met-

1. Perfectly smooth, rounded, sharply marginated homogeneous lesions.
2. No enhancement.
3. At least one-fourth of the lesion's circumference should extend outside the kidney so that the smoothness of the wall can be evaluated.
4. Size < 4 cm.

Cystic RCC may Rarely Show Similar CT Features

Hemorrhagic cysts on MRI – Increase T1-WI,
                              increase T2-WI
                         – Do not enhance
                         – Fluid-iron levels

Category 3: Should undergo surgical exploration.

- Thick, irregular mural or septal calcification.
- Numerous or thick (> 1 mm) irregular septa.
- Uniform or slightly nodular wall thickening.

- Some category 3 lesions are benign, e.g. Multilocular cystic nephromas, Hemorrhagic renal cysts.
- Others are cystic RCCs

Category 4: Clearly malignant lesions with large cystic components, may show marginal irregularity or solid vascular elements.

POLYCYSTIC KIDNEY DISEASE

Autosomal Recessive Polycystic Kidney Disease (ARPKD—1980-81)

Presents in childhood
1. B/L Large smooth kidneys with dense striated nephrogram.
2. Markedly hyperechoic kidneys on USG with loss of CMD (small 1-2 mm cysts)
3. Associated with Congenital hepatic fibrosis and portal HT.
   - Dilated collecting ducts in renal medulla with relative preservation of the renal cortex.

Autosomal Dominant Polycystic Kidney Disease (ADPKD)

Presents in 3rd-4th decade and terminal renal failure occurs in 10 years.
1. B/L but asymmetrical lobulated enlargement of kidneys.
2. Multiple smooth defects in the nephrogram, with elongation and deformity of calyces giving a "spider leg", appearance, cysts may produce filling defects in the renal pelvis. Calcification in cyst walls.
3. Associated with
   - Liver and Pancreatic cysts.
   - Berry aneurysms (Intracranial)
   - Colonic diverticulae.
   - Increased incidence of RCC.

Diagnostic Criteria : (Ravine et al 1994)
< 30 year : Two cysts U/L or B/L
30-59 year : Two cysts in each kidney } > 6 0
year : > Four cysts

UNILATERAL (LOCALIZED) RENAL CYSTIC DISEASE (URCD)

- Most of one kidney is replaced by multiple cysts. However, the other kidney is normal.
- No family history, No liver cysts, No renal failure.
- Affected kidney is enlarged and may show normal function.

ACQUIRED CYSTIC DISEASE OF KIDNEY (ACKD)

It is characterized by the development of multiple renal cysts in patients without a history of hereditary renal cystic disease. Diagnosis is based on detection of at least 3-5 cysts in each kidney in a patient with CRF not due to hereditary renal cystic disease.

Affected kidneys are usually small, however, nephromegaly eventually develops.

Hemorrhagic cysts occur in about 50% of these patients. (40-100 HU on non-enhanced scans)

Increased incidence of small RCCs (< 3 cm)

EXTRAPARENCHYMAL RENAL CYSTS

Parapelvic Cyst (Lymphatic in origin)

- Located in or near the hilum.
- Does not communicate with the renal pelvis.
- Simple (Multilocular; single/Multiple : U/L or B/L
- May compress renal pelvis and cause hydronephrosis.

DDx

Dilated or Extrarenal pelvis.

Perinephric Cyst

- Secondary to trauma.
- May compress the kidney, pelvis or ureter, leading to hydronephrosis or causing renal displacement.

Multilocular Cystic Nephroma

Cystic renal mass derived from metanephric blastoma, males < 4 year; females 5th/6th decades; presents as abdominal mass.

Spectrum: Benign (Multilocular renal cyst)—Malignant (Multilocular cystic Wilms')

No associated anomalies.

USG: Multilocular renal mass with multiple cysts and septations.

Nonfunctioning on isotope imaging.

Hallmark on imaging is presence of a capsule.

MULTICYSTIC DYSPLASTIC KIDNEY (MDK)

2 types < Pelvico-infundibular atresia
Hydronephrotic type.

In the classic. Pelvico-infundibular type—no discernible renal pelvis. Seen on imaging, kidney may be small or normal in size, or enlarged containing multiple variably sized non-communicating renal cysts—No perfusion on renal scintigraphy.

In the Hydronephrotic form of MDK—dilatation of renal pelvis and calyces is seen with multiple non-communicating cysts.

The affected kidney may remain unchanged, but it frequently undergoes spontaneous regression.

T2-W pulse sequence can be used to diagnose MDK, esp in utero.

MEDULLARY CYSTS

Calyceal Cyst (Diverticulum)—small, solitary cyst communicating via an isthmus with fornix of a calyx.

Medullary Sponge Kidney—B/L in 60-80% cases.

Multiple, small, mainly pyramidal cysts which opacify during excretory urography and contain calculi.

Juvenile Nephronophthisis (Medullary Cystic Disease)—Normal or small kidneys, presents with polyuria. USG shows few medullary or corticomedullary cysts with loss of CMD and increased echogenicity.

Table 7.14.1: Comparison of renal cystic disease

	ADPKD	Cystic TS	ARPKD	MCDK	Simple cyst
Inheritance	AD	AD	AR	None	None
Unilateral / Bilateral	Unequal-Bilateral	Bilateral	Bilateral symmetrical	Unilateral	Unilateral
Kidney size	N/L	N/L	Very Large	Large	Normal
Extrarenal manifestations	Cysts in liver, spleen, pancreas Intracranial aneurysms Colonic diverticulae	Intracranial Tubers, cardiac Rhabdomyo-sarcomas	Congenital hepatic Fibrosis, portal hypertension	None	None
Age at presentation	Third decade	<18 months	Neonate, childhood	Antenatal diagnosis	Rare in children onset in adult life
Cyst size	Kidney size increases with number of cysts	Variable	Generally small occasionally - 1 to 2 cm	Large, involute with time	Variable
Diagnosis	USG, genetic linkage	USG, cardiac echo, Cranial MRI	USG, IVU, liver biopsy	USG, ^{99m}TC, MAG3	USG, IVU
Malignancy	No	Yes	No	Rare	No

7.15 CARCINOMA OF THE BLADDER

- Most common tumor of the GUT.
- TCC 90%; SCC 5%; Adenocarcinoma 2%
- Peaks in the seventh decade.
- Males predominate by 3:1.
- Hematuria, most common clinical presentation.
- Chemical agents such as Aniline, biological agents (coffee, artificial sweeteners), radiation, chronic urothelial irritation, and nicotine are associated with bladder carcinogenesis. Bilharziasis is an independent risk factor.
- Squamous cell carcinoma and adenocarcinoma have poor prognosis.
- The lateral wall of the bladder and bladder diverticulae are more frequently involved.
- Only 60% of known bladder tumors are detected on urograms.
- Bladder tumors cause nonspecific intravesical filling defects.
- The "Stipple sign" (Contrast trapped within interstices of tumor) suggests transitional cell carcinoma. Fungus balls or mycetoma may also occasionally entrap contrast material, but the pattern is lamellar and frequently associated with gas formation.
- CT cannot accurately depict the depth of invasion of the bladder wall and cannot distinguish edema or inflammatory changes from tumor. CT can accurately evaluate perivesical and local pelvic extension.
- MRI is superior to CT in determining local growth and detection of bone marrow infiltration.
- *Stage of tumor*—single most important prognostic parameter. Synchronous upper tract urothelial lesions must be excluded.

- Clinical staging has an accuracy of 50% when compared with that with CT (32-80%) or MRI (73%)
- Overstaging commonly occurs as a result of edema after endoscopy and/or endoscopic resection and as a result of fibrosis from radiation therapy.
- A staging classification that incorporates the TMN and Jewett-Strong-Marshall (JSM) system is useful.
- T1A—indicates lesions involving the mucosa and submucosa.
- T2B1—invasion of the superficial muscle layer.
- T3aB2—invasion of the deep muscular wall.
- T3bC—invasion of perivesical fat.
- T4aD1—extension to perivesical organs.
- T4b—invasion of the pelvic and/or abdominal wall.
- D2—distant metastases.
- Metastases occur in approximately 11% of cases, retroperitoneal nodes (34%); distant lymph nodes (17%); lumbar vertebrae (13%); lungs (9%); kidneys (8%); adrenals (4%)
- Plain radiographic findings are nonspecific, particularly the presence of calcification. The calcification is on the surface in TCC. Intrinsic calcifications suggest an adenocarcinoma or the unusual cell type.
- Irregular filling defects with broad base and fronds in the bladder is seen with IVU, CT and MRI. Increased thickness of the bladder wall in the region of the tumor should indicate infiltration. Unusually the tumor may present as diffuse thickening of the bladder wall.
- Both CT and MRI have been shown to perform better than cystography in the diagnosis of tumors in the bladder diverticula that are not depicted on cystograms because of obstruction at the diverticular orifice.

- Ultrasonography is inaccurate for diagnosing early tumor, and it is useful in the diagnosis of obstructive uropathy. Vesical US can be performed endoscopically during cystoscopy or suprapubically. Tumor is echopoor relative to the vesical wall. As the staging modality US is invasive.
- *On NECT, the TCC is iso*—to hyper attenuating relative to urine. TCCs demonstrate mild-to-moderate enhancement on CECT, and they become hypoattenuating relative to opacified urine.
- On MRI, the tumor is hyperintense than urine but hypointense than fat on both T-1 and PD WI; the tumor is hypointense than urine on T2WI. Post-GD T1WI within the first two minutes can identify early tumors.

Differential Diagnosis

- Nonneoplastic lesions—calculi, blood clot, fungus balls, inflammatory pseudosarcoma, cystitis.

Primary

- *Epithelial tumors*—Papilloma, SCC, adenocarcinoma, carcinosarcoma, undifferentiated tumors.
- *Mesodermal tumors*—Smooth muscle—leiomyoma, leiomyoblastoma, leiomyosarcoma; neural tumors—neurofibroma, neurilemoma; vascular-hemangioma, lymphangioma, hemangiosarcoma; fibrous - fibroepithelial polyp, mixed tumours—fibromyoma, fibrolipoma, fibromyxoma; Lymphoma.
- Metastases or direct invasion of the uroepithelial by tumors.

Flow Chart 7.15.1: Filling defect in bladder on IVU, CT, MRI

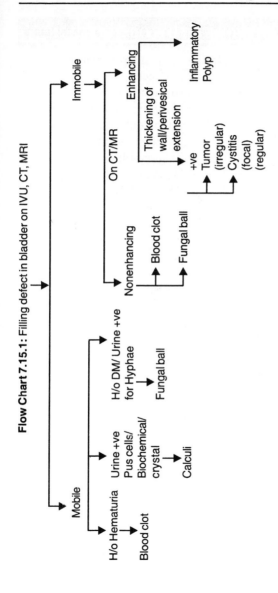

7.16 BLADDER OUTFLOW OBSTRUCTION

1. Prostate
   - Benign prostatic hyperplasia
   - Prostate cancer
   - Other prostatic lesions—
     Wegener's granulomatosis
     - Lymphomatoid granulomatosis
     - Malignant lymphoma

2. Urethral
   - Congenital urethral valves
   - Urethral atresia
   - Urethral dysplasia
   - Anterior urethral diverticulum
   - Urethral stricture
   - Calculus
   - Meatal stenosis

3. Vesical
   - Acquired bladder neck stricture
   - Bladder calculi
   - Fungus ball
   - Bladder tumors
   - Neurogenic bladder
   - Bladder sphincter dys-synergia

4. Miscellaneous
   - Ectopic ureterocele
   - Prune-belly syndrome
   - Hydrocalpos
   - Cervical/lower uterine segment leiomyoma
   - Vaginal carcinoma, rhabdomyosarcoma
     Phimosis

BPH (Benign Prostatic Hyperplasia)

Most common cause of vesical neck obstruction in adult males.

On MCU the prostatic urethra appears elongated and compressed.

Cystogram—Floor of urinary bladder is. elevated with a rounded defect.

Trabeculations and distention of urinary bladder with/ without Bladder deverticula/bladder calculi

IVU—Hydronephrosis /Hydroureter in advanced cases.

Distal ureters form a 'J' (fishhook) deformity.

US—Diffusely altered inhomogenous echopattern.

Demonstrate size and shape of gland.

Concomitant prostatic calculi + other feature of obstruction.

CT—Unequivocal enlargement—prostate is seen 2-3 cm or more above the symphysis and is surrounded by the bladder.

MR—Appearance of prostate varies depending on the type of hyperplasia

Nodular hyperplasia—Enlarged gland with nodules of decrease signal intensity on T1WI and of varying intensity on T2WI

Diffuse hypertrophy—Enlarged gland with decrease signal intensity on T1WI and homo/inhomogenous medium to high SI on T2WI.

Carcinoma of the Prostate

95% are Adenocarcinoma; Rarely squamous or transitional cell carcinoma.

70% originates in periphery—C zone; 20% in transitional zone and 10% in central zone.

Screening for primary carcinoma is by Digital Rectal Examination and Serum PSA.

MCU—Narrow prostatic urethra. Irregularity of urethra/floor bladder laterosuperior of urethra.

Seminal vericulogram—Medial portion of seminal vesicles are reduced is size and the lateral portion may be dilated.

US—Carcinoma is seen as hypoechoic area within the peripheral zone which warrants a TRUS guided needle biopsy

Feature of extracapsular invasion—contour deformity of capsule irregularity and duct tumor extension into periprostatic fat

CT—Used for tumor staging (nodal, visceral, bony)

Radionuclide bone scintigraphy—Accurately detects small and early metastatic lesion.

MR—Major role is in tumor staging esp. extracapsular extension seminal, vesicular and bladder invasion.

Signal intensity of prostate carcinoma has been variously repeated as being of decreased, increased, and/or heterogeneous.

Congenital Urethral Valves

Almost exclusively in males.
Anterior urethral valves—Rare; Posturethral valves are more common.

Posturethral Valves

Type:
1. Two mucosal folds extending from lower aspect of verumontenum to distal posturethra—most common
2. Two folds extending from cephalad aspect of verumontenum to bladder neck.
3. Horizontal membrane in region of verumontanum with central/eccentric opening.

Antenatal ultrasound—Dilated bladder with thickened walls with dilated posturethra. Dilated pelvi calyceal system and ureter (50%).

Urinary tract rupture—Urinary ascites, paranephric urinoma.

Oligohydroamnios and pulmonary hypoplasia.

Cystic dysplasia

MCU—Dilatation of prostatic urethra upto valves.

Valves may be seen as their crescenteric filling defect.

Unilateral or bilateral VUR.

Ring like constriction of vesical neck (Detrusar muscle hypertrophy).

UB—Thick wall with trabeculation/sacculation.

Urethral Atresia

Exceedingly rare and is usually associated with renal dysplasia.

Urethral Dysplasia

- Entire urethra is dysplastic and this is associated with dysplasia of kidneys.
- Suprapubic catheter is required to outline the urethra on *MCU*—thin line of contrast in the region of urethra but no normal anatomical landmarks can be destinguished.

Anterior Urethral Diverticulum

- Saccular, wide necked ventral expansion of the anterior urethra, usually at the penoscrotal junction.
- During micturation, the diverticulum expands with urine and obstructs the urethra.

Urethral Stricture

Causes—infective, trauma, instrumentation
- Most common infective cause is Gonorrhea. Post-gonococcal strictures are several cm in length and involve bulbous urethra. Associated filling of glands of Littre and cowpers is seen during MCU.

Traumatic Stricture

Most common site is both—prosta..c and membranous urethra. Usually associated with pelvic fractures.

Urethral Calculus

- Rare and happens to be present in urethra during passage from the bladder.
- Urethral calculus is so characteristic in position that the triangle is made from plain radiograph.
- RGU and MCU provide definitive information as to the relationship of the radiopacity to urethra.
- 'Hour glass' calculus—occupies bladder and prostatic urethra.

Acquired Bladder Neck Stricture

Formation of scar tissue at vesical neck can occur following. Suprapubic/previous/transurethral prostatectomy.

RGU—Shows dilatation of the distensible unscarred segments of the anterior and posterior urethra and visualization of contracted neck of bladder.

Bladder Calculi

- Arise as a result of stasis, infection, FB or can descend from the kidney.

- There are usually triple phosphate stones or uric acid mixed with urate.
- X-ray—Faceted/starshaped/laminated calculus.
- US—echogenic focus with post-acoustic shadowing. Feature of obstructive uropathy—thickened, trabeculated urinary bladder with hydroureteronephrosis.

Fungal Ball

In immunocompromized and diabetic patients numerous hyphae within the urinary bladder unite to form a fungus ball. Leading to bladder outlet obstruction.

- Fungus ball is associated with alternating lucent and opaque irregular laminations owing to gas formation.
- It may be seen as mobile filling defect during IVU or cystography.

Bladder Tumors

1. *Epithelial:* Most common is transitional cell carcinoma squamous cell carcinoma and adenocarcinoma are rare
2. *Nonepithelial:*

   Benign—Leiomyoma, fibroma

   Malignant—Leiomyosarcoma, rhabdomyosarcoma.

   Most common site—Around trigone and posterolateral wall of urinary bladder

   Cystogram—Well demarcated filling defect with lobulated margins

   US—Nonmobile mass lesion/focal wall thickening.

   CT—Useful for detection of perivesical extension, invasion,

   MRI—Visceral and pelvic lymph node involvement.

Rhabdomyosarcoma

Constitutes about 1/8th of the childhood solid tumors
- Peak period of incidence is 1 to 8 years.
- Bladder is the most common site of rhabdomyosarcoma.
- In males tumor typically arises from the bladder wall or prostate; In females from vagina.
- These tumors are quite large at the time of diagnosis and the exact site of origin of these tumors is difficult.

Radiological Features

Lobulated soft tissue density mass in the bladder base or as echogenic soft tissue projecting into urinary bladder on US.

Once diagnosed—Chest X-ray, 99^m Tc-MDP bone scan and CT for staging.

Bladder—Sphincter Dys-synergia

Caused by asynchronous opening of the bladder neck with the detrusor contraction producing characteristic high voiding pressure and low flow rates.

Diagnosis Established by Videocystometrography (VCMG)

- Bladder neck opens slightly at first, but then widens further as the detrusor pressure falls.
- Eventually patients develop hypertrophied bladder which is unable to overcome bladder outlet obstruction. Decompensated obstruction.

Neuropathic Lesions of Bladder
1. Suprasacral cord lesion
   - Injuries to cerebral/pontine micturation area.

Loss of voluntary detrusor control and uncoordinated voiding. If bladder dysurea is also positive—Detrusor contracts against a closed sphincter.
- Diagnosis made by VCMG. On cystogram—UB is contracted, trabeculated and thick walled "Fircone bladder".

2. Damage to sacral/peripheral nerves—disrupts the vesical parasympathetic nerve supply
   - Underactive /Acontractile bladder muscles.
   - Large capacity bladder with smooth wall.
     Need to be evacuated by manual compression/ abdominal straining and intermittent catheterization

Complication

VUR, Recurrent UTI, stone formation.

Prune-Belly Syndrome

Caused by triad of deficient abdominal musculature, undescended testes and urinary tract dysplasia.

Proposed etiology   :   ? Fetal urethral level obstruction which resolves in later gestation.
                      :   ? Early mesenchymal developmental arrest.

- Protuberant abdomen.
- Small kidneys with minimal dilatation of pelvi calyceal system.
- Upper ureters are mildly dilated; lower ureters are tortous and show disproportionate dilatation.
- Posterior urethra is markedly dilated prominantly with a typical conical narrowing with poor stream in the distal urethra.
- Urinary bladder is of large volume, irregularly shaped, thin walled and with wide neck.

Ectopic Ureterocele

- This is a saccular dilatation of the intramural portion of the ureter as it passes through the bladder wall which results because of the narrowed opening of the ectopic ureter.
- Ectopic ureter most commonly occurs with the upper moiety of a kidney.
- An ectopic unterocele opening into the urethra, bladder neck, on vestibule—results in bladder outlet obstruction.

Radiological Features

Dilated ureter with small hydronephrotic upper pole moiety
- Ureteroceles can be seen on ultrasound and on IVU show a characteristic 'Cobra head' sign—caused by contrast medium pooling in the ureterocele, which is surrounded by halo of radiolucent ureterocele wall of bladder mucosa.

Flow Chart 7.16.1: Bladder outflow obstruction

Adults

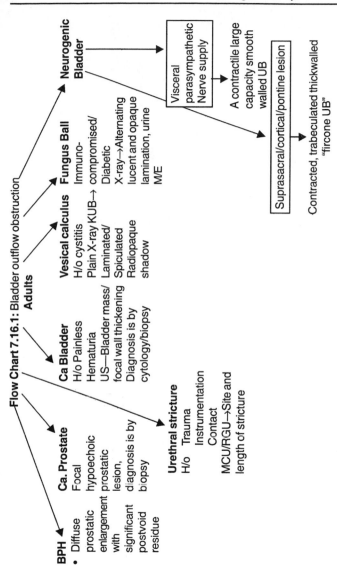

BPH
- Diffuse prostatic enlargement with significant postvoid residue

Ca. Prostate
Focal hypoechoic prostatic lesion, diagnosis is by biopsy

Urethral stricture
H/o Trauma
Instrumentation
Contact
MCU/RGU→Site and length of stricture

Ca Bladder
H/o Painless Hematuria
US—Bladder mass/ focal wall thickening
Diagnosis is by cytology/biopsy

Vesical calculus
H/o cystitis
Plain X-ray KUB→ Laminated/ Spiculated Radiopaque shadow

Fungus Ball
Immuno-compromised/ Diabetic
X-ray→Alternating lucent and opaque lamination, urine M/E

Neurogenic Bladder

Visceral parasympathetic Nerve supply

→ A contractile large capacity smooth walled UB

Suprasacral/cortical/pontine lesion

→ Contracted, trabeculated thickwalled "fircone UB"

Flow Chart: 7.16.2: Bladder outflow obstruction Children

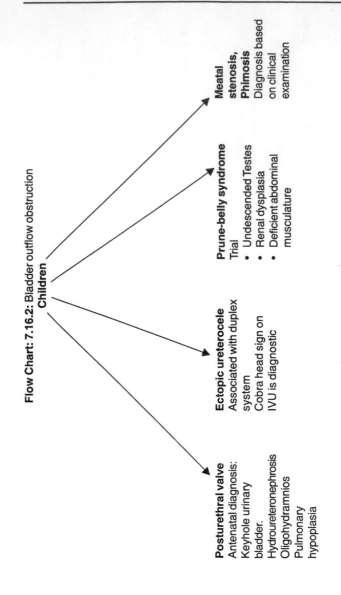

Posturethral valve
Antenatal diagnosis:
Keyhole urinary
bladder.
Hydroureteronephrosis
Oligohydramnios
Pulmonary
hypoplasia

Ectopic ureterocele
Associated with duplex
system
Cobra head sign on
IVU is diagnostic

Prune-belly syndrome
Trial
• Undescended Testes
• Renal dysplasia
• Deficient abdominal
  musculature

**Meatal
stenosis,
Phimosis**
Diagnosis based
on clinical
examination

7.17 TESTICULAR TUMORS

- Adult testes are ovoid glands measuring 3-5 cm in length, 2-4 cm in width and 2-3 cm in anteroposterior diameter. Weight ranges from 12.5 to 19 gm.
- Epididymis is—Posterolateral to testis, 6 to 7 cm in length divided into head (10-12 mm diam), body (4 nm) and tail.

DD of Testicular Tumors

1. Primary Testicular Tumors:
   - A. Germ cell tumors : Seminoma
     - : Nonseminomatous germ cell tumors (NSGCT)
     - : Embryonal carcinoma
     - : Choriocarcinoma
     - : Teratoma
     - : Yolk sac/Endodermal sinus tumor
     - : Tumors of more than one histological type
     - : Teratoma and embryonal cell carcinoma
     - : Choriocarcinoma and any other type
   - B. Tumors of gonadal stroma : Sertoli cell
     - : Leydig cell
     - : Granulosa cell
     - : Undifferentiated
     - : Combination
2. Secondary Testicular Tumors : Lymphoma
   - : Leukemia

: Nonlymphoma metastasis
(Lung and Prostate)

3. Benign/Miscellaneous Lesions of Testis
- Tunica albuginea cyst
- Intratesticular cyst
- Tubular ectasia of rete testis
- Cystic dysplasia
- Epidermoid cyst
- Abscess.

Germ Cell Tumors (95%)

Clinically patient presents with a palpable painless mass, chronic pain or sense of heaviness. 15% cases have acute symptoms of pain following traumatic hematoma. Rarely patient presents with signs of distant metastasis (NSGCT)

- *Seminomas:* Accounts for 40% of testicular tumors. Peak prevelance is in the 4th decade.
- *Ultrasound:* Well circumscribed homogenous hypoechoic mass
- *Multiple calcification (1-2 mm):* May be seen in 1/3rd cases.
- As tumor enlarges it become heterogeneous (hemorrhage/necrosis)
- *Burnt outseminoma:* Primary testicular tumor is not identified as a discrete mass despite a large tumor burden elsewhere in the body.
- Seminomas are most common tumor type in cryptorchid testis.
- *MR:* Lobulated homogenous, intermediate SI on T2 WI:
- *NSGCT:* Peak prevalence is in the 2nd to 3rd decade.
- More likely to occur as combination of different histotypes rather than as isolated pure form.

- More likely to be locally advanced and have a higher likelyhood of metastases than seminomas.
- *Ultrasound:* Heterogeneous and poorly defined.
- *Calcification:* 50% cases.
- *MR:* Hetrogeneous with areas of high and low SI or T2 WI.
- Endodermal sinus tumor and Teratomas are the most common tumors of infancy and early childhood.

Stromal Tumors (3-5%)

- 20% of these occur in children. Rest occur between 20-50 years.
- It is not possible to differentiate between the different stromal or between stromal and germ cell tumors radiologically.
- Most common stromal tumor is Leydig cell tumor.
- Associated with gynecomastia (30%) (Androgen/estrogen production)
  - Impotence
  - Loss of libido
  - Precocious puberty.

On ultrasound these tumors are usually small, solid and hypoechoic.

Spread of Testicular Tumors

- *Lymphatic:* Upper retroperitoneal, retrocrural, mediastinal and supraclavicular lymph node
- Pelvic lymphadenopathy is less common and is suggestive of penetration of testicular capsule.
- *Hematogenous:* Lung, Liver, Brain and Bone.

Lymphomas

- Most common secondary testicular neoplasm: Peak age of diagnosis is:60-70 years.
- Testicular involvement occurs in 0.3% cases of lymphoma (NHL)
- Most common cause of bilateral testicular tumor.
- Majority of lymphomas are homogenous, hypoechoic and diffusely replace the testis. Focal hypoechoic lesions are rare.

Leukemia

- Second most common testicular metastatic tumor.
- Testis acts as a sancturay site for leukemic cells during chemotherapy because of blood gonadal barrier that inhibits concentration of chemotherapeutic agents 64% cases of acute leukemia and 25% chronic leukemia show testicular involvement.
- *Characterized by:* Diffuse infiltration producing diffusely enlarged hypoechoic testes.

Other Metastases

Uncommon occurs from; lung and prostate and rarely kidney, stomach colon, pancreas and melanoma.
- Commonly multiple and bilateral (15%)
- Hypoechoic but may be echogenic /complex in appearance.

Cyst of Tunica Albuginea

- Located within the tunica; usually on anterior and lateral aspects of testes
- 5th and 6th decade
- Patient is asymptomatic, cystic, lesion is 2 to 5 mm in size.

Intratesticular Cyst

- Simple cyst filled with clear serous fluid that vary in size between 2-18 mm.
- Probably originate from the rete testis possibly secondary to post-traumatic /post-inflammatory stricture formation.

Tubular Ectasia of Rete Testes

- Usually associated with epididymal obstruction secondary to inflammation or traumatic lesions.
- Characterized by variable sized cystic lesion in the region of the mediastinum testis with no associated soft tissue abnormality and no flow on color flow Doppler imaging.
- May be B/L and associated with spermatocele.

Cystic Dysplasia

- Rare; Seen in infants and young children.
- Embryologic defect preventing connection of the tubules of the rete testes and efferent ductules.
- Characterized by multiple interconnecting cyst of varying size and shape separated by fibrous stroma.
- Renal agenesis/Dysplasias frequently coexist with cystic dysplasias.

Epidermoid Cyst

- Benign tumor of germ cell origin.
- Occurs at any age, most frequently 2nd to 4th decade.
- Well-defined hypoechoic solid masses with echogenic capsule, internal echogenic contents may be present.

Abscess

- Results from—Complication of epididymo-orchitis, missed testicular. Torsion, gangrenous /infected tumor, primary pyogenic orchitis.
- Common infectious causes are—mumps, smallpox, scarlet fever, influenza, typhoid, sinusitis, osteomyelitis, appendicitis.
- Ultrasound—Enlarged testicle containing a fluid filled mass with hypoechoic/mixed echogenic areas.
- Complications—Rupture-pyocele/Fistula to the skin.

Flow Chart 7.17.1: Testicular tumors

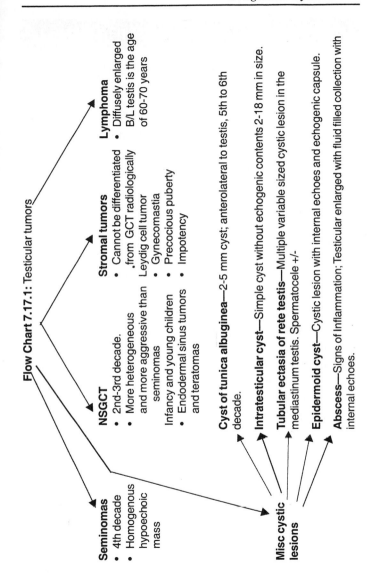

Testicular tumors

Seminomas
- 4th decade
- Homogenous hypoechoic mass

NSGCT
- 2nd-3rd decade.
- More heterogeneous and more aggressive than seminomas
- Infancy and young children
- Endodermal sinus tumors and teratomas

Stromal tumors
- Cannot be differentiated from GCT radiologically
- Leydig cell tumor
- Gynecomastia
- Precocious puberty
- Impotency

Lymphoma
- Diffusely enlarged B/L testis is the age of 60-70 years

Misc cystic lesions

Cyst of tunica albuginea—2-5 mm cyst; anterolateral to testis, 5th to 6th decade.

Intratesticular cyst—Simple cyst without echogenic contents 2-18 mm in size.

Tubular ectasia of rete testis—Multiple variable sized cystic lesion in the mediastinum testis. Spermatocele +/-

Epidermoid cyst—Cystic lesion with internal echoes and echogenic capsule.

Abscess—Signs of Inflammation; Testicular enlarged with fluid filled collection with internal echoes.

7.18 SEMINAL VESICLE CALCIFICATION

Seminal vesicles are paired symmetric organs, present along the posterior aspect of prostate being separated from it by a fat plane. These are accessory reproductive organs of males and there duct fuse with the Vas to make the ejaculatory duct which opens on the veru montanum of posterior urethra.

Methods of Investigation

Plain X-ray: These may sometime show calcifications in the seminal vesicles, which may be confused to be of bladder origin. The calcifications may be seen as either specks of scattered calcification or mushroom shaped.

USG: They appear as bilaterally symmetrical structure on the posterior and superior aspect of prostate and are normally heterogeneous in appearance.

CT: They are seen as lobulated extraperitoneal pouches located superior to the prostate gland between the bladder and the rectum.

MRI: They are seen as convoluted tubular structures. The seminal fluid within their lumen results in high signal intensity on T2 weighted images; these lumens are surrounded by low signal intensity of the tubular walls. MR imaging with endorectal coils provide excellent images.

Differential Diagnosis

Diabetes mellitus: This is seen either as an incidental finding in a known case of DM or may masquerade as obstruction and subsequent enlargement of the gland leading to either to subfertility or infertility.

Chronic Infections: These include:

1. Tuberculosis.
2. Schistosomiasis.
3. Chronic UTI
4. Syphilis

Calcification of seminal vesicle may be seen in either of the above disease and is usually secondary to the involvement of either the urinary system, i.e. the kidneys, ureters and bladder or secondary to prostatitis. The primary changes in the above organs gives a clue to the real etiology of the calcification.

- Tubercular seminal vesicle calcifications may present with changes of renal TB (calcifications, calyceal cut off sign, calyceal diverticulae, putty kidney, multiple ureteric strictures and a small capacity thimble bladder). Changes of tubercular prostatitis may also be seen (abscesses, hypoechogenicity, hemospermia calcifications).

- Schistosomiasis classically present as bladder wall calcification, which may extend to involve the ureters but never the PCS(Pelvi calyceal system). This calcification may secondarily also involve the prostate and seminal vesicle.

- *Idiopathic:* This is by far the commonest cause of seminal vesicle calcification but may, however, present clinically as either hemospermia, ejaculatory duct obstruction, sub-fertility or infertility. The diagnosis is that of exclusion.

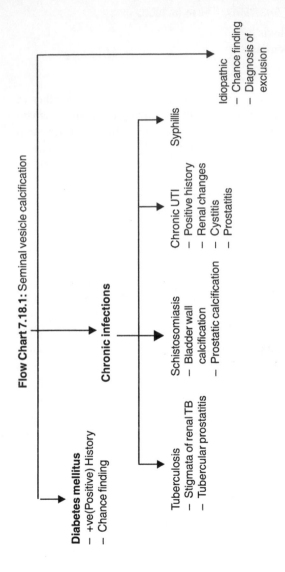

Flow Chart 7.18.1: Seminal vesicle calcification

Diabetes mellitus
– +ve (Positive) History
– Chance finding

Chronic infections

Tuberculosis
– Stigmata of renal TB
– Tubercular prostatitis

Schistosomiasis
– Bladder wall calcification
– Prostatic calcification

Chronic UTI
– Positive history
– Renal changes
– Cystitis
– Prostatitis

Syphillis

Idiopathic
– Chance finding
– Diagnosis of exclusion

7.19 DIFFERENTIAL DIAGNOSIS OF ABNORMAL NEPHROGRAMS

1. **Dense persistent nephrogram with slow onset:**
   A. Acute ureteral obstruction
   B. Acute renal failure
   C. Systemic hypotension
   D. Renal vein thrombosis
   E. Partial renal artery occlusion
2. **Dense persistent nephrogram with rapid onset:**
   A. Acute renal failure
   B. Hypotension secondary to contrast injection
3. **Persistent faint nephrogram:**
   A. Acute renal failure
   B. Chronic renal failure
   C. Acute pyelonephritis
4. **Persistent dense nephrogram:**
   A. Contrast nephropathy
5. **Rim nephrogram:**
   A. Severe hydronephrosis
   B. Acute complete arterial occlusion
6. **Striated urographic nephrogram:**
   A. Acute ureteral obstruction
   B. Infantile polycystic kidney disease
   C. Medullary sponge kidney
   D. Medullary tubular ectasia
7. **Absent nephrogram:**
   A. Sudden complete arterial occlusion
   B. Sudden complete venous occlusion
   C. Sudden complete long standing ureteral occlusion
   D. Acute renal failure
   E. Acute cortical necrosis

8. **Inhomogenous arteriographic nephrogram:**
   A. Catheter induced arteriospasm
   B. Small vessel disease
      – Nephrosclerosis
      – Necrotizing angiitis
      – Wegener's granulomatosis
      – PAN-polyarteritis nodosa
         PAN
         ↓
         moth-eaten nephrogram
   C. Scleroderma
   D. Acute renal failure
   E. Acute pyelonephritis
   F. Early adult polycystic kidney disease
   G. Renal vein thrombosis

7.20 FILLING DEFECT IN THE BLADDER

1. **Neoplasm:** Majority are—transitional cell carcinoma. Other masses simulating carcinoma of bladder include:
   A. Ca prostate or rectum or seminal vesicle
   B. Metastasis
   C. Phaeodromocytoma
   D. Leiomyoma
   E. Lymphoma
   F. Malacoplakia
2. **Prostate: Seen as impression on the floor of bladder**
3. **Blood clot:**
   – Usually post-traumatic
   – Seen as filling defect

4. **Instrument:**
   - Urethral or suprapubic catheter
   - Can be confirmed sonographically
5. **Calculus:**
   - Many are non-opaque
6. **Ureterocele:**
   - Is the saccular dilatation of the intrarenal portion of a ureter as it passes through the bladder wall. Resulting from a narrowed opening of the uretric orifice
7. **Schistosomiasis:**
   - There is calcification of the bladder wall which is about 1-3 mm wide
8. **Fungal ball:**
   - Appearance of a gas-filled, laminated rounded mass is diagnostic
9. **Malacoplakia:**
   - It is an inflammatory condition usually due to *E.coli* infection. Radiographically a smooth, oval or round filling defect is seen in the bladder.
10. **Endometriosis**

7.21 CARCINOMA PROSTATE

Anatomy

Prostate is a male accessory reproductive organ situated below the base of the bladder and surrounds the prostatic urethra, which runs through the peripheral zone. It is a pyramidal organ with its base directed upwards. The normal gland consists of glandular and non-glandular elements surrounded by a fibromuscular capsule. The basic architecture of prostate can be divided as follows:

- *Lobar anatomy:* The prostate is said to be composed of anterior, posterior and median lobes.
- *Zonal anatomy:* This is the anatomy revealed after anatomic dissection of prostate. It describes prostate to be composed of the following four glandular zones surrounding the prostatic urethra:
- *Peripheral zone* is the largest glandular zone containing approx. Seventy percent of the prostatic glandular tissue and it is this zone that is the source of most prostatic cancers. It surrounds the distal urethral segment and is separated from the transition zone and central zone by the surgical capsule.It occupies the posterior, lateral, and apical region of the prostate.
- *Transition zone* contains approx. 5% of prostatic glandular tissue. It consists of two small glandular areas located adjacent to the proximal urethral segment. It is the site of origin of BPH. The verumontanum bounds the transition zone caudally.
- The Central zone constitutes approx. 25% of the glandular tissue. It is located at the prostatic base. The ducts of the vas deferens and seminal vesicles enter the central zone, and the ejaculatory duct pass through it. It is relatively resistant to disease processes.
- The Periurethral glands form about 1% of the glandular volume. They are embedded in the longitudinal smooth muscle of proximal urethra.
- The prostaticovesical arteries arising from the internal iliac arteries supply the prostate. The prostate is a very vascular structure. The lymphatic drainage of the prostate is thus via the pelvic nodes to the internal iliac group.
- *Incidence:* The prostate cancer is the second most common malignancy in males being superseded only by the carcinoma bronchus. It is said to be recognized in

35% of males above 45 years of age at autopsies. One out of 11 males will develop prostate cancer.

- *Risk factors:* Advancing age, presence of testes, cadmium exposure, animal fat intake.
- *Histopathology:* The prostatic carcinoma is usually an adenocarcinoma.

Premalignant Changes

- PIN or prostatic intraepithelial neoplasia is the lesion frequently associated with invasive carcinoma either next to it or elsewhere in the gland.
- Atypical adenomatous hyperplasia leading to frank adenocarcinoma.
- *Spread:* Mainly blood-borne along the neurovascular bundle.
- *Grading:* (Gleason score 2-10). This is histopathological grading of prostatic carcinoma
  - 1,2,3 glands surrounded by 1 row of epithelial cells.
  - 4 Absence of complete gland formation.
  - 5 Sheets of malignant cells.
- Low numbers on Gleason's score refers to well differentiated, high numbers to anaplastic tumors.

Categories

- *Latent:* Discovered at autopsy of a patient without signs or symptoms referable to the prostate (26-73%).
- *Incidental:* Discovered in 6-20% of specimens obtained during TURP for clinically benign BPH.
- *Occult:* Found at biopsy of metastatically involved bone lesions/lymph nodes in a patient without symptoms of prostatic disease.
- *Clinical:* Cancer detected by digital rectal examination based on induration, irregularity or nodule.

- *Prostate specific antigen:* (PSA) is a glycoprotein produced by prostatic epithlium and it may be elevated in cases of carcinoma. Monoclonal radioimmunoassay is most commonly used and the normal values range from 0.1 to 4 ng/ml.
  - Cancers of less than 1ml volume usually do not elevate PSA.
  - Cancers with PSA levels of <10 ng/ml are usually confined to gland.
  - 19% of prostate cancers do not elevate PSA.
  - 16% of normal men have PSA >4 ng/ml.
  - Benign conditions may also elevate PSA like BPH, prostatitis, PIN.
  - PSA levels may also be used in post-treatment screening of patients for disease recurrence.

Staging

American urological association system modified Jewitt-Whitmore staging is used most commonly:

A. *No palpable lesion*
   A1 focal well differentiated tumor <1.5 cm or < 5% of resected tissue
   A2 diffuse poorly differentiated tumor >5% of chips from TURP
   Specimen
B. *Palpable tumor confined to prostate*
   B1 lesion < 1.5 cm in diameter confined to one lobe
   B2 lesion > 1.5 cm involving more than one lobe
C. *Localized tumor with capsular involvement*
   C1 capsular invasion
   C2 capsular penetration
   C3 seminal vesicle involvement

D *Distant metastasis*

  D1 involvement of pelvic nodes

  D2 distant nodes involved

  D3 metastasis to bones, soft tissue, organs.

American joint committee on cancer staging: AJCC or TNM staging

T0 No evidence of primary tumor

T1 Clinically inapparent non-palpable non-visible tumor

  T1a <3 microscopic foci of cancer /<5% of resected tissue

  T1b >3 microscopic foci of cancer /> 5% of resected tissue

  T1c tumor identified by needle biopsy

T2 Tumor clinically present + confined to prostate

  T2a tumor involves half of a lobe or less

  T2b tumor involves more than half of one lobe

  T2c tumor involving both lobes of any size but confined to prostate

T3 Extension through prostatic capsule

  T3a unilateral extracapsular extension

  T3b bilateral extracapsular extension

  T3c invasion of seminal vesicle

T4 Tumor fixed / invading adjacent structures other than seminal vesicles

  T4a invasion of bladder neck, external sphincter, rectum

  T4b invasion of levator ani muscle and/or fixed to pelvic wall

N Involvement of regional lymph nodes

  N1 metastasis in single lymph node < 2 cm

  N2 metastasis in single node > 2 and < 5 cm / multiple lymph nodes

  Affected

  N3 metastasis in lymph nodes > 5 cm

M   *Distant metastasis*
     M1a non-regional lymph nodes
     M1b bone
     M1c other sites

DIAGNOSTIC WORK UP

Diagnosis is usually established by prostate biopsy guided by:
A. *Digital rectal examination*
B. *Transrectal US*

   In most cases, however, the diagnosis is established by histopathological examination of prostatic tissue obtained after TURP. After the establishment of the diagnosis the standard staging work up includes-

A. *Digital rectal examination*
B. *Serum acid phosphatase*
C. *PSA levels*
D. *Cell ploidy*
E. *Bone scan*
F. Cross-sectional imaging: which includes US, CT, MRI, are used to determine the local extent of the tumor and identify the operative candidates.

PROSTATE IMAGING

Ultrasound

- With the advent of high frequency transducers (5-8 MHz) and trans rectal approach the zonal anatomy of the prostate can be identified.
- On sonography it is more useful to separate the prostate into a peripheral zone and inner gland which encompasses

the transition and central zone and the periurethral glandular area.

- A non-glandular region on the anterior surface of the prostate is termed the anterior fibromuscular stroma.
- The surgical capsule that separates the peripheral zone from the inner gland is identified as a hyperechoic band.
- The seminal vesicles are identified as paired, relatively hypoechoic, multiseptated structures surrounding the rectum cephalad to the base of the prostate gland.
- The anterior urethra and its surrounding smooth muscle and glandular area appear relatively hypoechoic.
- On coronal imaging, the junction of the hypoechoic periurethal area with the verumontanum creates an appearance resembling the Eiffel tower.
- The peripheral zone has a uniform echogenicity.
- The ejaculatory ducts are seen often coursing through the central zone from the seminal vesicles and joining the urethra at the verumontanum.
- The prostate with the periprostatic fat is usually sharply defined. Hyperechoic structures within are most characteristic of fat, corpora amylacea, or calculi.
- The sonographic appearance of most prostatic cancers is usually hypoechoic or mixed. Small cancers are usually hypoechoic.
- The hypoechoic lesions have less stromal fibrosis and grade lower on the Gleason grades.
- Hyperechogenecity in a cancer is the result of desmo-plastic reaction, few extensive large cancers may also have hyperechoic appearance.
- A significant number of prostatic cancers are isoechoic and thus difficult to detect and so the indirect signs like glandular asymmetry and capsular bulging may be indicative.

- When the tumor replaces the entire peripheral zone, it will often be less echogenic than the inner gland which is the reversal of normal echo pattern.
- When the entire gland affected by hyperplasia is replaced by tumor, the echogenicity becomes very inhomogenous.
- Sonographic staging allows for separation of those patients with macroscopic local extension into the periprostatic fat, seminal vesicle, or local lymph nodes from those with disease confined to the prostate gland.
- Large tumors can be easily seen to extend outside of the capsule as a result of loss of symmetry and capsular irregularity.
- Seminal vesicle extension is defined sonographically by enlargement, cystic dilatation, asymmetry, anterior-displacement, hyperechogenicity, and loss of seminal vesicle beak.
- Sonographic staging is more sensitive than CT for both local and periprostatic structures and lymph nodes.

CT SCAN

- Oral contrast opacification of small and large bowel is essential.
- Positive contrast in the form of either 2% oral barium suspension or diluted water soluble contrast media can be used.
- Negative contrast in the form of plain water can also be used.
- The oral contrast can be given night before to opacify large bowel or an on table contrast enema may also be used to opacify the rectum and large bowel.
- Contrast is also given 45 min. before examination to opacify small bowel. Both plain non I/V and post I/V contrast scans are taken in spiral mode.

- Prostate is visualized as a musculoglandular organ situated between the bladder base above and the pelvic diaphragm below.
- CT cannot reliably differentiate stage A from stage B tumors, CT stage criteria are thus stage B or less, tumor confined to prostate; stage C, extracapsular tumor extension to involve the periprostatic fat, seminal vesicles, bladder, rectum, obturator internus muscle; stage D1, pelvic nodes greater than 1.5 to 2.0 cm in diameter; stage D2, enlarged lymph nodes above aortic bifurcation, bone metastasis, or extrapelvic metastases.
- CT is also not an effective technique to differentiate stage B from stage C tumors. CT is most useful in evaluating advanced bulky disease (stage D1 to D2) with gross objective findings.
- The most common signs of advanced disease are extraprostatic soft tissue masses invading the posterior bladder base or seminal vesicles (stage C). Associated pelvic (stage D1) and para aortic (stage D2) lymph node metastases are usually easy to detect because they are large and multiple. Bone metastases should be evaluated on appropriate window and level settings.

MRI

- The prostate gland is best studied by using endorectal coils or by using pelvic multi coil arrangement.
- T2 weighted images display the zonal anatomy of the prostate to best advantage; aquisition in the axial and coronal or oblique coronal planes is usually most desirable.
- T1 weighted images are important for the assessment of the integrity of the periprostatic fat and neurovascular bundle, and for the identification of sites of hemorrhage.

- The normal prostate has a homogenous low to intermediate signal on T1 weighted images.
- Zonal anatomy can be demonstrated on T2 images comprising a low signal central zone and a higher signal peripheral zone.
- The transition and central zone appear of similar signal intensity and are thus termed as central gland.
- The periprostatic venous plexus can be visualized as a thin rim of higher signal intensity anterolateral to the peripheral zone.
- Denonvillier's fascia can be observed on sagittal images separating the prostate from the rectum.
- The neurovascular bundle is sited posterolaterally at 5 and 7'o clock position on transverse section of prostate.
- A normal appearing prostate gland on MRI does not exclude the presence of tumor and heterogeneity of the gland is a common nonspecific finding.
- MRI is often undertaken for staging after a positive biopsy, which can lead to artifacts from hemorrhage and edema.
- On T1 weighted images a carcinoma is usually isointense to the normal gland.
- On T2 weighted images (including fat suppressed) the majority of tumor appears low signal contrasted by the high signal from the peripheral zone, but this is not a specific finding.
- Macroscopic capsular penetration can be assessed on MRI as focal thickening or bulging of capsule.
- Periprostatic infiltration can be demonstrated on T1 images as a low signal within the periprostatic fat or as an intermediate signal using T2 fat suppressed scans.
- Extension to seminal vesicles is best demonstrated on T2 transverse and coronal scans and to rectum and bladder on transverse and sagittal scans.

- For the detection of adenopathy T1 images are required. MRI can detect bone metastases also.
- Post-contrast (Gd-chelate) enhanced imaging shows prostatic ca. as enhancing more than the surrounding tissue but becoming isointense on delayed scans.
- MR spectroscopy also known as chemical shift imaging is an emerging tool in the early detection of prostatic cancer. This relies on the changes in the emitted signal produced by a higher level of choline in carcinomas as compared to BPH.
- *Bone scintigraphy:* This is the most sensitive method of detecting occult bone metastases.
- *Screening:* It is postulated that all men above the age of 50 years should be screened yearly for the presence of carcinoma prostate by digital rectal examination and PSA levles.

Treatment

- Watchful waiting in patients with incidentally discovered carcinoma on TURP specimens and ages above 80 years.
- Radical prostatectomy for disease confined to capsule + life expectancy of more than 15 years.
- Radiation therapy for either to patients with disease confined to capsule and life expectancy of less than 15 years or to disease outside capsule but with no spread.
- Hormonal therapy (orchidectomy, diethylstilbesterol, leuprolide acetate) for widely metastatic disease.
- Cryosurgery
- Chemotherapy

CONCLUSION

Prostatic carcinoma is the second most common carcinoma affecting males. It is thus desirable to have an effective screening program to identify the disease in its early stages. Digital rectal examination and PSA levels in the serum are currently used as screening procedures. Imaging only plays a secondary role in the management in deciding the correct line of treatment and identifying the cases fit for surgery. MRI currently is the imaging modality of choice for staging of carcinoma prostate with USG especially TRUS being the second choice and CT only useful in advanced disease and for identifying bony metastasis.

7.22 THE PROSTATE

NORMAL ANATOMY

Prostate gland is a flattened conical structure oriented in the coronal plane.
- Length of normal prostate is 2.5-3 cm.
- Transverse diameter at base 4-4.5 cm.
- Thickness 2-2.5 cm.
- Normal weight 20-25 gm.

Prostatic Anatomy

Lobar Anatomy
- 5 lobular divisions
  - One anterior lobe
  - One median lobe
  - One prostatic lobe
  - Two lateral lobes
- The concept of median lobe is useful in evaluation of patients termed with BPH but this lobar anatomy is not useful for evaluating CA prostate.

Zonal anatomy
- 4 glandular zones
  - Peripheral zone
  - Transition zone.
  - Central zone.
  - Periurethral glandular area
- A non-glandular region on anterior surface of prostate is anterior fibromuscular stroma

SONOGRAPHIC ANATOMY

- USG can differentiate prostate into a peripheral zone and inner gland comprising transition zone. Central zone and periurethral glandular area.

Peripheral Zone

- Contains 70% of prostatic glandular tissue.
- Occupies posterior, lateral and apical regions of prostate and surrounds distal urethral segments.
- Ducts of peripheral zone drain in distal urethra.
- It is the source of most prostate cancers.
- It is separated from inner gland by the surgical capsule which is often hyperechoic due to carpora amylacea or calcifications.

Transition Zone

- Contains 5% of prostetic glandular tissue.
- Located adjacent to proximal urethral segment.
- Its ducts and in proximal urethra at the level of verumontanum.
- Site of origin of benign prostatic hyperplasia.

Central Zone

- Constitutes 25% of glandular tissue.
- Located at prostatic base.
- Its ducts drain in proximal urethra.
- Relatively resistant to disease process.

Periurethral Glands

- Form 1% of glandular tissue.
- Also known as internal prostatic sphincter.

Adjacent Structures

- Seminal vesicles
  - Seen in bow tie configuration on transaxial view.
  - Echogenicity is similar to or less than that of peripheral zone.
- Vas deferens
  - Located arteromedial to seminal vesicle.

Volumetric Measurement of Prostate

$V = \frac{1}{2} (l \times AP \times W)$ Where V = Volume
$$L \quad = \text{Length}$$
$$AP \quad = \text{Anteroposterior diameter}$$
$$W \quad = \text{Width}$$

CT Anatomy

- Prostate gland is located just posterior to symphysis pubis and anterior to rectum.
- Homogenous soft tissue density on NCCT.
- CECT—Peripheral zone may enhance to or lesser degree than central gland.
- Zonal anatomy is more evident in older patient and in patients with enlayed gland.

MR Anatomy

- On T1 weighted segments:-
  - Prostate has homogenous low signal intensity similar to skeletal muscle.
  - Neurovascular bundles are seen posterolateral to prostate gland at 5 o'clock and 7 o'clock position.
  - Zonal anatomy is not well demonstrated on T1W segments.

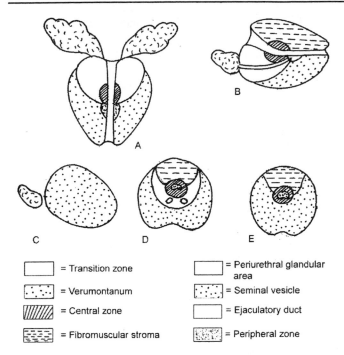

Fig. 7.22.1: Diagram of prostate zonal anatomy. **A.** Coronal section, midprostate. **B.** Sagittal midline section. **C.** Sagittal section, lateral prostate and seminal vesicle. **D.** Axial section, prostatic base. Paired ejaculatory ducts are seen posterior to urethra and periurethral glandular area. Peripheral zone encompasses most of posterior and lateral aspect of gland. **E.** Axial section, apex of gland showing mostly peripheral zone, and urethral and periurethral glandular area

- In post-gadolinium T1 weighted images, peripheral zone has a more uniform and cause intense enhancement than central gland.
· T2 weighted sequence
- Best for visualizing zonal anatomy.
- Peripheral zone has a higher signal than central gland

      due to its more abundant glandular component and more loosely intervening muscle bundles.
- Anterior fibromuscular band seen as low signal structure.
- True (anatomic) capsule of prostate and Denonvilliers' fascia are seen as low signal intensity bands.
- Surgical pseudocapsule can be seen in older patients at the interface between transition and peripheral zones.
- Periprostatic venous plexus seen as high signal structure around prostate.
- Seminal vesicles look like grapes with high signal intensity fluid and low signal intensity walls.

PROSTATIC LESIONS

Agenesis/Hypoplasia

Prostatic and seminal vesicle cysts

Congenital

- Prostatic utricle cyst.
- Müllerian duct cyst.
- Seminal vesicle cyst.

Acquired

- Ejaculatory duct cyst.
- Retention cyst.

Infection of Prostate

- Acute prostatitis.
- Chronic prostatitis.
- Prostatic abscess.
- Granulomatous prostatitis.

Prostatic Calculi

Tumors of prostate
- Benign
- BPH
- Malignancy
- Carcinoma.

A. PROSTATIC AGENESIS/HYPOPLASIA

- Associated with hypospadias, epispadias, extrophy.
- The only tissue visualized anterior to rectum is urethra with a thick periurethral muscle.

B. PROSTATE AND SEMINAL VESICLE CYSTS

- Well-defined smooth walled anechoic structure with posterior acoustic enhancement.
- Has septations/debris if secondarily infected.

PROSTATIC CYST

Prostatic Utricle Cyst

- Always present in midline
- Usually small
- Rarely contain spermatozoa
- May contain calculus
- Associated with other anomalies
  E.g. Prune belly syndrome
     Hypospadias
     Renal agenesis.

Müllerian Duct Cyst

- May extend lateral to midline

- Can be large
- Never contain spermatozoa
- Not associated with other anomalies.

Ejaculatory Cyst

- Usually small
- May contain spermatozoa
- Associated with infertility.

Retention Cyst

- Secondary to benign prostatic hypoplasia.

C. PROSTATIC INFECTIONS

Acute Prostatitis

- Narrowing, elongation or straightening of prostatic urethra on MCU.
- Enlarged hypoechoic gland with periprostatic inflammation and increased vascularity.

Chronic Prostatitis

- Reflux can be seen in prostatic ducts.
- Focal areas of varying echogenicity are present with ejaculatory duct calcification.

Prostatic Abscess

- Localized hypoechoic in peripheral gland.
- Peripheral rim enhancement present on CT.

Granulomatous Prostatitis

Nonspecific

- Prostatic urethra elongated in infraverumontanum portion (cf. BPH) is widened (cf. CA prostate).

Specific (Tubercular)

- Features of associated genitourinary tuberculosis in other viscera.
- Cavity formation in prostate with hypoechoic areas.

D. PROSTATIC CALCULI

- Bright echogenic foci in prostate with ± posterior acoustic shadowing.
- Corpora amylacea are thought to be precursor

Types

True or Endogenous	Urinary calculi	Exogenous calculi
↓	↓	↓
Develop from acini and ducts of prostate gland	Lodged in prostatic urethra	Form in preexisting abscess cavities

E. BENIGN PROSTATIC HYPERPLASIA

- Criteria—Prostate gland weighing more than 40 gm in older men.
  - Prostate is visualized in CT sections 2-3 cm or more above pubic symphysis.
- Involves transition zone and periurethral glandular tissue.

- Prostatic urethra elongated and slit like.
- Enlarged prostate bulges in bladder floor with J (fish hook) deformity of ureters on IVU.
- Secondary changes are:
  - Bladder trabeculation ± diverticulae and calculi.
  - Hydronephrosis and hydroureter.

F. CARCINOMA PROSTATE

- Involves peripheral zone in 70% cases.
- Presents as hypoechoic area in peripheral zone of prostate.
- Criteria for extracapsular extension
  - Contour deformity of capsule.
  - Irregularity.
  - Obliteration of rectocapsular extension–
  - Asymmetry or direct involvement of neurovascular bundle.
  - Focal capsular retraction or thickening.
  - Direct tumor extension in periprostatic fat.
- Criteria for seminal vesicular invasion.
  - Loss of angle between seminal vesicle and prostate.
  - Direct tumor extension to seminal vesicle.
- Higher chlorine and lower citrate levels are seen in cancerous prostate tissue on proton MR spectroscopy.
- Radionuclide bone seen is useful to detect skeletal metastases.

Table 7.22.1: TRUS, CT and MRI staging criteria following the Jewett and TNM classifications of prostatic cancer

Jewett	TNM	System	TRUS	CT	MRI
A	T_1a	<5% of gland	NA*	NA*	NA*
	T_1b	>5% of gland			
B	T_2a	<1/2 lobe	Hypoechoic mass <1/2 lobe		On T2WI low-signal-intensity focus in the peripheral zone (PZ) <1/2 lobe
	T_2b	≥1/2 lobe	Hypoechoic mass ≥ 1/2 lobe	Normal CT of the prostate gland	On T2WI low-signal-intensity focus in the PZ ≥ 1/2 lobe
	T_2c	Both lobes	Hypoechoic mass, both lobes		On T2WI low-signal intensity PZ bilaterally
C	T_3a	Unilateral extracapsular extension	Irregular margin, localized bulge or tumor stranding in the periprostatic Region—unilateral	Irregular margin or asymmetrical shape—unilateral	On T1 or T2WI localized bulge, irregular margin or step-off sign. Unilateral
	T_3b	Bilateral extracapsular extension	Bilateral	Bilateral	Bilateral
	T_3c	Seminal vesicle	Loss of seminal	Loss of tissue	On T2WI low-signal-intensity

Contd...

Contd...

Jewett	TNM	System	TRUS	CT	MRI
		Invasion	vesicle angle, asymmetrical enlargement hyperechoic gland	planes between the seminal vesicle and the prostate gland	of the seminal vesicles accompanied by enlargement of the SV and prostate gland
	T_4	Tumor Invades Neighboring Tissue, e.g. Bladder, Rectum, Levator ani Muscle	TRUS limited	Thickened and/or irregular posterior bladder wall; unilateral enlargement of levator ani and irregular thickening of anterior rectal wall	Bladder base: direct tumor extension; loss of low-intensity bladder wall on T2WI. Rectum: tumor extension demonstrated in two planes; disruption of rectal wall intensity. Levator ani: localized increase on T2WI
D1	N	Any size of Local tumor Plus Metastases Pelvic Lymph nodes	NA	Any or all of the above and pelvic nodes > 10 mm	Any or all of the above and nodes > 10 mm
D2	M	Bone Metastases	NA	Any or all of the above and bony metastases	Any or all of the above and bony metastases

7.23 D/D OF ADRENAL MASS

A Neoplastic

1. Cortical
   - Carcinoma
   - Adenoma

2. Medullary
   - Neuroblastoma
   - Ganglioneuroma
   - Pheochromocytoma

3. Stromal
   - Lipoma
   - Myblipomas

4. Metastasis.

B Others

1. Granulomas
   - Histoplasmobis
   - Tuberculosis
   - Blastomylosis

2. B/L Hyperplasia

3. Cysts

4. Hematoma

5. Amyloid

CT Features S/O Adernal Mass

1. Absence of normal adernal gland
2. Mass at superior level of kidneys
3. Downward displacement of kidneys.
4. Anterior displacement of IVC, pancreas and splenic vessels. Positive biochemical test indicating hyper-functioning adrenal mass.

Structures Mimicking Left Adrenal Mass

1. Upper pole of left kidney
2. Gastric Diverticulum—Give oral contrast
3. Splenic lobulation/Accessory splecn —on intravenous contrast it enhances to the same level as body of spleen.
4. Large mass in Tail of pancreas.

Give intravenous contrast. Pancreatic mass usually displaces splenic vein posteriorly whereas adrenal mass displaces it anteriorly.

SALIENT FEATURES

1. Adrenal Cortical Carcinoma

- Slow growing tumor
- 50% nonfunctioning, 50% Cushing's, Conn's or virilizing syndrome.
- Average size 8-10 cm at diagnosis.
- Average Age at onset 45 years.
- X-ray and IVP-   Show soft tissue shadow of mass, downward displacement of kidney calcifications±
- USG—Mixed echogenicity mass with calcifications +–
- CT—Large mass with heterogeneous enhancement
- Area of central necrosis
- Thin capsule rim, calcifications +-
- Liver and LN metastasis
- MRI—Mixed intensity on T1 and hyperintense on T2

2. Adrenal Cortical Adenoma

- Usually non-functioning and symptomless.
- U/L, 2-5 cm
- Variable density
- Half have soft tissue density and half have low attenuation due to higher lipid content.
  (d/d with cysts which do not enhance)

MEDULLARY TUMORS

1. Neuroblastoma

– Occur in children mostly < 3 years
– Present as abdominal mass or with secondaries
– X-ray and IVP—Soft tissue mass with downward displacement of kidney
– Downward drooping of pelvis and calyces.
– USG—Mixed density to echogenic tumor calcifications +
  Cystic areas of necrosis and hemorrhage
  Encasement of aorta and IVC
– CT—Irregularly shaped solid mass
– Soft tissue density with necrosis, calcifications and hemorrhage
– Local, distant invasion.
– Crossing of midline is higly suggestive.
– MIBG scan shows increase uptake by primary as well as metastatic tumor.

2. Ganglioneuroma

– More mature form of neurogenic tumor.
– Children, 60% < 20 years.
– Soft tissue mass with calcifications.
– May invade spinal canal.

3. Pheochromocytoma

– Commonest adrenal tumor in clinical practice
– 90% arise in adrenal medulla
– 10% ectopic
  – Hilum of kidney
  – Aortic bifurcation
  – Bladder wall
  – Mediastinum

- S/S—Paroxysmal attacks of hypertension headache, sweating, palpitation, anxiety 50% have sustained hypertension.
- Elevated urinary VMA or metanephrine level.
- Usually solitary and located on right
- 10% cases are familial

	Bilateral
"RULE OF TEN"	Multiple
	Extra-adrenal
	Children
	Malignant

- Size 2-20 cm   avg-7cm.
- X-ray and IVP—Soft tissue mass with renal displacement.
- CT—U/L homogenous mass >2cm and of soft tissue density.
- Solid with or without cystic areas or entirely cystic
- Inhomogenous with denser periphery with central necrosis.
- Enhance markedly to the point of becoming isodense with vascular structures.
- MIBG method of choice in ectopic or recurrent pheochromocytoma.
- Metastasis can occur in LN, bones liver and chest in malignant tumor.

3. Stromal Tumors

1. Lipomas and Myelolipomas
   - Rare nonfunctioning tumors.
   - 1 to 2% incidence.
   - Usually small
   - Highly echogenic on USG.
   - Varying proportion of myeloid and fat tissue
   - Well circumscribed mass with attenuation −30 to −140 HU with frequent foci of calcification.

4. Metastasis

- Fourth most frequently involved site of blood-borne metastasis.
- Lung > Breast > Thyroid > colon > Metastasis.
- B/L adrenal masses in a patient with known primary in absence of hyperfunction suggests metastasis.
- In a patient with known malignancy U/L adrenal mass could be Mets, carcinoma or adenoma so FNAC is must.
- Metastasis produce U/L or often B/L circumscribed soft tissue density mass.

Granulomas

- Infections like TB, histoplasmosis and blastomycosis result in solid or cystic mass with calcification.
- U/L or B/L

Adrenal Cysts

- Endothelial
- Pseudocyst
- Epithelial
- Parasitic (hydatid)
- Smooth marginated, well circumscribed usually U/L, low density mass, non-enhancing.
- Rim of calcification in 15%.

Adrenal Hemorrhage

- Abdominal mass or B/L masses
- Marginal calcification
- B/L adrenal hyperplasia
- Diffuse enlargement of adrenals.

Flow Chart 7.23.1: Adrenal mass

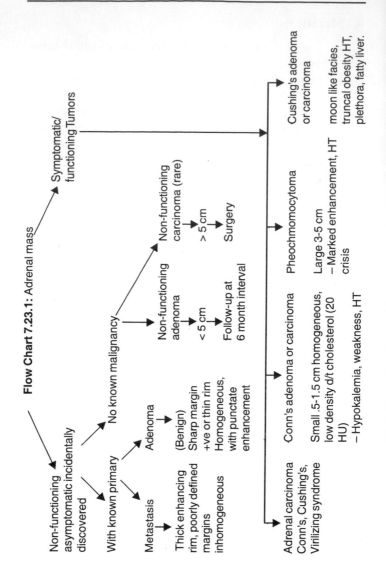

Adrenal mass

Non-functioning asymptomatic incidentally discovered

Symptomatic/functioning Tumors

Non-functioning asymptomatic incidentally discovered

With known primary → Adenoma → (Benign) Sharp margin +ve or thin rim Homogeneous, with punctate enhancement

With known primary → Metastasis → Thick enhancing rim, poorly defined margins inhomogeneous

No known malignancy → Non-functioning adenoma → <5 cm → Follow-up at 6 month interval

No known malignancy → Non-functioning carcinoma (rare) → >5 cm → Surgery

Symptomatic/functioning Tumors

Adrenal carcinoma Conn's, Cushing's, Virilizing syndrome

Conn's adenoma or carcinoma
– Small .5-1.5 cm homogeneous, low density d/t cholesterol (20 HU)
– Hypokalemia, weakness, HT

Pheochmomocytoma
– Large 3-5 cm
– Marked enhancement, HT crisis

Cushing's adenoma or carcinoma
moon like facies, truncal obesity HT, plethora, fatty liver.

7.24 PAINLESS HEMATURIA

DEFINITION

Blood cells in urine whether occult or frank constitutes hematuria.

Hematuria is mostly PAINLESS; PAIN is caused whenever there is obstruction to outflow of urine (mainly by blood clot or stone, etc).

• To define hematuria >3 R.B.C /HPF.

ETIOLOGY

A. Lesions in the Urinary Tract

1. *Causes in kidney and pelvicalyceal system*
   • Polycystic kidney disease.
   • Acute nephritis; Tuberculosis; Filariasis
   • Angioma; Papilloma;(Transitional cell carcinoma) TCC; (Renal cell carcinoma) RCC; Wilms' tumor.
   • Essential hematuria.
2. *Causes in Ureters*
   • Papilloma
   • TCC
   • Pyeloureteritis cystica
3. *Causes in bladder*
   • TCC
   • Papilloma
   • TB
   • Bilharzia
   • Filaria
4. *Causes in Prostate*
   • Varices caused by BPH
   • Malignancies.

5. *Causes in Urethra*
   - TCC
   - Angioma

B. Lesions in Adjacent Organs

- CA cervix invading the bladder.
- CA rectum
- PID
- Retroperitoneal masses pressing over renal vessels.
- Several vesicle tumors.

C. Systemic Causes with Secondary Renovascular Effects

Hematopoitic causes:	Hemophilia; scurvy; Malaria; Purpura; Sickle cell disease.
Congestive:	Renal vein thrombosis; Right—Heart failure.
Infarcts:	Subacute infective Endocarditis. Myocardial infarction.

- Collagen vascular diseases.

D. Drugs

- Sulfonamides
- Salicylates (in large doses)
- Anticoagulants
- Phenolphthalein
- Urates
- DFM
- Chloroquine
- Pyridium

E. Hematuria Like Conditions

- Porphyrinuria
- Myoglobinuria

CLINICAL FEATURES

1. Urine normal in appearance
   Known as Microscopic Hematuria, i.e. > 5 RBC/HPF in 2-3 urinanalysis.
2. Urine of altered color
3. Fever
4. Lump and other signs and symptoms
5. Outflow obstruction.

PATHOLOGY

Hematuria

Medical
(Renal/Glomerular)

- Associated with cast
- Associated with Proteinuria
- Dysmorphic RBC (Esp if glomerulus)
  Ig A nephropathy—Child
  MPGN—Adult
- Eumorphic Rounded RBC
- RBC if tid
- Upto 10 6/24 hrs—Normal
- But >2/Hpf-Abnormal

- Dysmorphic
  - Acanthocytes

Urological
(Surgical epithelial)

- Associated with no cast
- No proteinuria.

- Rounded eumorphic
- RBC
- > 1/Hpf
- Abnormal
- Eumorphic.
- Round
- Regular
- Smooth.
- Even Hb distribution

- Schistocytes
- Amylocytes
- Echinocytes
- Somatocytes
- Codocytes
- Knizocytes
- It is basically the urological hematuria which is more accessible to radiological diagnosis as the nephrological causes are usually evaluated by laboratory methods.

Radiological Evaluation

Always ask a small question
- *Is the urine bright red*—Lower urinary tract origin—Gross
- *Is the urine smoky*—Upper urinary tract origin—Occult

Keep in mind the major causes
1. Malignancies
2. Infections
3. Stone
4. BPH
5. Renal parenchymal lesions
6. Trauma
7. Benign idiopathic

Always try to reach to two or three possibilitis before starting investigation.

X-ray abdomen—28
- CXR = 1.4 MSV = 28 weeks radiation

X-ray Pelvis—24
- CXR = 1.2 MSV = 24 weeks

I.V.U—88
- CXR = 4.4 MSV = 88 weeks

C.T abdomen—176
- CXR = 8.8 MSV = 176 weeks

A. Plain X-ray Abdomen

- Calcified Nodes—TB.
- Cyst Wall Calcification—Polycystic kidney disease
  -Evidence of mass lesion.

Chest:

- For cardiac evaluation as Rt. heart failure is a cause.
- For looking any tubercular focii

Bones:

- To evaluate and correlate for hemophilia; sickle cell anemia; scurvy; cardiovascular disease; renal osteodystrophy.

B. Intravenous Pyelography

- Is always the imaging modality of choice in any patient presenting with hematuria whether painful or painless.
- Gives a gross global idea about the structure and function of urinary tract
- Gives a baseline investigation for further comparison.
- Polycystic kidney disease-Swiss cheese nephrogam
- Spider web pyelogram
- Renal cell carcinoma—Distorted/Destroyed/Displaced/ Delayed — Pyelogram — Nephrogram
- Transitional cell carcinoma—role of IVP is to r/o multicentricity, to comment on function, to evaluate back pressure.
- Renal vein thrombosis—increasingly dense nephrogram with delayed pyelogram.
- Tuberculosis—thimble bladder; corkscrew/pipestem ureter; renal cavities/perirenal collection/pyelonephritis.

C. Barium Examinations

- E.g. T.B
- E.g. Ca Rectum

D. USG +- C.D

- For general survey of KUB even before IVP
- In renovascular diseases.

E. CT Scan

- For retroperitoneal evaluation.
- For landmarking masses.
- For renovascular evaluation.

G. MRI

- Better imaging modality due to multiplanner capabilities.

H. Renal Scan

- Has only minimal corroborative role.

I. Arteriovenography

- Esp when intervention is contemplated.

J. Newer Modalities

   A. MR Urography
   B. CT
   C. Endovesicle USG
   D. Sonourethrography
   E. PET

K. RGU/MCU

Definitive modality for evaluation of UB and urethral lesions

CT Urography

- Perlman. 1966
1. Protocol—Projectional technique
    A. • Conventional
       • Digital
       • CT scanned projectional images.
3. Protocol—Reconstructional technique.
    B. • 2-D
       • 3-D
- Phases almost similar to liver.
- For urothelial lesions conventional > CT URO.

MR Urography

1. An MRCP like Technique- I.C. T2w Single/Multislice
2. Gad+T1 W.
3. Fusion.
   - At present reserved for patients who cannot undergo CT URO/IVP—pregnant, pediatric, allergy, poor renal function
   - Calculus detection is a limitation.
     - FNAC
     - BX

CONCLUSION

Flow Chart 7.24.1

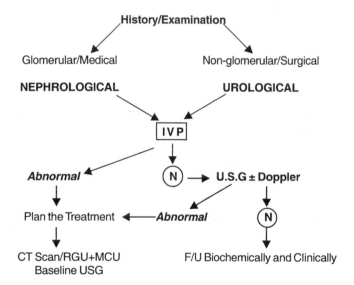

In Conclusion

↓

Patient with Painless Hematuria

↓

Biochemical Evaluation

and

History/Examination

Glomerular/Medical   Non-glomerular/Surgical

NEPHROLOGICAL   **UROLOGICAL**

IVP

Abnormal   (N) → **U.S.G ± Doppler**

↓   *Abnormal*   (N)

Plan the Treatment ◄ ─── *Abnormal*

↓   ↓

CT Scan/RGU+MCU   F/U Biochemically and Clinically
Baseline USG

Head, Neck and Spine

8.1 LUCENCY IN THE SKULL VAULT—WITHOUT SCLEROSIS

1. Neoplastic	Traumatic	Metabolic	Infective
Multiple myeloma	-Burr hole	Hyperpara-thyroidism	TB
Mets	-Lepomeningeal		Hydatid
Hemangioma	Cyst		syphilis
Neurofibroma			Pyogenic osteo-myelitis
Paget's sarcoma			

Idiopathic—Osteoporosis Circumscripta

Multiple Myeloma

> 40 years, Males : Females 2 : 1, increase of total serum protein because of production of abnormal Ig. Leukopenia, anemia, abnormal urine protein - Bence Jones protein - 50% of hypercalcemia, Hypercalciuria, Amyloidosis.

RF

Generalized decrease in bone density, localized area of lucency in Red marrow, lesion also seen in mandible, clavicle and scapula.

Adjacent soft tissue mass.

Spine—collapse with paravertebral soft tissue mass (I/V disc are not affected)

Pedicle and post arches are less frequently affected, proximal end of humerus and femur are also affected.

Hemangioma

- Well circumscribed area of punctate or stellate rare faction without expansion.
- Prominent vascular grooves may present in the vicinity and External carotid arteriography shows a blush.

Neurofibroma

Lucent defect in occipital bone (Adjacent to it—Lambdoid suture).

Paget's disease male more than females, elderly.

Most common site -   Sacrum and lumbar spine

Skull → pelvis → femur

Osteoporosis circumscripta = occurs in the active lytic phase of Paget's disease.

It starts in the lower part of the frontal and occipital region and can cross suture line.

Destructive process affecting the outer table and sparing the inner table.

Hyperparathyroidism

Usually pepper pot skull. Rarely severe enough to cause overt-lytic lesions.

Mandible is a common site for "Brown tumors", there may be a loss of lamina dura.

"Basilar invagination" is a common findings.

Traumatic

"Burr hole" - H/O surgery.

Laptomeningeal cyst: Develop after head injury. If dura is torn the arachnoid membrane can prolapse and the pulsation of CSF can cause progressive widening and scalloping of the fracture line.

Langerhans Cell Histiocytosis

Proliferation of histiocytic cells particularly in the bone marrow, the spleen, liver and lymphatic gland and lungs. Later cells become swollen with lipid deposit.

Eosinophilic Granuloma

Most mild expression of histiocytosis.

age = 3 to 12 years. Especially boys.

Site any bone (1/4th in skull)

2/3rd = pelvis, skull and femur.

RF = translucent - areas of bone destruction with sharply difined margins—in active phase. Peripheral sclerosis seen in healing phase.

The lesion is having bevelled edges difficult to differentiate destruction of the inner and outer tables.

- Button sequestrum may be seen.
- Other RF - spine - solitary lesion in spine, may collapse - leading to vertebra plana.

Most common site is thoracic spine.

Para vertebral soft tissue mass present.
Disc space - maintained.

Long bones - predilection for diaphysis.
Mandible and lamina dura - osteolytic lesion leading to 'floating teeth' appearance.

Metastasis - in adult

Most common site for metastasis - spine, pelvis and ribs with proximal ends of humerus and femur and less often skull areas corresponds to sites of persistent hematopoiesis.

Primary tumors in male - carcinoma prostate, lung and kidney.

In female = breast –2/3rd of cases of bronchial carcinoma develop secondaries - lab finding—

Serum Alkaline phosphatase increase in metastasis but normal in multiplemyeloma. Serum ca++ increase.

Ca prostate PSA and Acid phosphatase increase.

RF = Mainly osteolytic, develop in medulla and extended in all directions, destroying the cortex- not much periosteal reaction.

Soft tissue extension uncommon, multiplicity in pediatric age - Esp. neuroblastoma and leukemia.

+/– wide suture

Infective: TB - osteomyelitis - skull is a rare site.

Pyogenic OM - usually direct infection from a frontal sinus or secondary to a compound fracture.

Syphilis = moth eaten appearance.

Flow Chart 8.1.1

Differential Diagnosis

Lytic lesions in skull vault with no surrounding sclerosis

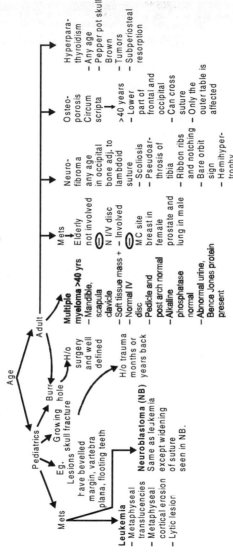

Age

Pediatrics

Adult

Mets

Leukemia
– Metaphyseal translucencies
– Metaphyseal cortical erosion
– Lytic lesion

Neuroblastoma (NB)
Same as leukemia except widening of suture seen in NB.

Growing hole
Eg. Lesions skull fracture have bevelled margin, vertebra plana, flooting teeth

Burr hole
H/o surgery and well defined

H/o trauma months or years back

Mets
Elderly not involved
N I/V disc – Involved
MC site breast in female prostate and lung in male

Multiple myeloma >40 yrs
– Mandible, scapula clavicle
– Soft tissue mass +
– Normal IV disc
– Pedicle and post arch normal
– Alkaline phosphatase normal
– Abnormal urine, Bence Jones protein present

Neuro-fibroma
any age in occipital bone adj, to lambdoid suture
– Scoliosis
– Pseudoar-throsis of tibia
– Ribbon ribs and notching
– Bare orbit sign
– Hemihyper-trophy

Osteo-porosis Circum scripta
>40 years
– Lower part of frontal and occipital
– Can cross suture
– Only the outer table is affected

Hyperpara-thyroidism
– Any age
– Pepper pot skull
– Brown Tumors
– Subperiosteal resorption

8.2 LUCENCY IN THE SKULL VAULT—WITH SURROUNDING SCLEROSIS

Fibrous Dysplasia (FD) - Unknown pathogenesis.

Replacement - of medullary bone by fibrous tissue.

Age = 3 to 15 years.

Most common site - femur, pelvis, skull, mandible, ribs.

Two types = monostotic, polyostotic - lesion tend to be unilateral.

RF = Cyst like lesion in the diaphysis or metaphysis with endosteal scalloping +/- bone expansion.

No periosteal new bone.

Rind sign - thick sclerotic border, ground glass appearance.

Common site in skull = In skull FD takes 2 main forms—sclerotic and cystic.

Sclerotic form - more common, involves the base or facial skeleton which are expanded and dense and sometime showing ground glass appearance. Most common cause of leontiasis ossea.

Cystic form - produces a small lesion in skull vault expanding the outer table and giving a blistered appearance.

DEVELOPMENTAL

Epidermoid: thin sclerotic margins with scalloping.

Most common site - squamous portion of occipital or temporal although can involve any region.

Intramedullary in origin, so can expand and both inner and outer bones. More homogenous radiolucent centre.

Meningocele: Midline defect

Smooth and sclerotic margins with an overlying soft tissue mass.

Most common site = occipital bone, may occur in the frontal, parietal or basal bones.

Neoplastic Hemangioma - Rarely has sclerotic margin. Radiating spicules of bone within it.

Langerhans cell histiocytosis - only a sclerotic margin of it is in the healing phase.

Infective - Chronic osteomyelitis: Brodie's abscess-intra-osseous abscess surrounded by intense sclerosis.

Mucocele of Frontal Sinus

If the ostium of sinus becomes blocked and infection does not supervene, the sinus fills with mucus - Mucus acts as slow growing mass lesion, expanding the sinus and thinning the sinus wall - can give rise to proptosis.

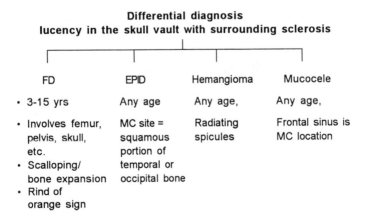

Differential diagnosis
lucency in the skull vault with surrounding sclerosis

FD	EPID	Hemangioma	Mucocele
• 3-15 yrs	Any age	Any age,	Any age,
• Involves femur, pelvis, skull, etc.	MC site = squamous portion of temporal or occipital bone	Radiating spicules	Frontal sinus is MC location
• Scalloping/ bone expansion			
• Rind of orange sign			

8.3 THICKENING OF THE SKULL VAULT

Generalized

1. Marble bone disease
2. Dystrophia myotonica
3. Acromegaly
4. Paget's disease
5. Cooley's anemia

Localized

1. Meningiomas
2. Primary osteosarcoma
3. Osteomas
4. Ossifying fibromas
5. Fibrous dysplasia
6. Leontiasis ossia
7. Hyperostosis frontalis interna

Generalized Hyperostosis

1. *Marble bone disease*
   - The bones of the skull base are mainly affected with sclerosis and thickening, mainly in the anterior cranial fossa.
   - The cranium is affected to a lesser degree
   - The sphenoid and frontal sinuses and mastoids are underpneumatized or not at all.
   - Neural foramina may encroached upon and blindness results in serious cases.
2. *Dystrophia myotonica*
   - They show a thickened skull vault with a small pituitary fossa.
3. *Acromegaly*
   - Thickened skull vault in association with the enlarged sinuses and prognathous jaw

- The vault thickening involves both table and the diploe is encroached on and difficult to distinguish.

4. *Paget's disease*
   - Vault becomes widened and thickened, with alterations in its bony texture, there are also osteomalacic changes and the bones becomes softer and more pliable, giving rise to platybasia with basilar invagination.
   - Skull shows a typical irregular mottled texture to the thickened bone.

5. *Cooley's anemia*
   - Generalized thickening of the skull with a characteristic and diagnostic appearance.
   - Widening of the diploe.
   - It's texture becomes abnormal with radiating linear spicules of the sunray or hairbrush type. Sometimes the bone change in this type of anemia may be more localized, affecting mainly the frontal region.

Localized Hyperostosis of the Skull

1. *Meningiomas*
   These commonly invade the bony skull and produce a localized hyperostotic reaction. The diagnosis is often suggested by the classic meningioma site, i.e. parasagittal or sphenoidal ridge.

   - Originally the hyperostosis is confined to the inner table but later it may grow through the diploe and outer table and present as a palpable lump.
   - When protruding externally the lesion can sometimes show sunray spicules.
   - Other radiological evidence of meningioma such as enlarged vascular markings leading to the lesion or signs of raised intracranial pressure may also be present.

– If the meningioma grows from the sphenoidal ridge into the orbit it can present with proptosis.

2. *Primary osteosarcoma*

It is very rare but can give rise to localized hyperostosis often with sun ray spicules. It is commonest as a complication of Paget's disease.

3. *Osteomas*

These can occur in the skull vault when they appear as dense flat ivory nodules growing from the surface.

– More commonly they present as chance findings growing from the wall of the frontal sinus.

– They are usually small-under 1cm in size.

4. *Ossifying fibroma*

These are relatively rare.

– They most frequently commence in the paranasal sinuses, particularly the antrum.

– They can produce large density calcified masses.

5. *Fibrous dysplasia*

– It is an important cause of localized hyperostosis involving the skull vault, facial bones or skull base.

– It may occur as an isolated lesion or in association with lesions in other bones (polyostotic fibrous dysplasia and Albright syndrome).

6. *Leontiasis ossia*

It is a form of hyperostosis affecting the frontal bones and facial bones and giving rise to severe facial deformity.

7. *Hyperostosis frontalis interna*

– Mysterious condition frequently seen in adult skulls

– Occurs almost exclusively in postmenopausal women.

– It is characterized by irregular nodular thickening of the inner table of the skull vault, mainly the frontal bone. The lesion are characteristically bilateral and symmetric and spare the midline.

Flow Chart 8.3.1

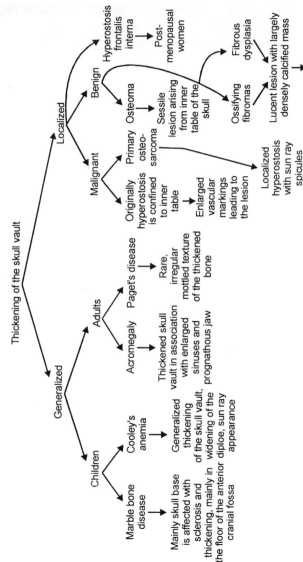

Thickening of the skull vault

- Generalized
  - Children
    - Marble bone disease
      - Mainly skull base is affected with sclerosis and thickening, mainly in the floor of the anterior cranial fossa
    - Cooley's anemia
      - Generalized thickening of the skull vault, widening of the diploe, sun ray appearance
  - Adults
    - Acromegaly
      - Thickened skull vault in association with enlarged sinuses and prognathous jaw
    - Paget's disease
      - Rare, irregular mottled texture of the thickened bone
- Localized
  - Benign
    - Hyperostosis frontalis interna
      - Post-menopausal women
    - Osteoma
      - Sessile lesion arising from inner table of the skull
  - Malignant
    - Primary osteosarcoma
      - Localized hyperostosis with sun ray spicules
    - Originally hyperostosis is confined to inner table
      - Enlarged vascular markings leading to the lesion
  - Ossifying fibromas
  - Fibrous dysplasia
    - Lucent lesion with largely densely calcified mass
      - Usually differentiated histologically

8.4 GENERALIZED INCREASE IN DENSITY OF SKULL VAULT

Idiopathic	– Paget's disease Fibrous dysplasia, myelosclerosis
Congenital	– Osteopetrosis pyknodysostosis Pyle's disease.
Metabolic	– Renal Osteodystrophy Fluorosis
Neoplasm	– Sclerotic mets Meningioma
Endocrinal	– Acromegaly
Hematological	– Chronic hemolytic anemia, phenytoin therapy

- *Idiopathic – Myelosclerosis-* Peak age = 6th decade, cause is unknown.

  Sex = Both sexes are equally affected.

  Pathologically = obliteration of marrow by fibrosis or bony sclerosis-leading to normochromic and normocytic anemia.

  – Hemopoiesis in spleen and liver so they enlarged.

  RF = Bone sclerosis in 40% of cases.

  Most common pattern - diffuse but may be patchy.

  Marrow diameter decreased and blurred CMD.

  Lucent areas due to fibrous tissue.

  1/3rd cases show periosteal new bone.

Fibrous dysplasia - Two form - sclerotic and cystic form, sclerotic form-commoner of the two, especially in the polyostotic version.

Site - base and facial skeleton which are expanded and dense. Most common cause of leontiasis ossea.

Lower density areas (cyst or fibrotic masses) with in the sclerotic bones-strong with evidence of fibrous dysplasia.

Paget's Disease

Male more than female, > 40 yrs.
Skull is involved in 2/3rd of cases.

Mixed pattern of sclerosis and lysis is common. An early change is a spotty cotton wool. Increase density of bone and also thickening of vault.

Middle and outer Tables are most affected and thickened with coarse trabeculation.

Meningioma

Sclerosis is more marked than expansion and extension from the sphenoid bone into the facial skeleton is much less common.

Metastasis

Irregular lysis or sclerosis and multiplicity prostate and breast are most common. Diffuse osteosclerosis is also seen in occasionally in Hodgkin's lymphoma and leukemia and very rarely with multiple myeloma.

Congenital

Osteopetrosis - several types. More severe types are autosomal recessive.

RF = Generalized increase density.

Skull base are initially affected with sclerosis and thickening.

Cranium is affected to a lesser degree /sphenoid, frontal and mastoid are underpneumatized or not at all.

Neural foramina encroached upon and blindness result in serious cases.

Pyknodysostosis

Autosomal recessive in inheritance. Patients are usually short, (<150 cm).

Skull - brachycephaly with wide suture and persistence of open fontanells into adult life.

Wormian Bones

Site - Calvarium, base of skull and orbital rims are very dense. Facial bones are small and maxilla is hypoplastic.

Mandible has no angle, it is obtuse.

Other Feature

Limbs	– Increase density of bones. Thorax lat. ends of clavicle are hypoplastic. Ribs are dense.
Spine	– Failure of fusion of neural arches, spondylolisthesis.
	– Spool shaped V bodies
Hand	– Acroosteolysis with irregular distal fragments of distal phalanges.

METABOLIC

Renal Osteodystrophy

Bony changes in patients suffering from chronic anemia due to long standing renal disease.

Osteosclerosis occurs in 25%.

Skull and spine are commonly involved and can look similar to Paget's disease.

Other Features

Secondary hyperparathyroidism-subperiosteal resorption, subchondral resorption, brown tumors.

- Osteomalacia/rickets.
- Osteoporosis.
- Al. toxicity.
- Soft tissue calcification (vascular and periarticular).
- Fractures.

FLUOROSIS

Chronic ingestion of excessive amount of fluoride results in fluorosis.

Osteosclerosis is seen with conc. of 8 PPM in drinking water, calvarium is rare site.

Other Feature

Osteosclerosis predominantly in axial skeleton.

- Calcification or ossification of ligaments.
- Enthesiopathy.

Acromegaly

Enlarged frontal sinus, prognathism, enlarged sella, thick vault.

Flow Chart 8.4.1

D/D - Generalized increase density in skull vault

	Paget's	Fibrous dysplasia	Renal osteodystrophy	Fluorosis	Mets	Osteopetrosis	Myelosclerosis	Pyknodysostosis
Age	> 40 years	3 - 16 years	–	–	Old age	Young	6th decade	Young
Sex	Male and female	–	–	–	–	–	Male-female	–
Other feature	Mixed pattern of sclerosis and lysis is common	Sclerotic form in 2/3rd	Sclerotic in 25%	–	Ca breast and prostate sclerotic E/o primary tumors	–	–	–
Clavicle wormian bone mandible - maxilla	–	–	–	–	–	N	–	Lat-end hypoplastic ++
EG	–	–	Less feature of secondary hyperparathyroidism Al. toxicity rickets ST Ca++	H/o ingestion of water of increased Fl. content +Ca++ of ligament	–	Hypopneumatization of sphenoid and frontal sinus and mastoid Liver and spleen enlarged	Liver and spleen enlarged. +1/3rd show periosteal new bone formation	Obtuse angle of mandible and hypoplastic maxilla

8.5 LOCALIZED INCREASE IN DENSITY OF THE SKULL VAULT

IN BONE

1. Neoplasm
   a. Sclerotic mets
      - Most common prostate and stomach.
   b. Ivory osteoma
      - Commonly affect the PNS. Slow growing dense lesion- well-defined spherical or hemispherical shape.

   Mostly < 1cm in diameter, rarely exceed 2-3 cm.

   Complication—Large osteoma may interfere with drainage of the sinus, CSF rhinorrhea, pneumocephalus or even meningitis.

   c. Treated lytic mets - Esp. breast - primary.
   d. Treated brain tumors.
2. Paget's disease
3. Fibrous dysplasia
4. Depressed fracture due to overlapping bone fragments.
5. Hyperostosis frontalis interna - seen in postmenopausal female, involves the Frontal bone.

   B/L and symmetrical.

   Thickening of inner table-"choppy sea appearance."

   Adjacent to bone.
1. *Meningioma* -Mainly involves the inner table but if breaks through the outer table it may cause a "hair-on-end" appearance.

   15% -show calcification.

   Abnormal increase in vascular channel and signs of raised intracranial pressure.

Ch. site - parasagittal/olfactory grove, sphenoid ridge and tentorium.
2. Calcified sebaceous cyst.
3. *Old cephalhematoma* - Usually seen in the parietal region and may be bilateral in neonate.
   Caused by subperiosteal bleeding during birth, does not cross suture.
4. *Tumors*
   – Gliomas are the most common tumors
   – 5% show calcification
   Oligodendroglioma
   – 50% cases calcification
   Craniopharyngioma - mainly in children, calcification in 75% cases.
   Position of calcification - midline and just above the sella.

Ch.subdural Hematoma

Calcification in the membrane.
Characteristics position adjacent to skull vault.

Basal Ganglia Calcification

B/L and symmetrical, seen in the region of basal ganglia, primary or idiopathic - related to age, secondary - hypoparathyroidism, pseudohypoparathyroidism, Fahr's syndrome.

Button Sequestra

EG (Eosinophilic granuloma), tends to Erode both tables of skull. The outer table is more extensively destroyed at time producing a characteristic. Double contour, with radiodense focus within the lytic area termed a button sequestra.

Flow Chart 8.5.1

Localized increase in density in skull

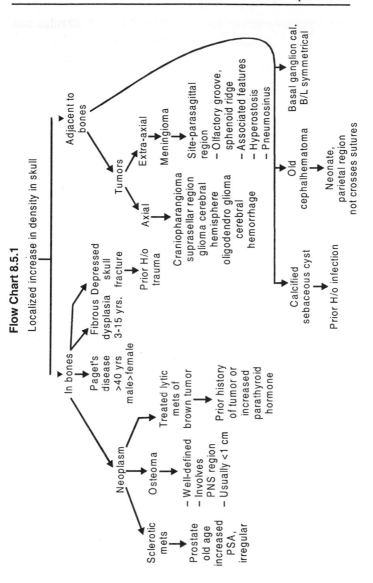

8.6 DESTRUCTION OF PETROUS BONE (APEX)

Acoustic Neuroma

Arising from 8th nerve, increase in size of Internal Auditory Meatus (>1 cm in diameter or > 2 cm asymmetric between the two sides (1mm in height and 2 mm in length).

- Erosion of crista transversalis and apparent shortening of the Internal Auditory Meatus may occur.
  B/h in NF 2.
- CT = Iso to brain, CECT = more enhancement.
  MR = FSE T2 -Intermediate SI.
- Congenital cholesteatoma - In the petrous apex they form a well demarcated expanded cystic lesion which may enlarge to erode the IOC and bony labyrinth.
  No IV contrast enhancement.
  MRI = T1 = low signal T2 = high signal
  Chelesteatoma tend to encase arteries without causing obstruction.
- *Cholesterol granuloma* is a cystic granulomatous lesion containing hemosiderin and cholesterol deposits.
  CT appearance = similar to congenital cholesteatomas.
  MRI= high signal on both T1 and T2 due to presence of meth Hb and other Hb break down products and increase of protein content.
- *Meningioma* - Tend to excite a bony proliferative response and produce narrowing of pons acousticus internus rather than erosion.
  CT = local hyperostosis and erosion of petrous bone.
- Density similar to brain tissue, often surrounding zone of low density.
  CECT and MR = Contrast uptake in most cases. MR may show a "dural tail" adjacent of dural infiltrate.

Typically a meningioma does not enter the IOC.

- *Metastasis* - particularly breast, kidney and lung. Irregular cystic defect.

  Pain and nerve paresis are common.

- Vth nerve neuroma - are rare.

  If arising from the intracanalicular or intracranial segments cannot be distinguished radiologically from the acoustic neuroma.

  CT = Expansion of facial nerve canal.

  CECT = Enhancement.

  MR = Sensitive.

- *Nasopharyngeal angiofibroma*

  Usually large area of destruction in the floor of the middle cranial fossa.

Flow Chart 8.6.1

	Acoustic neuroma	Congenital cholesteatoma	Ch granuloma	Meningioma	Vth Nerve neuroma	JNA
Age	Middle age	Any age	–	40-60 yrs	–	Young boy
Sex	–	–	–	F > M	–	Male
Plain film	Perorbital view widening of IOM with petrous apex erosions	Enlarge and erode the IO canal and bony labyrinth	Same as congenital cholesteatoma	Hyperostosis, narrowing of pons, acousticus internus rather than erosion	Expansion of IOM and facial canal	Lateral radiograph -sessile mass is naso-pharynx more anteriorly than adenoid
NCCT	Diff of 1 mm Height and 2 mm is length of the two auditory hiatia	Expanding cystic lesion may enlarge and erode the IOC and bony labyrinth	Cystic granulomatous	Hyperdense mass, narrowing of pons acoustic internus, less commonly erosion of petrous apex	Chronic erosion of facial canal	Soft tissue mass in nasopharynx • Forward displacement of post wall of maxillary antrum • Widening of pterygoid fossa • Late cases show intra-cranial extension
CECT	Iso to brain – Enhancement seen with a large dose of contrasts	Bone erosion irregular, fossa, no enhancement	–	Honogenous contrast	++	++
MR T1	Decrease signal intensity	Decrease signal	Increased signal	Iso-iso-hypo	Hypo to iso	Low to intermediate, flow void due to vascular channel
T2	Intermediate SI	Increase on T2, tend to encase arteries	Increased	May show dural tail D/to adjacent dural infiltration	Intermediate to hyper	Low to intermediate
CEMR	Intense uptake	–	–	–	–	–

8.7 BASILAR INVAGINATION

Elevation of the floor of the post-cranial fossa.

A. **Primary**

- Less with narrow foramen magnum + occipitalization of atlas.

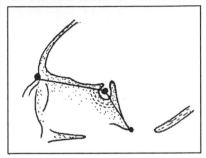

Fig. 8.7.1: Basal angle to measure platyplasia

B. **Secondary form**

Osteogenesis imperfecta, Paget's disease, osteomalacia.

Craniometric line used to diagnose basilar invagination or platybasia.

1. *Wachenheim's line (clivus canal line)*
   Line drawn along lines into cervical canal
   Normal odontoid tip is ventral and tangential to this line.
   Odontoid tip transects the line in basilar invagination.

2. *Chamberlain's line* - joins post-pole of hard palate to opisthion.
   Tip of dens lies 3-6 MM below this line. Odontoid process bisect the line in basilar invagination.

3. *MC Rae (FM line)* - joint anterior and posterior edges of foramen magnum (basion to opisthion).
   Tip of dens does not exceed this line.

4. *Fishgold's bimastoid line* - Line connecting tip of mastoid process.
   Odontoid tip may be 10 mm above the line.

Osteogenesis Imperfecta

Due to disorder of collagen.

4 Types

Type 1 = Gracile, osteoporotic bones.
          Rapid fracture healing +/- exuberant callus.
Type 2 = Lethal perinatal.
          Extremely severe osseous fragility.
Type 3 = Moderate to severe osseous fragility, severe deformity of long bones and spine results in severe dwarfing.
          – Cystic expansion of ends of long bones.
          – Wormian bones.
Type 4 = Osseous fragility with normal sclerae with severe deformity of long bones and spine.

- *Paget's disease* - Caused by excessive abnormal remodelling of bones.
  Site - spine -75%, prox. femur-75%
  Skull - 65%
  Pelvis - 40%
Three stages of the disease
1. Active (osteolytic)-skull-osteoporosis circumscripta.
2. Osteolytic and osteosclerotic areas.
3. Inactive (osteosclerotic)
- *Osteomalacia* - Increased uncalcified osteoid in the mature skeleton.
  Decrease bone density.
  Looser's zone - Common sites are the scapula, femoral neck and shafts, pubic rami and ribs.
  Bilateral symmetrical transverse lucent bands of uncalcified osteoid which, later in disease have sclerotic margin.
  – Coarsening of trabecular pattern.
  – Bone softening, protrusion acetabuli, bowing of long bones, biconcave vertebral bodies and basilar invagination.

Flow Chart 8.7.1

Differential diagnosis

Basilar Invagination

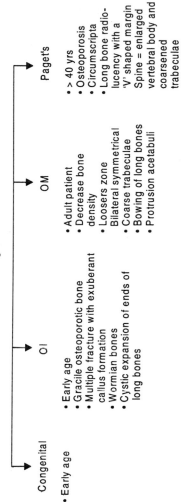

Congenital
- Early age

OI
- Early age
- Gracile osteoporotic bone
- Multiple fracture with exuberant callus formation
- Wormian bones
- Cystic expansion of ends of long bones

OM
- Adult patient
- Decrease bone density
- Loosers zone Bilateral symmetrical
- Coarse trabeculae
- Bowing of long bones
- Protrusion acetabuli

Paget's
- > 40 yrs
- Osteoporosis
- Circumscripta
- Long bone radio-lucency with a 'V' shaped margin
- Spine = enlarged vertebral body and coarsened trabeculae

Platybasia

Flattening of base of skull does not always accompany basilar invagination but occur in similar situation.

The index is basal angle or sphenoid angle. Angle b/n roof of sphenoid and clivus > 180.

Causes

1. Osteomalacia
2. Rickets
3. Hypoparathyroidism
4. FD
5. Paget's disease
6. Arnold-Chiari malformation

8.8 HAIR ON END SKULL VAULT

A. Hemolytic Anemia

Sickle cell anemia: Develops due to abnormal hemoglobin.

RF = Deossification due to marrow hyperplasia.

– Decrease in density of bones with thickening of trabeculae.

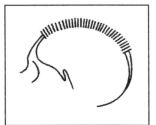

Fig. 8.8.1: Hair-on-end appearance on skull vault

– "Hair-on-end" skull vault seen in 5%, begins in the frontal region and can affect all the calvarium except that which is below the internal occipital protuberance since there is no marrow in this area.

The diploic space is widened due to marrow hyperplasia.

Other Features

1. Thrombosis and infarction in diaphysis of small tubular bones in children and in metaphysis and subchondrium of long bones (adults).
2. Sec-osteomyelitis.
3. Abdomen—splenomegaly and splenic sequestration.

Thalassemia

- Marrow hyperplasia in thalassemia major is more marked than in any other anemia.
- Severe hair on end appearance.
- Impediment of pneumatization of maxillary antrum and mastoid sinus.
- Lateral displacement of orbit, Rodent facies.

Other Features

Earliest changes in small bones of hands and feet, widened Medullary spaces with thinning of cortices.
- Erlenmeyer flask deformity.
- *Chest:*
  - Cardiac enlargement.
  - Paravertebral masses.
- *Abdomen*
  - Hepatosplenomegaly
  - Gallstones
- *Others*
  - Hereditary spherocytosis.
  - Elliptocytosis.
  - Pyruvate kinase deficiency
  - G-6 PD deficiency

B. Neoplastic

1. *Hemangioma*
   - Mostly cavernous
   - *Age:* 4th or 5th decade. M:F = 1:2
   - *Location* = Vertebral body and calvarium.

RF   = < 4 cm round osteolytic lesion.
   Sunburst or hair on end and without definite margin may occur in diploe, producing palpable lump secondary to widening of diploe.

2. *Meningioma*
   Only rarely, when it break through outer table.

3. *Metastasis*
   Prostatic carcinoma, retinoblastoma, neuroblastoma (skull) and GI tract.

C. Cyanotic Heart Disease

- Due to erythroid hyperplasia. Hypertrophic pulmonary osteoarthropathy may occur.
- Iron deficiency anemia = severe childhood cases.

Flow Chart 8.8.1

Hair on End" appearance on skull vault

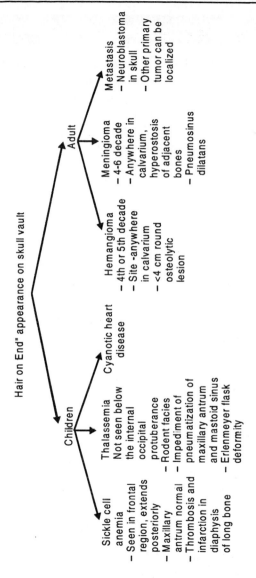

Children

Sickle cell anemia
– Seen in frontal region, extends posteriorly
– Maxillary antrum normal
– Thrombosis and infarction in diaphysis of long bone

Thalassemia
Not seen below the internal occipital protuberance
– Rodent facies
– Impediment of pneumatization of maxillary antrum and mastoid sinus
– Erlenmeyer flask deformity

Cyanotic heart disease

Adult

Hemangioma
– 4th or 5th decade
– Site - anywhere in calvarium
– <4 cm round osteolytic lesion

Meningioma
– 4-6 decade
– Anywhere in calvarium, hyperostosis of adjacent bones
– Pneumosinus dilatans

Metastasis
– Neuroblastoma in skull
– Other primary tumor can be localized

8.9 MULTIPLE WORMIAN BONES

Common in infancy but only considered significant when 6×4 mm or larger in size, >10 in number and with a tendency to be arranged in a mosaic pattern.(PORKCHOPS)

1. *Pyknodysostosis:* Abnormal recessive
   - Short limbed dwarf with some features of osteopetrosis and cleidocranial dysplasia.
2. Osteogenesis imperfecta.
3. Rickets in healing phase.
4. Kinky hair syndrome.
5. Cleidocranial dysplasia.
6. Hypothyroidism/hypophosphatasia.
7. Otopalatodigital syndrome.
8. Primary acro-osteolysis/pachydermoperiostosis.
9. Down syndrome

Osteogenesis imperfecta = Heterogenous group of a generalized connective tissue disorder leading to a micromelic dwarfism, caused by bone fragility, blue sclera and dentinogenesis imperfecta.

2 types $\Big\langle$ < Congenita
Tarda -4 types—1 to 4 (I to IV)

RF   Diffuse demineralization, cortical thickening, multiple fracture, pseudoarthrosis with bowing.
- Normal exuberant callus formation.
- Rib thining or notching.
- Wormian bones persisting into adulthood.
- Basilar impression.
- Biconcave vertebral bodies with Schoff nodes.
- Rickets in healing phase.
  - *Age group:* 4-18 months.

- Location metaphysis of long bones subjected to stress are particularly involved (wrists, knee, ankles)
- RF cupping + fraying of metaphysis.
- Poorly mineralized epiphyseal centers with delayed appearance.
- Coarse trabeculation.
- Deformities common.
- Frontal bossing.
- Multiple wormian bones.

Cleidocranial Dysplasia-AD

- Delayed ossification of midline structure.
  - a. *Skull:* Decrease ossification of skull.
    - – Wormian bones.
    - – Widened fontanelle + sutures
    - – Large mandible
    - – Hypoplastic PNS.
  - b. *Chest and upper extremity*
    - – Hypoplasia or absence of clavicle (10%)
    - – Supernumerary ribs, short radius, hemivertebrae
  - c. Pelvis and lower extremity.
    - – Delayed ossification of bones at symphysis pubis, hypoplastic iliac bones.

Hypothyroidism

- Delayed skeletal maturation, fragmented stippled Epiphysis.
- Wide sutures /fontanelle with delayed closure.
- Delayed dentition.
- Delayed pneumatization of sinuses.
- Wedging of D-L vertebral bodies.

Hypophosphatasia

- Autosomal recessive.
- Low activity of serum, bone, liver alkaline-phosphatase resulting in poor mineralization.
- Phosphoethanolamine as a precursor of alkaline phosphatase.
- Normal serum Ca^{++} and phosphorus.
- RF moderate to severe dwarfism
- Resembles rickets
- Separated cranial sutures.

Flow Chart 8.9.1

Differential Diagnosis
wormian bones

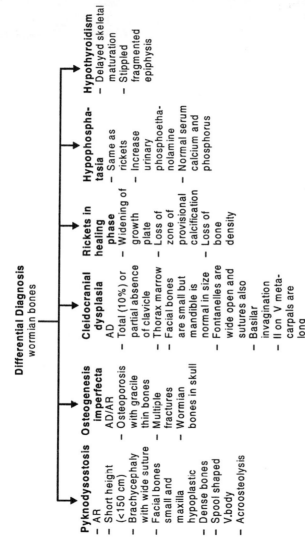

Pyknodysostosis
– AR
– Short height (<150 cm)
– Brachycephaly with wide suture
– Facial bones small and maxilla hypoplastic
– Dense bones
– Spool shaped V.body
– Acroosteolysis

Osteogenesis imperfecta
– AD/AR
– Osteoporosis with gracile thin bones
– Multiple fractures
– Wormian bones in skull

Cleidocranial dysplasia
– AD
– Total (10%) or partial absence of clavicle
– Thorax marrow
– Facial bones are small but mandible is normal in size
– Fontanelles are wide open and sutures also
– Basilar invagination
– II on V metacarpals are long

Rickets in healing phase
– Widening of growth plate
– Loss of zone of provisional calcification
– Loss of bone density

Hypophosphatasia
– Same as rickets
– Increase urinary phosphoethanolamine
– Normal serum calcium and phosphorus

Hypothyroidism
– Delayed skeletal maturation
– Stippled fragmented epiphysis

8.10 POSTERIOR FOSSA CYSTS AND CYSTS LIKE MASSES

- Dandy-Walker malformation (DWS) and variant
- Mega cisterna magna
- Posterior-fossa arachnoid cyst
- Enterogenous cyst
- Inflammatory
- Dermoid
- Epidermoid
- Cystic neoplasm.

Dandy-Walker Malformation

- Atresia of embryonic roof of 4th ventricle—caused by cystic dilatation of 4th ventricle and enlarged post fossa with upward displacement of lateral sinuses, tentorium and torcular herophili associated with varying degree of vermian hypoplasia or aplasia.

  Floor of 4th ventricle is present, cystically dilated 4th ventricle balloons posteriorly.

  Complete vermian absence in 25% and mild hypoplasia. The vermian remanant typically appear as rotated and elevated above the post fossa cyst.

Cerebellar hemisphere – Varying degree of hypoplasia. Brainstem = hypoplastic or compressed.

Associated Feature

CCA. (corpus callosum agenesis)
Gray matter heterotopia
Clefts, polymicrogyria
Occipital cephalocele
Polydactyly and cardiac anomalies.

Mega Cisterna Magna

- Vermis and cerebral hemisphere, IVth ventricle normal

- Enlarged posterior fossa cyst can cause scalloping of occipital and squamous base.

Posterior Fossa Arachnoid Cyst

- CSF filled masses enclosed within split layer of arachnoid.
- IVth ventricle and vermis normal but displaced.
- Nonenhancing mass, parallel in CSF attenuation.

Enterogenous Cyst

- Developmental cyst (The notochord and foregut may fail to separate during formation of definitive alimentary canal)
- Anterior to brainstem
- IVth ventricle and vermis normal
- Equal or slightly higher attenuation.

Inflammatory

- IVth ventricle - Normal but may be distorted
- Enhancement after contrast administration
- Calcification common
- Slightly hyperdense to CSF

Dermoid and Epidermoid

Both epidermoid and dermoid cysts are ectodermal inclusion cysts.

Epidermoid-IVth ventricle is most common intraaxial site.

Dermoid-Vermis and IVth ventricle most common infratentorial site.

Calcification is common in dermoid.

Cystic Neoplasm

- Site-vermis and cerebellum.
- Vermis and IVth ventricle— normal but distorted.
- Calcification common.
- Common tumors – Cerebellar astrocytoma and ependymoma.

Table 8.10.1

	DW malformation	DW variant	Mega cisterna	Post. fossa arachnoid cyst	Entero-genous cyst	Inflamma-tory cyst	Dermoid	Epider-moid	Cystic neoplasm
Location	Most of the post. fossa	Midline post.	Midline post.	Midline post c-p angle	Ant-to-brainstem	Any location	Midline	C-P angle	Ventricle cerebellum
IVth ventricle	Floor present, open dorsally to large cyst	Keyhole appearance	N	Normal but displaced	Normal	Normal but distorted	Normal but distorted/displaced	Normal but distorted/displaced	Normal but distorted/displaced
Vermis	Absent hypoplastic, everted over cyst	Inferior lobules hypoplastic	N	Normal but distorted	Normal	Normal	Normal but distorted	Normal but distorted	Normal
Obstructive hydrocephalus	Common	Absent	Absent	Variable	Absent	Variable	Variable	Variable	Common
Contrast enhancement	-ve	-	-	-	-	+	-	-	+
Calcification	Negative	-	-	-	-	+	+	-	+
Cyst density	- CSF	CSF	CSF	~CSF	=or ↑ than CSF	> CSF	Hypo on NECT due to fat	= or > CSF	Hyperdense to CSF
Margin	Smooth	Smooth	Smooth	Smooth	Smooth	Smooth	Smooth/lobulated	Irregular or round	Smooth/lobulated
Skull	Large post. fossa, lambdoid, torcular inversion	N	Scalloping of inner table	N	N	N	May have sinus tract	Normal	Normal

8.11 ENLARGED SYLVIAN FISSURE/ MIDLINE CRANIAL FOSSA OF CSF DENSITY

1. Schizencephaly open lip.
2. Arachnoid cyst.
3. Epidermoid.
4. Cystic neoplasm.
5. Infarct.
6. Loculated hygroma.
7. Porencephalic cyst.

Schizencephaly—(split-brain) - is a gray matter lined CSF filled cleft that extends from the ependymal surface of the brain, through the white matter to the pia.

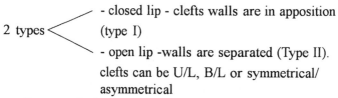

2 types
- closed lip - clefts walls are in apposition (type I)
- open lip -walls are separated (Type II).

clefts can be U/L, B/L or symmetrical/ asymmetrical

- *Porencephalic cysts*—results from insults to otherwise normally developed brain.
  CSF space is lined by gliotic white matter not by dysplastic heterotopic cortex.
- *Arachnoid cysts* are benign, congenital, intra-arachnoidal space occupying lesions that arc filled with clear CSF like fluid.

Age incidence—all ages, 75% occur in children 3:1 M.F.

Location—supratentorial -50-60% = Middle cranial fossa, 10% - suprasellar and quadrigeminal region.

CT—smoothly demarcated noncalcified extra-axial mass that does not enhance.

Pressure erosion of adjacent calvarium.

Ipsilateral pneumosinus dilatans.

MR—Sharply demarcated extra-axial mass. Displaces or deform adjacent brain.

• Parallel to CSF signal intensity on all pulse sequence.

Epidermoid (i) Congenital nonneoplastic inclusion cyst.

            (ii) Acquired-result of trauma.

Age and sex = peak = 4th decade, No gender predilection.

90% = intradural-10% intra-axial.

Most common site-basal subarachnoid space-

40-50% - C-P angle cisterns.

NECT = attenuation similar to CSF, lobulated margin.

        Calcification = 10-25%

Occasionally = appear hyperdense -due to hemorrhage, high protein, etc.

        CECT = Most do not enhance.

MR—Confined and insinuate along basilar CSF cistern, similar to CSF.

        SSFP, MR and DWMR - to differentiate from a cyst. Engulf the main vessels and nerve while arachnoid cyst displaces.

Cystic neoplasm—contrast enhancement is common.

Infarct—old chronic infarct

• At any age.

• Lined by gliotic white matter.

• Changes of volume loss present

• *Loculated Hygroma*

   – CSF density.

   – membrane can be seen on CE MR study.

Flow Chart 8.11.1

Differential Diagnosis

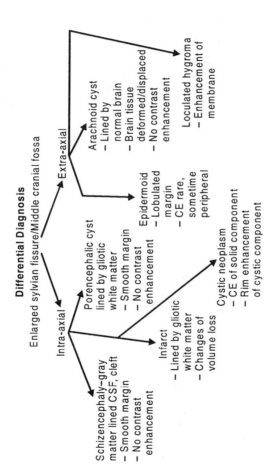

Enlarged sylvian fissure/Middle cranial fossa

Intra-axial

Extra-axial

Schizencephaly–gray
matter lined CSF, cleft
– Smooth margin
– No contrast
  enhancement

Porencephalic cyst
lined by gliotic
white matter
– Smooth margin
– No contrast
  enhancement

Infarct
– Lined by gliotic
  white matter
– Changes of
  volume loss

Cystic neoplasm
– CE of solid component
– Rim enhancement
  of cystic component

Arachnoid cyst
– Lined by
  normal brain
– Brain tissue
  deformed/displaced
– No contrast
  enhancement

Epidermoid
– Lobulated
  margin
– CE rare,
  sometime
  peripheral

Loculated hygroma
– Enhancement of
  membrane

8.12 SKULL BASE AND CAVERNOUS SINUS

Skull base is composed of the ethmoid, sphenoid, occipital bone and paired frontal and temporal bones.

Anterior Skull Base Lesion

Anterior skull base lesion consists of orbital plates of ethmoid bones.

Cribriform plate of ethmoid bone.

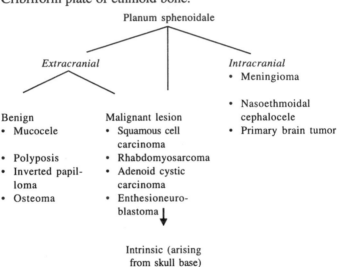

Extracranial

Most arise from nose and PNS.

Benign

Mucocele—Accumulation of impacted mucus secondary to occluded draining sinus osteum.

If a mucocele becomes infected it is termed mucopyocele.

In descending order of frequency mucocele are found in frontal, ethmoid, maxillary and sphenoid sinus.

Imaging—They are usually of soft tissue density mass with bone expansion and remodelling.

Inverted papilloma (IP)—Benign, slow growing.

IP arise in the nasal vault near the junction of ethmoid and maxillary sinuses, in the region of middle turbinate.

Imaging—A unilateral polypoidal nasal fossa soft tissue mass widens the nasal vault, sometime destroying the bone and extending into the adjacent ethmoid and maxillary sinuses.

• Focal erosion of cribriform plate with cephalad extension sometime.

Osteoma—Benign bone tumor made up of mature cortical bone. Frontal sinus is most common site.

Osteoma can expand and erode the sinus wall.

Malignant sinonasal masses can cause extradural intracranial extension.

In children—Most common extracranial malignant that involves the skull base is rhabdomyosarcoma.

Most common soft tissue sarcoma in children.

Imaging—Bulging soft tissue mass with areas of bone destruction T1 = similar to mass. T2 = Hyperintense meningeal and perineural spread are common.

Adult—98% of nasopharyngeal tumors in adult are carcinoma.

SCC = 80%

Adenocarcinoma = 18%

Nasopharyngeal Ca = spread directly into the skull base, as well as along muscle.

They extend intracranially along neural and vascular bundles via osseous foramina.

ENB

Enthesioneuroblastoma or olfactory NB arise from bipolar sensory receptor cells is the olfactory mucosa.

- Can occur at any age—Bimodal distribution

$$< \begin{array}{l} \text{2nd} \\ \text{4th decade} \end{array}$$

- ENB often confined to the nasal cavity but may extend to the PNS, orbit or brain through the cribriform plate.

Imaging— high nasal vault mass. MR—variable signal.
            moderate to inhomogenous enhancement.

- Bacterial/fungal sinusitis.
- Sarcoidosis.
- Sinonasal lymphoma.
- Wegner granulomatosis.

Intrinsic Lesion

Fibrous dysplasia
Paget's disease
Osteopetrosis.

Intracranial

- Most common lesion that involves the anterior skull base is meningioma.
- Planum sphenoidale or olfactory groove—site of origin
- Broad based, ant. basal subfrontal mass
- Strong and uniform enhancement
- Presence of tumor brain interface cleft
- Gray-white matter buckling
- Hyperostosis of adjacent bone.
- *Nasoethmoidal cephalocele*—complex masses of mixed soft tissue and CSF and are contiguous with intracranial sutures, typically through a widened calvarial opening. Cristagalli will be absent or eroded.
- Peripherally located brain neoplasm like ganglioglioma cause pressure erosion of adjacent skull.

Flow Chart 8.12.1

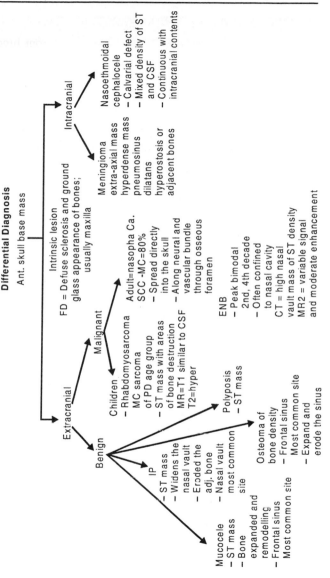

Differential Diagnosis

Ant. skull base mass

Intrinsic lesion
FD = Defuse sclerosis and ground glass appearance of bones; usually maxilla

Intracranial

Meningioma
extra-axial mass
hyperdense mass
pneumosinus
dilatans
hyperostosis or
adjacent bones

Nasoethmoidal
cephalocele
– Calvarial defect
– Mixed density of ST
and CSF
– Continuous with
intracranial contents

Extracranial

Malignant

Children
– Rhabdomyosarcoma
MC sarcoma
of PD age group
– ST mass with areas
of bone destruction
MR=T1 similar to CSF
T2=hyper

Adult=nasopha Ca.
SCC -MC=80%
– Spread directly
into the skull
– Along neural and
vascular bundle
through osseous
foramen

ENB
– Peak bimodal
2nd, 4th decade
– Often confined
to nasal cavity
CT = high nasal
vault mass of ST density
MR2 = variable signal
and moderate enhancement

Benign

Mucocele
– ST mass
– Bone
expanded and
remodelling
– Frontal sinus
Most common site

IP
– ST mass
– Widens the
nasal vault
– Eroded the
adj. bone

Polyposis
– ST mass

Osteoma of
bone density
– Frontal sinus
Most common site
– Expand and
erode the sinus

Nasal vault
most common
site

8.13 CENTRAL SKULL BASE LESIONS

Contents are –

Upper clivus, sella turcica, cavernous sinus and sphenoid sinus.

- *Osteomyelitis*
  - Predisposing factors—Immunocompromised states, diabetes, chronic mastoiditis, PNS infection, trauma.
  - Frontal sinusitis is very frequent leading to osteomyelitis.
  - RF loss of bone density, trabecular detail, sequestrum formation, blurring and loss of sinus outline.
  - Complication—Cerebral infarct, meningitis, subdural empyema and brain abscess.
- *Fungal Sinusitis*
  Imaging CT-multisinus nodular mucoperiosteal thickening high attenuation foci within the soft tissue masses.
  - Extensive lesion can produce skull base destruction.
    MR—lowsignal on both T1 and T2, surrounded by a high signal rim on T2.
    Complication—cavernous sinus thrombosis, blood, vessel invasion and rapid intracranial dissemination.
- Non-fungal granulomas = also have intracranial extension like Wegener's granulomatosis, LMG (lethal midline granulomas—lymphoma variant).
  CT—E/O mucosal ulceration and bone destruction in nasal cavity and PNS without the ST mass.
  Thus distinguishing from simple malignancy.
  MRI—Decrease signal on both T1 and T2.
  While simple inflammatory thickening will be bright on T2.
- *Primary neoplasm*—Common tumors that affect the central skull base are:

- Pituitary adenoma—slowly expanding that erode the sella turcica.

  Typically extend sup. through the diap. sella and laterally into the cavernous sinus.
- Some time may expend inferiorly and cause destruction of central skull base.
- *Meningioma*—of central skull base are located along the sphenoid wing, diaphragm, sella, clivus and cavernous sinus.

  Focal lobulated or flat 'En plaque' mass bony destruction or hyperostosis is occasionally.
- Nerve sheath tumors—In central skull base most often affect the cavernous sinus and Meckel's cave.

  Most common schwannoma to involve the central skull base and cavernous sinus is trigeminal and schwannoma.
  - They are encapsulated, well-delineated tumors.

    They are quite vascular and hemorrhage and necrosis may occur.
- JNA (juvenile angiofibroma)—highly vascular, locally invasive lesion that originate near the sphenopalatine foramen of adolescent.

  Spread along neural foramina and fissure into the pterygopalatine fossa, orbit, middle cranial fossa, sphenoid sinus and cavernous sinus.

  CT = ST density mass.

  highly vascular and strongly enhancing.
- *Chordoma*—slow growing, destructive tumor, histologically benign but locally invasive.

  1/3rd occur in spheno-occipital region.

  Most occur in midline and primarily involves the clivus.
- *Enchondroma*—Most common benign osteocartilaginous tumor in this location.

An expansile, lobulated ST mass with scalloped endosteal bone resorption and curvilinear matrix mineralization the Ch. findings.

MR—iso with muscle on T1,

hyper on T2

postcontrast T1 Wt- Enhancement of scalloped margin.

* *Metastasis*

Can arise via regional extension of head and neck malignancy or hematogenous spread from extracranial primary site.

prostate, lung and breast = MC

diffuse/focal cystic destructive lesion.

Mixed hyperostosis and bone destruction with an associated ST mass. } may resemble hemangioma

Lat. orbital wall is a favorite site for prostatic mets.

8.14 CEREBELLO PONTINE ANGLE MASSES

Cerebellopontine angle cistern lies between anterolateral surface of the pons and cerebellum and the post surface of the petrous temporal bone.

Important structures within the cerebellopontine angle cistern- 5th, 7th and 8th cranial nerves.

Superior and ant. inf. cerebellar arteries.

tributaries of superior petrosal veins.

Cerebellopontine angle masses—very common in adults.

Majority are extra-axial

* Arising in cerebellopontine angle cistern
  – Schwannoma (acoustic) - 75%

- meningioma – 8-10%
- Vascular ectasia/aneurysm-2-5%
- Epidermoid -5%

Other schwannoma.

- Arachnoid cyst.

4th ventricle/lateral recess

- Ependymoma.
- CP papilloma.

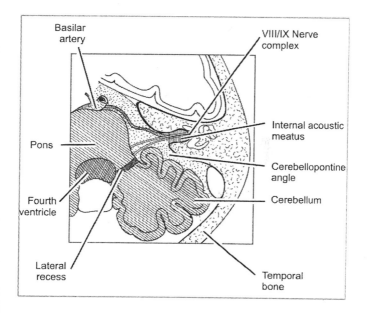

Fig. 8.14.1: Anatomic diagram depicts the cerebellopontine angle anatomy. Lesions that arise from each component are indicated

Brainstem/cerebellum
- Exophytic glioma metastasis
- Hemangioblastoma.

Temporal bone
- Cholesterol granuloma
- Gradenigo syndrome
- Paraganglioma
- Metastasis.

- Acoustic schwannoma—usually solitary, multiple seen in 5% of cases and characteristic of NF-2

  age =5-6th decade

  with NF-2 appear earlier

  Sex = M < F (1:1.5-2)

  plain X-ray = widening of IOC

  anteromedial petrous apex erosion may be enlarged foramen ovale/rotundum/sof [superior orbital fissure (CANAL).

CT = NECT = iso to hypodense.

CECT = almost all schwannoma enhances strongly, small tumors- uniform

Large - heterogenous pattern

Peripheral arachnoid cyst or pools of trapped CSF.

MRI = Characteristic findings of extra-axial mass.

- Distinct vascular/CSF cleft between tumor and brain.
- Larged CP < cistern.
- Corticomedullary junction of cerebellum appear displaced and brainstem rotated.
- Ice cream cone appearance due to intracanalicular component.

  T1 =2/3rd are hypo.

  T2 and PD = hyper = foci of cystic degeneration in larger lesion.

- All show enhancement.
- Peritumoral edema seen in 37% cases.

Angio-hypo to avascular tumor.

Drapping, stretching of vessels,

- Meningioma - Post.fossa meningioma accounts for approx. 10% meningioma -site - post surface of petrous temporal bone and clivus.

Arise from arachnoid cap cells.

Associated with NF-2

sex = F > M peak -4th to 6th decade.

Plain Film

- Bone erosion and hyperostosis
- Enlarged vascular channel.
- Tumoral calcification and expanded PNS (pneumosinus dilatans)

Angiography—Vascular tumor

Dual supply—meningeal and cerebral artery giving a characteristic radial or sunburst appearance.

CT—sharply circumscribed round or lobulated mass that abuts dural surface, usually an obtuse angle.

70-75% = homogenously hyperdense.

25% = isointense

Ca++ = 20-25%

Cystic changes or necrosis = 8-23%

Peripheral edema = 60%

CECT = intense and homogenous enhancement -in 90%

MR = gray-white interface 'buckling' or displacement cleft or pseudo capsule of CSF and vessels that surrounds the mass.

- T1 = Iso or slightly hypointense.

T2 = Variable.

- *Epidermoid tumor*—Intracranial epidermoid is cystic lesion that insinuate along CSF cistern.

  age—20-60 yrs.

  No gender predilection

  Location—40-50% occur at CP angle cistern.

  Imaging—plain film - round on lobulated well-delineated focal bone erosion with sclerotic margins.

  Angio—Avascular mass effect.

  NECT—Well-delineated lucent appearing lobulated masses with attenuation similar to CSF.

  $Ca^{++} = 10\text{-}25\%$

  Occasionally hyperdense on NECT.

  CECT—Most do not enhance although enhancement at the tumor margin. Epidermoid tumor encase vessel and engulf the intracranial nerves.

MRI—Most are confined to, and insinuate along the basilar CSF cisterns.

SI similar to CSF.

White epidermoid = iso or hyper to brain on T1 because of increased lipid content.

SSFP (steady-State Free precession and diffusion weight MR are helpful in differentiating the lesion with arachnoid cyst.

- *VB dolichoectasia*—on elongation and dilatation of vertebrobasilar artery.
- *Elongation of basilar artery*—if any portion of it extends lateral to the margin of the clivus or dorsum sellae or if the artery bifurcates above the plane of suprasellar cistern.
- Ectasia is diagnosed if the Diameter of the basilar artery is greater than 4-5 millimeter on CT.
  - Angiography—non-selective angiography demonstrates well.
  - MRI and MRA = gives signal void on MR.

- *Arachnoid cyst*—are benign, congenital, intra-arachnoidal space occupying lesions that are filled with clear CSF-like fluid.

  age—75% occur in children. F:M = 3:1. 5-10% of arachnoid cyst occur in post. fossa < CP angle and cistern magna

  NECT—CSF density extra-axial masses do not enhance on contrast administration.

  Pressure erosion of adjacent calvarium.

  Ipsilateral pneumosinus dilatans.

MRI—They parallel CSF SI on all sequences.

- Ependymoma - are slow growing lobulated neoplasm that are often partly cystic.

  age—6 times more common in children.

  peak—1-5 yrs and mid 30 yrs.

  location -rarely arise in C-P angle cistern.

  imaging—angiography =hypovascular to extremely hypervascular lesion.

CT—iso on NECT, 50% exhibit Ca++

  mild to moderate enhancement.

MRI—lobulated ST mass hypo or iso on T1 and hyper on T2WI cystic portion =hypor on T1 and hyper to brain on T2WI.

- *Pilocystic astrocytoma* - (juvenile or cystic cerebellar)

  age—children and young adults.

  location around the 4th ventricle and cerebellar hemisphere.

  angio—avascular.

  NECT—hypo or isodense mass / Ca++ seen in 10%

variable but strong enhancement.

Sometimes having mural nodule in a large cysts.

MR—hypo or iso on T1 and hyper on T2.

- Metastasis – 1-2% of CP mass

  Usually have multiple or B/L cranial nerve and lepto-meningeal lesions coexisting parenchymal lesion are identified in 75% of these cases.

Table 8.14.1: Cerebellopontine angle masses

	AC Schwannoma	Meningioma	Epidermoid	VB ectasia aneurysm	Arachnoid cyst	Ependymoma
Plain X-ray	Widening of IOC	Hyperostosis of adjacent skull hypervascular channels	Focal bone erosion with sclerotic border	Pressure erosion of bone	Pressure erosion of adjacent calvarium	–
Ca++	–	+	10-25%	Frequent	–	+
Margins	Irregular/regular	Sharp, round/lobulated	Lobular, insinuate along the CSF cistern	Will-defined	Regular	Extrudes along the CSF cistern
4th ventricle	Compressed	Compressed	Compressed	Not affected	May compress	Enlarged
Angio	Hypo to avascular	Vascular tumor, dual blood supply	Avascular	Shows the ectatic vessel	Avascular	Variable
NCCT	Iso-hypodense Enlargement of IOC	Most hyperdense Ca++ pneumosinus dilatans	Lucent - similar to CSF	Iso dense	Similar to CSF density	Iso dense Ca++ seen
CECT	Strong enhancement	Strong	No enhancement	Varies	No enhancement	Mild to moderate
MRI	Characteristic feature of extra-axial mass T1 = 2/3rd hypo T2 hyper	T1 = iso to slightly hyperintense T2 = variable	Similar to CSF	MRA is useful IAC-N	Similar to CSF	Hypo-to-iso on T1 and hyper on T2

8.15: MAJOR APERTURES OF THE SKULL BASE

Aperture	Location	Transmitted structure(s)	Connects
Cribriform plate	Medial floor of anterior cranial fossa	Olfactory nerve (CN* I) Ethmoidal arteries (anterior and posterior)	Anterior fossa to superior nasal cavity
Optic canal	Lesser wing of sphenoid bone	Optic nerve (CN II) Ophthalmic artery Subarachnoid space, cerebrospinal fluid, and dura around optic nerve	Orbital apex to middle cranial fossa
Superior orbital fissure	Between lesser and greater sphenoid wings	CNs III, IV, V_1, VI Superior ophthalmic vein	Orbit to middle cranial fossa
Foramen rotundum	Middle cranial fossa floor inferior to superior orbital fissure	CN V_2 Emissary veins Artery of foramen rotundum	Meckel's cave to pterygo-palatine fossa
Foramen ovale	Floor of middle cranial fossa lateral to sella	CN V_3 Male Emissary veins from cavernous sinus to pterygoid plexus Accessory meningeal branch of maxillary artery (when present)	Meckel's cave to nasopha-ryngeal masticator space (infratemporal fossa)
Foramen spinosum	Posterolateral to foramen ovale	Middle meningeal artery Recurrent (meningeal) branch of mandibular nerve	Middle cranial fossa to high masticator space (infratem-poral fossa)
Foramen lacerum	Base of medial pterygoid plate at petrous apex	Meningeal branches of ascending pharyngeal artery (not internal carotid artery)	Not a true foramen; filled with fibrocartilage in life

Contd...

Contd...

Aperture	Location	Transmitted structure(s)	Connects
Vidian canal	In sphenoid bone below and medial to foramen rotundum	Vidian artery	Foramen lacerum to ptery-gopalatine fossa
Carotid canal	Within petrous temporal bone	Internal carotid artery Sympathetic plexus	Carotid space to cavernous sinus
Jugular foramen	Posterolateral to carotid canal, between petrous temporal bone and occipital bone	Pars nervosa, inferior petrosal sinuses (CN IX and Jacobson's nerve) Pars vascularis internal jugular vein, CNs X and XI, nerve of Arnold, small meningeal branches of ascending pharyngeal and occipital arteries	Posterior fossa to naso-pharyngeal carotid space
Stylomastoid foramen	Behind styloid process	CN VII	Parotid space to middle ear
Hypoglossal canal	Base of occipital condyles	CN XII	Foramen magnum to naso-pharyngeal carotid space
Foramen magnum	Floor of posterior fossa	Medulla and its meninges Spinal segment of CN XI Vertebral arteries and veins Anterior and posterior spinal arteries	Posterior fossa to cervical spinal canal

8.16 SUPRASELLAR MASS

INTRASELLAR LESIONS (PITUITARY)

1. Common
   a. Pituitary hypertrophy
   b. Microadenoma
   c. Cyst (Rathke cleft cyst and pars intermedia cyst)
2. Uncommon
   a. Craniopharyngioma
   b. Metastases
   c. Aneurysm

INFUNDIBULAR LESIONS

I. Uncommon
   a. Astrocytoma
   b. Germinoma
   c. Histiocytosis
   d. Lymphoma/leukemia
   e. Meningitis
   f. Metastasis
   g. Sarcoidosis

II. Rare
   a. Hypophysitis
   b. Choristoma
   c. Pituicytoma

SUPRASELLAR LESIONS

I. Common
   1. Aneurysm

   2. Craniopharyngioma
   3. Glioma

II. Uncommon
   1. Cyst (Arachnoid, inflammatory)
   2. Dermoid/epidermoid
   3. Ectopic neurohypophysis

4. Meningioma
5. Macroadenoma

4. Hamartoma
5. Lipoma

ANTERIOR 3RD VENTRICLE/OPTIC CHIASMATIC LESIONS

I. Common
1. Glioma

II. Uncommon
1. Colloid cyst
2. Germinoma
3. Glioependymal cyst ˙
4. Metastases

SPHENOID SINUS/CAVERNOUS SINUS LESIONS

I. Common
1. Osteomyelitis
2. Meningioma
3. Metastasis

II. Uncommon
1. Chordoma
2. Histiocytosis
3. Lymphoma
4. Osteoma/ osteosarcoma/ osteochondrosarcoma
5. Sarcoid
6. Schwannoma
7. Thrombus

Common Masses are:

- Macroadenoma (upward extension)
- Meningioma
- Aneurysm
- Craniopharyngioma.
- Glioma (usually pilocystic astrocytoma).

Uncommon

- Lipoma
- Dermoid/Epidermoid
- Cysts (Arachnoid, Rathke cleft)
- Focal meningitis
- Metastasis
- Ectopic neurohypophysis.

Macroadenoma—upward extension of pituitary adenoma through the diaphragmatic sella accounts for 1/3rd to 1/2 of all suprasellar masses in adults.

Pituitary adenoma with suprasellar extension typically have a figure of 8 appearance.

Most enhances strongly but inhomogenously.

Calcification is rare.

MRI—similar to gray matter on T1 and T2 sequences.

Hemorrhage, Cyst formation can complicate the MR appearance.

Meningioma

Second most common suprasellar neoplasm in adults.

Most parasellar meningioma originate from the sphenoid ridge, diaphragm or tuberculum sella.

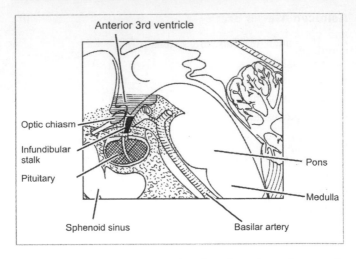

Fig. 8.16.1: Anatomic diagram depicts the sella turcica and suprasellar region as seen from the lateral view. Common lesions and their differential diagnosis by location are indicated

NECT slightly hyperdense.

Strong uniform enhancement, but not as intense as adjacent pituitary gland and cavernous sinus, allowing most meningioma to distinguish from adjacent pituitary adenoma.

Craniopharyngioma

Half of all suprasellar tumors in children.

2nd peak = 4th-6th decade

90% of craniopharyngioma—exhibit calcification.

Enhance and at least partially cystic. MRI signal intensity varies with cyst content on T1 seq. but majority of craniopharyngioma are hyperintense on T2WI.

Astrocytoma—of the visual pathway, optic nerve, chiasma and optic tracts account for 25% of pediatric suprasellar neoplasm.

CT—Iso or hypodense mass and frequent enhancement following contrast administration.

MRI—Hypointense on T1 but hyper on T2WI.

Hypothalamoneurohypophyseal Axis Germinoma

Most are both intra and suprasellar.

Age—most patients are <30 yrs. MR—An infiltrating mass isoin-tense to brain on T1, moderately hyperintense on T2 wt images.

Enhances strongly and homogenously after contrast administration.

CSF dissemination throughout the ventricular system and subarachnoid space is common.

Epidermoid Tumor

Occasionally occur in the suprasellar cistern.

On imaging = lobulated, irregular, frond-like surface Appearance similar to CSF on imaging studies.

Dermoid Tumor

Well-delineated, lobulated masses that typically occur in or near the midline. Suprasellar dermoids are uncommon.

On imaging—Usually appear similar to fat.

Ruptured dermoids may spill their contents throughout the CSF spaces and elicit severe chemical meningitis.

Metastasis—to the hypothalamic—pituitary axis represents approx. 1% of sellar—suprasellar masses. Breast cancer is the most common site in female followed by lung, stomach and uterus.

In men, common primary tumor are neoplasm of the lung, followed by prostate, bladder, stomach and pancreas.

MRI—ISO intense on T1 and hyperintense on T2WI. Moderate enhancement following contrast administration.

Vascular Lesion

Vascular ectasias and supraclinoid ICA. Aneurysms are the most common suprasellar nonneoplastic masses in adults.

Imaging appearance of aneurysm is variable, depending on the presence and age of thrombus and various flow parameters.

Congenital

Suprasellar arachnoid cyst

Ten percent of arachnoid cysts occur in the suprasellar region.

On imaging appear as smoothly marginated mass that is similar to CSF density.

SSAC—Neither calcify nor enhance.

A displaced, compressed III ventricle can be seen on MR studies.

- *Rathke's cleft cyst* (RCC) is a benign epithelium lined cyst that probably arises from remnants of Rathke's pouch.
  RCC usually have both supra- and intrasellar component-
  CT and MR = Varies with cyst content.
  Calcification is absent.

Table **8.16.1:** Suprasellar masses

	Pituitary adenoma	Meningioma	Craniopharyngioma	Glioma	Patent aneurysm	Partially thrombosed
Ca++	Rare	Common	90% Ca++	Rare	Rim Ca++	—
Unenhanced CT	Iso	Slightly hyperdense	Heterogenous cystic hypodense. Solid-iso or slighty hyperdense	Iso or slightly hypodense	Slightly hyper D	Slightly hyperdense
Enhanced CT	Modest uniform enhancement	Strong uniform enhancement	Variable cystic =rim enhancement. Solid = enhancement	+/–	Strong uniform enhance	Non-enhancing in areas of thrombus, enhancing patent tumor
T1WI	Iso	Iso	Variable cystic hypo. Solid-isointense	Iso	Flow void	Rim enhancement. Thrombus variable
T2WI	Iso-to slightly hyper	Variable hypo, iso or slightly hyperintense	Variable-cystic-hyperintense. Solid hyperintense	Slightly hyperintense	Flow void	Variable

8.17 SELLAR AND SUPRASELLAR MASSES

Common Causes
1. Pituitary adenoma
2. Craniopharyngioma
3. Aneurysm

4. Suprasellar meningioma.

Rare Causes
1. Rathke's cleft cyst
2. Arachnoid cyst
3. Visual pathway glioma (VPG)
4. Chordoma
5. Metastasis
6. Epidermoid and dermoid
7. Teratoma
8. Germinoma

PITUITARY ADENOMA

- Fifteen percent of all intracranial tumors.
- Microadenoma – <10 mm in height.
- Macroadenoma – 10 or >10 mm.

Classification

- Endocrine Active—80% (Like prolactinoma, acromegaly/gigantism, hepatosplenomegaly.
- Endocrine inactive -20%

Plain X-ray

Macroadenoma

- Pituitary fossa increases in size, expand and erode. In classic case give "ballooned sella" appearance with backward bowing of dorsum, under cutting of anterior clinoid and downward protrusion of floor and extension to sphenoid sinus.

Microadenoma

It produces local bulging of sellar floor or "Double floor" appearance.

In case of acromegaly—other features like thickening of skull vault, grossly enlarged sinuses and prognathous jaw seen.

CT

The most common microadenoma, prolactinoma typically produce some enlargement of pituitary and a discrete hypodense region within the enhanced gland-on CECT.

Other imaging findings are thinning or asymmetry of the sellar floor, displacement of infundibulum from the midline (infundibulum sign) and displacement of capillary tuft (tuft sign).

The macroadenoma are: isodense or slightly hyperdense mass and enhance uniformly on CECT. Cystic or necrotic areas may be seen within it. In some cases calcification is seen in the rim of the tumor or less commonly throughout the tumor matrix. The adenoma usually enlarges the sella, compress the sphenoid sinuses or encroaches on the suprasellar cistern and may displace the chiasm or temporal lobes. Some time it extend into the anterior end of 3rd ventricle and cause hydrocephalus, rarely it destroy the skull base degenerate to carcinoma.

MRI

The normal pituitary yields a homogenous brain like signal in most pulse sequences and is best shown in sagittal and coronal images. The normal optic chiasm, carotid vessels and sphenoid sinus are also highly conspicuous. Macroadenoma are usually of relatively lower signal than normal brain on T1 WIS of higher signal or T2 weighted images. Regions of lower signal on T1 and higher signal on T2 are seen within the tumor and usually represent cyst when rounded and circumscribed and necrosis when more irregular. Area of recent hemorrhage found frequently and seen as high signal on T1 wt. images.

- Microadenoma on T1 weighted images with IV gadolinium showing delayed enhancement of the adenoma compared to the normal gland.

PITUITARY APOPLEXY

Pituitary tumors occasionally undergoes ischemic necrosis and hemorrhage if the blood supply to tumor is impaired and leads to rapid expansion of tumor is known as pituitary apoplexy.

- It may also occur as a complication of pregnancy in postpartum period called Sheehan's syndrome.

CT

Shows hyperdensity due to hemorrhage or may show only hypodensity in the sella with a rim or enhancement.

MRI

It is more sensitive than CT. A subacute hemorrhage in the pituitary gland has hyperintensity on T1 wt. and T2 wt. images.

EMPTY SELLA

A varying amount of CSF within the sella with the pituitary gland occupying less than 50% of the volume of sella is defined as empty sella.

Classification

1. *Primary (Idiopathic):* Common in females, patients are often obese, multiparous and hypertensive.
2. *Secondary:*
   I. After hypophysectomy or tumor removal.
   II. After radiation therapy of sellar contents.
   III. After infarction of pituitary gland.

X-ray

The sella often appears enlarged. The enlargement however is more globular and symmetric and the cortex of the sella remains intact.

CT (EMPTY SELLA)

Pituitary fossa to be occupied largely by tissue of CSF or water density rather than a normal gland. The "infundibulum sign" can be used to differentiate an empty sella from other low density process, such as cystic tumor or an infrasellar 3rd ventricle which displace the infundibulum.

CRANIOPHARYNGIOMA

It is the 2nd most common sellar tumor and account for 3% of all intracranial tumor. 70% of cases occur before 20 yrs of age.

X-rays

Shows suprasellar calcification, expansion of sella and/or erosion of dorsum sellae. Such finding in a child are highly suggestive of craniopharyngioma. However, there is often a typical deformity of the sella which can be helpful in cases without calcification—mostly in adults. The sella appears elongated and the dorsum may be short and bowed forward as if pressed on from above.

CT

Suprasellar calcification is more readily identified by CT and always suggest the diagnosis. The tumor are often cystic or partly cystic and the cyst may be multiple or single. Calcification occur frequently in the wall or solid portion. After contrast injection. There is enhancement of the outer walled solid portion. The cystic component does not enhance.

MRI (CRANIOPHARYNGIOMA)

On MR with T1WI, The cystic contents are of variable signal intensity, most often hypointense but occasionally hyperintense. On T2WI, the cystic contents may be slightly or markedly hyperintense. On CEMR, the solid portion and the wall enhance.

SUPRASELLAR MENINGIOMA

It arises on dural surface of the anterior clinoid process, diaphragm sella, tuberculum, dorsum sellae or cavernous sinus.

X-ray

Localized hyperostotic reaction seen. Other evidence such as enlarged vascular markings and sign of raised intracranial pressure seen. With meningioma arising in the region of anterior clinoid, a rare manifestation is local bone extension with pneumatization, so called "BLISTERING" seen.

CT

Shows a well-defined and smoothly marginated iso to hyperdense mass which enhance homogenously intensely on CECT. Perilesional edema may be present. Rarely meningioma have cystic hypodense area within it. Globular calcification seen in 10% of cases.

Hyperostotic bone adjacent to tumor is characteristic.

MRI

It is isointense with brain on T1WI. So this can be missed unless a contrast enhanced study is done. After IV gadolinium, most meningioma are homogeneously enhanced in T1WI.

ANEURYSM

X-ray

Calcification are rare and when seen as characteristic arc like or circular marginal calcification.

CT

It is seen as a high density suprasellar or parasellar mass and enhance strongly related to circles of Willis on CECT. They may have calcification in the rim. When an organized thrombus is present. The aneurysm appears non-homogenous in CECT because the thrombus enhance less than do the lumen and the vessel wall.

MRI

In T1 T2 wt. serial images, flowing blood within the aneurysm has very low signal intensity.

Turbulent flow may produce a heterogenous signal. A thrombus within an aneurysm usually has signal intensity higher than that of flowing blood.

In T1 wt. gradient echo images, the lumen of an aneurysm typically has high signal intensity. The vascular anatomy in the sellar region and the presence of suspected aneurysm can be confirmed with magnetic resonance angiography (MRA).

RATHKE'S CLEFT CYST

CT

Shows a rounded mass in the suprasellar cisterns with no calcification. The values of density varies from that of CSF to more solid looking.

MRI

Shows a homogenous high signal on both T1 and T2 weighted images possibly due to altered blood in the cyst fluid.

ARACHNOID CYST

CT

The characteristic CT appearance of the cyst is a mass with CSF density (5-15 HU) and no solid or enhancings structure. In MR the cyst has an intensity similar to or slightly higher than the CSF in spin density and T2WI images.

EPIDERMOID AND DERMOID

CT

The tumors usually of fatty density. But the density can be as high as that of CSF or higher, depending on the contents. The margin may be ill-defined and that don't enhance with contrast medium. The presence of calcification or fat in a predominantly cystic lesion suggest a dermoid rather than epidermoid.

MRI

They are usually isointense with CSF on T1 wt. and isointense or slightly brighter on T2 weighted images.

TERATOMA

X-ray

Calcification is present in 50% of mature teratoma.

Very rarely presence of dental element seen and that is the true diagnostic feature.

CT

Shows cystic or multicystic tumor. The specific diagnosis will depend upon recognition of multiple tissues like fat, calcified element and dental element.

GERMINOMA (ATYPICAL TERATOMA)

CT

On CT germinoma may hypodense or hyperdense, homogenous or non-homogenous, enhancing or non-enhancing and frequently calcified. Presence of a pineal as well as suprasellar mass, which enhances homogeneously when seen in a young male, is characteristic of germinoma.

MRI

Germinoma is typical isointense with brain in T1WI and sometimes hyperintense in T2WI. Fat within it has high and low signal intensity in T1WI and T2WI respectively. Intense enhancement is common after IV gadolinium.

VISUAL PATHWAY GLIOMA (VPG)

Usually seen in first decade of life. 6-45% of patients with VPG have neurofibromatosis type I.

CT

It appears as an expansile mass involving the optic nerve, chiasm and tract and/or a mass that infiltrate and expand the hypothalamus. They are isodense to hypodense before contrast and usually show enhancement. The optic nerve may be uniformly enlarged with peripheral enhancement.

CHORDOMA

Commonly occur between 4th and 6th decade of life. They are locally invasive, slow growing involving the clivus and the sphenoid bone.

CT

Characteristic finding are destruction of bone in skull base and a soft tissue mass that is often calcified and may extend to nasopharynx.

MRI

The tumors appears as a lobulated inhomogenous mass, generally isointense with brain on T1 wt. and of higher signal on T2-weighted images. Calcification seen as focal areas of signal void.

METASTASIS

Metastasis to sellar region most commonly arise from lung, breast, kidney, GI tract, lymphoma, leukemia and naso-pharyngeal tumor.

Imaging

MRI effectively demonstrating the mass that may be invading the pituitary fossa, cavernous sinus, sphenoid sinus and sellar cortex. Bone destruction is better evaluated with CT.

NEUROSURGEON'S QUERIES

When a neurosurgeon preoperatively reviews a pituitary CT scan or MRI, his interest is focused on several anatomic features possible considered insignificant by the Radiologist. If transsphenoidal surgery is anticipated, imaging consideration include the degree of pneumatization of sphenoid sinus, location of sinus, septa and sinonasal inflammatory disease, bony dehiscence of the optic and carotid canals and vascular anomalies like anterior communicating artery aneurysms or the "kissing" carotids. So the additional information required from imaging to help plan surgery.

8.18 EXPANDED PITUITARY FOSSA

Size   -N range is   Ht   = 6.5-11 mm.
                       length   = 9-16 mm
                       breadth   = 9-19 mm.

Causes

1. Para/intrasellar mass
    – Pituitary adenoma
    – Craniopharyngioma

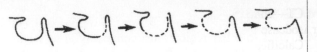

Fig. 8.18.1: Erosion and osteoporosis of
the sella, with no expansion

- Prolactinoma
- Meningioma
- Aneurysm
2. Raised intracranial pressure -d/to dilated 3rd ventricle
3. Empty sella.
   Primary-defect in diaphragm sella allows pulsating CSF to expand the sella.
   Patients are usually obese with hypertension and headache.
   Associated with benign intracranial hypertension.
   S×R = abnormal in 85%—shows symmetric expansion with no erosion.
   Secondary—pituitary tumor at treatment of a pituitary lesion may distort the diaphragmatic sellae.

POSTERIOR FOSSA NEOPLASM IN CHILDHOOD

50-60% of pediatric cerebral tumors.
1. Cerebellar astrocytoma.
2. Medulloblastoma.
3. Ependymoma.
4. Brainstem glioma.
5. Choroid plexus papilloma.

Cerebellar Astrocytoma

Most common posterior fossa tumor in pediatric age group. peak at age 10.
Location—around the 3rd or 4th ventricle.
Angiography—only an avascular mass effect.
   Occasionally a mural module shows neovascularity.

CT—sharply demarcated and smoothly marginated hypo- or isodense masses.

Calcification in 10% obstructive hydrocephalus.

CECT—strong but variable.

Some show enhancing mural nodule in a large cyst.

MR—Most cerebellar astrocytomas are cystic so hypo- or iso on T1 and hyper on T2.

Mural nodule and solid T—Enhance.

Pontine and medullary glioma—are usually diffusely infiltrating neoplasm that are inhomogenous hypodense on T1 and hyperdense on T2WI.

Obstructive hydrocephalus is mild or absent.

Medulloblastoma—arise from bipotential embryologic cells located in the roof of the IVth ventricle.

Incidence—15-25% of primary brain tumor in children, 75% occur before 15 yr and rest at age of 24-30 yrs.

Site—75%—in vermis

Less common location—is lateral cerebellum seen in older children and adults.

Extension—tend to metastasize early, widely and massively through CSF.

Brain parenchyma mets through virchow robin perivascular space.

Imaging

Angio - hypo or avascular.

CT = midline vermain mass that displaces the IVth ventricle anteriorly and cisterna magna posteriorly.

Hyperdense on NECT.

Obstructive hydrocephalus.

Calcification in 15%.

CECT = strong and homogenous E.

Atypical changes = cystic changes – 65%

isodense to brain – 3%

absent CE = 3%

MRI—Typical medulloblastoma fills the 4th ventricle and extending inferiorly through foramen of magendie into the cisterna magna. Heterogenous hypo on T1.

Heterogenous contrast enhancement.

Ependymoma

A rise from floor or roof the IVth ventricle and protrude through the outlet foramina into adjacent cisterns.

Incidence = 15% of posterior fossa neoplasm is childhood.
Peak age = 1-5 yrs, 2nd smaller peak-mid 30 yrs.
Site – 60% located below the tentorium.
40% above the tentorium.
90% of infratentorial occur in 4th ventricle.

Angio	= variable.
CT	= iso to NECT.
50%	= calcification
CECT	= mild to moderate inhomogenous enhancement
MRI	= solid component hypo or iso on T1WI and hyper on T2WI.

Choroid plexus papilloma—are one of the most common brain tumor in children under 2 yrs.

Location—Most common location is lateral ventricle, trigone in children. 4th ventricle is most common site in adults.

Imaging—angiography—highly vascular neoplasm.
Enlarged choroidal artery.

CT	= 75% are iso or hyperdense to brain on NECT. Calcification in 25%

Tumor margins are irregular and frond like CECT
= Intense and heterogenous enhancement.

MRI	= lobulated mass isointense to brain on T1 and iso on slightly hyper on T2WTI.

Table 8.18.1: Posterior fossa neoplasms in childhood

	Medulloblastoma	Cerebellar astrocytoma	Ependymoma	CPP
1. Age/sex	75% before 15 yrs, 25% at 24-30 yrs.	At age 10	1-5 yrs	< 2 yrs
2. Location	75% in vermis rest cerebellar hemisphere.	Around the 3rd/4th ventricle	Floor or roof of 4 ventricle	Lateral ventricle trigone in child 4th ventricle in adults
3. Angio	Hypo/avascular	Avascular mass effect	Variable	Highly vascular
4. Ca^{++}	15%	10%	50%	25%
5. NECT	Hyperdense midline vermian mass	Sharply defined iso or hypodense mass	Iso to brain	Iso or hyperdense and frond like T margin
6. CECT	Strong and homogenous enhancement	Strong but variable and show mural nodule in some cases	Mild to moderate inhomogenous enhancement	Intense and heterogenous
7. T1 MR	Hypo	Hypo	Solid part hypo on T1	Iso to brain on T1
8. T2 MR	Hyper	Hyper	Hyper	Slightly hyper on T2

8.19 RING ENHANCING LESIONS ON CECT

1. Primary neoplasm—GBM, meningioma, leukemia, pituitary macroadenoma, craniopharyngioma.
2. Metastatic Ca and sarcoma.
3. Abscess—Bacterial, fungal and parasitic.
4. Empyema of epidural/subdural or intraventricular space.
5. Resolving infarction.
6. Aging hematoma.
7. Thrombosed aneurysm.
8. Radiation necrosis.

1. *Primary Neoplasm*
   High grade astrocytoma
   - *Anaplastic Astrocytoma*
     age –40-60 yrs
   Location—Cerebral white matter most common.
   CT—Inhomogenous/mixed density tumors on NECT. After contrast injection they enhance strongly but nonuniformly and irregular rim enhancement is common.
   - Peripheral edema is present
   - GBM—Most common of all primary intracranial CNS tumors age = 75 yrs
   Location—Deep cerebral white matter of frontal and temporal lobes in most cases.
   NECT—Heterogenous in appearance.
   Ca^{++}—Rare
   Peripheral edema
   - Striking
   Enhancement
   - Strong but very inhomogenous thick, irregular rim enhancement.

2. *Parenchymal metastasis*

   Most common tumors to metastasize to brain are:

   Lung

   Breast

   Malignant melanoma.

   Age—>40 yrs.

   Location—Anywhere, gray white matter junction.

   NECT—Most metastasis are isodense to brain, hyperdense metastasis occur in round cell tumor. Edema associated with metastasis is striking.

   CECT—both solid and ring like enhancement with irregular wall.

3. *Abscess*—Most abscesses are caused by pyogenic bacteria.

   But sometime Mycobacterium tuberculosis and fungi such as actinomycosis and parasites can cause abscess.

   Location—gray white matter junction—Most common location frontal and parietal lobes are most frequent.

   Multiple abscesses are uncommon except in immunocompromised.

   CT—In late cerebritis stage—An irregular enhancing rim surrounds a central low density area edema+.

   Delayed scan show contrast 'fill in' in the central low density region.

   An abscess rim is typically thicken near the cortex and thinnest near the ependyma.

   ^{99m}Tc HMPAO—A new radionuclide imaging label for leukocytes and radiolabeled polyclonal.

   IgG (immunoglobulin/antibodies may be helpful in selected case.

4. *Epidural or subdural empyema*

   Fifty percent of cases are caused by sinusitis, frontal sinus is the most common site.

CT—Crescentic or lentiform extra- axial fluid collections that are increase density on CT, and mildly hyperintense to CSF on T2 Wt images.

Location—The cerebral convexities and interhemispheric fissure are common site.

CECT—A surrounding membrane that enhances intensely and uniformly following contrast administration.

5. *Resolving hematoma*—Between 1-6 wks subacute ICH become virtually isodense with adjacent brain parenchyma on NECT.

Subacute ICH show peripheral enhancement after contrast administration because there is blood brain barrier breakdown in the vascularized capsule that surrounds the hematoma.

6. *Thrombosed aneurysm*—Partially thrombosed aneurysm have a patent lumen inside a thickened often partially calcified wall that is lined with laminated clot.

The residual lumen and outer rim of the aneurysm may enhance strongly following contrast administration.

Radiation necrosis—Extensive radionecrosis and recurrent -or persistent neoplasm produce a similar picture, i.e. an expanding contrast enhancing mass.

PET may be helpful for determining the extent of cerebral gliomas as well as distinguishing radiation necrosis from residual neoplasm.

Table 8.19.1: Ring enhancing lesions on CECT

	Neoplasm	Mets	Abscess	Resolving hematoma	Thrombosed partial aneurysm
Location	Cerebral white matter	Gray-white matter junction	Cortico-medullary junction	Any	At the site of major arterial region
Age	40 onwards	> 40 yrs	Any	Any	Middle to late
Multiplicity	Usually single	Single/multiple	Single/multiple In immuno compromised	Single	Usually single
NECT	Heterogenous	Most are iso-dense to brain	Low density with thinner wall toward the epen-dyma	Subacute-iso-dense to brain	–
Edema	++	++	+	+	
CECT	Thick and irregular rim enhance	Thick and irregular rim enhance	In early stage thin later-thick and thinner wall towards the ependyma	Enhancing rim	Rim enhancement
Other investigation	MRI	MRI	^{99m}Tc HMPAO-radionuclide labelled for leuko-cyte	MRI	MRI and angio-graphy

8.20 SUPERIOR ORBITAL FISSURE ENLARGEMENT

It's large foramen, which connects orbit with the middle cranial fossa.

Between greater and lesser wing of sphenoid bone approximately 22 mm long, comma-shaped.

Inferomedial portion is wider, superolateral portion-thinner. Right muscle origin divide into superior and inferior part.

Sup. division—LFT [Lacrimal, frontal, trochlear] nerves.
Inf. division—Superior and inferior div. of CN III
V, Cranial nerve and nasociliary branch
Inferior and superior ophthalmic vein
Sympathetic nerve plevus

SOF is directed towards the cavernous sinus and a small amount of fat protrudes through the SOF into the region of ant. cavernous sinuses.

CAUSES

A. *Congenital/Developmental*
 – Neurofibromatosis
 – Hypoaplasia of GW of sphenoid
 – Spheno-orbital encephalocele
 – Orbital cysts ⟨— Enterogenous cyst
 Congenital
 – Dermoid/teratoma
 – MFD (mandibular-fascial dysostosis)
B. Infective
 Tolosa Hunt syndrome/ophthalmoplegia.
C. Trauma
D. Vascular causes
 – Aneurysm

- AVM/CCF
- CST [cavernous sinus thrombosis]

E. Neoplasm

Extraorbital—Neurogenic tumor

Orbital—lymphoma

Capillary hemangiomas.

- Parasellar chordoma
- Meningioma
- Juvenile angiofibroma
- Metastasis.

A. Neurofibromatosis-Phakomatoses

NF-1-AD—Ch.17

NF-2-AD—Ch.22

Skull and dural lesions are common in NF 1

- Hypoplasia of GW of sphenoid with spheno-orbital
  Encephalocele temporal lobe herniation-
  Proptosis (often pulsatile).

BARE ORBIT SIGN

- Calvarial defect due to lamboid suture
- Dural ectasia
- Enlargement of IOC
- Plexiform neurofibromas-hallmark of NF and 1/3rd of all
  patients with NF 1.
  Multiple tortuous wormlike masses that arise along the
  axis of a muscle or nerve.
  V_1 -Most common site in head and neck.
- *Enterogenous cysts*—Rare, congenital. Cyst lined by
  single layer of epithelial cells.
  Cyst may be seen in anterior cranial fossa and orbit.

CT—Homogeneous, well-circumscribed, hyperdense lobular, non-enhancing.

Extension through SOF may seen.

MR — hyper on T1
variable on T2

Dermoid/Teratoma

Dermoid and epidermoid—among the most common orbital tumor of childhood.

Most frequent location-superior and temporal aspect.

Although congenital, but many appears in 2/3rd disease.

Both have fibrous capsule.

CT—Well-circumscribed lesion with decrease diameter large one can extend through SOF.

Dermoid	*Epidermoid*
Calcification +ve characteristic	No Ca^{++}
if signal of fat present	– ve
Fat fluid level	

MR—Decrease signal on T1 and increase on T2/FLAIR/DW. MR.

Teratoma—Rare congenital germ cell tumor having all 3 elements.

No bony invasion, but causes orbital enlargement.

Congenital Cystic Eye

Present as complex cyst occupying the orbit. CT and MR-Enlarged orbit containing a rounded/ ovoid septated cyst. ipsilateral SOF increased.

MR—SI of the cyst is same as of normal vitrous.

A rudimentary connection to a thinned opposite nerve

• Primitive ectopic lens

- In corobomatous orbital cyst-globe and optic nerve are seen on CT and MR.
- *MFD*—orbital defect

Due to developmental defect affecting 1st and 2nd branchial arches.

Maxilla and molar bones are poorly developed

Downward slopping floor of orbit

CT—Defective lateral orbital floor.

GW of sphenoid may be hypoplastic.

B. Infective

- Tolosa Hunt syndrome: painful Ext. ophthalmoplegia U/L immediate relief following steroid treatment
  Imaging- occlusion of the superior ophthalmic vein on affected side with partial/complete obliteration of ipsilateral. C.S.
- *Carotid angio/MRA*—in excluding the aneurysm as a cause of syndrome.

C. Trauma

GW of sphenoid bone—is a thinner bone- offers least resistance to fracture.

- Neural foramina- represents weak points in the bones and nerve within the foramen may be crushed, contused or lacerated.
  Severe trauma can result in SOF synd. including a dilated pupil, ptosis with sometime extraocular muscle dysfunctioning.

D. Vascular

1. Aneurysm of the intracavernous part of the ICA.
   - Spontaneous

- Post-surgical (psuedo)
- Sphenoid sinus infected -esp. fungal, can extend into the cavernous sinus
- Large aneurysm -1.widening of SOF- may erode into the floor of middle cranial fossa.
2. Pressure in nerves of caverous sinus cause- ophthalmo plegia.
3. Can rupture into the sp. sinus or SA space → erosion of ant. clinoid process.
   MRA/CA- can be helpful in diagnosis.

AVM/CCF

Arteriovenous shunts in orbit are rare.

CCF- proptosis, chemosis, venous engorgement, pulsatile exophthalmos and an auscultable bruit.

CT/MR =   Proptosis
           Engorgement of SOV
           Increase of ipsilateral EOM.

CST (Cavernous sinus thrombosis)- arises from an infection in an area having venous drainage to the CS.

Source of infection

CST may develop from a septic thrombophlebitis arising in the ophthalmic vein.

Proptosis and ophthalmoplegia, meningitis, B/L CN palsies.

Thrombosed CS- Decrease attenuation non-enhancing lateral border bow laterally.

Carotid artery within the cavernous sinus

SOV = markedly enlarged and often thrombosed.

MR- Enlarged vein that appears less hyperintense than the vein on normal side.

CST= causes- Engorgement of cavernous sinus and ophthalmic veins and enlargement of EOM.

NEOPLASM

Orbital Tumors

Capillary Hemangioma

Infants, during the 1st year of life. Increase size for 6-10 M through the gradually involutes may extend.

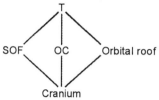

CT—poorly to well-marginated, irregular, enhancing lesions.
• Most are extraconal
Dynamic CT—intense homogeneous enhancement
MR—hypo on T1 and hyper on T2

Lymphoma

Seventy five percent of orbital lymphoma will have systemic lymphoma.
• Seen in adults.
• CT/MR—Homogeneous areas of high density, having a sharp margin seen either in the anterior portion of orbit, retrobulbar area. Sup. orbital compartment.
• *Extension of Extracranial Tumor*
• *Neurogenic Tumor*
 Schwannoma (nerve sheath tumor) arise from nerve sheath. The nerves most common affected in the central skull base trigeminal nerve.
 Tumor can extend through the SOF into the orbit.
 CT—obliteration of fat of SOF—if small.
 Expanded foramen with smooth margin if large.

Enhances after contrast administration.

Similarly neurofibroma can affect the mass.

- *Parasellar chordoma* arising from embryonic notochord, at any age between 30-50 yrs
  - > [Male > Female]
- CT—bone destruction as well as soft tissue mass
  Radiodense- present-represents remaining fragment of bones.
  ST—Enhances
  MR—T1 wt-ST mass- hypo to isocystic areas (hemorrhage/mucoid material)-increase on T1 bony fragment-signal void.
  T2 = High SI.

Meningioma

Can arise from any part of the sphenoid bone, from the initial site of origin, the tumor extends along the dural surface.

Tumor grows into the orbit, causes widening of SOF-patient presents with proptosis.

On CT—Enhancement of the soft tissue component of tumor.

Ca^{++} may be seen

Hyperostosis may be seen

Pneumosinus dilatans

MR—iso to brain parenchyma

GD-DTPA—Enhances homogenously

Dural tail.

Nasopharyngeal Angiofibroma-Benign Tumor

Arising adjacent to sphenopalatine foramen
- Adolescent male boy
- Nasal obst./epistaxis.
- Very vascular.

CT/MR
Enhances intensily
MR = T1 = Intermediate SI, high SI on T2.

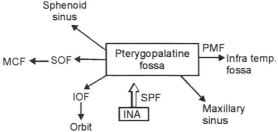

Metastasis

Direct Encroachment

Perineural spread: Tumor can selectively follow a nerve or the sheath of a nerve to reach and ultimatly pass through a foramen.

- Adenoid cystic Ca.
  lymphoma
  melanoma
  SCC.
- Trigeminal nerve and its branches travel from the brain-stem to many areas of the face, sinus and oral cavity. This nerve is primary route for peripheral spread of tumor of head and neck.
- Perineural spread along vein rare but lacrimal gland and skin malignancy can extend along with nerve through SOF.
  - Enlargement of nerve and foramen.
- Effacement/obliteration of the fat plane.
- Enhancement of a normal sized nerve on a Gd. enhancement suggestive of tumor spread.

Flow Chart 8.20.1

SOF enlargement
Pediatric population

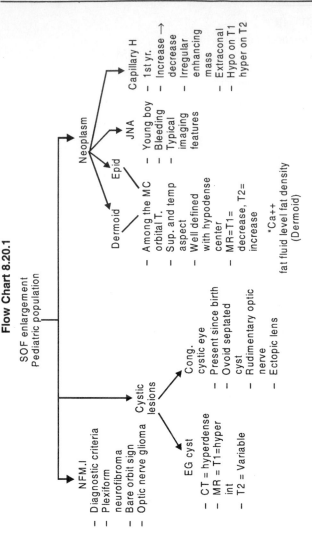

NFM.I
- Diagnostic criteria
- Plexiform neurofibroma
- Bare orbit sign
- Optic nerve glioma

Cystic lesions

EG cyst
- CT = hyperdense
- MR = T1=hyper int
- T2 = Variable

Cong. cystic eye
- Present since birth
- Ovoid septated cyst
- Rudimentary optic nerve
- Ectopic lens

Neoplasm

Dermoid
- Among the MC orbital T.
- Sup. and temp aspect
- Well defined with hypodense center
- MR=T1= decrease, T2= increase
   *Ca++
   fat fluid level fat density (Dermoid)

Epid

JNA
- Young boy
- Bleeding
- Typical imaging features

Capillary H
- 1st yr.
- Increase → decrease
- Irregular enhancing mass
- Extraconal
- Hypo on T1 hyper on T2

Flow Chart 8.20.2

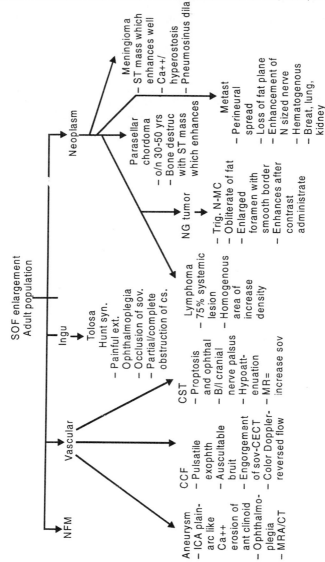

SOF enlargement
Adult population

- NFM

- Vascular

  - Aneurysm
    - ICA plain-arc like
    - Ca++ erosion of ant clinoid
    - Ophthalmo-plegia
    - MRA/CT

  - CCF
    - Pulsatile exophth
    - Auscultable bruit
    - Engorgement of sov-CECT
    - Color Doppler-reversed flow

  - CST
    - Proptosis and ophthal
    - B/l cranial nerve palsy
    - Hypoatt-enuation
    - MR= increase sov

- Ingu

  - Tolosa Hunt syn.
    - Painful ext. Ophthalmoplegia
    - Occlusion of sov.
    - Partial/complete obstruction of cs.

- Neoplasm

  - Lymphoma
    - 75% systemic lesion
    - Homogenous area of increase density

  - NG tumor
    - Trig. N-MC
    - Obliterate of fat
    - Enlarged foramen with smooth border
    - Enhances after contrast administrate

  - Parasellar chordoma
    - o/n 30-50 yrs
    - Bone destruc with ST mass which enhances

  - Meningioma
    - ST mass which enhances well
    - Ca+/ hyperostosis
    - Pneumosinus dila

  - Metast
    - Perineural spread
    - Loss of fat plane
    - Enhancement of N sized nerve
    - Hematogenous
    - Breat, lung, kidney

Hematogenous mets—lung, bronchus, kidney, prostate usually causes lytic destruction.

If GW of sphenoid is affected—metastasis tends to grow in all directions.

8.21 TEMPORAL BONE SCLEROSIS

- Otospongiosa/otosclerosis
- Fibrous dysplasia
- Paget's disease
- Osteogenesis imperfecta
- Osteopetrosis
- Progressive diaphyseal dysplasia
- Endosteal hyperostosis
- Osteopathia striata
- Ossifying fibroma
- Meningioma
- Metastasis
- Inflammatory lesion-chorionic mastoidis
- Hyperparathyroidism
- Labyrinthine ossification.

D/D Temporal Bone Sclerosis

- Otosclerosis/otospongiosa
  Disorder of bony labyrinth stapes.
  Adult male, peak is 2nd-3rd decade
  B/L in 80% cases
- Tinnitus and hearing loss (conductive).

Pathology

Type: Fenestral or retrofenestral (cochlear)

Fenestral: Progressive connective hearing loss.

Normal tympanic membrane, No E/O middle ear inflammation.

HRCT= Early-small, dimineralized focus anterior to oval window- protrudes slightly into the middle ear cavity.

- Narrowing of the oval window, thickening of the post. Piece of the stapes, small decrease density lesion in the lateral wall of the labyrinth.

Cochlear

Combined sensory nerve and conductive hearing loss.

CT = Demineralization of cochlear capsule and area just anterior to the oval window- B/L symmetrical.

- 'Double ring' or 4th turn sign—low density demineralized endochondral defect around the cochlea.
- Chronic/sclerotic phase—these lesion can under go remineralization and become indistinguishable from the normal dense cochlear capsule.

  MR- Both T1 and T2—Very subtle signal changes in demineralized cochlear capsule.

Fibrous Dysplasia

- Unknown etiology. Female more than male in the ratio of 2:1.
- Pathologically: It basically involves the cancellous bone.
- Mono-ostotic—at puberty
- Oligo-ostotic
- Polyostotic—Unilateral—May seen beyond the 3rd or 4th decade.

  R/F—pagetoid—Most common >30 yrs- bony expansion, area of opacity and lucency, sclerotic- temporal bone, younger, expansile, ground glass appearance.

  Cystic—younger, cystic lesion with sclerotic border.

Present as conductive hearing loss, increase size of temporal bone, obstruction of external auditory canal, etc.

CT—Increase in bone thickness and density.

Loss of trabecular pattern.

Obliteration of the mastoid air cells and external auditory canal, cochlear capsule may involved.

MR—low to intermediate signal on both T1 and T2WI images moderate to marked enhancement.

Paget's Disease

Chronic inflammatory disorder that result in the eventual replacement of normal bone by thickened less dense weaker bone.

> 40 yr

Temporal bone-most often B/L.

Petrous pyramid, external auditory canal, middle ear, otic capsule ossicles are rarely involved.

+– Hearing impairment-conductive or sensory nerve or mixed.

HRCT—Decrease density of bone areas may show of mixed appearance of bone thickening and sclerosis.

Mastoid process—Bone thickening, demineralization or a mosaic pattern.

MR = Variable, T1 = decrease signal intensity.

Heterogenous high signal primary hemorrhage.

Osteogenesis Imperfecta (van der Hoeve's Syndrome)

Genetic disorder of connective tissue caused by an error in type I collagen formation.

CT of temporal bone—proliferation of undermineralized, thickened bone around the otic capsule.

Narrowing of middle ear cavity, obstruction of windows, facial canal narrowing.

Demineralization is much more extensive D/D-cochlear ossification.

Osteopetrosis

Defect in the mechanism of bone remodeling.

Generalized increase in bone density.

Temporal bone CT-

Increase density of petrous pyramid and mastoid bone, lack of pneumatization of mastoid air cells.

IOC- shortened and trumpet shaped, ossicles may be thickened and enlarged.

Progressive Diaphyseal Dysplasia

Rare, autosomal dominant.

Diagnosed in childhood.

CT—middle ear may be completely encased by sclerotic bone with wide spread neural foramen narrowing.

Endosteal Hyperostosis

Van Buchem's Disease: Autosomal Recessive:

Temporal bone shows a marked increase in overall size, Extensive sclerosis
Narrowing of EOC and IOC.
Osteopathia striata (Voorhoeve syndrome)—Autosomal dominant generalized temporal bone sclerosis.

Meningioma—Most meningioma arise outside the middle ear from the meninges covering the postpetrous bone. Some meningioma may subsequently invade the temporal bone.

C-P angle < meningioma—can cause temporal bone sclerosis.

CT—Semicircular dural base lesion

Partially calcified and usually enhance, hyperostosis of post. margin of temporal bone is different but air space changes are very sensitive.

MRI—Isointense to brain (gray matter).

Metastasis

Temporal bone is susceptible to any neoplasm that typically metastasizes to bone.

Tumor of breast, lung, stomach, prostate, kidney.

Prostatic and stomach tumors—cause osteoblastic metastasis.

CECT = Enhancement.

Chronic Mastoiditis and CSOM

Following repeated bouts of osteomyelitis and accompanying mastoid infection.

Gradual reduction in the number of mastoid aircells with thickening of mastoid and reactive sclerosis of the bony septa.

Labyrinthine ossification: Ossification of the membranous labyrinth may occur as a result of a previous inflammatory process, trauma, surgery such as labyrinthectomy.

Ossification may be localized and limited to the basilar turn of cochlear or round window niche.

Flow Chart 8.21.1

D/D of temporal bone sclerosis

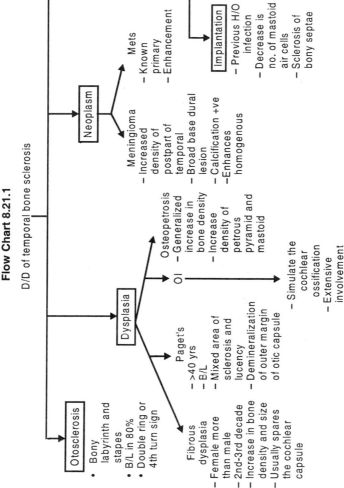

Otosclerosis
- Bony labyrinth and stapes
- B/L in 80%
- Double ring or 4th turn sign

Dysplasia

Fibrous dysplasia
- Female more than male
- 2nd-3rd decade
- Increase in bone density and size
- Usually spares the cochlear capsule

Paget's
- >40 yrs
- B/L
- Mixed area of sclerosis and lucency
- Demineralization of outer margin of otic capsule

OI
- Simulate the cochlear ossification
- Extensive involvement

Osteopetrosis
- Generalized increase in bone density
- Increase density of petrous pyramid and mastoid

Neoplasm

Meningioma
- Increased density of postpart of temporal
- Broad base dural lesion
- Calcification +ve
- Enhances homogenous

Mets
- Known primary
- Enhancement

Implantation
- Previous H/O infection
- Decrease is no. of mastoid air cells
- Sclerosis of bony septae

8.22 IV DISC SPACE CALCIFICATION

1. *Degenerative spondylosis.*
   Seen in nucleus pulposus.
   Confined to dorsal region.
   Other signs of degenerative spondylosis
   - Disc space narrowing
   - Osteophytosis
   - Vacuum sign
2. *Alkaptonuria*
   Onset of arthropathy—4th decade.
   - Osteophytosis.
   - Disc space narrowing.
   - Osteoporosis.
   Calcification is in the inner fibers of annulus fibrosus
   Severe changes progress to ankylosis.
3. *CPPD*
   Calcification seen in outer fibers of annulus fibrosus.
   Associated conditions—
   hyperparathyroidism.
   hemachromatosis, gout, Wilson's disease.
   - Osteophyte formation.
4. *Ankylosing spondylitis*
   - Calcification in outerfibers of annulus fibrosus.
   - Square vertebral bodies.
   - Syndesmophytes formation.
   - Ankylosis.
5. *Juvenile chronic arthritis* may mimic anykylosing spondylitis.
6. *DISH* (Diffuse idiopathic skeletal hyperostosis.)
   - Elderly male.

Flow Chart 8.22.1

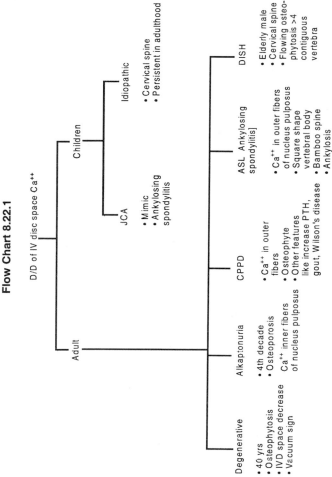

D/D of IV disc space Ca⁺⁺

- **Adult**
  - **Degenerative**
    - 40 yrs
    - Osteophytosis
    - IVD space decrease
    - Vacuum sign
  - **Alkaptonuria**
    - 4th decade
    - Osteoporosis
    - Ca⁺ inner fibers of nucleus pulposus
  - **CPPD**
    - Ca⁺⁺ in outer fibers
    - Osteophyte
    - Other features like increase PTH, gout, Wilson's disease
  - **ASL Ankylosing spondylitis]**
    - Ca⁺⁺ in outer fibers of nucleus pulposus
    - Square shape vertebral body
    - Bamboo spine
    - Ankylosis
  - **DISH**
    - Elderly male
    - Cervical spine
    - Flowing osteophytosis >4 contiguous vertebra
- **Children**
  - **JCA**
    - Mimic
    - Ankylosing spondylitis
  - **Idiopathic**
    - Cervical spine
    - Persistent in adulthood

Common location—Cervical spine.

Anterior flowing osteophytes involving >4 contiguous vertebra.

7. *Gout*

May show IVD calcification

Predilection of joints of lower extremity esp. 1st metatarsophalangeal joints.

8. *Idiopathic*—Seen in children.

Cervical spine—Most often affected, may be asymptomatic or associated with fever/neck pain persistent in adults.

9. Following spinal fusion.

8.23 IVORY VERTEBRAL BODY

Single or Multiple Very Dense Vertebrae
1. Lymphoma
2. Osteopetrosis
3. Osteoblastic metastasis
4. Paget's disease
5. Low grade infection
6. Hemangioma
7. Trauma
8. Fluorosis
9. Myelosclerosis
10. Sickle cell disease

1. *Lymphoma* - MC is HD(Hodgkin's).
   - Normal size vertebral body.
   - Disc space intact.
   - Mediastinal, retroperitoneal RP and mesenteric lymphadenopathy.
2. *Osteopetrosis*
   Defective osteoclast function with failure of proper reabsorption.
   - Rugger jersy spine—Sclerosis of both endplates of vertebra or sandwich spine.
   - Diffuse osteosclerosis.
3. *Osteoblastic metastasis*
   - Usual primary site are prostate, stomach and carcinoid.
   - Initial lytic metastasis which after treatment has become sclerotic.
   - Normal vertebral body size.
   - IVD space preserved until late.
4. *Paget's disease*
   - Usually a single vertebral body is affected.

- Expanded vertebral body with a thickened cortex and coarsened trabeculation.
- IVD space normal
5. *Low grade infection*
   - End plate destruction.
   - IVD space narrowing.
   - Paraspinal soft tissue mass.
6. *Hemangioma*
   - Sclerosis is accompanied by coarsened trabecular pattern with prominent vertical striation.
   - Expansion may or may not be .
   - IVD space - normal
7. *Trauma*
   With H/O trauma.
   - Vertebral height is usually decrease with anterior wedging.
   - IVD space - normal
8. *Fluorosis:* Due to chronic fluoride poisoning.
   - Generalized increase in bone density.
   - Characteristics feature is calcification in the interrosseous membrane.
   - Thorn spine.
9. *Myelosclerosis*
   Hematologic disorder of unknown etiology with gradual replacement of bone marrow elements by fibrosis.
   - > 50 yrs.
   - Lumbar spine - most common spine to be involved.
   - Rugger jersy spine.
   - Diffuse increase in density in almost all bones.
10. *Sickel cell disorder*
    - Hematological disorder.
    - Biconcare vertebral due to depression of the central portion of the vertebral end plate and 'H' shaped vertebrae.
    - Due to infarction of vertebral body.

Flow Chart 8.23.1: Ivory vertebral body

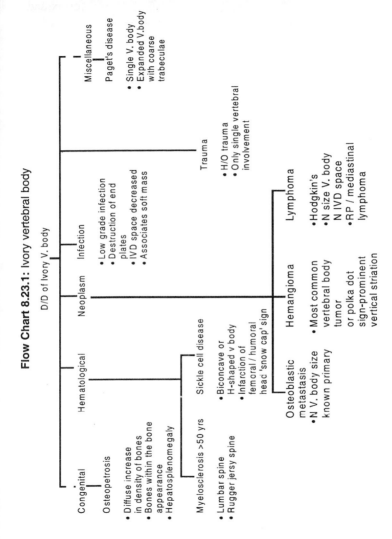

D/D of Ivory V. body

Congenital

Osteopetrosis

• Diffuse increase in density of bones
• Bones within the bone appearance
• Hepatosplenomegaly

Hematological

Myelosclerosis >50 yrs

• Lumbar spine
• Rugger jersy spine

Sickle cell disease

• Biconcave or H-shaped v body
• Infarction of femoral / humoral head 'snow cap' sign

Neoplasm

Osteoblastic metastasis

• N V. body size known primary

Hemangioma

• Most common vertebral body tumor or polka dot sign-prominent vertical striation

Lymphoma

• Hodgkin's
• N size V. body
• N IVD space
• RP / mediastinal lymphoma

Infection

• Low grade infection
• Destruction of end plates
• IVD space decreased
• Associates soft mass

Trauma

• H/O trauma
• Only single vertebral involvement

Miscellaneous

Paget's disease

• Single V. body
• Expanded V.body with coarse trabeculae

8.24 ATLANTO AXIAL SUBLUXATION

When the distance between the post aspect of anterior arch of atlas and anterior aspect of the odontoid process exceed 3 mm in adults and older children or 5 mm in younger children.

Causes

1. *Trauma*
   - Usually associated with odontoid fracture.
2. *Congenital*
   Occipitalization of atlas—fusion of basion and anterior arch of atlas.
   - Congenital insufficiency of transverse ligament.
   - OS odontoideum/aplasia of dens.
   - Down's syndrome.
   - Morquio's syndrome
   - Bone dysplasia.
3. *Arthritis*
   Due to laxity of transverse ligament or erosion of dens.
   - Rh. arthritis—associated erosion of odontoid.
   - Psoriasis.
   - Reiter's syndrome
   - AS - usually a late features.
4. *Inflammatory process*
   Pharyngeal infection in childhood, retropharyngeal abscess, coryza, otitis media, etc.
   - Destruction occur after 8-10 days of onset of symptoms.

8.25 POSTERIOR SCALLOPING OF VERTEBRAL BODY

1. Tumors in the spinal canal.
   Ependymoma—most common
   dermoid, lipoma/neurofibroma and less commonly meningioma, these lesion causes raised intraspinal pressure which leads to scalloping of vertebral body.
   - Ependymoma—Usually site is lower spinal cord, conus medullaris well demarcated/diffusely infiltrating tumor.
   - Local mass with extensive areas of cystic degenerates, hemorrhagic and Ca^{++} calcification.
2. *Chronic-hydrocephalus* (Communicating/-also known as extraventricular hydrocephalus.
   R/F = symmetric enlargement of lateral 3rd and 4 ventricle.
   - Dilatation of subarachnoid cisterns.
   - Normal or effaced.
   - Transependymal flow of CSF.

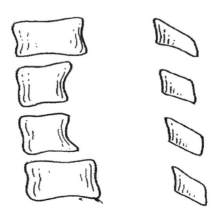

Fig. 8.25.1: Posterior scalloping of vertebral bodies

3. *Neurofibromatosis*—Scalloping is due to mesodermal dysplasia and is associated with dural ectasia.
   May be enlargement of an intervertebral foramen and flattening of one pedicle - "Dumb-bell" tumor.
4. *Acromegaly*
   - Increase AP transverse diameter of vertebral body.
   - Osteoporosis.
   - Spur formation.
   - Calcified discs
   - Increase heel pad thickness, prognathism, spade-like fingers.
5. *Achondroplasia*
   - Spinal stenosis
   - Anterior vertebral body peaks in upper lumbar spine, wide intervertebral foramen.
   - Lumbar angulation kyphosis+sacral lordosis.
6. *Mucopolysaccharidoses*
   In Hurler and Hunter disease
   In Hurler = Dorsolumbar kyphosis with lumbar gibbus
   Anterior-beak at T12/L1/L2
   Long slender pedicle
   - Spatulated rib configuration
7. *Morquio's syndrome*
   - Hypoplasia/absence of odontoid process of C1-C2 instability with anterior subluxation.
   - Platyspondyly-
   - Ovoid vertebral body with central anterior beak. at lower thoracic and upper lumbar vertebral.
   - Widened I/V disc spaces.
- *Osteogenesis imperfecta*
   - Biconcave vertebral body.
       Schmorl's nodes.
       Increase height of I/V disc space.
- *Marfan's syndrome*

Flow Chart 8.25.1: Post scalloping of vertebral body

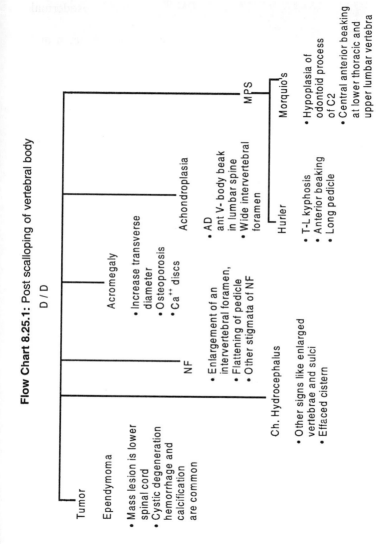

D / D

Tumor

Ependymoma
- Mass lesion is lower spinal cord
- Cystic degeneration hemorrhage and calcification are common

Ch. Hydrocephalus
- Other signs like enlarged vertebrae and sulci
- Effaced cistern

NF
- Enlargement of an intervertebral foramen,
- Flattening of pedicle
- Other stigmata of NF

Acromegaly
- Increase transverse diameter
- Osteoporosis
- Ca^{++} discs

Achondroplasia
- AD ant V- body beak in lumbar spine
- Wide intervertebral foramen

Hurler
- T-L kyphosis
- Anterior beaking
- Long pedicle

MPS

Morquio's
- Hypoplasia of odontoid process of C2
- Central anterior beaking at lower thoracic and upper lumbar vertebra

8.26 ANTERIOR SCALLOPING OF VERTEBRAL BODIES

1. *Aortic aneurysm*
   - IVD space remain intact.
   - Well defined anterior vertebral margin.
   - Calcification may or may not be seen.
   - Usually seen in elderly patient M:F = 5:1.
   - Widening of aorta. Twice the size of normal aorta.
2. *Tubercular spondylitis*
   - Marginal erosion of effected vertebral-bodies.
   - Ivory vertebrae - Reossification as healing response to osteonecrosis.
   - IVD space destruction.
   - Widening of paraspinal soft tissue mass.

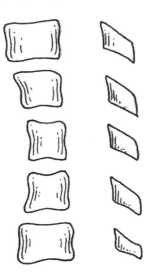

Fig. 8.26.1: Anterior scalloping of vertebral bodies

- Calcification may or may not be seen.
- Usually seen is children and adults.
- Dorsolumbar region is the most common to be involved. Multiple contiguous involvement of multiple segments.
- Angular kyphotic deformity in adults.

3. *Lymphadenopathy*
   - Pressure resorption of bones results in a well defined anterior vertebral body margin unless there is a malignant infiltration of bones.
   - IVD space maintained.

4. *Delayed motor development*
   (*Down's syndrome*)
   Also k/a mongolism – Trisomy-21.
   - Atlantoaxial subluxation
   - "Squared vertebral-bodies" – Center high and narrow.
   - Positive lateral lumbar index – (ratio of horizontal to vertical diameter of L2).

Flow Chart 8.26.1

D/D of ant. Scalloping of vertebral bodies

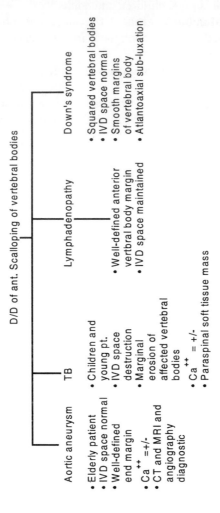

Aortic aneurysm
- Elderly patient
- IVD space normal
- Well-defined end margin
- $Ca^{++} = +/-$
- CT and MRI and angiography diagnostic

TB
- Children and young pt.
- IVD space destruction
- Marginal erosion of affected vertebral bodies
- $Ca^{++} = +/-$
- Paraspinal soft tissue mass

Lymphadenopathy
- Well-defined anterior vertebral body margin
- IVD space maintained

Down's syndrome
- Squared vertebral bodies
- IVD space normal
- Smooth margins of vertebral body
- Atlantoaxial sub-luxation

8.27 ANTERIOR VERTEBRAL BODY BEAKS

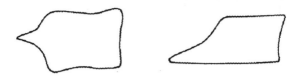

Central **Lower 1/3rd**

Diagrame-involves 1-3 vertebral bodies at the dorsolumbar junction and usually associated with kyphosis.

Hypotonia is probably the factor with leads to an exaggerated dorsolumbar kyphosis, anterior herniation of the nucleus pulposus and subsequently an anterior vertebral body defect.

- *Central beaking*
  1. Morquio's syndrome
  2. Psuedoachondroplasia.
- *Lower 1/3rd*
  1. Hurler's syndrome
  2. Achondroplasia.
  3. Cretinism.
  4. Down's syndrome
  5. Neuromuscular disorder.

1. MPS

   Morquio's—central beaking at dorsolumbar vertebral body. Hypoplasia/absence of odontoid process.

   C1-C2 instability with anterior subluxation.

   Platyspondyly.

   Widened IVD space

Hurler Syndrome

Beaking in lower 1/3rd of vertebral body
Anterior beaking at T12 /L1/L2.
Long slender pedicle.
IVD space - N
Spatulated rib configuration.

Achondroplasia

Beaking in the lower part of lumbar vertebral bodies, spinal stenosis.
Wide intervertebral foramen.
Lumbar angular kyphosis + sacral lordosis.
Psuedochandroplasia
Cretinism or hypothyroidism
- Demineralization
- Dense vertebral margins
- Delayed skeletal maturation
- Fragmented, stippled ossification
- Wide sinuses /fontanelles with delayed closure.

Down's syndrome

- Trisomy 21
- Atlantoaxial subluxation
- Squared vertebral bodies
- Positive lateral lumbar index (ratio of horizontal to vertical diameter of L2)
- IVD space N.

Flow Chart 8.27.1

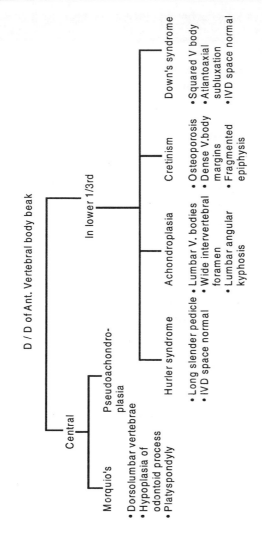

D / D of Ant. Vertebral body beak

Central

In lower 1/3rd

Morquio's
• Dorsolumbar vertebrae
• Hypoplasia of odontoid process
• Platyspondyly

Pseudoachondro-plasia

Hurler syndrome
• Long slender pedicle
• IVD space normal

Achondroplasia
• Lumbar V. bodies
• Wide intervertebral foramen
• Lumbar angular kyphosis

Cretinism
• Osteoporosis
• Dense V.body margins
• Fragmented epiphysis

Down's syndrome
• Squared V body
• Atlantoaxial subluxation
• IVD space normal

8.28 BLOCK VERTEBRA

- Congenital
- Kippel-Feil syndrome
- Rheumatoid arthritis
- Ankylosing spondylitis
- Tuberculosis
- Operative fusion
- Post traumatic

1. *Congenital*
   - Segmentation failure
   - Most common site—lumbar and cervical spine
   - The ring epiphysis of adjacent vertebrae do not develop and thus the AP diameter of the vertebral at the site of the segmentation defect is decreased.
   - Anterior concavity.
   - The articular facet, neural arches or spinous process may also be involved.
   - A faint lucency can be seen, sometimes representing vestigeal disc.

2. *Kippel-Feil syndrome*
   - Segmentation defect in cervical spine.
   - Feil's triad -   low hairline
                       short neck
                       limited cervical movement.
   - C2-C3 and C5-C6 are most common involved.
   - Scoliosis >20 in >50% of pts.
   - Sprengel's shoulder –30%
     +/– omovertebral body.
   - Cervical ribs.
   - Facial asymmetry.
   - Genitourinary abnormality –66%
   - Renal agenesis in 33%
   - Deafness in 33%.

3. *Rheumatoid arthritis*
   Esp. juvenile chronic arthritis, juvenile onset rheumatoid arthritis.
   – Angulation at fusion site.
   – Posterior element usually do not fuse.
4. *Ankylosing spondylitis*
   Middle aged patient
   – Squaring of vertebral body because of fusion of anterior concavity of vertebral body.
   – Calcification in IVD space and ant. and post- long-ligament.
   – Syndesmophyte formation—extending from one vertebral margin to another.
5. *TB*
   – Usually affects young patients
   – Vertebral body collapse.
   – Destruction of IVD space.
   – Paraspinal soft tissue mass.
   – Paraspinal calcification
   – May be angulation of spine.
6. *Postoperative fusion*
   H/O operation.
7. *Post traumatic*

Flow Chart 8.28.1

D / D Block vertebra

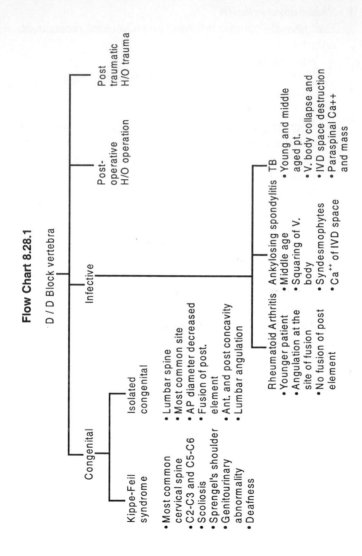

Congenital

Kippe-Feil syndrome
- Most common cervical spine
- C2-C3 and C5-C6
- Scoliosis
- Sprengel's shoulder
- Genitourinary abnormality
- Deafness

Isolated congenital
- Lumbar spine
- Most common site
- AP diameter decreased
- Fusion of post. element
- Ant. and post concavity
- Lumbar angulation

Infective

Rheumatoid Arthritis
- Younger patient
- Angulation at the site of fusion
- No fusion of post element

Ankylosing spondylitis
- Middle age
- Squaring of V. body
- Syndesmophytes
- Ca^{++} of IVD space

TB
- Young and middle aged pt.
- V. body collapse and
- IVD space destruction
- Paraspinal Ca^{++} and mass

Post-operative
H/O operation

Post traumatic
H/O trauma

8.29 ENLARGED VERTEBRAL BODY

Gereralized

1. Gigantism
2. Acromegaly

Local—Single or Multiple

1. Paget's disease
2. Benign bone tumor.
   a. ABC.
   b. Hemangioma
   c. GCT
3. Hydatid

   Gigantism - Excess of growth hormone before skeletal maturity results in gigantism.

   Acromegaly - Results from excessive GH production by an eosinophilic adenoma after skeletal maturity.
   - Enlargement of spine or vertebral bodies with characteristic posterior scalloping.

Other characteristic features are:
- Enlarged mastoid air cells and sinuses.
- Pituitary fossa enlargement.
- Spade like fingers.
- Increase thickness of heel pad.

Paget's disease - Esp. involves the lumbar spine. Age >40 yrs.
- Enlargement and coarsened trabeculae.
- Cortical thickening producing picture framing.
- Can also involves the appendages and neural arch.

ABC

Age = 10-30 yrs.

- Usually lytic and expansile lesion but cortex intact.
- Involves both the anterior and posterior elements, more commonly shows rapid growth.
- Thin internal strands of bone.
- *Hemangioma*
  - Most common benign tumor of vertebral body.
  age - 10-50 yrs.
  Site - dorsal or lumbar.
  Usually affects the vertebral body, but rarely involves the posterior elements.
  Prominent primary trabeculae with lytic vertebral body- "Accordion sign".

GCT

Involvement of the body alone is most common. Expansion is minimal.

Hydatid

Over 40% of cases of hydatid disease in bones occur in vertebra.
- Thoracic region is most common site.
- Disease tends to involve adjacent vertebrae and ribs and to spare the I/V discs.
- Cysts cause bubble-like round or lobulated circumscribed lytic lesions in the bones with virtually no sclerotic reaction.
- Adjacent soft tissue mass which tend to be extensive and cause extradural compression.

Flow Chart 8.29.1: Enlarged vertebral body

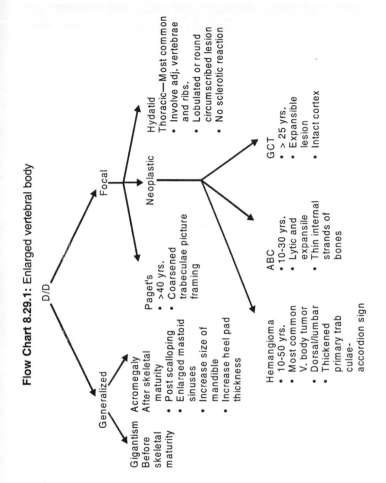

D/D

Generalized

- Gigantism
  Before skeletal maturity

- Acromegaly
  After skeletal maturity
  - Post scalloping
  - Enlarged mastoid sinuses
  - Increase size of mandible
  - Increase heel pad thickness

Focal

Paget's
- >40 yrs.
- Coarsened trabeculae picture framing

Neoplastic

- Hemangioma
  - 10-50 yrs.
  - Most common V. body tumor
  - Dorsal/lumbar
  - Thickened primary trabeculae-accordion sign

- ABC
  - 10-30 yrs.
  - Lytic and expansile
  - Thin internal strands of bones

- GCT
  - > 25 yrs.
  - Expansible lesion
  - Intact cortex

Hydatid
Thoracic—Most common
- Involve adj. vertebrae and ribs.
- Lobulated or round circumscribed lesion
- No sclerotic reaction

8.30 SOLITARY COLLAPSED VERTEBRA

D/D

1. Langerhans' cell histiocytosis
2. Neoplastic disease
   Malig.
   - Metastasis
   - Multiple myeloma/plasmocytoma.
     Lymphoma

Benign

- Hemangioma
- GCT
- ABC
3. Osteoporosis
4. Trauma
5. Infection
6. Paget's disease

Langerhans' Cell Histiocytosis

Eosinophilic granuloma is the most frequent cause of a solitary vertebral plana in childhood.
- Vertebral plana is osteochondritis of vertebral body causes increase density and collapse of vertebral body.
- Adjacent disc spaces are normal or increase.
- Posterior elements are usually spared.
- *Neoplastic Disease*

Benign

Hemangioma

Most common benign tumor of spine.
Age = 10-45 yrs.

Site - Lumbar spine is the most common site.

Fifty percent only in the vertebral body and half may extend into the post-element.

Size of vertebral body—Normal

Soft tissue mass is seen in small number of patients.

R/F = Increase translucency with a characteristic fine vertical striation.

GCT-Rarely seen in spine.

Age = 20-40 yrs (Mature skeleton)

R/F—A zone of radiolucency without evidence of calcification or new bone formation.

Site = Neural arch is more commonly involved than body.

Age = 10-20 yrs in immature skeleton.

R/F = Area of bone resorption with slight or marked expansion.

Malignant Lesion

Metastasis

Breast, bronchus, prostate, kidney and thyroid account for the majority of patients with a solitary spine metastasis.

- Focal areas of bone destruction.
- Disc spaces are preserved until late.
- Destruction of pedicle = +
- The bone may be lytic, sclerotic or mixed.

Multiple Myeloma/Plasmacytoma

- Common site for plasmacytoma
- Age = Elderly
- Osteopenia with discrete lucencies—The lucencies are usually widely disseminated at the time of diagnosis -seen in spine, pelvis, skull, ribs and shafts of long bones uniform in size and are well defined.

- Vertebral body collapse occasionally with disc destruction paravertebral shadows may or may not be seen.
- Involvement of pedicle is late.
  Normal Alk. phosphatase level.
  - Osteoporosis
  Usually seen in older population.
  - Generalized osteopenia.
  - Coarse trabecular pattern due to resorption of secondary trabeculae.
  - Preserved I/V disc space.
3. *Trauma*
  - IV disc spaces are usually preserved.
4. *Infection*
  Destruction of vertebral end plates and adjacent disc spaces.
  Collapse is usually accompanied by soft tissue mass.
  Blurring or displacement of psoas shadows.
5. *Eosinophilic granuloma*
  Most common cause of a solitary vertebral plana in childhood.
  Adjacent disc spaces are usually normal or increase in height. Post elements are usually spared.
6. *Paget's disease*
  - Neural arch is affected in most cases, sclerosis and expansion is seen.
  - Width of body increase. Increase in interpedicular distance. Characteristic finding of picture framing is seen due to thickened vertebral end plates.
  Collapse is common and may cause spinal nerve compression. Vertebral enlargement distinguishes this from osteoporotic or malignant disease.

8.31 MULTIPLE COLLAPSED VERTEBRAE

1. Osteoporosis
2. Neoplastic disease
3. Trauma
4. Scheuermann's disease
5. Infection
6. Langerhans' cell histiocytosis
7. Sickle cell anemia.

Osteoporosis

Decrease in bone mass
Trabeculae loss → Pencilling of vertebral by the more radiographically dense plates.
Biconcave vertebral bodies (codfish vertebrae)

Neoplastic Disease

Usually wedge fracture are seen.
Seen in osteolytic metastasis and osteolytic marrow tumors e.g. multiple myeloma, leukemia and lymphoma.
R/F = Altered or obliterated normal trabeculae.
Disc space are usually preserved until late.
Paravertebral soft tissue mass is more common.

Trauma

- H/O of trauma, usually lower cervical, lower dorsal or upper lumbar.
- Discontinuity trabeculae.
- Sclerosis of fracture line due to compressed and overlapped trabeculae.
- Disc spaces are preserved.
- Usually without soft tissue mass.

Infection

- Usually starts anteriorly beneath the end plates.
- Extends beneath the anterior longitudinal ligament or into the disc which is rapidly destroyed and loses height.
- Vertebral destruction in the body above or below.
- In most cases two vertebral bodies are involved.
- Collapse of vertebral body is usually accompanied by soft tissue masses.
- Blurring or displacement of psoas shadows.
- Kyphosis and cord compression may also seen.
- Radiologically it is not possible to differentiate between pyogenic and tubercular but few signs are said to be helpful. Pyogenic is rapidly progressive while TB is slow in progress. Pyogenic infection shows marked osteoblastic response and TB usually associated with large para-vertebral abscess.
- Scheurmann's disease
  - Age—onset at puberty.
  - Location—LT or UL (Lower thoracic or upper lumbar)
  R/F= Ant. wedging of vertebral body of >5.
      Increase AP diameter of vertebral body.
      Slight narrowing of I/V disc space.
      Schmorl nodes—upto 30% of cases.
      End plate irregularity.

Infection

Both tubercular and pyogenic can cause collapse of vertebrae.
  In Indian setting TB is more common than pyogenic.
  R/F = Destruction of end plates adjacent to a destroyed discs. Paravertebral soft tissue abscess with or without calcification.

Langerhans' Cell Histiocytosis

Most common site is thoracic
- Disc spaces preserved.
- Rare involvement of post. elements.
- No kyphosis.

Sickle Cell Anemia

Characteristic step like depression in the central part of the end plate.

8.32 INTRASPINAL MASSES

Can be classified into 3 category:
1. Extradural masses
2. Intradural extramedullary
3. Intramedullary

i. Extradural Mass

1. *Prolapsed or sequestered IVD*
   Occur at all levels - Most common L4-L5, L5-S1 in cervical spine—C6-C7 is most common.
   Usually extradural but occasionally penetrates dura, especially is thoracic region.
   - NECT = soft tissue mass with effacement of the epidural fat and displacement of the thecal sac.
   - MR - will delineate the extent of Herniated nucleus pulposus.
2. *Metastasis*
   Myeloma and lymphoma deposits are common.
   - Associated vertebral infiltration.
   - Destruction in body or neural arch may lead to collapse.

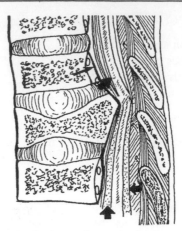

Fig. 8.32.1: Imaging features of an extradural mass—The dura (small arrow) and spinal cord (large arrows) are displaced

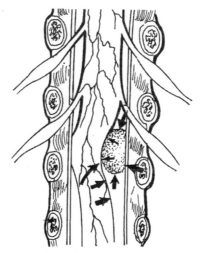

Fig. 8.32.2: Imaging findings of an extramedullary intradural mass—Mass displaces the spinal cord and enlarges the lateral subarachnoid space. A sharp crescenteric interface formed between mass and contrast column

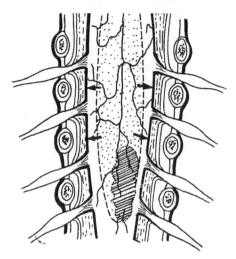

Fig. 8.32.3: Imaging features of an intramedullary mass—shows diffuse cord enlargement

- Paravertebral mass
- E/O primary tumor.

3. *Neurofibroma*

   Solitary or multiple in neurofibromatosis.

   Lateral indentation of theca at the level of the intervertebral foramen.

   - Enlarged neural foramina.

4. *Tumors*

   Hemangioma—Most common benign tumor of vertebral body. Focal or diffuse.

   Lytic lesion with prominent vertical striation.

   Neuroblastoma or *ganglioneuroma-*

   - Common in pediatric population.
   - Arising from sympathetic chain in paraspinal location.

   Meningioma

   In 85% cases they are intradural.

15%—Extradural.

Sex = F > M, middle aged.

Site = thoracic spine.

5. *Hematoma* - May be due to trauma, dural AVM.

Anticoagulant therapy

CT and MRI show signal characteristic of blood on MR—hyperintense on both T1 and T2 Wt. images.

6. *Abscess* - *Epidural abscess*

Secondary to disc or vertebral sepsis, long segment extradural mass with marginal enhancement (usually involves >6 vertebra).

Plain film—Osteomyelitis disc space narrowing. Myelogram, CT myelogram-extradural soft tissue mass.

MR = Extradural soft tissue mass iso to hypo on T1 hyper on T2

CEMR = Diffuse homogenous or slightly heterogenous enhancement is seen is 70% cases—phlegmonous stage or thick/thin enhancing rim that surrounds a liquified low signal pus collection.

7. *Extradural arachnoid cysts*

Are CSF fluid out pouchings of arachnoid that protrude through a dural defect.

2/3rd in lower thoracic spine.

– Long segment CSF density extradural mass.

– Widening of interpedicular distance.

– Scalloping of vertebral bodies.

– Pedicle thinning, erosion.

Flow Chart 8.32.1

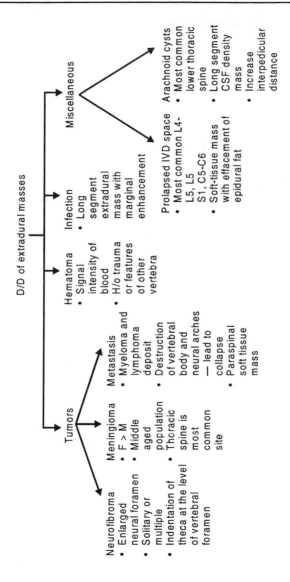

D/D of extradural masses

Tumors

Neurofibroma
- Enlarged neural foramen
- Solitary or multiple
- Indentation of theca at the level of vertebral foramen

Meningioma
- F > M
- Middle aged population
- Thoracic spine is most common site

Metastasis
- Myeloma and lymphoma deposit
- Destruction of vertebral body and neural arches — lead to collapse
- Paraspinal soft tissue mass

Hematoma
- Signal intensity of blood
- H/o trauma or features of other vertebra

Infection
- Long segment extradural mass with marginal enhancement

Miscellaneous

Prolapsed IVD space
- Most common L4-L5, L5 S1, C5-C6
- Soft-tissue mass with effacement of epidural fat

Arachnoid cysts
- Most common lower thoracic spine
- Long segment CSF density mass
- Increase interpedicular distance

ii. Intramedullary Masses

A. Tumors

1. *Ependymoma*—Most common intramedullary tumor in adults.

   Mean age = 43 yrs.

   Location—conus medullaris and filum terminale

   plain film—wide canal or bone destruction.

   Myelography—Nonspecific cord widening multi-segmental lesion.

   CT = Nonspecific canal widening.

   Scalloped post vertebral body.

   Enlarged neural foramina.

   MR = iso to cord on T1 and hyper on T2

2. *Astrocytoma*—Low grade tumors.

   Most common intramedullary tumor in children.

   Cervical spine is most common site.

   Multisegmental involvement is the rule.

   Plain film – Widened interpedicular distance with mild scoliosis.

   NECT   –   Widened canal, multisegmental cord enlargement

   MR   –   Iso or slighty hypo on T1 wt images
                 hyperintense on T2 wt images
                 Enhances following contrast administration.

3. *Hemangioblastoma*

   75% intramedullary.

   50% occur in thoracic cord.

   Imaging - Dilated tortuous feeding artery and veins.

   MR = Diffuse cord expansion with high signal on T2 wt images

   Cyst formation or syrinx = 50-70% of cases.

4. *Dermoid*—Including lipoma, teratoma
   Most common site—conus medullaris.
   CT and MR signal—lipomatous tissue -decrease signal on CT, bright on T1.
   Cystic space—Decrease on CT, increase on T2.
   Soft tissue—Intermediate on CT and T1, WMRI.
   Enhance after contrast administration.
5. *Cysts*
   – Congenital and acquired hydrosyringomyelia.
   – Inflammatory cysts.
   – Hematomyelia.
   MRI = With contrast enhancement is helpful in differentiating these from cord neoplasm.
   All cord neoplasm will enhance while cysts do not.
6. *Hematoma/contusion*
   on CT = Only E/O cord swelling.
   MR = Blood signal - Increase on T1 and T2
7. *Myelitis/cord edema*
   CT = Nonspecific
   MR = T1 = isointense T2 = hyperintense.
8. *Infarct*—Expanding in acute phase.

Flow Chart 8.32.2

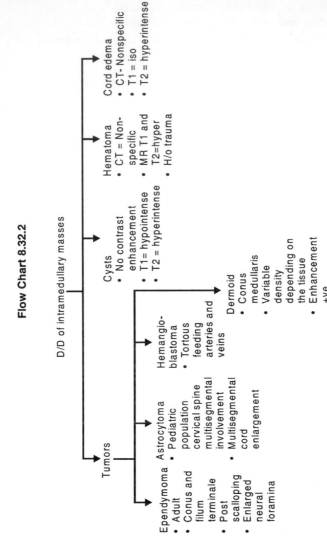

D/D of intramedullary masses

Tumors

Ependymoma
- Adult
- Conus and filum terminale
- Post scalloping
- Enlarged neural foramina

Astrocytoma
- Pediatric population
- cervical spine multisegmental involvement
- Multisegmental cord enlargement

Hemangio-blastoma
- Tortous feeding arteries and veins

Dermoid
- Conus medullaris
- Variable density depending on the tissue
- Enhancement +ve

Cysts
- No contrast enhancement
- T1 = hypointense
- T2 = hyperintense

Hematoma
- CT = Non-specific
- MR T1 and T2=hyper
- H/o trauma

Cord edema
- CT- Nonspecific
- T1 = iso
- T2 = hyperintense

8.33 DIFFERENTIAL DIAGNOSIS OF POSTERIOR FOSSA CYSTS

- Dandy-walker malformation
- Dandy-walker variant
- Mega cisterna magna
- Posterior fossa arachnoid cyst
- Enterogenous cyst
- Inflammatory cyst
- Cystic neoplasm
- Dermoid
- Epidermoid

Dandy-Walker Malformation

- Failure of development of the anterior medullary velum, atresia of the 4th ventricle outlet foramina

Skull and Dura

- Large posterior fossa
- High tentorial insertion (Lambdoid - torcular inversion)
- High transverse sinuses

Ventricles and CSF Spaces

- Fourth ventricle open dorsally to large posterior fossa cyst
- Hydrocephalus in 80%

Cerebellum, Vermis and Brainstem

- Vermian and cerebeller hemispheres hypoplasia
- Vermian remanant anterosuperiorly everted above cyst
- Cerebeller hemispheres winged anterolaterally in front of cyst.
- Brainstem may be hypoplastic, compressed
- Heterotopias, cerebellar dysplasias common

Associated CNS anomalies
Corpus callosum agenesis in 20-25%
Heterotopias, gyral anomalies, schizencephaly.
Cephaloceles.

Dandy-Walker Variant

- Mild vermian hypoplasia with a variably sized cystic space caused by open communication of the posterior fourth ventricle and cisterna magna through an enlarged vallecula. (Key-Hole) (deformity).
- 4th ventricle is often enlarged but the posterior fossa is typically normal size.
- The inferior vermian lobules are variably hypoplastic.

Mega Cisterna Magna

- A large cisterna magna is present and may extend above the vermis to the straight sinus.
- Occasionally, posterior fossa appear enlarged with scalloping of occipital square.
- An enlarged normal cisterna magna is easily opacified following contrast instillation into the lumbar arachnoid space.

Arachnoid Cyst

- Benign, congenital, intra arachnoidal, space occupying lesions that are filled with CSF like fluid.
- Occur in all ages but 75% occur in children
- 50-65%- in mid. cranial fossa
  5-10%- posterior fossa (cerebellopontine angle and cisterna magna)
  CT- Smoothly demarcated, noncalcified extraaxial mass that does not enhance.
- Unless hemorrhage occurs, arachnoid cysts are similar to CSF in attenuation.

- Pressure erosion of the adjacent calvarium can occurs
- Cyst may displace vermis and 4th ventricle.

Enterogenous Cyst (Neurenteric Cyst)

- Are rare intraspinal masses and even less frequent intra-cranial lesions.
- Typically intradural extramedullary posterior fossa masses
- Cerebellopontine angle and craniocervical junction.
  CT- well defined, noncalcified, nonenhancing lobulated mass and are typically hypodense compared to adjacent brain parenchyma.
  MR- Most lesions are iso or mildly hyperintense compared to CSF on T1 weight images and moderate hyperintense on proton density and T2 weight images.

Pilocystic Astrocytoma

- 5-10% of all glioma's
- Children, young adults
- Located typically around 3rd and 4th ventricle.
  – optic chiasma hypothalamus—Most common
  Cerebellar vermis/hemispheres-Next.
  CT- Round or oval sharply demarcated and smoothly marginated hypo or isodense masses.
- Calcification occurs in 10%
- Some lesions enhance homogeneously and solidly others have a small enhancing mural nodule in large cyst.
- Wall does not show enhancement (Non-neoplastic)
- In some the cyst fluid enhances, with dependent layering that creates a contrast-fluid level, particularly if delayed scans are obtained.
- Hydrocephalus may occur relatively early and moderate. Severe if in vermis.
MR- Hypo or isointense on T1
       Hyperintense on T2
  Mural nodules and solid tumors enhance strongly but somewhat inhomogeneously.

Table 8.33.1: D/D Post fossae cysts

	Dandy-Walker malformation	D-W variant	Mega cisterna magna	PFAC	Enterogenous cyst	Inflam. cyst	Dermoid	Cystic neoplasm
Location	Occupies most of the post fossa	Midline posterior	Midline, posterior	Post midline CP angle	Anterior to brainstem	Any location	Midline 4th vent.	Vermis cerebellum
4th vent.	Floor present, open dorsally to large cyst	Key hole appearance	N	N but displaced	N	N	N but distorted/displaced	N but displaced
Vermis	Absent hypoplastic everted over cyst	Inf. lobules hypoplastic	N	N but distorted	N	N	N but distorted	N but distorted
Obstructive hydrocephalus	+	–	–	Variable	–	Variable	Variable	+
Contrast enhancement	–	–	–	–	–	+	±	+
Calcification	–	–	–	–	–	+	+	+
Cyst density	CSF	CSF	CSF	~CSF	Equal or slightly higher than CSF	Slightly higher than CSF	Iso/hypodense on NECT like fat on MR	Often higher than CSF
Margins	Smooth	Smooth	Smooth	Smooth	Smooth	Smooth	Smooth/lobulated	Smooth/lobulated
Skull	Large post. fossa: Lambdoid toricular inversion	N	Inner table may be scalloping	Usually N scalloping may be seen	N	N	May have sinus tract	N

8.34 ENLARGED OPTIC FORAMEN

- Normal size—4.4-6mm.
- Increased size, if diameter >7mm
- A diff. of >1mm is diagnostic

Concentric Enlargement

1. Optic nerve glioma.
2. Neurofibroma.
3. Extension of retinoblastoma.
4. Vascular-ophthalmic artery aneurysm AV malformation.
5. Granuloma- very rarely in sarcoidosis or pseudotumor.

Local Defect

Roof

1. Adjacent neoplasm- meningioma, metastases, glioma.
2. Raised intracranial pressure- due to thinning of floor of anterior cranial fossa.

Medial Wall

1. Adjacent neoplasm-carcinoma of ethmoid/sphenoid.
2. Sphenoid mucocele.

Optic Nerve Glioma

- Occur in children, most often in association with neurofibromatosis-1.
- Slow growing, non-aggressive with a benign course.
- Fusiform enlargement of optic nerve.
- Enhance after contrast administration with variable pattern.

Optic Nerve Sheath Meningioma

- Most common in middle aged females.
- Tubular appearance on CT and MR.
- Enhance more than gliomas with 'Railroad track' appearance.

• Calcific within mass /hyperostosis around optic canal may be seen.

NF-1 (Neurofibromatosis –1)

• In addition to optic nerve glioma may have orbital flexiform neurofibroma.
• Orbital bone changes of sphenoid, dysplastic egg shaped enlargement of orbital rim, bony defects in posterior orbit, AP enlargement of middle cranial fossa, enlargement of other cranial foramina.

Retinoblastoma

• Most common intraocular tumor in children.
• Presents in first 2 years of life.
• High density areas arising from retina.
• Calcification common, subretinal fluid on MR.

AV Malformation

• Isolated anomalies rare, usually associated with intracranial AV malformation.
• Usually present with orbital congestion and proptosis.
• Bright enhancement on CECT, serpiginous flow, void on MR

Orbital Pseudotumor

• Non-specific inflammation of orbital fissures involving predominantly fissures behind the globe.
• On CT, seen as area of soft tissue density with poorly defined margins.
• MR with fat suppression, most sensitive to detect early changes.
• If discrete mass-lymphoma must be considered.

Sarcoidosis

• Rarely involves orbit
• May mimic pseudotumor.

Flow Chart 8.34.1

Lesions leading to optic foramen enlargement

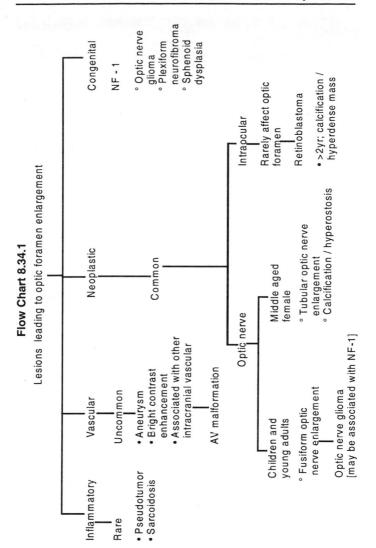

8.35 BARE ORBIT/HYPOPLASIA OF GREATER WING OF SPHENOID

Causes

- Meningioma
- Optic glioma
- Relapsing hematoma
- Metastasis
- Aneurysm
- Retinoblastoma
- Idiopathic
- Neurofibromatosis
- Eosinophilic granuloma.

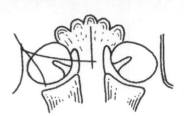

Fig. 8.35.1: 'Bare' orbit

Meningioma

- Most common below 40-60 years of age in females.
- Arises from arachnoid granulations. Extra-axial dural based mass.
- Associated with neurofibromatosis.
- Sites
  - 25% parasagittal
  - 20% convexity
  - 15 to 20% sphenoid ridge
  - 5 to 10% olfactory grooves.
- Plain film
  - Hyperostosis
  - Erosion
  - Enlarged vascular channel
  - Tumor calcification
  - Pneumosinus dilatans
- *CT*: Enhancing hyperdense mass with areas of calcification and cystic areas with peritumoral edema.

MR: Strongly enhancing typically isointense mass with grey matter.

Optic Glioma

- Usually a tumor of childhood (2-6 years).
- Presents with unilateral loss of vision and rapidly progresses to bilateral blindness and death with in 1 or 2 years.
- CT shown homogenously enhancing well-defined fusiform enlargement of the optic nerve. It shows characteristic kicking and buckling (sinusoid) appearance.

MRI: Enlarged fusiform and kicked optic nerve. T1 weighted and proton weighted images, the optic glioma will appear isointense or slightly hypointense compared to the white matter.

On T2 weighted images, the lesion may show greater variability in intensity, however, it may appear hyperintense compared to the white matter.

Retinoblastoma

- Most common intraocular tumor of childhood

CT: Moderate to markedly enhancing mass with calcification within it.

MRI: Slightly or moderately hyperintense in relation to normal vitreous on T1 weighted or proton weighted MR images.

On T2 weighted images, they appear as areas of markedly to moderately low signal intensity.

Neurofibromatosis

- Two type
  1. NF-1/von Recklinghausen's disease/peripheral NF chromosome no 17.

2. NF-2/Central NF/B/L acoustic schwannoma, chromosome no 22
- Autosomal dominant.
- Ossous dysplasia in particular bony orbit is associated with von Recklinghausen's disease.
- Partial or complete absence of the greater or lesser wing of the sphenoid; the body of the sphenoid bone may be involved producing an abnormal and dysplastic sella turica.
- Herniation of the temporal lobe of the brain of pulsating exophthalmos.
- Associated hypoplasia of frontal and maxillary sinuses as well as of adjacent ethmoid air cells.

Eosinophilic Granuloma

- Children especially boys below 3 and 12 years of life are most commonly affected.
- The skull, pelvis and femora are most commonly affected.
- There are usually solitary lytic lesions in these areas.
- Spine
  - Thoracic spine is usually affected.
  - Vertebra plana is usually present.

Metastasis

- Lung, breast, kidney, GIT are usually affected.

Aneurysm

- Large retro-orbital aneurysm can erode the bony structures at the back of the orbit or adjacent to the sella.
- Erosion of the inferolateral margin of the optic foramen is characteristic.
- An anterior clinoid process can also be eroded, as can the bone adjacent to it or sella.

Flow Chart 8.35.1

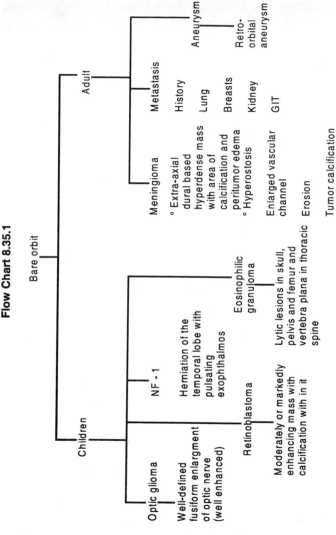

Bare orbit

Children

Optic glioma
Well-defined fusiform enlargment of optic nerve (well enhanced)

NF - 1
Herniation of the temporal lobe with pulsating exophthalmos

Retinoblastoma
Moderately or markedly enhancing mass with calcification with in it

Eosinophilic granuloma
Lytic lesions in skull, pelvis and femur and vertebra plana in thoracic spine

Adult

Meningioma
° Extra-axial dural based hyperdense mass with area of calcification and peritumor edema
° Hyperostosis
Enlarged vascular channel
Erosion
Tumor calcification

Metastasis
History
Lung
Breasts
Kidney
GIT

Aneurysm
Retro-orbital aneurysm

8.36 ORBITAL HYPEROSTOSIS

Causes

- Meningioma
- Sclerotic metastasis
- Fibrous dysplasia
- Paget's disease
- Osteopetrosis
- Chronic osteomyelitis
- Lacrimal gland malignancy
- Langerhans cell histiocytosis
- Radiotherapy
- Hyperostosis frontalis interna

Meningioma (Optic Nerve)

- Most often seen in middle-aged women
- Visual loss, papilledema and pallor of optic nerve head.

Plain Film

Calcification (common)
Widening of optic canal
Hyperostosis of sphenoid wing

CT: Dense sharply defined tubular mass surrounding and paralleling the optic nerve with enhancement (Tram Track appearance).

- *Metastasis*
  - Uncommon
  - Neuroblastoma, carcinoid, stomach and colon
- *Fibrous Dysplasia*
  - Monostotic or polyostotic (McCune-Albright)
  - Skull shows mixed lucencies and sclerosis mainly on the convexity of the calvarium, floor of anterior cranial fossa sometimes affecting orbit.

- Usually involvement of other bones like femur, pelvis, mandible, ribs is seen.

Paget's Disease

- Rare below 40 years old
- Generalized hyperostosis of skull. Vault becomes widened and thickened. Osteomalacic changes lead to platybasia and basilar impression (Geographic skull)
- Orbital involvement may be seen.
- Picture frame vertebral body, ivory vertebrae
- Widening and coarsened trabeculation of pelvic bones.

Osteopetrosis

- Generalized bone thickening
- Skull- sclerosis and thickening is more prominent in anterior cranial fossa affecting the orbital roof. Cranial nerve compression.
- Sinuses-under pneumatized.
- Erlenmeyer flask deformity
- 'Bone with in bone' appearance.
- Rugger jersey spine

Lacrimal Gland Malignancy

- Middle aged females
- S-shaped upper lid with eyeball displaced down and in
- Lateral rectus involvement may cause restriction of movement
- Erosion or sclerosis of orbital lateral wall may be seen.
- Spread along muscle or nerve is characteristic.

Langer Cell Histiocytosis

- Long bones, pelvis, skull and flat bones
- Punched out lesions in skull with little or no surrounding sclerosis, bevelled edges (geographic skull).

- Orbital involvement leading to exophthalmos seen in clinical subgroup (Hand-Schüller-Christian disease).
- Other findings like vertebral plana, rib expansion.
- Hepatomegaly, lymphadenopathy, skin lesions, pulmonary disease.

Hyperostosis Frontalis Interna

- Postmenopausal females
- Irregular nodular thickening of inner table of skull mainly affecting frontal bones, bilateral.
- May sometimes involve orbit.

Flow Chart 8.36.1

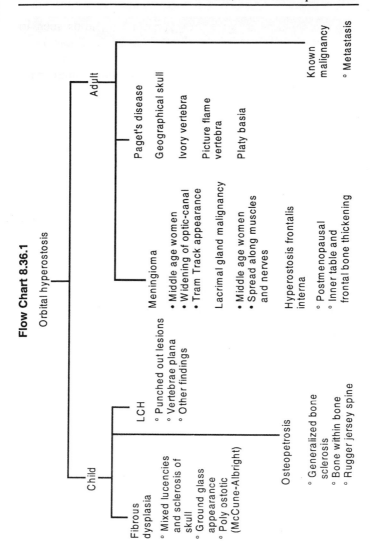

8.37 CEPHALOCELES

- A skull defect in association with herniated intracranial contents is termed a cephalocele.
- If the herniation contains solely leptomeninges and CSF, it is termed a meningocele.
- Cephaloceles in which the protruding structures consists of leptomeninges, CSF and brain are termed as mening-encephalocele.
- Incidence: Cephaloceles occur approx. 1 to 3 times in 10,000 lives births.
- Occipital cephaloceles predominate in individuals of white europeans or North American origin.
- Sincipital (Frontoethmoidal) lesions are more common in south east Asians and aboriginal Australians.
- Basal encephalocele are the rarest form of encephalocele.

OCCIPITAL AND PARIETAL CEPHALOCELES

- Occipital cephaloceles originate between the foramen magnum and lambda.
- Brain within these cephaloceles is usually dysplastic and gliotic cerebellum.
- In severe cases the midbrain and part of ventricular system may also be contained within these cephaloceles.
- Occipital cephaloceles can be associated with neural tube defect such as Chiari II and III malformations, Dandy-Walker malformations, cerebellar dysplasias, diastomato-myelia, Klippel-Feil syndrome.
- *Parietal cephaloceles* arise from a skull defect between the lambda and bregma.
- They are commonly associated with midline anomalies such as absent corpus callosum, Dandy-Walker malfor-

mations, lobar holo prosencephaly and Chiari II malformations.

SINCIPITAL AND SPHENOPHARYNGEAL CEPHALOCELES

- Sincipital (fronto ethmoidal) cephaloceles lie between the nasal and ethmoid bones.
- They typically show no association with neural tube defects.
- Trans-sphenoidal (sphenopharyngeal) Meningoencephalocele

  Occur in association with numerous distortions of the sellar and parasellar structure as well as endocrine abnormalities.
- They are frequently associated with callosal agenesis.

NASAL CEPHALOCELES, DERMOIDS AND GLIOMAS

- Nasal cephaloceles as well as nasal dermoids and nasal gliomas occur when a dural diverticulum that traverses the prenasal space and normally connects the superficial ectoderm of the developing nose with the developing brain fails to regress.
- Resulting anomalies range from dermal sinus, dermoid and epidermoid to nasal cephaloceles and so called nasal gliomas (which are usually sequestrations of dysplastic or heterotopic glial tissues).
- The crista galli is very importants in D/D of congenital nasal masses. If it is present but split, the mass is typically a dermoid. If it is absent or eroded and the foramen caecum is enlarged, the lesion is a cephalocele.

ATRETIC CEPHALOCELES /
MENINGOCELE

- They consist of a skin covered subcutaneous lesions that consist of meningeal and ectopic foci of glial or other CNS tissue such as anomalous blood vessels.
- They are associated with cerebro-oculomuscular (Walker-Warburg syndrome).

Table 8.37.1

Type	Site	Associated anomalies
Occipital	Between foramen magnum and bregma	Dysplastic and gliotic cerebellum Chiari II and III malformations Dandy-Walker malformation Diastematomyelia Klippel-Feil syndrome
Parietal	Between lambda and bregma	Absent corpus callosum Dandy-Walker malformation Lobar holoprosencephaly Chiari II malformation
Sincipital	Between nasal and ethmoid bones	No association with neural tube defects
Trans-sphenoidal	Numerous distortion of sellar and parasellar structures and endocrine abnormalities	Callosal agenesis

8.38 PATHOLOGICAL INTRACRANIAL CALCIFICATION

1. *Neoplasms*
   - Glioma
   - Craniopharyngiomas
   - Meningioma

- Ependymoma
- Papilloma of the choroid plexus
- Pinealoma
- Chordoma
- Dermoid, epidermoid and teratoma
- Hamartoma
- Lipoma
- Pituitary adenoma(rarely)
- Metastasis (rarely)

2. *Vascular*
   - Atheroma
   - Aneurysm
   - Angioma
   - Subdural hematoma
   - Intracranial hematoma

3. *Infections*
   - Toxoplasmosis
   - CMV inclusions
   - Herpes
   - Rubella
   - TB
   - Pyogenic abscess
   - Cysticercosis
   - Hydatid cyst
   - Paragonimus abscesses
   - Trichinosis
   - Torulosis
   - Coccidioides

4. *Metabolic and Miscellaneous*
   - Idiopathic basal ganglia calcifications
   - Hypoparathyroidism
   - Pseudo hypoparathyroidism
   - Tuberous sclerosis

- Sturge-Weber syndrome
- Neurofibromatosis
- Lissencephaly
- Fahr's syndrome
- Cockayne's syndrome
- X-radiation and methotrexate
- Hemodialysis
- Lead poisoning
- Co-poisoning

Normal Intracranial Calcification

1. Pineal
2. Habenula
3. Choroid plexus
4. Dura (Falx; Tentorium; over vault)
5. Ligaments (Petroclinoid and interclinoid)
6. Basal ganglia and dentate nuclei
7. Pituitary gland
8. Lens

Tumors

Gliomas

Commonest cerebral tumor
- Calcification is visible on skull films as little as 5%.
- Slow growing and less malignant tumor are most likely to calcify.
- Oligodendroglioma calcify in 50% of cases.
- Posterior fossa gliomas calcify in 20% of cases.
- Few punctate dots to a large calcified nodule or linear streaks to large amorphous calcification.

Craniopharyngiomas

- Present mainly in children
- Calcification
  - Midline and just above the sella
  - Few punctate dots to a densely calcified mass
  - Sella is bent forward
  - If the tumor is cystic, curvilinear calcification may be seen.

Meningiomas

- Calcification on plain film in about 10% of cases.
- Calcification is ball like and amorphous and in a characteristic parasagittal or other typical meningioma site.
- Other radiological organs include bony hyperostosis where the tumor is involving the vault or sphenoid ridge and increased meningeal vascular markings leading upto the site of attachment.

Dermoids

- Commonest in the posterior fossa or near the base of the skull.
- Arcs of calcification.
- Associated with a characteristic small central defect in the occipital bone.

Epidermoids

- These are much less likely to calcify
- Occasionally show small arc calcifications which can be multiple

Teratomas

- Found mainly in the pineal and suprasellar regions in children.
- They frequently contain calcification and rarely the recognition of a dental element may establish on the plain film.

Pineal Tumors

- Calcification in the pineal area, abnormal in extent, particularly in a child.

Ependymomas

- Occur mainly in posterior fossa in children
- In adults occur in supratentorial compartment.
- Calcification is unusual but can occur and be quite dense.

Choroid Plexus Papilloma

- Mainly in children
- Show calcification in one case in 4.
- Characteristic site is lateral or 4th ventricle.

Lipoma

- Occur in relation to corpus callosum
- Large lesions show a highly characteristic marginal calcification ('bracket sign').

Chordomas

- Irregular calcification in minority of cases.
- They grow from the clivus and other radiological features such as a soft tissue mass projecting into the nasopharynx or basal erosion.

VASCULAR LESIONS

Aneurysms

- Characteristic arc like or circular marginal calcification.
- Most occur in the region of the circle of willis and a linear ring or arc of calcification.
- Mostly small (under 1cm in diameter).
- Occasional calcification is seen in the margins of fusiform carotid siphon or basilar aneurysms.

Angioma

- Consists of scattered flecks of calcium associated with the presence of one or more ring or arc shadows.
- The latter arc in the walls of aneurysmal dilatations of vessel on the venous side of the angioma.

Chronic SDH

- Calcification in membrane.

Intracerebral Hematoma

Irregular calcification but has no diagnostic features.

Atheromas

- Linear fleck in atheromatous carotid siphons and may be quite extensive.
- Atheromatous calcification at the carotid bifurcation in neck.

Infections and Infestations

Tuberculoma

- Calcification on plain film is rare.
- Seen in patients successfully treated for TB meningitis.

- Small nodules in the healed basal exudate at the base of the brain.

Toxoplasmosis

- Most human infestation is derived from cats.
- Pregnant carrier can infect the fetus *in utero*.
- Widespread granuloma with calcifications, severe brain atrophy with ventricular dilatation and bilateral choroido-retinitis.
- Calcification in congenital toxoplasmosis is characteristic consisting of multiple scattered fleck in the cortex and linear streak in the basal ganglia.

CMV

- There is a severe intrauterine brain, infection.
- Microcephaly, a characteristic widespread periventricular calcification.
- Calcification is stippled, bilateral and symmetric.

Cysticercosis

- Human autoinfection with the tapeworm *Taenia solium*
- Muscle mass is mainly affected and the calcified cysts present a diagnostic picture.
- There is characteristic picture of scattered calcified nodules.

Paragonimus Westermani

- This trematode infection is acquired from crabs or crayfish.
- Brain lesions are usually in the parietal region and give rise to extensive 'roof bubble' calcification in cyst measuring 3 to 4cm in diameter.

Metabolic and Miscellaneous

Basal Ganglia Calcification

- Chance finding in the X-ray of adult skull.
- B/L and symmetrical and commences in the region of the head of caudate muscles. The globus pallidus, putamen and lateral part of thalamus may be involved. The dentate nuclei in the posterior fossa may be affected with or without supratentorial calcification. The latter is hazy or punctate in type.
- Most cases are primary or idiopathic and the condition is related to age.
- Secondary cases are due to hypoparathyroidism, either spontaneous or following thyroidectomy.

Hyperparathyroidism

- Extensive calcification in falx and tentorium in patients with CRF and on long-term hemodialysis.

Neurofibromatosis

Extensive calcification of the choroid plexus of the 3rd and lateral ventricles.

Tuberous Sclerosis

- Multiple areas of dysplasia in the brain may contain calcifications.
- On the plain film there appear as scattered discrete nodule of varying size.

Sturge-Weber Syndrome

- Occipital cortical calcification described as 'Tram line'

Flow Chart 8.38.1

Intracranial calcification

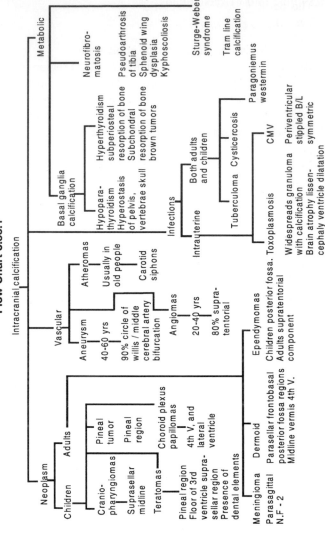

- The parallel lines represent the sulci seen end on since the calcification lies in the atrophic cortex.
- Calcification is U/L and occipital region.

Lissencephaly

- Rare anomaly
- Characteristic small (3 mm) calcified nodule in the septum pellucidum and just behind the foramen of monro.

8.39 J-SHAPED SELLA

Common

- Normal variant
- Mild arrested hydrocephalus
- Optic chiasm glioma

Less Common

- Achondroplasia
- Congenital hypothyroidism
- Hurler's syndrome
- Neurofibromatosis
- Pituitary tumor
- Intrasellar arachnoid cyst
- Suprasellar tumor.

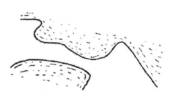

Fig. 8.39.1: J-shaped sella

The normal pituitary fossa in lateral skull radiography can vary considerably in size. A length of 11-16 mm and a depth of 8-12 mm are regarded within normal limits.

J- shaped sella is an elongated sella with a shallow anterior convexity which represents an exaggeration of the normal slight impression of sulcus chiasmaticus.

Optic Nerve Glioma

- Appear as fusiform enlargement of optic nerve with secondary involvement of the chiasm or may envelop the chiasm and spread secondary to the optic nerve.
- X-ray—Classically demonstrate a J-shaped sella, optic foramina > 7mm or a diff of > 2mm
  CT and MRI—provide the exact localization
- Usually isodense, may show enhancement especially the posterior lesions.
- Calcifications can be seen.
- Eighty five percent cases seen before 15 years of age

Hurler's Syndrome

- Caused by deficiency of enzyme alpha-1-uronidase
- Excess urinary excertion of dermatan sulphate and heparan sulphate
- Macrocephaly, thick vault with ground glass opacity, J-shaped sella
- Chest- Wide ribs. wide, short clavicles
- Spine- odontoid hypoplasia, ovoid hook shaped vertebral bodies inferior beaking of vertebral bodies
- Pelvis- iliac wings flared with constricted iliac bones, small irregular tumoral capital epiphysis
- Metacarpals- short and wide with proximal coning
- Genu valgum.

Hydrocephalus

- Bulging fontanelles, sutural diastasis
- Copper beaten skull
- Usually seen in arrested hydrocephalus, i.e. when the enlargement of ventricles stops due to compensatory mechanisms but they may undergo decompensation.

Hypothyroidism (Cretinism)

- Delayed skeletel maturation
- Fragmented, stippled epiphysis
- Wide sutures, fontanelles with delayed closure
- Delayed dentition
- Hypertelorism, wormian bones
- Delayed/decreased pneumatization of sinuses and mastoides
- Calvarial thickening/sclerosis-Adulthood
- Hypoplastic phalanges of 5th finger

Achondroplasia (Autosomal Dominant)

- A skeletal dysplasia with short limbs and a characteristic facial appearance and body habitus.
- Skull—Large skull vault, brachycephaly, short skull base, small foramen magnum, hydrocephalus.
- Spine—Platyspondyly, wide disc spaces, narrow spinal canal with lumbar spinal canal stenosis, thoracolumbar kyphus.
- Square iliac wings, horizontal acetabular roofs.
- Long bone shortening particulary femur and humerus.
- Trident hand.

Neurofibromatosis

- One or more relatives primary with NF
- Optic glioma's (MC CNS tumor in NF-1)
- Typical bone lesions-sphenoid dysplasia or tibial pseudo-arthrosis
- Twisted ribbon ribs; splaying of ribs
- Heavy calcification of choroid plexus
- Cafe au lait spots.

Arachnoid Cyst (Heptomeningeal Cyst)

- Benign, congenital, intra-arachnoidal SOL, i.e. filled with clear CSF like fluid.
- Mainly seen in middle cranial fossa but may involve sella.
- CT- Smoothly demarcated, non-calcified extra-axial mass that does not enhance.

Findings on Skull X-ray

- Copper beaten skull
  Bulging fontanelle, sutural   – Hydrocephalus
  diastasis
- Optic foramina >7mm
  or a diff. of >2mm   – Optic glioma
- Associated sphenoid dysplasia   – Neurofibromatosis
- Large skull vault, brachycephaly,
  short skull base, small   – Achondroplasia
  foramen magnum
- Macrocephaly, thick
  vault with ground glass
  opacity, odontoid hypoplasia   – Hurler's syndrome
- Wide sutures, fontanelle's with
  delayed closure, wormian   – Hypothyroidism
  bones, Hypertelorism, calvarial
  thickening decreased pneumatization of mastoid and sinuses.

8.40 CEREBELLAR MALFORMATIONS

Differential Diagnosis

1. Chiari IV malformations.
2. Joubert's syndrome

3. Rhombencephalosynapsis
4. Tecto-cerebellar dysraphia
5. Lhermitte-Duclos disease

Chiari IV Malformations

- Absent or severely hypoplastic cerebellum
- Small brainstem
- Large posterior fossa, CSF fluid spaces.

Joubert's Syndrome

- Autosomal recessive presents with marked global developmental delay and neonatal breathing abnormalities.
- Dysgenetic vermis that appears split, segmented or disorganized.
- The inferior and superior cerebellar peduncles are often small.
- The fourth ventricle roof appears superiorly convex on sagittal MR scans.
- No hydrocephalus.
- Associated with callosal dysgenesis, congenital retinal dystrophy, occulomotor abnormalities, polydactyly, cystic kidney.

Rhombencephalosynapsis

- Presentation is with mental retardation and severe ataxia
- Vermain agenesis or hypogenesis
- Midline fusion of cerebellar hemispheres and peduncles
- Apposition or fusion of dentate nuclei
- Variable fusion of colliculi
- Key hole fourth ventricle
- Associated with ventriculomegaly, absent septum pellucidum, anterior commissure hypoplasia, fused thalami, schizencephaly, cephalocele.

Tecto-cerebellar Dysraphia

- Vermian hypoplasia or aplasia
- Occipital cephalocele
- Dorsal traction of brainstem
- The hypoplastic cerebellar hemispheres are rotated lying ventrolateral to brainstem.

Lhermitte-Duclos disease: Also known as dysplastic ganglio-cytoma of cerebellum.

- Gross thickening of cerebellar folia with or without mass effect.
- Mimics posterior fossa neoplasms.
- On CT there are poorly delineated hypo or isodense posterior fossa lesions that does not enhance.
- Mass effect and displacement of fourth ventricle may occur.
- Calcification and hydrocephalus may be present.
- On MR decreased signal non-enhancing mass is seen on T1 weighted images and a very characteristic laminated folial pattern of increased signal intensity is seen on T2.
- Usually an isolated abnormality.

Miscellaneous

Dandy-Walker Complex

- Failure of development of anterior medullary velum (roof of fourth ventricle) or atresia of foramina of luschka and magendie
- Large posterior fossa
- High tentorial insertion
- High transverse sinus
- The fourth ventricle communicates with a posterior fossa cyst
- Hydrocephalus
- Vermian or cerebellar hemispheric hypoplasia

Flow Chart 8.40.1

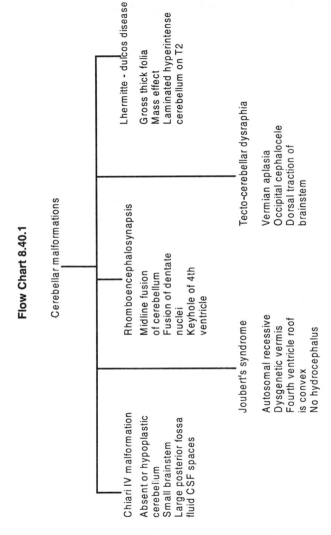

Cerebellar malformations

Chiari IV malformation
Absent or hypoplastic cerebellum
Small brainstem
Large posterior fossa fluid CSF spaces

Joubert's syndrome
Autosomal recessive
Dysgenetic vermis
Fourth ventricle roof is convex
No hydrocephalus

Rhomboencephalosynapsis
Midline fusion of cerebellum
Fusion of dentate nuclei
Keyhole of 4th ventricle

Tecto-cerebellar dysraphia
Vermian aplasia
Occipital cephalocele
Dorsal traction of brainstem

Lhermitte - dulcos disease
Gross thick folia
Mass effect
Laminated hyperintense cerebellum on T2

- Anterolaterally winged cerebellar hemispheres in front of the cyst
- Brainstem may be hypoplastic and compressed
- Heterotopias and cerebellar dyplasias are common
- Associated with corpus callosum agenesis.

Dandy-Walker Variant

- Mild vermian hypoplasia
- Communication of fourth ventricle to cisterna magna with enlargement of fourth ventricle
- Posterior fossa size is normal.

8.41 DEMYELINATING DISORDERS

- Two main categories
  - Dysmyelinating disorders- Primary abnormality of formation of myelin
  - Demyelinating- result of myelin loss after its normal formation.
- General imaging features
  - Hypodense on CT
  - Hypointense on T1 WI
  - Hyperintense on T2 WI
  - Acute lesions may show focal contrast uptake.

Demyelination

- Multiple sclerosis
- ADEM (Acute disseminated encephalomyelitis)
- Infections
  - Congenital or perinatal
  - CMV
  - Rubella
  - HSV

- Acute encephalitis
  - HSV
  - Mumps
  - Rubella
  - Measles, chicken pox
  - AIDS encephalitis
  - PML
  - SSPE
  - CJD
- Toxic/Metobolic
  - Osmotic demyelination
  - Wernicke's
  - Marchiafava-Bignami
- Vasculer
  - Subcortical arteriosclerosic encephalopathy
  - HIE

Radiation and Chemotherapy

Dysmyelination

- Metachromatic leukodystrophy
- Krabbe's disease

Paroxysomal Disorders

- ALD
- Zellweger's syndrome

Amino Acid Metabolism

- Canavanis disease

Mitochondrial Dysfunction

- Leigh's disease
- MELAS

- MERRF
- Kearns- Sayre syndrome

Unknown

Alexander's disease
Pelizaeus-Merzbacher disease

DEMYELINATION

- Multiple sclerosis
- Unknown etiology, - Autoimmune mediated demyelination.
- Most common demyelinating disorder, except for age-related vascular demyelination.
- 20-40 years F > M, 1.7-2:1
- *Location*: Ovoid periventricular lesions, oriented parallel to long axis of the brain and lateral ventricles.
  Demyelination around subependymal and deep white matter medullary veins.
  – Calloso-septal interface.
- Infratentorial with 10% in adults.
  (Posterior fossa) - more commonly involved in children and adolescents.
- C/F
  – Prolonged relapsing-remitting disease

Imaging

- CT
  – May be normal
  – Iso to hypodense lesions on NC CT
  – Variable contrast enhancement-both nodular and rim like

- MRI, iso to hypointense on T1 WI, lesion with in lesion appearance (beveled appearance)
  - Hyperintense on T2 WI
- Criteria
  - Presence of three or> discrete lesions, > 5mm in size, characteristic location with compatible clinical H/O
  - Oblong lesions at colloso-septal interface is typical with characteristic periventricular extension into adjacent white matter, called, Dawson's finger.
  - Variable and transient CE, only during active demyelinating stage.

Acute Disseminated Encephalomyelitis

- Immune mediated response to a preceding viral infection or vaccination.
- Any age, mostly children and young adults.
- Abrupt onset, with monophasic course, neurological symptoms characteristically develop 1 to 3 weeks after infection.
- Multifocal subcortical hyperintense foci on T2 WI.
- Deep white matter, brainstem and cerebellum can be affected.
- Occasionally basal ganglia involvement occur.
- Typically bilateral, but asymmetric.
- Usually non-hemorrhagic.
- Some but not all lesions enhance often CE.

INFECTIOUS

Congenital and Perinatal Viral Infections

CMV
- Most common cause of congenital infections.
- >60% of infected fetuses have multisystem involvement.

- Most common intracranial abnormalities 70%.
- Cardiac abnormalities and hepatosplenomegaly- (HCM) 1/3rd cases.
- C/F
  - Prematurity, hepatosplenomegaly, Jaundice, thrombocytopenia, chorioretinitis, during newborn period.
  - Seizures, mental retardation, optic atrophy, sensorineural hearing loss.
  - Hydrocephalus—Later manifestations.
- Imaging
  - X-ray—Microcephaly with egg shell like periventricular calcification, due to widespread periventricular tissue necrosis with subsequent dystrophic calcification.
- USG
  - Ventriculomegaly with periventricular calcification.
- CT
  - Hydrocephalus, atrophy, periventricular calcification.
- MRI
  - Migrational anomalies, encephalomalacia, ventriculomegaly, delayed myelination, subependymal periventricular cysts and calcification.
- Rubella
  - Interferes with multiplication of cells located in germinal matrix- Microcephaly, delayed myelination, vasculopathy with perivascular necrosis in basal ganglia, periventricular region and cerebral white matter.
- Parenchymal calcification.
- Other
  - Cataract, glaucoma chorioretinitis, microphthalmia cardiac malformations.
  - Deafness.

Herpes Simplex Encephalitis (HSE)

Most common viral encephalitis
- Neonatal HSE is caused by HSV-2
- In older children and adults HSV-1
- HSV causes fulminant hemorrhagic necrotizing meningoencephalitis.
- Neonatal HSV-2 infection is a diffuse non-focal infection. HSV-1- Limbic system predilection.
  - Temporal lobe, insular cortex, subfrontal area, the cingulate gyri.
  - "Sequential bilaterality"
- C/F
  - Altered mental states, seizures, fever, headache
- CT
  - Normal Or Low density lesion in temporal lobe with mild mass effect.
  - Hemorrhage-if present highly s/o HSE -usually seen later in the course of disease
- CECT
  - Ill-defined patchy or gyriform CE
- Neonatal HSE-2
  - Strikingly increased density of cortical grey matter, and diffuse low attenuation in the white matter.
- MR
  Decrease-T1
  Increase-T2
  - In limbic system, with sequential bilaterality with variable CE and subacute hemorrhage
- Encephalomalacia, atrophy and dystrophic calcification late sequelae.

HIV ENCEPHALOPATHY

Progressive subcortical dementia-subacute encephalitis
- Develops in 60% of AIDS patients
- CT
  - Most common finding-Atrophy
  - Multifocal hypodense areas in deep white matter
- MR-T2 WI
  - Ill-defined diffuse or confluent patches of increased signal intensity in the deep white matter
  - Most common site- frontal lobes, often-B/L and symmetric
  - Grey matter-typically spared
  - No contrast inhancement
- *PML*

  Group B human papovavirus (JC virus)
  - Infects and destroys oligodendroglia-Demyelination.
  - Adults immunocompromised patients, extremely rare in children.
  - Periphery to central progression, subcortical areas first to be affected.
  - Typically bilateral and asymmetic
  - Posterior centrum semiovale -most common site.
  - Rarely, unilateral, thalamic and basal ganglia lesions.
- *SSPE*
  - Rare progressive encephalitis that develops several (Subacute sclerosing panencephalitis)
  - Years after measles infection.
  - Affects, children and young adults.
- C/F
  - Behavioral abnormalities, myoclonus, tremors and seizures.
    NCCT- hypodense lesion in subcortical and periventricular white matter basal ganglia.
  - Generalized atrophy.

- T2W MRI
  Multifocal hyperintensifies in cerebral white matter and basal ganglia

Osmotic Demyelination

- Alcoholics
- Malnourished or chronic debilitated adults.
- Rapid correction of hyponatremia
- Hypernatremia.
- Myelinolysis with selective neuron sparing.
- MC site- central pons. (CP myelinolysis)
- Extrapontine sites:
  - Putamina, caudate, Midbrain, Thalami, subcortical white matter.
- NCCT- hypodense, hypointense on T1WI, hyper on T2WI
- CE- Most lesions do not enhance, some show variable CE.
- Transverse pontine fibers are most severely affected with sparing of corticospinal tracts.

Marchiafava-Bignami Disease

- Chronic alcoholism.
- Corpus callosum demyelination and necrosis, with or without- cerebral hemispheric white matter and other commissural fibers may be affected.
  Wernicke's encephalopathy - Nutritional thiamine deficiency-chronic alcoholics
- TRIAD- Ophthalmoplegia, ataxia, confusion
- Involves both grey and white matter
- Characteristic topographic distribution. Periventricular regions, mammillary bodies.
- Periaqueductal grey, mid brain reticular formation and tectal plate

- Post contrast enhancement- may or may not be present. Radiation and chemotherapy- cyclosporin A, methotrexate, cytarabine, 5-FU
- Small and medium sized vessel injury
- Predominant involvement of deep white matter with relative sparing of the cortex and underlying subcortical arcuate fibers.
- Widespread perivascular calcification condition known as mineralizing angiopathy (MA), typically occur in children receiving irradiation and chemotherapy for acute leukemia.
- MC site- basal ganglia, and junction of the cortex with subcortical white matter.

Vascular Lesions

HIE: Premature infants- Periventricular leukomalacia (PVL) ischemic infarction
- Isolated PVL-reflects-second or early third trimester injury.
- CF- spastic diplegia, non-progressive but permanent.
- MR-peritrigonal hyperintensities focal ventricular enlargement with irregular ventricular contour, atrophy of posterior corpus callosum.
- B/L, and asymmetric.
- Term infants: Predominant involvement of cortex and subcortical white matter, with common involvement of deep grey matter nuclei.
- Children and adults: Watershed infarction, with B/L selective neuronal necrosis in basal ganglia, thalami, hippocampus, parahippocampal gyrus, cerebellum and brainstem.

Sub-cortical Arteriosclerotic Encephalopathy: (Binswanger's disease)
- Patients with chronic HTN
- Dementia, spasticity, seizures, gait apratia, incontinence
- Multifocal white matter lesions in periventricular and deep white matter,-extending peripherally with increasing severity.
- Associated with lacunar infarcts in central grey matter and atrophy.

DYSMYELINATION (LEUKODYSTROPHIES)

- Disorders of children
- Present with variable mental retardation

Metachromatic Leukodystrophy

Most common hereditary (AR) leukodystrophy.
- Lysosomal disorder, deficiency of -Aryl sulfatase-A, AR
  - Symmetric demyelination with subcortical U-fiber sparing.
  - Cerebellum-often atrophic
- Anterior white matter is most severity affected.
- CT
  - Moderate ventricular enlargement
  - Hypodensity in white matter progressing anterior to posterior with no contrast enhancement.
- MR
  - Increase T2, with arcuate fiber sparing initially
  - Increase intensity in cerebellar white matter
  - Thalamic hypointensity mild to extreme.

Krabbe's Disease(Globoid Cell Leukodystrophy)

- Deficiency of galactocerebroside β galactosidase, AR.
- Cerebral atrophy with small brain, extensive symmetric demyelination of the centrum semiovale and coronaradiata with subcortical arcuate fiber sparing.
- Cerebellar white matter is affected to a lesser degree.
- Parieto-occipital lobes may be selectively involved early in disease.
- NCCT
  - Periventricular white matter hypodensity.
  - Thalami and basal ganglia-hyperdense
  - Corona radiata, cerebellum- also are hyperdense
- MR
  - Periventricular white matter hyperintensity on T2 WI
  - Late onset disease may show changes limited to posterior hemispheric white matter.
- Cerebral atrophy.

Adrenoleukodystrophy

Single paroxysomal enzyme deficiency- Acetylcoenzyme-A synthease
- X-linked recessive.
- Three types
  - ALD
    - Rare neonatal form
  - AMN
    neonatal ALD-AR
  - ALMN
    - Multiple enzyme deficiency
- Ventricular enlargement, cerebral atrophy.
  - First involvement of occipital lobes and splenium-B/L
  - Centrifugal and anterior extension symmetrical.

- ALD-3 months-1 years of age,
  - Sparing of subcortical white matter early in disease.
- AMN- 20-30 years
  - Auditory pathway involvement common.
  - Typically three zones:
    - Innermost central and posterior zone with necrosis, gliosis and sometimes calcification.
- Intermediate zone of active demyelination and inflammatory change.
- Peripheral zone of demyelination with inflammatory change.

  CT

  Large symmetric hypodensity in parietoccipital region ± calcification (peritrigonal)
  - After contrast- enhancement in advancing rim with more peripheral non-enhancing edematous zone.
- MR
  - Central necrosis, zone of decrease T1 and increase T2
  - Intermediate zone show CE
  - Peripheral zone of decrease T1 and increase T2
  - Abnormal signal in lateral geniculate bodies, auditory pathways, corpus callosum splenium and corticospinal tracts.
- AMN

  Symmetric hyperintensity in posterior limb of internal capsule

Zellweger's (cerebrohepatorenal syndrome)—Autosomal recessive, multiple paroxysomal enzyme deficiency.
- Neuronal migration disorders with heterotopic grey matter pachygria, polymicrogyria, with white matter hypomyelination

Leigh's disease: (Subacute necrotizing encephalopathy)
- Multiple mitochondrial enzyme deficiencies, automatic recessive
- Involvement of both grey and white matter.
- C/F—hypotonia, seizure, vomiting, loss of head control, respiratory failure.
- CT—hypodensity in caudate and putamen, no contrast enhancement
- MR—symmetric hyperintensity in globus pallidus putamen, caudate, periventricular white matter and peri-aqueductal grey.

MELAS

Cerebral infarcts-occipital lobes most common site
- Focal cortical and brainstem white matter changes with basal ganglia calcification with or without-cerebral and cerebellar atrophy.

MERRF

Kearns-Sayre syndrome
- Childhood/adolescence AD
- Progressive external ophthalmoplegia
- Pigmentary retinal degeneration
- Heart block/increase CSF protein/cerebellar dysfunction.
- White matter disease with cortical and/or cerebellar atrophy, and calcification in basal ganglia or deep white matter.

LEUKODYSTROPHIES—DISTINCTIVE FEATURES

- Complete/near complete lack of myelination-Canavan's disease
  - Pelizaeus-Merzbacher disease

- Frontal white matter most involved-Alexander's disease
- Occipital white matter most involved-ALD
- Macrocephaly
  - Alexander disease
  - Canavan's disease
- High density basal ganglia-Krabbe disease
- Enhancement following CE
  - Alexander's disease
  - ALD
- Stroke
  - Leigh's syndrome
  - MELAS
  - MERRF

Flow Chart 8.41.1
Demyelination

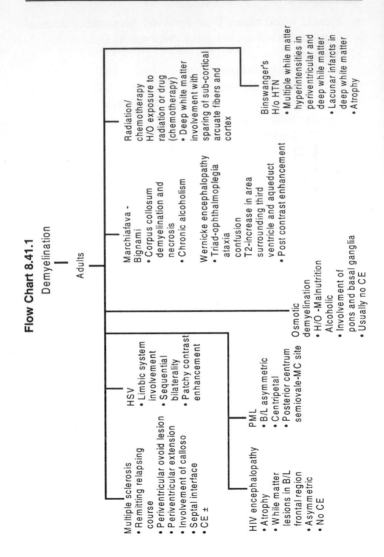

Adults

Multiple sclerosis
- Remitting relapsing course
- Periventricular ovoid lesion
- Periventricular extension
- Involvement of calloso
- Septal interface
- CE ±

HIV encephalopathy
- Atrophy
- White matter lesions in B/L frontal region
- Asymmetric
- No CE

HSV
- Limbic system involvement
- Sequential bilaterally
- Patchy contrast enhancement

PML
- B/L asymmetric
- Centripetal
- Posterior centrum semiovale-MC site

Osmotic demyelination
- H/O -Malnutrition Alcoholic
- Involvement of pons and basal ganglia
- Usually no CE

Marchiafava - Bignami
- Corpus collosum demyelination and necrosis
- Chronic alcoholism

Wernicke encephalopathy
- Triad-ophthalmoplegia ataxia confusion
- T2-increase in area surrounding third ventricle and aqueduct
- Post contrast enhancement

Radiation/ chemotherapy
- H/O exposure to radiation or drug (chemotherapy)
- Deep white matter involvement with sparing of sub-cortical arcuate fibers and cortex

Binswanger's
- H/o HTN
- Multiple while matter hyperintensities in periventricular and deep while matter
- Lacunar infarcts in deep white matter
- Atrophy

Flow Chart 8.41.2

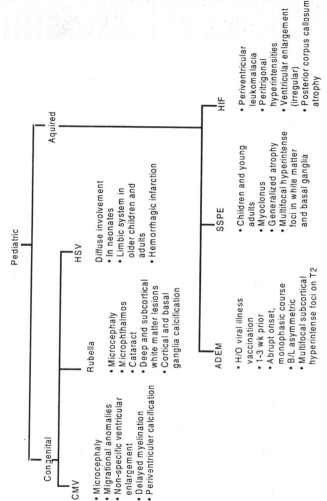

Pediatric

Congenital

CMV
- Microcephaly
- Migrational anomalies
- Non-specific ventricular enlargement
- Delayed myelination
- Periventricular calcification

Rubella
- Microcephaly
- Microphthalmos
- Cataract
- Deep and subcortical white matter lesions
- Cortical and basal ganglia calcification

Aquired

HSV
Diffuse involvement
- In neonates
- Limbic system in older children and adults
- Hemorrhagic infarction

ADEM
- H/O viral illness vaccination
- 1-3 wk prior
- Abrupt onset, monophasic course
- B/L asymmetric
- Multifocal subcortical hyperintense foci on T2

SSPE
- Children and young adults
- Myoclonus
- Generalized atrophy
- Multifocal hyperintense foci in white matter and basal ganglia

HIF
- Periventricular leukomalacia
- Peritrigonal hyperintensities
- Ventricular enlargement (irregular)
- Posterior corpus callosum atrophy

8.42 PREVERTEBRAL SOFT TISSUE THICKENING

(Cervical Region)

Normal Values of Prevertebral Soft Tissue

Level	Thickness(in mm)
C1	10
C2	5
C3	7
C4	7
C5	20
C6	20
C7	20

- Weight and age variation
- Flexion and extension < 1 mm variation

FASCIAL SPACES IN PREVERTEBRAL REGION

Retropharyngeal space between buccopharyngeal fascia anteriorly and alar fascia posteriorly.
Laterally- Cloison sagittal.

Retroesophageal space: Continuation of the above space in mid and lower neck surrounds the esophagus.

Danger space—   Ventrally-   alar fascia
                Dorsally-   prevertebral fascia
From skull base down to posterior mediastinum.
Prevertebral space between prevertebral fascia and vertebrae from skull base to coccyx.

Causes of Prevertebral Soft Tissue (Cervical Region)

- Retropharyngeal space
  - Lymphadenopathy
  - Abscess

- Cellulitis
- Edema
- Hematoma
- Lipoma
- Hemangioma
- Tortous carotid artery
- Extension of goiter
- Prevertebral space
  - Abscess
  - Phrenic nerve-Schwannomas
  - Mesenchymal tumors of muscles
- Extension of tumors like nasopharyngeal or esophageal carcinoma or lymphoma.

Retropharyngeal Lymph Adenopathy

- Lateral group is involved more than median group.
- Reactive, suppurative, metastatic, lymphoma –4 main categories
- Metastasis- nasopharynx, oropharynx, nasal cavity, and hypopharynx (Unresectability of primary tumor)
  CT—Inflamed lymphoid tissue enhance homogeneously or heterogeneously or may appear edematous with decreased attenuation and mild delayed peripheral enhancement, nodal edema or suppuration.

Retropharyngeal Cellulitis and Abscess

- Retropharyngeal infections result from suppurative lymph-adenitis, associated tonsilitis, pharyngitis, sinonasal infection, otitis media, etc.
- Fever, sore throat, swelling, stridor, odynophagia, trismus.
- Plain film
  - Widening of retropharyngeal soft tissue
  - Loss of cervical lordosis
  - Occasionally air in retropharyngeal soft tissue.

CT- is used to differentiate adenitis, abscess and cellulitis.

- Like lymphadenopathy, abscess is also characterized by low attenuation and ring enhancement but the margins no longer confine to nodal morphology (skull base to T4).
- So (CT gives invaluable information but it is not entirely accurate.
- US
  - Differentiate between abscess and adenitis
  - Guidance for intraoperative aspiration and drainage
- Diagnosis of cellulitis on CT is made when edema of soft tissues and obliteration of fat planes without rim enhancement.
- *Necrotizing cellulitis*: Extensive stranding of subcutaneous fat planes.
- Complications
  - Airway obstruction
  - Displacement and compression of internal carotid artery.
  - Internal jugular vein-compression/thrombophlebitis

Retropharyngeal Edema

- Usually seen following radiation therapy in patients with head and neck cancer.
- May also follow trauma or infection of oropharynx or vertebral column.

Hemangioma

Are vascular nests subdivided in 3 types
1. Capillary
2. Cavernous
3. Mixed type

On CT and MRI
- Intensively enhance after contrast injection
- Phleboliths

Lipoma

- Predominantly found in posterior cervical space but may occur in RPS.
- Seen as fat density, well-defined encapsulated on CT and MR.
- Lipomas tend to enlarge with weight gain but do not decrease with weight loss.

Tortous Carotid Artery

- A tortous common or internal carotid artery may present submucosal mass displacing the posterior pharyngeal wall.
- Palpation may not be feasible, pulsation overlooked.
- CT diagnosis is straightforward.

Extension of Thyroid Masses

Pretracheal space communicating with retropharyngeal space between levels of thyroid cartilage and inferior thyroid artery thyroid can extend through this space.

Prevertebral Abscess

- Abscess in prevertebral space is usually from osteomyelitis of vertebral bodies.
- Displace RPS anteriorly and carotid sheath laterally.

Tumors

- Masses arising from prevertebral muscles are mesenchymal in origin.
- Erosion of vertebral body- malignant
- Rhabdomyosarcoma- mostly from pharyngeal mass.
- In children- Rhabdomyosarcoma and neuroblastoma.
- Nasopharyngeal lymphoma or minor salivary gland malignancy may directly invade.

Flow Chart 8.42.1
Prevertebral soft tissue mass

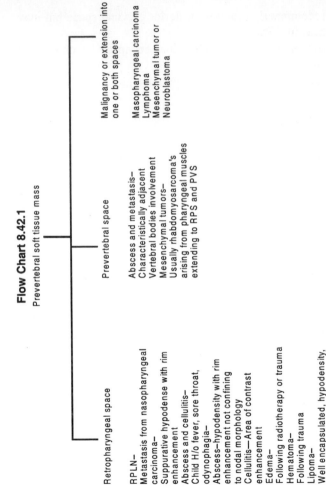

Retropharyngeal space

RPLN—
Metastasis from nasopharyngeal carcinoma—
Suppurative hypodense with rim enhancement
Abscess and cellulitis—
Child H/o fever, sore throat, odynophagia—
Abscess—hypodensity with rim enhancement not confining to nodal morphology
Cellulitis—Area of contrast enhancement
Edema—
Following radiotherapy or trauma
Hematoma—
Following trauma
Lipoma—
Well encapsulated, hypodensity, homogeneous
Tortous carotid artery—
CE CT diagnostic

Prevertebral space

Abscess and metastasis—
Characteristically adjacent
Vertebral bodies involvement
Mesenchymal tumors—
Usually rhabdomyosarcoma's arising from pharyngeal muscles extending to RPS and PVS

Malignancy or extension into one or both spaces

Masopharyngeal carcinoma
Lymphoma
Mesenchymal tumor or
Neuroblastoma

8.43 NASOPHARYNGEAL MASSES

Nasopharynx is a space situated posterior to the posterior nares and bounded superiorly by the floor of the middle cranial fossa and posteriorly by the base of skull and laterally by the pharyngeal musculature, the mandible and the parotid.

Methods of Investigations

Plain X-ray soft tissue neck: This is now only some time used as a lateral projection of the pharynx. The film is placed against the shoulder and the central ray is centered at the angle of the mandible.

Computed tomography: CT is now the optimum method of imaging; it shows not only the outlines of the nasopharynx but also the soft tissue structures of the infratemporal fossa and parapharyngeal space. The scan can be done in axial views and sagittal and coronal reconstructions can be done or direct coronal scanning can be done. Both pre and post-contrast scans should be undertaken. The role of CT for lesions in this region may be defined as:

1. As a complement to direct examination.
2. To assess the size, situation and relations of a well-defined mass for prospective surgical removal, or the extent of local and deep infiltration for radiotherapy planning.
3. To assess the relationship of the mass with great vessels and the parotid gland on post-contrast scans.

Magnetic resonance imaging: Now the imaging investigation of choice, but careful selection of cases is necessary. It shows the major vessels of neck without contrast enhancement and clearly depicts the soft tissue anatomy in multiplanar projections. T1 weighted sequences have the best spatial resolution and give a strong signal from fat in the tissue planes.

However, T2 weighted protocols are most useful for showing muscle invasion by carcinomas. A standard head coil is all that is used for the assessment of nasopharynx.

Differential Diagnosis of Nasopharyngeal Masses

1. Meningoceles
2. Adenoid hyperplasia
3. Antrochoanal polyps
4. Infections
5. Juvenile angiofibroma
6. Chordomas
7. Carcinomas
8. Lymphoma
9. Extension of neoplasms (sphenoid/ethmoid carcinoma, parotid tumor).

Meningoceles

Presents as a smooth well-defined mass in an infant or a young child posterior to and projecting into the nasopharynx. These are rare manifestations and are usually associated with a defect in the skull base. These masses may show fluid or CSF density of intracranial contents. These are best shown by coronal CT or MRI, which will differentiate meningocele from an encephalocele.

Adenoid Hyperplasia

- Presents in younger age group with nasal blockage and recurrent attacks of rhinitis.
- There is a verrucoid polypoidal mass in the nasopharynx with no evidence of bone involvement or mucosal invasion.

- CT and MRI best delineate the size, volume and extent of the lesion.

Antrochoanal Polyp

- These are antral polyps which outgrow from the antrum and presents in the nasopharynx.
- They are smoothly outlined pear shaped masses in the nasopharynx.
- They are associated with partial or complete opacification of the antrum but with no evidence of bone destruction or erosion, however, thinning of bones, secondary to the expansile nature of the mass, may be seen.
- One CT they presents as hypodense soft tissue masses, on MR they have high homogenous signal on T2 weighted sequences. CT and MR can elegantly define the origin of mass from the maxillary antrum and will also define the extent of the mass.

Infections

- Abscess in the parapharyngeal spaces may present in the nasopharynx posterior to the mucosal lining presenting clinically as masses in the nasopharynx with or without associated changes of inflammation on the overlying mucosa and the patient may show signs of toxemia.
- The abscess are usually secondary to infection extending either from the parotid glands, the sinuses and hematogenous spread from a distant location.
- On CT they are seen as well-defined walled of necrotic masses with enhancement of walls on CECT. Associated changes may be seen in the near by structures from which the abscess has originated.

Juvenile Angiofibroma

- Commonest benign tumor in pubescent males presents classically with epistaxis and nasal obstruction and a dark red or ulcerated mass in the nasal cavities and postnasal space.
- CT and MR clearly define the extent and origin of the lesion.
- The mass arises at or close to the base of the pterygoid lamina, thus bone erosion at this site is probably a pathognomic feature.
- The tumor not only spreads into the nose and PNS but has a special tendency to spread laterally through the pterygomaxillary fissure and anterior bowing of the posterior wall of the antrum, an important differentiating feature. It causes destruction of the adjacent bones.
- Neglected cases may also show extension into the orbit, sphenoid sinus and the cranial cavity.
- There is considerable contrast enhancement on CECT and MR may show presence of flow voids as well as marked enhancement after gadolinium, which is charac-teristic to the tumor.

Chordomas

- These are midline tumors arising from commonly the clivus, but may also arise from basisphenoid and present as postnasal mass.
- They are usually found in patients of older age group.
- They present on CT as a large soft tissue mass in the postnasal space associated with destruction of the basisphenoid and flecks of calcifications. There is usually an associated intracranial mass.

Carcinomas

- Eighty percent of the carcinomas are squamous cell type. When they are large and exophytic they present as a mass in the postnasal space. Usually, however, they infiltrate into the base of skull so that patient presents with a cranial nerve lesion or with enlarged neck glands. Serous otitis media due to blockage of Eustachian tubes may be another presenting complaint.
- There is erosion of the floor of middle cranial fossa.
- There is obliteration of the lateral pharyngeal recess (fossa of Rosenmüller).
- CT and MR may also show the obliteration of soft tissue planes suggestive of invasion.
- Extension in the cranial cavity and evaluation of neck glands by CT and MR helps in staging the tumor. In cases of adenocystic carcinoma. MR may also show perineural spread which is characteristic to the tumor.

Lymphomas

- In the postnasal space these tumors tend to grow in a bulky circumferential pattern without early invasion of the parapharyngeal spaces.
- CT and MR show bulky masses in the postnasal space with homogenous attenuation or intensity.

Extension from near by structures: This usually due to the spread of pathological process in near by structures like in cases of sphenoid or ethmoid carcinoma or parotid masses. CT and MR will show the presence of primary pathology elsewhere and its extension in the postnasal space.

Table 8.43.1: Nasopharyngeal masses

Mass	Age	Situation	Bone involvement	Infiltration	Contrast enhancement	Additional features
Meningo-cele	Infants and young child	Posterior to naso-pharynx	Defect in skull base	NA	NA	CSF density fluid or intracranial contents
Adenoids	Young patients	At the vault	NA	NA	NA	NA
A C polyp	Children and young adults	Nasopharynx proper	May cause thin-ning of bones	NA	NA	Extends from antrum
Infections	Any age group	Parapharyngeal spaces	NA	NA	Of the wall if an abscess	Primary infection in nearby organs
Angio-fibromas	Males near puberty	Arises from pterygoid lamina	Erosion of pterygoids and widened pterygo maxillary fissure	May extend intra-cranially or in the orbits	Intense with flow voids seen in MRI	Anterior bowing of posterior wall of maxillary sinus
Chordomas	Older	Posterior para-pharyngeal space	Destruction of basi- sphenoid	Usually has intra-cranial extension	Mild	Has flecks of calci-fications and is a midline tumor
Carcinomas	Older	Wall of naso-pharynx	Destruction and erosion of bones	Muscles and other structures including orbits, brain and parapharyngeal spaces	Mild to moderate	May present with CN palsy or enlarged neck glands
Lymphomas	Older	Bulky masses in the postnasal space	May cause pressure erosions	Later in paraphary-ngeal wall	Mild	May have enlarged neck gland

8.44 LARYNGEAL MASSES

Causes

Malignant
Carcinoma
Chondrosarcomas
Salivary gland tumors
Metastases
Miscellaneous

Benign
Papillomas/polyps
Laryngocele/mucocele
Hemangioma
Cartilage tumors
Salivary gland tumors

1. Malignant Lesions

- Carcinoma:Mass in the larynx are usually malignant, and virtually all are squamous cell carcinomas.
  - M:F is 5:1, almost always associated with tobacco and alcohol.
  - Peak incidence is 7th decade.
  - Divided into the supraglottic, glottic and subglottic (infraglottic) type.
  - Role of radiologist is to describe the deep extension, the relationship of the mass to surrounding structures, and lymphadenopathy. Pay perticular attention to: laryngeal cartilage invasion, transglottic extension, extension into adjacent fascial spaces especially parapharyngeal space and carotid space, regional lymph nodes including internal jugular chain of nodes and the midline Delphian node. Be observant for possible lung metastasis or secondary lung primary. Needle biopsy of suspicious deep masses may be necessary under imaging guidance.
  - Pitfalls of CT include the inability to reliably differentiate inflammation and edema from tumor, to accurately identify the subsite involvement in the presence of anatomic distortion from large tumors, and

to clearly define margins in the absence of well-developed fat planes.

– MRI has an advantage of multiplanar display especially in determining subglottic extension and in identifying the pre-epiglottic spread. MRI also has difficulty in differentiating edema from tumor but is superior to CT in detecting cartilage invasion.

- *Chondrosarcomas* are slowly growing neoplasms
  – Present usually in the 6th and 7th decade.
  – Cricoid cartilage is usually involved (80%) followed by thyroid cartilage.
  – Lesions in virtually all patients demonstrate coarse or stippled calcifications.
  – Features differentiating from carcinomas include older age at diagnosis, absence of smoking history, and predominately calcified tumor matrix.

- Minor salivary gland tumors as adenocystic carcinomas have been reported. They are indistinguishable from the laryngeal carcinomas but should be considered in patients with laryngeal mass and no history of smoking or drinking.

- Metastases to the larynx usually occur in the terminal stages of the disseminated malignancy. Primary tumors include melanoma (30%), renal cell carcinoma (15%). Site of deposit include supraglottic, (40%), subglottic (20%), glottic (5%) and multifocal (35%).

- Rare tumors include fibrosarcomas, liposarcomas and lymphomas.

2. Benign Lesions

- *Papillomas* constitute 80% of the benign mucosal tumors and are the commonest pediatric laryngeal tumors. These appear as multiple nodular excrescences on the false and true cords producing contour abnormalities of the mucosal surfaces.

- Small cystic lesions can arise in the vallecula or epiglottic surface secondary to the obstruction of minor salivary gland.
- *Vocal cord polyps* can arise secondary to vocal abuse.
- *Laryngoceles* are the air-filled diverticula arising from the saccule of the laryngeal ventricle. They are common in musicians who play wind instruments. They are associated with airway obstruction, pyoceles and vocal cord paralysis. 25% are bilateral. These are of three types:
  - Internal: when confined within thyroid lamina
  - External: lesions that pierce the thyroid membrane
  - Mixed: combination of the internal and external
- *Laryngeal mucocele* is a fluid-filled laryngocele that arises secondary to a small ventricular cancer obstructing the saccule.
- *Subglottic hemangioma* is the commonest laryngeal and upper tracheal neoplasm in the newborn and the young infant. It appears as a well-defined mass in the posterior or lateral portion of the subglottic airway.
- *Chondromas* arise from the hyaline or elastic cartilages of the larynx.
- *Chondrometaplasia* is a condition in which nodules of cartilage arise in the soft tissues of the larynx. Lesions arising in the close vicinity of the laryngeal cartilages may be difficult to differentiate from chondromas or chondrosarcomas on imaging.
- *Schwannomas* typically involve the sensory nerves such as the internal branch of the superior laryngeal nerve and usually arise in the 4th to 6th decade as a palpable mass.
- *Minor salivary gland* tumors as pleomorphic adenomas have been reported.
- Rare tumors include paragangliomas, atypical carcinoid tumor, amyloidosis, etc.

Table 8.44.1: Laryngeal masses

Mass	Location	CT density	Invasion	Comments
Carcinoma	Any part	Soft tissue	+	H/C of Tobacco/alcohol use
Chondrosarcoma	Cartilage (Cricoid)	Soft tissue mass with calcification	+	No H/O smoking with extensive calcification
Salivary gland tumor	Any part	Soft tissue	+ In malignant	No H/O smoking/alcohol devoid of calcification
Metastases	Any part	Soft tissue	NA	H/O primary
Papilloma	Cords	Soft tissue	–	Pediatric age and multiple
Cysts	Vallecula/Epiglottis	Fluid density	–	–
Polyps	Cords	Soft tissue	–	Common in orators, teachers
Laryngoceles/laryngeal mucocele	Vestibule	Air density/fluid density	–	May present as a lateral mass in neck
Hemangioma	Subglottis	Soft tissue	–	Intense enhancement on post-contrast images
Chondromas	Cartilage	Calcific mass	–	Rare

8.45 ORBITAL MASSES

The pediatric patient with an orbital tumor differs substantially from the adult patient with a much greater incidence of congenital lesions, higher frequency of infection, and unique benign and malignant tumors involving the orbit.

PEDIATRIC ORBITAL TUMORS

- Most common orbital masses are cystic lesions of the orbit, mainly dermoids
- Vasculogenic lesions are the second most common
- Others include inflammatory lesions, fat-containing lesions, lacrimal gland masses, lymphoid tumors and leukemia, optic nerve and meningeal tumors, osseous and fibro-osseous masses, rhabdomyosarcoma, and metastatic lesions
- Common malignant processes include rhabdomyosarcoma, metastatic disease, lymphomas and leukemia
- Most orbital tumors in children are benign.

CYSTIC LESIONS

Dermoid Cysts

- Arise from trapped embryonic ectoderm in the suture lines between the orbital bones
- Classified into juxtasutural, sutural, and soft-tissue types.
- Most common type—juxtasutural in the superotemporal and superonasal quadrants.
- Presents as painless mass in superotemporal area at the lateral portion of the eyebrow
- Usually unattached to overlying skin, mobile, smooth and non-tender.

- CT scan reveals a well-circumscribed lesion with a low density lumen.

Teratomas

- Congenital germ-cell tumors arise from primordial germ cells with ectodermal, mesodermal and endodermal components.
- Typically present at birth, with no bone invasion, often cause orbital enlargement.
- Large intraconal masses cause massive proptosis.

VASCULOGENIC LESIONS

Capillary Hemangioma

- One-third are diagnosed at birth, and over 90% are visible by 6 months of age.
- Most common presentation - superficial involvement appearing as tumor and telangiectatic vessels in the skin that with time develops the typical strawberry-like appearance.
- Deeper lesions may appear as raised soft, purplish nodules.
- Deep orbital involvement may present solely with proptosis and no skin changes.
- Orbital hemangiomas frequently produce proptosis, globe displacement and enlarge with Valsalva's maneuvers or crying.
- The typical course is—normal appearance at birth, lesion first noticed at one month, enlarging till 1 to 2 years followed by a stabilization and spontaneous involution by age 4 to 8 years of age.
- Best evaluated with CT or MRI—a diffusely infiltrating non-encapsulated mass, conforming to the surrounding

orbital structures. No bony erosion, although expansion of the orbit is possible.

- Ultrasonography is also a valuable noninvasive test.

Lymphangiomas

- Benign congenital malformation—may affect the conjunctiva, eyelids or deep orbit.
- Classically, viewed as separate from the vascular system, although some overlap has been noted
- Typically, the tumor is identified within the first two decades of life.
- Present as slow enlargement with increasing proptosis over many years, or one of sudden proptosis from intralesional hemorrhage (chocolate cyst).
- The classic lesion is a smooth, pink-orange mass (Salmon patch) under an intact conjunctiva.
- CT scan shows a homogeneous mass with well-defined borders that does not destroy surrounding structures or bone.
- Most lesions are extraconal and in the superior orbit.

ORBITAL MENINGIOMAS AND SCHWANNOMAS

- Most common during the fourth to seventh decade of life. *Primary orbital meningiomas* arise from the optic nerve, 70% invade the orbit from the cranium infiltrative, and enhancing. The classic *"railroad track"* describes calcifications of the tumor along the optic nerve in the subarachnoid space.
- MRI is used to evaluate intracranial extension, showing a hyperintense tumor after contrast administration. *Schwannoma*, or *neurilemmoma* is a benign, noninvasive, peripheral nerve tumor.

- They are relatively rare, usually occur in adults from age 20 to 70 years.
- CT shows well circumscribed, homogeneous, elongated ovoid mass displacing surrounding structures.
- MRI—tumor is hypointense on T1WI and hyperintense on T2-weighted images.
- The tumor is extraconal when associated with the IV cranial nerve, but is more commonly intraconal.

CAVERNOUS HEMANGIOMA (ENCAPSULATED VENOUS MALFORMATION)

- Most common vascular and the most common primary intraconal orbital lesion in adults.
- Average age of onset around 40 years.
- Commoner in women (70%) than men (30%) and is generally unilateral.
- Present with a slowly progressive painless proptosis over several years.
- These do not enlarge with Valsalva.
- CT or MRI reveals a well-defined mass with an oval shape.
- Most are intraconal, but occasionally extraconal.
- On CT they are homogeneous with increased density.
- On MRI they are homogeneous and isointense to muscle. on T1WI and hyperintense on T2WI.
- Following contrast addition, the lesions enhance inhomogeneously.

METASTATIC TUMORS

- Breast carcinoma is commonest metastatic tumor in women followed by lung carcinoma.
- In men, the most common are lung and prostate.
- The average age at presentation is the 7th decade, most being female (due to the higher incidence of breast metastasis).

- On CT, the most common finding is a well-defined, contrast enhancing, intraconal mass.
- The orbital bony walls are also a common site for metastasis, especially with prostate cancers.
- These tumors may show expansion during an acute upper respiratory infection.
- Superficial lesions are more common and have a better prognosis for vision than deeper lesions. No enlargement of the tumor with Valsalva maneuvers.
- Imaging studies include CT and MRI, which both show the multicompartmental nature of the venous-lymphatic malformations.
- MR imaging is preferred over CT because it delineates the internal structure of the cysts.

MISCELLANEOUS

Rhabdomyosarcoma

- Most common orbital malignant tumor found in children.
- Presents early in the first decade with rapid unilateral proptosis and displacement of the globe.
- CT scan shows an irregular tumor with moderately well-defined margins, soft tissue attenuation, and often evidence of bony destruction (50%).
- MR imaging demonstrates a signal similar to muscle on T1 and higher than muscle on T2 weighted images.

Optic Nerve Gliomas

- Often associated with neurofibromatosis type I (18 to 50% of cases), often bilateral.
- Mean age of presentation is about 8 years.
- Typical presentation is proptosis and visual loss or visual field changes.

- Appear as fusiform enlargement of the optic nerve which is isodense to brain on CT.
- Intracranial extension into the optic canal and chiasm is best evaluated with MRI.

Fibrous Dysplasia

- Most frequent fibro-osseous tumor seen exclusively in children in the first 2 decades of life.
- Replacement of normal bone with collagen, fibroblasts, osteoid and giant cells.
- Two types of fibrous dysplasia: polyostotic (Albright's syndrome) and monostotic.
- Polyostotic fibrous dysplasia involves multiple bones, not generally the orbit, abnormal skin pigmentation and precocious puberty.
- Monostotic fibrous dysplasia occurs most often in the bones of the face.
- The orbital roof is the most common site of orbital involvement.
- Usual presentation-adolescent child with proptosis, globes and orbit displacement and facial asymmetry.
- The CT shows thickened abnormal bone with sclerotic lesions with a "ground-glass" appearance.
- Biopsy is usually necessary to confirm the diagnosis and to rule out more aggressive lesions.

Metastatic Tumors

- Neuroblastoma is the most frequent metastatic orbital disease in children.
- Other include Ewing's sarcoma, leukemia, and lymphoma.
- Neuroblastoma is common in children, majority occurring before age 5 (median 22 months).

ADULT ORBITAL TUMORS

In the adult population, the more common types of orbital tumors vary significantly from children. The most common tumor includes carcinomas (paranasal sinus, secondary and metastatic), inflammatory masses (pseudotumor), lacrimal gland tumors, cysts, lymphomas, meningiomas, and vascular tumors (cavernous hemangiomas). Secondary tumors commonly invade the orbit and include mucoceles, squamous cell carcinoma, meningioma, vascular malformations and basal cell carcinoma.

PARANASAL SINUS MASSES

Mass in the paranasal sinuses has the potential to extend into the orbit. The most common mass lesion of the orbit originating in the sinus is the *mucocele.*

Mucocele result from obstruction of a sinus ostium leading to an enlarging fluid filled sinus, which eventually may erode through the orbital bony wall.

- The median age of presentation is around 50 years.
- Most arise from the ethmoid and frontal sinus.
- Patients will present with unilateral proptosis with globe displacement away from the mass, lid swelling and sometimes a palpable mass.
- CT scan reveals a well-defined homogencous mass extending into the orbit through a bony defect associated with an opacified sinus cavity.

Neoplasms of the Paranasal Sinuses

- Benign tumors push the periorbital structures aside, while malignant lesions invade the periosteum.

- Most common malignancy is squamous cell carcinoma.
- Disease is usually advanced at presentation with orbital invasion in almost 2/3rd of the patients.
- Adenocarcinoma arising from the ethmoid sinuses are frequently associated with wood workers.
- Adenoid cystic carcinomas show perineural spread via the infraorbital nerve.
- Locally invasive neoplasms as esthesioneuroblastoma and benign paranasal neoplasm as inverted papilloma may also extend into the orbit.
- Evaluation best done radiologically with CT scan, because of the ability to detect early lesions and note bony destruction with either orbital or intracranial extension.
- MRI scans are useful in detecting intracranial extension and distinguishing certain neoplastic diseases from one another.

ORBITAL PSEUDOTUMOR (IDIOPATHIC ORBITAL INFLAMMATION)

- An inflammatory condition of the orbit of unknown etiology.
- Common cause of proptosis from the 2nd to 7th decade of life.
- Multifocal involvement is common and any orbital structure may be involved.
- Onset of symptoms is acute, however, subacute or chronic forms have been described.
- The typical symptoms are dull orbital pain, which is worse with eye movement.
- Proptosis is the most common finding.
- CT findings show hazy enlargement of affected structures with enhancement after intravenous contrast injection.

- MR T1-weighted images show lesions with similar signal to muscle that enhance with contrast. T2-weighted images have increased signal similar or greater than fat.

LACRIMAL GLAND TUMORS

- About half are epithelial neoplasms, while the other half are lymphoproliferative disorder.
- Lymphoid lesions include benign lymphoid hyperplasia, malignant lymphoma and leukemias. Lymphoid lesions appear as smooth enlargement of the gland on CT scans.
- Epithelial neoplasms appear irregular on CT and include pleomorphic adenomas (benign), adenocystic carcinoma, adenocarcinoma, mucoepidermoid carcinomas, and undifferentiated carcinomas.
- The most common of epithelial leions is the pleomorphic adenoma (benign mixed tumor)which occurs primarily between the ages of 20 and 50 years.
- Most common malignant epithelial neoplasm is adenoid cystic carcinoma.
- CT scans will often show bony destruction and infiltration of the lacrimal mass.

LYMPHOID TUMORS

- Orbital lymphomas may be primary or associated with systemic disease.
- Most orbital lymphomas are localized to the orbit but many patients develop systemic lymphoma over time.
- Orbital lymphoma is an adult disease usually presenting between the age 50 and 70 years.
- Usually an anterior mass, enlarges slowly, causing progressive painless proptosis over months.

OCULAR MASSES

Melanoma

- Arise from choroid in elderly.
- Commonest malignancy in adults.
- Highly invasive with extraocular spread as well.
- Ultrasound typically shows raised echogenic focus along post wall of vitreous chamber (collar button).
- On MRI, melanotic type shows increase T1W and decrease T2W while amelanotic type is isointense to soft tissue.
- Trans-scleral and perineural spread is common.

Retinoblastoma

- Commonest malignancy in childhood.
- 1/3rd are B/L with autosomal dominant inheritance.
- Trilateral retinoblastoma when B/L tumor associated with pineal tumor.
- Highly malignant and aggressive with trans-scleral and hematogenous spread.
- US shows highly echogenic mass with DAS.
- CT is modality of choice and show dense calcification in a retinal based soft tissue mass.
- Any calcification within the globe on CT scans in pediatric patient should be considered retinoblastoma unless proved otherwise.
- MRI is superior to CT in evaluation of trans-scleral or perineural spread or in evaluation of pineal region for additional masses.

Table 8.45.1

Mass	Age	Location PS	Location EXC	Location INC	Orbital expansion	Bone dest[N]	Calcific[N]	ICEXT[N]	CT ATN	CT ENH	MRI T1W	MRI T2W
Dermoid	Newborn	++	++	+	+	−	+	−	Low	−	←→	←
Hemangioma	0-3 month	+−	++	++	+	−	+	+	Mixed	++	→	←
Lymphangioma	0-10 yr	++	++	+	++	−	+	−	Low	+	→	←
Rhabdomyosar	<15 yr	+−	−	+	−	++	−	++	Iso/↑	++	→	←
Op. N Glioma	<10 yr	−	++	++	+	−	−	+	Iso	++	→	←
Neuroblastoma	<4 yr	•+	++	−	−	++	++	++	Iso/↑	++	→	←
Leukemia	>10 yr	++	++	++	−	+	+	+	←	++	→	←
Lymphoma	>10 yr	++	++	+	−	+	−	+	←	++	→	←
PNS masses	>40 yr	−	++	−	+	+	+	+	Iso/↓/↑	+	→	←
Cellulitis/abscess	Any	++	++	+	−	−	−	+	Iso/↓	++	→	←
Pseudotumor	Any	++	++	++	−	−	−	+	Iso	++	→	←
Meningioma	>30 yr	−	−	++	+	+	+	+	Iso/↑	++	→	←
Schwannoma	>20 yr	−	−	++	+	−	−	+	Iso	+	→	←
Retinoblastoma	<10 yr	+	−	++	+	−	+	+	Iso/↑	++	→	←
Melanoma	>40 yr	−	−	++	+	−	−	−	Iso	+	←	→

8.46 INTRAORBITAL CALCIFICATION

Causes
1. Cataract
2. Retinoblastoma
3. Parasitic infection
   – Hydatid cyst
   – Cellulosae cysticercosae
4. Phlebolitis
   – Hemangioma
     Arteriovenous malformation
     Venous varix
5. Orbital meningioma
6. Others
   – Adeno and cystic carcinoma of lacrimal gland
     Neurofibroma
     Rhabdomyosarcoma.

- **Cataract**
  Immature cataract—scattered opacities are separated by clear zones: Mature cataract—totally opaque cortex is noted on US.
- **Retinoblastoma**
  – Most frequent intraocular tumor of childhood.
  – 85% are < 3yrs ; 20-40% have B/L tumors.

Classified as:

Grade-1:	Solitary/multiple, < 4 disc dram in size at or behind equator
Grade-2:	Solitary/multiple ; 4-10 disc dram
Grade-3:	Anterior to equator or solitary > 10 disc dram
Grade-4:	Tumors that are multiple and extend upto or a serrata
Grade-5:	Tumors that involve half of the retina or presence of vitreous seeds.

- Most children present with leukokoria/white pupillary reflex.

  R/F: Irregular intraocular mass, 90% cases show calcification on CT.

  Endophytic extension

  − Projects into vitreous

  Exophytic extension

  − Subretinal space - Radioopaque density

  Contrast enhancement is variable.

  Orbital and intracranial extension.

Orbital Meningioma

Primary: Optic nerve sheath

Secondary: Originates from greater wing of sphenoid with temporal and orbital extension.

Optic Nerve Meningioma

- Adults: 3-5th decades.

  R/F:

  − Tubular/Fusiform thickening of optic nerve.

  − Homogenous contrast enhancement.

  − Tram track sign: Hyperdense mass surrounding hypodense optic nerve.

  − Calcification +ve

  − Optic canal widened by mass or narrowed by hyperostosis

  − Intracranial ext +/-.

Hemangioma

Capillary Hemangioma

- Tumor of early childhood; involutes spontaneously by 6-7th year.
- Forms a soft bluish mass which may involve any part of orbit.

US—well-defined anterior soft lesion with small irregular echoes. Calcification +/−.
CDFI—high flow within immature vessels.

Cavernous Hemangioma

Commonest benign retrobulbar tumor 3-4th decade.

Usually it lies within the muscles core and displacing the optic nerve.

R/F: Honeycomb pattern of altered strong and weak signals on US.

CT: Homogenous mass (hyperdense) with smooth margin showing uniform contrast enhancement.

Phlebolitis +

Expansion of the orbital wall +

Arteriovenous Fistula (Carotid Cavernous Fistula)

Post traumatic/postsurgical

Spontaneous

- Atherosclerosis
  Osteogenesis imperfecta
  Ehlers-Danlos syndrome
  Pseudoxanthoma elasticum
- Clinically patient presents with pulsatile exophthalmos.

R/F: Dilated superior ophthalmic vein which cannot be compressed.

- Reverse flow in the superior ophthalmic vein which is arteralized
- Increased size of extraocular muscles
- Angiography required for endovascular treatment
- Phlebolitis +/−.

Orbital Varices

Varix becomes prominent on prone position, compression of jugular veins and Valsalva's maneuver.

- Ultrasound shows soft echofree lesion with phleboliths.
- CDFI may demonstrate movements of blood flow as malformation fills with blood or empties.
- Orbit may be expanded.
  CT show nodular/serpiginous mass, containing phleboliths, with marked contrast enhancement.
  MRI—Vase stream with signal void or flow related enhancement or echo rephasing due to slow flow.
  Permanent signal may indicate a clot.

Rhabdomyosarcoma

- Highly malignant tumor; most frequent in childhood.
  R/F- Seen as a well defined mass in a muscle or adjacent to it.
    - Mass may include the lacrimal gland with osseous and extraorbital invasion
    - Calcification are frequently seen after radiotherapy.
- *Adenocystic Carcinoma of Lacrimal Gland*
  Most common malignant lacrimal gland tumor.
  R/F—Enlarged gland with irregular serrated bodies, bony erosion of orbital roof.
  Presence of calcific deposit.
- *Hydatid Cyst*
  Can be seen in the retrobulbar region.
  R/F: Spherical/oval mass of low reflectivity/low density.
  Enhancement of walls +ve
  Calcification +ve
  Cellulosae cyst
- Intraocular (vitreous/subretinal space)
- Extraocular (EOMS, eyelid, lacrimal gland, optic nerve)
  R/F—Cystic lesion with an eccentrically placed hyperdense scolex showing ring enhancement.
  Later stages nodular calcification is seen.

Flow Chart 8.46.1

Intraorbital calcification

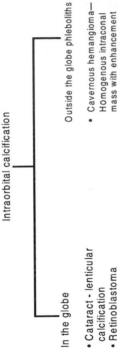

In the globe

- Cataract - lenticular calcification
- Retinoblastoma
  <3 yrs of age
  White pupillary reflex
  Intraocular mass with calcification

Outside the globe phleboliths

- Cavernous hemangioma—
  Homogenous intraconal mass with enhancement and phleboliths
- A-V fistula—
  Dilated SOV and reversal of flow pulsatile exophthalmos
- Orbital varix—
  Becomes prominent in prone position, Valsalva and on compression of jugular vein
- Meningioma—
  Tubular/Fusiform enlargement and optic nerve; tram track appearance 4-5th decade.
- Lacrimal gland carcinoma—
  Enlarged lacrimal gland with adjacent bony destruction
- Hydatid cyst—
  Unilocular/ multilocular retrobulbar cystic lesion

8.47 INNER EAR MASSES

* *The Temporal Bone*
  - Petrous Part 1
  - Squamous Part 2
  - Tympanic Part 3
  - Mastoid Part 4
  - Styloid Process 5
  - Zygomatic Process 6

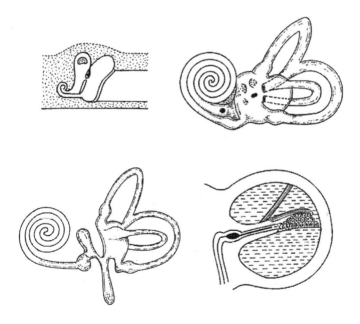

Fig. 8.47.1

- Houses The Structures of Middle and Inner Ears
    - Cochlear Apparatus
      (for Hearing)
      Vestibular Apparatus
      (for Equilibrium)
- The Bony Case is known as Ottic Capsule or Bony Labyrinth while the Funtioning Inner Organ System is known as Membranous Labyrinth.

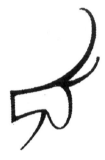

Fig. 8.47.2

METHODS OF IMAGING

1. Plain X-ray, e.g. Stenvers' view
2. Tomography of temporal bone
3. CT scan
    - Axial   especially bony
      Coronal   labyrinth
4. MRI
    - Axial   especially membranous
      Coronal   labyrinth

MASSES

Inflammatory

- Granulomatous labyrinthitis
- Labyrinthitis ossificans
- Sarcoid granuloma
  Cholesteatoma/cholesterol granuloma

Neoplastic

- Schwannoma
- Lipoma
- Arachnoid cyst
- Epidermoid cyst
- AVM
- Hemangioma
- Meningioma
- Lymphoma
- Metastasis
- Temporal bone tumors

Miscellaneous

- Intralabyrinthine hemorrhage
- Vestibular aqueduct syndrome (VAS)

SALIENT FEATURES

Inflammatory

- Labyrinthitis is a term used to describe inflammation of inner ear.
- Viral; Bacterial; Autoimmune.
- Tympanogenic; Meningogenic; Hematogenic; Post-traumatic; Iatrogenic; Tympanogenic may be associated with Cholesteatoma.

- B/L >> U/L: A cholesteatoma may occur here perse.
- On CT and Esp. MR, membranous labyrinth shows faint and segmental enhancement (as compared to schwannoma which shows complete and well-defined enhancement)- ACUTE and SUBACUTE.
- Associated enhancing granuloma and facial nerve enhancement maybe seen.
- In late stages when treatment failure occures a fibrous and very late bony labyrinth also known as labyrinthitis ossificans is seen. The imaging pattern corresponds accordingly, i.e.

Fibrous: hypo T1; minimal/No Enhancement; hypo T2 and GR.
            – iso CT.
Calcified   – hypo T1, T2 with no enhancement.
            – hyper CT.

Intralabyrinthine Bleed

- Coagulopathy, trauma, tumor
- Rare
- Hyper on CT and T1

Vestibular Aqueduct Syndrome

- Most common cause of congenital sensorineural hearing loss diagnosed by imaging.
- On imaging, a large endolymphatic duct and sac are seen. Associated deformity of chochleal medialus present.

Schwannoma

- Of 8th cranial nerve known as Acoustic Neuromas are usually combined intra-and extracanalicular (i.e. CP angle) but may sometimes be purely intracanalicular.

- Sometimes purely intralabyrinthine schwannomas may be seen.
- Slow-growing non-calcifying masses, larger in females
- When small are uniformly isodense [CT], isointense (T1 and T2) while enhance uniformly but as the size increases areas of necrosis and cyst formation may also be seen.

Other neoplasia: but these are not stressed as they are not primary inner ear conditions.

- The appearances are general with the epicentre of lesion being the only feature helping in predicting an inner ear origin, e.g.:

Lipoma: hyper T1, T2 hyper, hypo CT, no enhancement.
Arachnoid cyst: Follows fluid signal.
Epidermoid: Follows with specific changes.
Bone tumors: Bony changes
Vascular tumors: Extreme vascularity.

Flow Chart 8.47.1

Inner ear masses

Inflammatory
- Focal nodular enhancement of labyrinth, patchy
- Fibrous and few bony changes in later stages
- T2—increase, T1—decrease
- Ct—nondetectable in acute

Bleed
- MR is imaging of choice
  T1 - increased
  T2 - decreased
  GR - increased

Other mimicking neoplasm
- Epicentred elsewhere, e.g. bone tumors-temporal epidermoid, arachnoid-CP angle
- Vascular tumors show extensive vascularity, abnormal in nature
- Lymphoma and mets are diffuse conditions associated with known primary, etc.

V.A.S
- Bulky aqueduct with SAC

Schwannoma
- Intense definite nodular enhancement
- No signs of inflammation

8.48 MIDDLE EAR MASSES

A. CONGENITAL

- *Aberrant Internal Carotid Artery*
  - Vascular tympanic membrane.
  - Pulsatile tinnitus.
  - Imaging reveals a tubular soft tissue mass entering middle ear cavity posterolateral to cochlea, crossing mesotympanum along cochlear promontory, exiting anteromedially to become continuous with horizontal portion of carotid canal.
  - Protrusion into middle ear without bony margin.
- *Dehiscent Jugular Bulb*
  - Vascular tympanic membrane.
  - Pulsatile tinnitus.
  - Imaging reveals a soft tissue mass contiguous with jugular foramen and there is absence of a bony plate separating jugular bulb from posteroinferior middle ear.

B. INFLAMMATORY

- *Cholesteatoma*
  - Tumor-like mass of exfoliated keratin within a sac of stratified squamous epithelium.
  - Cholesteatoma is usually an acquired disease (secondary cholesteatoma), but can be congenital (primary cholesteatoma).
  - Acquired cholesteatoma result from in-growth of squamous epithelium through marginal tympanic membrane perforations, from retraction pockets or from in-growth into the middle ear of the basal layer

of the tympanic membrane and are usually related to chronic otitis media.

- High resolution CT is an excellent technique for showing the location and extent of the lesion prior to surgery.

- On CT-images cholesteatoma usually presents as a more or less rounded soft tissue mass, often centered within the epitympanic recess and lesions are commonly associated with erosion of the lateral epitympanic wall (more specifically the scutum) and the ossicular chain.

- Associated findings are thickening of the tympanic membrane and inflammatory polyps in the medial part of the external auditory canal.

- MRI may provide additional information, as the signal characteristics and/or enhancement pattern of cholesteatoma are characteristic being low signal intensity on T1-weighted and a high signal intensity on T2-weighted images.

- *Cholesterol Granuloma*
  - Expansile lesion arising from a pneumatized cavity which becomes closed; the subsequent decrease in air pressure causes edema, fluid accumulation and intralesional bleeding; that promotes granulomatous reaction leading to neovascularity and continuing hemorrhage.

  - In the middle ear cavity they usually arise in the context of chronic otitis media; on otoscopy, this may give rise to a blue tympanic membrane, suggesting the presence of a vascular mass lesion.

  - On CT-images a well-demarcated expansile lesion is seen, indistinguishable from cholesteatoma.

- MR characteristics of cholesterol granulomas are hyperintensity on both T1-and T2-weighted images (this being due to their hemorrhagic components).

- *Granulation Tissue*
  - Vascular reparative tissue, commonly seen in the middle ear and mastoid, in conjunction with other diseases (such as cholesteatoma) or in isolation.
  - It may produce a bluish discoloration of the tympanic membrane, causing clinical doubt as to the presence of a true hypervascular lesion.
  - On CT, granulation tissue causes opacification (linear stranding) of the middle ear and mastoid without erosive changes.
  - On MRI, pronounced enhancement is seen after injection of gadolinium.
  - In rare cases, granulation tissue itself may behave aggressively and cause bony erosion.

C. NEOPLASTIC

a. Benign Tumor

- *Glomus Tumor/Chemodectomas/Nonchromaffin Paragangliomas/Glomerulocytomas* (slow growing vascular lesion arising from glomus body).
  - *Glomus tympanicum* at the cochlear promontory.
- Appears as a globular soft tissue mass with intense post-contrast enhancement.
- It may cause erosion and displacement of the ossicles, however, the inferior wall of the middle ear cavity is left intact.
  - Glomus jugulare at the jugular foramen.
- It causes invasion of the middle ear from below and destroys the bony roof of the jugular fossa and bony spur separating vein from the carotid artery.

- There is intense post-contrast enhancement, destruction of ossicles (usually incus), otic capsule and posteromedial surface of the petrous bone.
- MR imaging show *'salt and pepper appearance'* due to multiple small tumor vessels.
- Angiography is also diagnostic.
- Malignant transformation with metastases to regional nodes is seen in 2-4% cases.
- *Facial Neuroma*
  - It appears as a tubular mass in enlarged/ scalloped facial canal.
- *Choristoma*
  - Ectopic mature salivary tissue.
- *Meningioma*
  - Extracranial meningiomas are rare.
  - Extracranial meningiomas are formed by direct extension outside the skull of a primary intracranial meningioma, by metastasis from a malignant intracranial meningioma, or from extracranial arachnoid cell clusters which accompany certain cranial nerves outside the cranium.
  - The imaging characteristics are similar to those of intracranial meningioma: An enhancing mass lesion with remodeling of the bone is seen; the neighboring bone may appear very sclerotic.

b. Malignant Tumor

- *Squamous Cell Carcinoma*
  - Appears a soft tissue mass with variable enhancement on post-contrast images.
  - Destruction and displacement of ossicular chain and adjacent bones.

- *Metastases*
- *Rhabdomyosarcoma*
  - Commonest soft tissue tumor in children.
  - Appears as a bulky soft tissue mass with uniform post-contrast enhancement producing bony destruc-tion as well.
  - MR is the imaging modality of choice with the tumor being intermediate in signal intensity on T1W images and hyperintense on T2W images.
- Adenocarcinoma (rare), adenocystic carcinoma.

Table 8.48.1: Middle ear masses

Tumor	Location	Imaging	Comments
Aberrant internal carotid artery	Posterolateral to cochlea crossing mesoty-mpanum along cochlear pro-montory	Enhancing mass on post-contrast images and continuous with carotid canal	Protrusion in middle ear cavity without a bony margin
Dehiscent jugular bulb	Posteroinferior middle ear	Enhancing mass contiguous with jugular bulb	Absence of bony plate between jugular bulb and middle ear
Cholesteatoma	Usually in the epitympanic recess	Hypointense on T1W and hyper-intense on T2WI	Erosion of the epity-mpanic wall esp. the scutum and ossicles
Cholesterol granuloma	Non-specific	Hyperintense on T1W and T2WI	Associated with CSOM
Granulation tissue	Non-specific	Linear stranding of middle ear cavity with enhancement on post-contrast images	No bony erosive changes
Glomus tympanicum	Cochlear promontory	Enhancing mass on post-contrast images with erosion and displacement of ossicles	Inferior wall of middle ear cavity remains intact

Contd...

Contd...

Tumor	Location	Imaging	Comments
Glomus jugulare	At the jugular foramen	Enhancing mass on post-contrast images with destruction of ossicles and posteromedial surface of petrous bone	Destruction of inferior wall of middle ear cavity, roof of jugular fossa and bony spur separating vein from carotid artery
Meningioma	Non-specific	Enhancing mass with remodeling of bone	Sclerosis of adjacent bone
Malignant masses as squamous cell carcinoma, rhab-domyosarcoma	Non-specific	Enhancing mass on post-contrast images with destruction of ossicles and other adjacent bones	Histopathology is confirmative

8.49 EXTERNAL ACOUSTIC MASSES

Causes

1. Keratosis obturans
2. Ext. auditory canal cholesteatoma
3. Malignant external otitis
4. Benign tumors
   - Exostosis
   - Osteomas
   - Epidermoidomas/primary congenital
   - Cholesteatoma.
5. Malignant tumors
   - Squamous cell carcinoma
   - Basal cell carcinoma
   - Ceruminoma
   - Rare

- metastasis, myeloma.
- osteosarcoma, chondrosarcoma.
6. Histiocytosis
7. Some middle ear masses may also extend.

Keratosis Obturans

- Usually occurs in individuals <40 yrs.
- H/O sinusitis/bronchiectasis [? Results in reflux sympathetic stimulation of ceruminous gland of external auditory canal (EAC)].
- Keratin plugs occlude the medial portion of EAC and the adjacent bony canal is diffusely widened (Reflux hyperemia).

EAC Cholesteatoma (0.1 to 0.5% in EAC)

- Usually occurs in individuals >40 yrs.
- Unilateral, chronic, associated with otorrhea.
- Localized erosion of the canal wall with elevation of epidermis by cholesteatoma embedded in the bony wall.
- Formation of sequestrum and sinus tracts may be present.
- Most common site is along the posteroinferior wall of EAC but lateral to temporomandibular joint.
- Exact cause-Unknown; periostitis of the bony canal.

Malignant External Otitis

- Disease of elderly who are diabetic/immunocompromised.
- Causative agent is usually pseudomonas. Staphylococcus and Aspergillus.
- Often begins in an insidious fashion at the osseocartilaginous junction as a focal area of ulceration and osteitis of EAC. TM is resistant to the infectious process.

- Infection may spread—Parotid gland, TMJ, soft tissue of neck, skull base/involvement of mastoid, petrous apex and middle ear may also occur.
- Intracranial extension can occur through the petro-occipital synchondrosis.

    CT: Bone destruction and sequestrum, soft tissue edema. Abscess in parapharyngeal spaces, intra-cranial invasion.

    MRI: Superior to CT for detection of marrow invasion and soft tissue changes.

    In-III WBC and Tc-99m SPECT- Best imaging approach to assess the post-therapeutic response.

EXOSTOSIS

- Most common benign tumor of EAC.
- Arises in the medial aspect of the osseous portion of the EAC near tympanic annulus.
- Seen in patients with prolonged exposure to cold sea water, swimming pool water.
- Seen as sessile multinodular bony masses. Unilateral or bilateral.

OSTEOMAS

- Less common than exostosis.
- Mastoid is the most common extracanalicular site.
- Seen as solitary, U/L pedunculated growths of mature bone located in the outer portion of the EAC.

Sq.Cell Ca. (Squamous Cell Carcinoma)

- Most common malignant tumor of the ear.
- H/O chronic external otitis is usually positive.

- Tumor destroys the adjacent bone in the EAC and middle ear and invades the surrounding tissue.
- The most important CT finding suspected of carcinoma is -erosion of the walls of EAC/middle ear by a soft tissue mass in a patient who does not have a history of cholesteatoma.
- Predictor of poor outcome
  - Extensive tumor, 8th nerve involvement, cervical/periparotid LN.

Ceruminomas

Apocrine gland within the EAC are known as ceruminous glands. Tumors arising from ceruminous gland.
- Ceruminous adenoma
  - Rare - 5th to 6th decade
- Pleomorphic adenoma
  CT: soft tissue mass without bony destruction.
- Adenoid cystic carcinoma
- Mucoepidermoid carcinoma
- Ceruminous adenocarcinoma
- Most common.
  CT findings are similar to squamous cell carcinoma except that metastases to regional lymph nodes is more common.

Metastasis

- Hematogenous: Breast, prostate, lung, kidney, thyroid.
- Direct spread: Skin, parotid, nasopharynx, brain, meninges.
- Systemic involvement: Leukemia, lymphoma, myeloma.
- These lesions present as diffuse/focal osteolytic destructive pattern.

Table 8.49.1: External acoustic mass

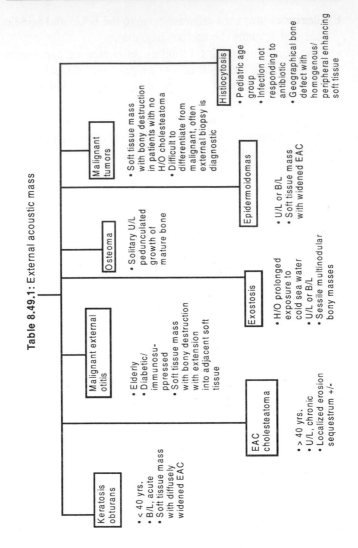

Keratosis obturans
- < 40 yrs.
- B/L, acute
- Soft tissue mass with diffusely widened EAC

EAC cholesteatoma
- > 40 yrs.
- U/L, chronic
- Localized erosion sequestrum +/-

Malignant external otitis
- Elderly
- Diabetic/immunosuppressed
- Soft tissue mass with bony destruction with extension into adjacent soft tissue

Exostosis
- H/O prolonged exposure to cold sea water
- U/L or B/L
- Sessile multinodular bony masses

Osteoma
- Solitary U/L pedunculated growth of mature bone

Malignant tumors
- Soft tissue mass with bony destruction in patients with no H/O cholesteatoma
- Difficult to differentiate from malignant, often external biopsy is diagnostic

Epidermoidomas
- U/L or B/L
- Soft tissue mass with widened EAC

Histiocytosis
- Pediatric age group
- Infection not responding to antibiotic
- Geographical bone defect with homogenous/peripheral enhancing soft tissue

Epidermoidomas (Primary Congenital Cholesteatoma)

- Consists of masses of ectodermal rests (different from true cholesteatomas whose formation is a reaction to inflammation and trapped squamous epithelium).
- Seen as a soft tissue mass with widening of EAC.

Histiocytosis

- Primarly affects the pediatric age group.
- In the temporal bone-EAC and mastoids are commonly involved.
- Patients presents with otalgia and draining ear.
- Cases are diagnosed only after treatment with antibiotic first to cure a suspected middle/ext. ear infection.
- Early imaging findings mimic inflammatory diseases beveled. Bone destruction pattern is usually geographical with edge enhancement of soft tissue may be homogenous or peripheral.

8.50 INTRAMEDULLARY LESIONS

- Intramedullary lesions are lesions of spinal cord.
- Tumors
  - Most are malignant.
  - 90-95%.
- Gliomas
  - >95%
- Ependymomas
  - Low grade astrocytomas
  - Oligodendroglioma
- Less common
  - Hemangioblastomas

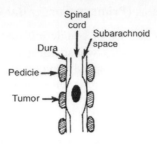

Fig. 8.50.1: Intramedullary lesions

- Paragangliomas
- Lipoma
- Epidermoid—rare
- Gangliocytoma
- Metastasis
- Non-neoplastic cystic lesions
  - Hydrosyringomyelia
  - Hematomyelia
- Inflammatory diseases
  - Multiple sclerosis
  - Transverse myelitis
  - Tuberculoma–rare
  - Cysticercosis
  - Intramedullary abscess
  - Sarcoidosis.
- Infarct

Ependymoma

- Most common spinal cord tumor overall.
- Most common intramedullary tumor in adults.
- Arise from ependymal cells.

Intramedullary

Most common- Cellular type- circumscribed, sharply.
- Most common site—cervical cord.
- Mean age 43 yrs
  - Cystic degeneration.
- F>M
  - Hemorrhage
- Typically—symmetric cord expansion.
- *Myxopapillary type* exclusively in conus and filum terminale.
- Mean age 28 yrs
  - Slow growing, filling and expanding lumbosacral spinal cord.
  - M > F hemorrhage and cystic degeneration-common.
- C/F- back or neck pain, leg or sacral pain.
- X-ray: Widened canal or bone destruction in -20%.
- Myelography
  - Nonspecific cord widening.
  - Multisegmented lesion.
  - Small conus medullaris or filum terminale lesions.
  - Well-delineated intradural mass with contrast meniscus.
- CT
  - Nonspecific canal widening.
  - Posterior scalloping.

- Neural foraminae enlargement.
- MRI
  - Iso on T1 and hyper on T2.
  - Hypointensity at tumor margin on T2WI.
  - Cyst formation, hemorrhage, necrosis.
  - Enhance strongly following contrast administration.

Astrocytomas

- Second most common spinal cord tumor overall.
- Most common cord tumor in children.
- Usually low grade-fibrillary astrocytomas.
- Anaplastic astrocytomas and glioblastoma multiforme.
- Mean age at presentation -21yrs (9 mth-70 yrs).
- M = F
- Most common site—Cervical cord, and thoracic cord.
  - Multisegmental involvement.
- Most common clinical feature—Pain
  - Sign and symptom of neurological dysfunction, often absent early in disease.

X-ray
- May be normal.
- Widened interpedicular distance.

Myelography
- Nonspecific cord enlargement.
- Canal widening.
  MRI—iso to hypo on T1, hyper on T2, enhance after contrast.
- Intratumoral cyst formation and associated syrinx are common.

Hemangioblastoma

- 1-5% of cord tumors
- Fourth decade

- 75% intramedullary
- 10-15% combined intra and extra medullary (intradural)

- Most common site (50%)
- Thoracic cord, cervical cord (40%)

- Highly vascular nodule with an extensive cyst that diffusely enlarges the cord with prominent leptomeningeal vessels.

C/F

- Sensory changes—typically impaired proprioception.
- 1/3rd- associated with VHL disease.
- Myelocord expansion with prominent dilated tortuous vessels seen in 50% patients.
- Angiography—highly vascular mass with dense prolonged tumor blush with prominent vessels.
  MR-cord expansion with high signal intensity on T2 WI with strong CE with prominent foci of high velocity signal loss.
- Cyst formation and syrinx—50-70%.

Oligodendroglioma

- Non glial neoplasms
  - Ganglioglioma
  - Schwannoma
    rare.

Lipoma

- Rare
- May be associated with dysraphism.

- CT- fat density.
- MR- high signal intensity on T1WI.

Epidermoid

- Rare.
- Congenital/ or iatrogenic.
- Usually oval shaped lesions with variable signal intensity depending upon contents.

Syringohydromyelia

- Fluid-filled cavity usually centered on the central canal $\pm$ extending into dorsal column through the white commissure.
- Cylindrical—Involve most of the cord. May enlarge the cord.
- Fusiform—usually segmental.
  - 80% associated with Chiari-I malformation.
  - Most of the rest are idiopathic.
    - Post-traumatic.
    - Post-arachnoiditic.
    - Above and below intramedullary tumors especially hemangioblastoma.
- Well shown by MRI-signal characteristics similar to CSF.
- IVGd may be necessary to exclude tumor in idiopathic cases.
- Plain CT—May or may not reveal dilatation of central canal.
- CT myelo early and delayed imaging after contrast administration.
  (6 or 10 hours)- Helps in diagnosis.

Hematomyelia

± May or may not be associated with subarachnoid hemorrhage.

- Trauma
- SVM
  - Spinal cord AVM most common course of non-traumatic spinal hemorrhage.
- Anticoagulant therapy
- Hemorrhage into cord tumor, syrinx, or hemorrhagic area may be associated with inflammatory myelitis.

MRI—Aside from intramedullary hematoma and their primary causative lesions, may show superficial hemosiderosis, seen as a coat of marked hypointensity on T2WI.

Intramedullary Abscesses

- Very rare
- Usually associated with dermal sinuses
- Enhancement of the meninges after IV gadolinium contrast can be helpful to indicate inflammation in some of the rare condition.
- Enhancement not seen with multiple sclerosis or acute transverse myelitis.
- Metastatic disease to the cord-
  - Rare
  - Variable incidence-0.9% -8.5%
  - Most common primary lung 40-85% of total metastatic lesions.
- Breast carcinoma, melanoma, lymphoma, colonic Ca, kidney Ca.
- Thoracic cord > cervical >lumbar.

C/F- Pain, weakness, paresthesias, bowel and bladder dysfunction.

- Rapid clinical progression as compared to primary cord tumors.
- Plain X-ray and myelography—usually normal.
- Vertebral metastasis may or may not be associated.
- MR—hypointense on T1 and hyperintense on T2 -with or without cord widening.
- Usually central—hypointensity, on T1 which may be confused with syrinx.
- Contrast enhancement is present.

Note: Size of metastasis is disproportionately small compared to the amount of the edema.

Infarction

- Usually involve long segment of the cord.
- Shown only by MRI.
- Usually intensified centrally.
- Particular clinical setting.
  MC-after
    - Thoracoabdominal aortic aneurysm repair.
    - Thrombosis of dural AVF and their draining veins.

Table 8.50.1: Intramedullary lesions

Lesion	X-ray	Myelo	CT	MRI	Comments
• Ependymoma	• Canal widening	• Cord expansion	• Canal widening	• Iso on T1	• Most common site→conus
	• Posterior scalloping		• Post scalloping	• Hyper on T2	• Cervical cord
			• Neural foramen enlargement	± cyst	• Mean age for intra-medullary lesion – 43 yrs
			• Focal lesion with contrast enhancement	• Intense homogenous, sharply marginated contrast enhancement	
			± cyst		
• Astrocytoma	–do–	–do–	–do–	• hypo on T1	• Most common site-cervicothoracic
				• hyper-T2	• Mean age-21 yrs
				• More patchy irregular CE	
• Hemangio-blastoma	–do–	• Prominent dilated tortous vessels 50%	• Cystic lesion with mural nodule showing CE	• Cystic lesion	• Angiography shows highly vascular mass with prolonged tumor blush
				• Hyperintense T2 with strongly enhancing nodule	± Dysraphism
• Lipoma	• Normal	• Cord expansion	• Fat +	• Flow void	• H/o primary malignancy
				• ↑T1 and ↑T2	
• Metastasis	• Canal widening ± normal ± vertebral lesions	• ± Cord expansion	• ± Normal	• ↓T1 and ↑↑T2 with CE ± cord widening	
			• Focal hypodensity with CE focus		
• Multiple sclerosis	• Normal	• ± Normal, ± Cord enlargement	• Normal	• Focal T2 hyperintense with CE	• Clinical H/o relapse or remission
				• Posterolaterally	• oligoclonal band on CSF examination
				• Pencil shaped ± CNS (intracranial) lesion	
• Transverse myelitis	• Normal	• Normal	• Normal	• ↓T1 and ↑T2 with CE	• Cervicothoracic
				• Effects both half of cord	• H/o Inf vaccination
• Syringohydromyelia	• Normal	• ± Cord enlargement	• ± widened central cord	• Cystic lesion with signal intensity parallel to CSF	• 80% Chiari-I malformation
			• Delayed CT myelography		

8.51 INTRADURAL EXTRAMEDULLARY MASSES

Intradural extramedullary masses arise inside the dura but outside the spinal cord. Nerve sheath tumors and meningiomas account for 80-90% of such masses. Other tumors are uncommon and include paraganglioma, epidermoid, dermoid, arachnoid cysts and meningoceles, lipoma, sarcoma, metastases and non-Hodgkin's lymphoma.

From a *radiological point of view* the classical myelographic criteria are:
- Widening of the subarachnoid space on the side of the mass
- Contralateral displacement of the cord and nerve roots away from the mass.
- Delineation of the mass by a sharp meniscus of contrast abutting the lesion.

Nowadays, MRI is the modality of choice and clearly shows not only the signs of cord displacement and CSF space widening but also the lesion itself. Plain films may show bony changes when the tumor has enlarged the spinal canal, erosion of the pedicle with widening of the neural foramen, scalloping of the vertebral body.

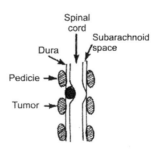

Fig. 8.51.1: Intradural extramedullary masses

NERVE SHEATH TUMORS

Nerve sheath tumors usually arise from dorsal roots, rarely are entirely intramedullary presumably from aberrant nerve roots. They include schwannomas, neurofibromas and rare ganglioneuromas and neurofibrosarcoma.

Clinical symptoms are often similar to those of a disk herniation, with pain and radiculopathy. When they compress the spinal cord myelopathic signs may be present.

- *Nerve sheath tumors* are the commonest intradural extramedullary mass (25-30%) and are primarily seen in middle-aged adults between the ages of 20 and 50 years, with no predilection for either sex.
- *Schwannomas* (Synonyms-neurinoma/neurilemmoma)are typically lobulated, encapsulated masses; nerve fibers do not course through them. They are slightly more common than neurofibromas.
- Neurofibromas are unencapsulated, typically fusiform and less well-defined lesions. Nerve fibers course through them.
- Nerve sheath tumors are variable in location: 70% are intradural extramedullary, 15% are "dumb-bell" shaped tumors, and 15% are extradural.
- These lesions typically enlarge the adjacent neural foramen; calcification within them is rare.
- They are typically (75%) isointense on T1WI and the vast majority are hyperintense on T2WI; virtually all exhibit marked and homogeneous enhancement with Gadolinium.
- Other nerve sheath tumors such as ganglioneuroma or neurofibrosarcoma are rare.
- Multiple intraspinal neurofibromas and schwannomas are pathognomonic of NF1 and NF2 respectively. Malignant degeneration of neurofibromas and rarely schwannomas may occur in NF.

MENINGIOMAS

Meningiomas arise from arachnoid cluster cells located at exit zones of nerve roots or entry zones of arteries. Slowly progressive myelopathy is the most common clinical presentation with motor and sensory deficits, sphincter dysfunction and pain.

- Meningiomas are second to nerve sheath tumors, in frequency, accounting for 25% of all spinal tumors. They are, however, much less common than intracranial meningiomas, the ratio being 1:8.
- Peak incidence is in the fifth and sixth decades. More than 80% occur in women.
- The thoracic spine is the most common site (80%) followed by the cervical spine (15%). The lumbar spine is an uncommon location.
- Meningiomas may rarely calcify and can be seen also on plain films and at CT
- On MRI they are isointense on both T1-and T2-weighted images and enhance markedly
- Most spinal meningiomas are benign and slow-growing neoplasm. Ninety percent of spinal meningiomas are intradural, whereas 5% each are "dumb-bell" or extradural lesions.
- Plain films are usually normal. Bone erosion is uncommon (15%). Calcification is rare (1-5%).
- MR scans may demonstrate broad-based dural attachment; a "dural tail" sign in some cases. Occasionally, densely calcified meningiomas are markedly hypointense on MR and show only minimal contrast enhancement.
- A rare variant of spinal meningioma is meningiomatosis characterized by diffuse involvement of the meninges by the tumor. MR imaging demonstrates thick or nodular enhancement, but is nonspecific. This variant carries a dismal prognosis.

- Another rare type of meningioma is angioblastic meningioma, a significantly more aggressive type that carries the potential for extraneural metastases and possibly subarachnoid seeding. These contain a dense capillary bed and varied cellular element including xanthomatous features with intracellular fat. This results in varied signal intensity on T1WI, depending on the amount of fat present, and generally increased signal on T2WI because of the rich capillary bed.

EMBRYONAL TUMORS

Embryonal tumors are a less common group, with the exception of lipomas, which are probably the most common. Lipomas, dermoids and epidermoids may present as primary intramedullary mass lesions at the level of the spine. They are most frequently recognized as intradural intramedullary lesions at or near the conus medullaris in conjunction with dysraphic complexes.

- *Lipomas*
    - Are characterized by the high signal intensity on T1 weighted images which is less intense with more T2 weighting.
- *Epidermoid cysts*
    - Are lined only by superficial epidermal contents of the skin and are filled with keratinized debris and cholesterol
    - They are congenital or may be acquired as a result of subarachnoid implantation of epidermal elements following lumbar puncture or spinal surgeries.
    - They are found in thoracic spine.
    - They have signal characteristic that follow CSF on T1 and T2WI and are detected on PD and FLAIR images on the basis of their 'cottage cheese' appearance.

- *Dermoid cysts*
  - Are lined by simple or stratified squamous epithelium containing hair follicles, sweat glands, and sebaceous cysts that secrete fatty material into the cyst.
  - Approximately 80% are isolated masses and the rest are associated with dorsal dermal sinuses.
  - They display a variety of noncharacteristic signal intensity patterns with MR not only among different lesions but also within the same tumor. This may be related to the physical state (solid *Vs* liquid) and lipid content (cholesterol *Vs* fatty acid) of the cyst.

PARAGANGLIOMAS

- Usually found in the cauda equina and filum terminale
- They are usually isointense to spinal cord on T1WI and hyperintense on T2WI. MRI may show a 'salt and pepper' appearance because of multiple areas of flow voids secondary to hypervascularity.

ARACHNOID CYSTS

- Are common in mid and lower thoracic region, most commonly located posterolaterally, displacing the cord anteriorly and compressing it.
- They are believed to result from the proliferation of arachnoid adhesions caused by trauma, hemorrhage, inflammation or congenital abnormalities. They are accurately characterized noninvasively by MRI.

METASTASES

- May be in form of single or multiple nodules or diffuse subarachnoid seeding.
- Medulloblastoma in pediatric age group and ependymomas and glioblastoma in adults are the commonest intracranial tumors producing CSF seeding followed by

pineoblastoma, germinoma, retinoblastoma and choroid plexus carcinoma. Extracranial tumors seeding the meninges include the carcinoma of the lung and breast, leukemia, lymphoma and melanoma.

- The overall sensitivity of unenhanced and enhanced MRI in detecting intradural extramedullary metastases is only 19% and 36% respectively in patients with CSF cytological findings positive for neoplasia, so the CSF examination remains the gold standard (despite the fact that the single CSF specimen is only 50% sensitive to drop metastases).

CYSTICERCOSIS

- A parasitic infestation that can result in cysts within the subarachnoid space
- Most cases are associated with extraspinal involvement.
- These are most commonly seen in the thoracic region.
- MRI reveals lesion with typical cyst-like intensity.
- In addition, nonspecific cord changes resulting from arachnoiditis can be seen characterized by an enlarged cord with irregular margins on T1WI and focal increased signal on T2WI.

LATERAL THORACIC MENINGOCELES

- Seen in association with NF-1 and Marfan's syndrome
- They represent CSF outpouchings that extend into and enlarge the neural foramina, containing both the dura and arachnoid, and follow CSF signal intensity on MRI. No enhancement is seen on postcontrast images.

SPINAL SUBDURAL EMPYEMA

- Collection of pus in the subdural space
- It is very rare event.

Flow Chart 8.51.1: Intradural extramedullary masses

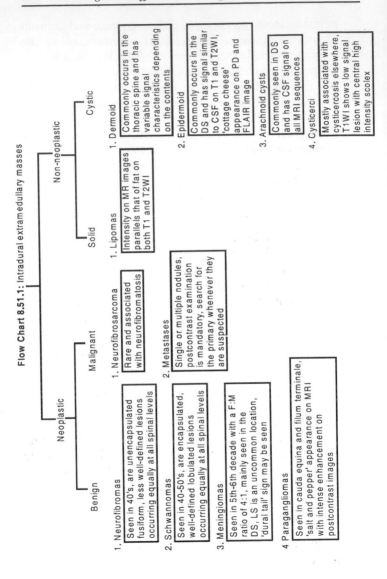

Intradural extramedullary masses

- **Neoplastic**
  - **Benign**
    1. **Neurofibromas** — Seen in 40's, are unencapsulated fusiform, less well-defined lesions occurring equally at all spinal levels
    2. **Schwannomas** — Seen in 40-50's, are encapsulated, well-defined lobulated lesions occurring equally at all spinal levels
    3. **Meningiomas** — Seen in 5th-6th decade with a F:M ratio of 4:1, mainly seen in the DS, LS is an uncommon location, 'dural tail' sign may be seen
    4. **Paragangliomas** — Seen in cauda equina and filum terminale, 'salt and pepper' appearance on MRI with intense enhancement on postcontrast images
  - **Malignant**
    1. **Neurofibrosarcoma** — Rare and associated with neurofibromatosis
    2. **Metastases** — Single or multiple nodules, postcontrast examination is mandatory, search for the primary whenever they are suspected
- **Non-neoplastic**
  - **Solid**
    1. **Lipomas** — Intensity on MR images parallels that of fat on both T1 and T2WI
  - **Cystic**
    1. **Dermoid** — Commonly occurs in the thoracic spine and has variable signal characteristics depending on the contents
    2. **Epidermoid** — Commonly occurs in the DS and has signal similar to CSF on T1 and T2WI, 'cottage cheese' appearance on PD and FLAIR image
    3. **Arachnoid cysts** — Commonly seen in DS and has CSF signal on all MRI sequences
    4. **Cysticerci** — Mostly associated with cysticercosis elsewhere, T1WI shows low signal lesion with central high intensity scolex

- Different factors including the absence of veins, the filter action of the epidural spinal space, and the centripetal direction of spinal blood flow have been suggested to explain the rarity of this event as compared to spinal epidural empyemas on the one hand and to intracranial subdural empyemas on the other.

8.52 EXTRADURAL EXTRAMEDULLARY LESION

Epidural Space

- Space between dura mater and bone.
- Contains epidural venous plexus, lymphatic channels connective tissue and fat.
- Classic myelographic feature is displacement of the thecal sac away from bony walls of the spinal canal with extrinsic compression.
- If block-interface between lesion and contrast column is poorly defined with "feathered" appearance of level of obstruction.
- MR scan clearly show the dura draped over the mass.
- Crescent of epidural fat can be seen capping the lesion.

D/D's

- Disk Disease
  - Bulging disk

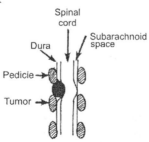

Fig. 8.52.1: Extradural extramedullary lesions

- – Disk protrusion
- – Herniated nucleus pulposus
- – Sequestrated nucleus pulposus
- Inflammation
  - – Epidural abscess
- Hematoma
  - – Post-traumatic
  - – Spontaneous
- Tumors
a. Benign
   Nerve sheath tumor
   Meningioma
   Hemangioma
   Epidural lipomatosis
   Angiolipoma
   Cysts
   - – Arachnoid cysts
   - – Synovial cysts
b. Malignant
   Metastasis
   - – Adult
     - o Breast
     - o Lung
     - o Prostate
   Lymphoma
   - – Children
     - o Ewing's sarcoma
     Neuroblastoma
   Ewing's sarcoma

Disk Bulge

- Loss of turgor of nucleus pulposis and loss of elasticity of annulus fibrosis → disk bulges.
- Decrease height of intervertebral disk space

X-ray

- Vacuum sign
- Endplate sclerosis/osteophyte

NECT/MR

- Loss of (normal) posterior disk concavity.
- Diffuse, non-focal protrusion of disk material beyond the adjacent vertebral endplate.

Disk protrusion → Focal incomplete extension of contents of nucleus pulposus through an incomplete tear of annulus fibrosis.

Disk herniation → Herniation of nucleus pulposus through an annular defect causes focal protrusion of disk material beyond the adjacent endplate.

Free disk or sequestrated disk → Disk material migrates inferiorly, superiorly, medially or laterally.

Epidural abscess

- Hematogenous dissemination → staphylococcus access
  I. Phlegmonous stage: Thickened inflamed tissue with granulomatous material and embedded micro-abscesses.
  II. Frank abscess—with collection of liquid pus

Clinical features → Fever, local tenderness

- Predisposing condition → diabetes, i.v. drug abuse

Imaging → X-ray →

- Osteomyelitis
- Disk space narrowing

CT/MR/Myelo/CT myelo → extradural soft tissue mass with extradural block

CE → Diffuse homogenous or slightly heterogenous → 70% → Phlegmonous stage.

- Thick/thin rim enhancement, 30% frank necrotic abscess

Epidural Hematoma

- Most common cause
  - Trauma
- Spontaneous →
  - Anticoagulation
  - Vigorous exercise
  - Hypertension
  - Vascular malformation
  - Postsurgical
  - Collagen vascular disorders
- Most common site → Upper thoracic region, in dorso-lateral aspect of spinal canal.
  CT → high density lentiform collection located adjustment to neural arch
  MRI → investigation of choice.

Hemangioma

- Slow growing benign neoplasm, 4th to 6th decade
- Most common site vertebral body, 10-15% → Posterior elements
- Most epidural → secondary to expansion of intraosseous lesion
- 1% → completely extraosseous

C/F

- Most → asymptomatic
- Pain → Due to pathological fracture
- Epidural mass

X-ray → Lytic lesion with honeycomb trabeculation or thick vertical striation.

NCCT → Lytic lesion with typical Polka-dot densities in medullary space

Myelo/CT myelo → Epidural mass

MR → Hyperintensity on T1 and T2 with foci of very low SI, suggestive of thickened vertical trabeculae.

Show—Contrast enhancement.

Epidural Lipomatosis

- Excessive deposition of unencapsulated fat in epidural space
- Part of—Morbid obesity
  - Associated with central or truncal lipomatosis
- M>>f
- 60% thoracic spine 40% in lumbar spine

Clinical features—weakness back pain
- Redicular pain, numbness

Myelo → (Normal) to extradural blocks.

CT/MR→ Increased extradural fat with diminished subarachnoid space.

Spinal Angiolipoma

Very rare—Mature adipose tissue with blood vessels
- Fifth decade, F > M
- MC → Thoracic spine
- Dorsal or dorsolateral to cord

Myelo → Extradural mass or block

CT → Low to intermediate density, epidural mass showing contrast enhancement

MR → Iso to hyper on T1 and hyper on T2
- Diffuse homogenous contrast enhancement → Typical.

Cysts

Extradural arachnoid cysts: → CSF filled out pouching of arachnoid that protude through dural defect.

- 2/3rd → Mid to low thoracic level
- 20% → Lumbosacral region
- Imaging studies show → long segment CSF equivalent extradural mass that causes spinal cord

Compression or myelographic block
- Secondary bony changes → Widened interpedicular distance
- Scalloping of vertebral bodies
- Pedicle thinning/erosion
- Synovial (Juxta-articular) cysts—Rare
  - Associated with facet degeneration

Malignant Lesions

Metastasis
- In adults from → Breast
  - Lung   → 50%
  - Prostate

Other from → lymphoma, Melanoma, Renal cancer, Sarcoma and Multiple myeloma

In children
- Ewing's sarcoma
- Neuroblastoma
- Pediatric tumors → invade via neural foramen causing a circumferential cord compression
- Adult → initial site is in invertebral body with secondary involvement of epidural space
- Lower thoracic and lumbar spine

X-ray →
- Pedicle destruction
- Multifocal lytic vertebral body lesion
- Sclerotic lesion → Breast/prostate
- Indistinct posterior vertebral body margin

- Paraspinal soft tissue mass.
- Myelography—extradural blocks
- Bone scintigraphy → Sensitive
- NCCT → Lytic/blastic lesion, with epidural soft tissue mass.
- Intrathecal contrast required to delineate precise extent of lesion
- MR → exquisitely delineates epidural and paraspinal soft tissue involvement
- Low signal on T1 and high on T2.

Lymphoma—NHL → 85%

- HL → Less common
- –40-60 yrs, M>>F
- Spinal extradural mass with nonspecific imaging findings
- NHL → can cause bone destruction and hyperostosis
- Epidural extension best delineated on MRI.
- Ewing's sarcoma → Children second decade M>F
- Nonspecific findings
- Eroded vertebral body with paraspinal soft tissue mass
- Hypo- to isointense T1 and hyper on T2WI.

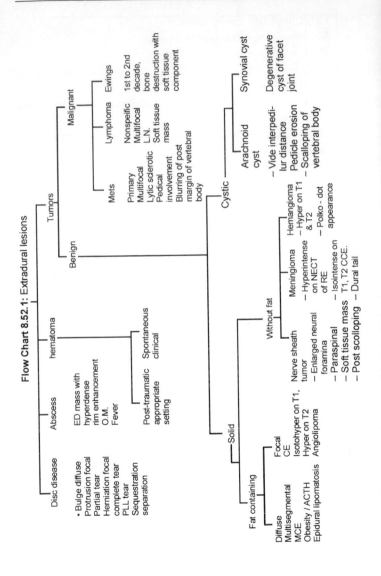

Flow Chart 8.52.1: Extradural lesions

Extradural lesions
- Disc disease
  - Bulge diffuse
  - Protrusion focal
  - Partial tear
  - Herniation focal complete tear
  - PLL tear
  - Sequestration separation
- Abscess
  - ED mass with hyperdense rim enhancement O.M. Fever
- hematoma
  - Post-traumatic appropriate setting
  - Spontaneous clinical
- Tumors
  - Benign
    - Solid
      - Fat containing
        - Diffuse Multisegmental MCE Obesity / ACTH Epidural lipomatosis
        - Focal CE Isotohyper on T1, Hyper on T2 Angiolipoma
      - Without fat
        - Nerve sheath tumor
          - Enlarged neural foramina
          - Paraspinal
          - Soft tissue mass
          - Post scolloping
        - Meningioma
          - Hyperintense on NECT of RE
          - Isointense on T1, T2 CCE.
          - Dural tail
        - Hemangioma
          - Hyper on T1 & T2
          - Polko - dot appearance
    - Cystic
      - Arachnoid cyst
        - Vide interpedicular distance
        - Pedicle erosion
        - Scalloping of vertebral body
      - Synovial cyst
        - Degenerative cyst of facet joint
  - Malignant
    - Mets
      - Primary
      - Multifocal
      - Lytic sclerotic
      - Pedical involvement
      - Blurring of post margin of vertebral body
    - Lymphoma
      - Nonspeific
      - Multifocal
      - L.N.
      - Soft tissue mass
    - Ewings
      - 1st to 2nd decade, bone destruction with soft tissue component

Extradural Masses

Feature	Nerve sheath tumor	Meningioma	Hemangioma	Extradural lipomatosis	Angiolipoma
1. Age	Middle decades	5th to 6th decade	4th to 6th decade	Adult	Fifth decade
2. Sex distribution	M = F	F > M	M = F → Asymptomatic cases	M > F	F > M
3. Distribution	Uniform distribution with slight lumbar predominance	Thoracic spine ≈ 80% Cervical spine ≈ 15%	F>M symptomatic cases Twice thoracic than lumbar spine	60% thoracic spine 40% lumbar spine	Thoracic spine
4. Usual location	70% intradural 15% extradural 15% dumb-bell	90% intra dural 5% extra dural 5% dumb bell	Part or all of vertebral body with sec. extradural space ext.	Primarily in extradural space	Primarily in extradural space
5. C/F	Pain, Rediculopathy	Motor and sensory deficit	60% Asymptomatic 20% pain 20% progressive neurologic deficit	• Weakness • Body pain	Weakness body pain, paresthesia, numbness
6. X-ray	• Pedical erosion • Enlarged neural foramen • Paravertebral soft tissue mass • Posterior scalloping of vertebral body	Usually normal	Cystic lesion with prominent vertical trabeculation	Normal	Normal

8.53 D/D OF FLOATING TOOTH

DEFINITION

The term "floating tooth" applies to a state where there is no supporting bone or periodontal structures, the tooth however, maintaining it's normal position.

Causes

A. Infective Pathology
   - Chronic osteomyelitis
   - Acute osteomyelitis
B. Osteonecrosis
C. Malignant Pathology
   - Osteosarcoma.
   - Local extension of malignancy in nearby structures.
   - Burkitt's lymphoma
   - Histiocytosis
   - Metastasis esp. from lung, breast, kidney.
   - Multiple myeloma.
D. Others
   - Fibrous dysplasia
   - Cementoma and cemento-ossifying dysplasia
   - Ossifying fibroma
   - Hyperparathyroidism
   - Severe periodontal disease.

Salient Features

A. *Acute Osteomyelitis*
   - Iatrogenic, traumatic, extension of pulpal infection or acute exacerbation of chronic process.

- Various forms may be seen as acute periapical abscess, subacute abscess or Gum boil or chronic apical infection
- On Imaging: Earliest feature seen is widened periodontal space (but this is nonspecific)
- After 7-14 days definitive features like blurring of trabecular pattern, loss of lamina dura and finally a periapical abscess are seen. Associated sequestra and periosteal reaction may be seen. MR shows marrow changes early or in association to bony changes.

B. *Chronic Osteomyelitis*
- A persistent low grade infection or an untreated inadequately treated infection.
- It is usually the chronic suppurative osteomyelitis that leads to "floating tooth".
- This is simply a more protracted form of the above disease process and shows similar features.

C. *Osteonecrosis*
- Irradiation of developing tooth leads to hypoplasia of both primary and secondary dentition. Also it leads to an associated mandibular hypoplasia.
- It further leads to reduction in salivary gland function and more acidic, dry environment leading to increased chances of dental infection.
- Direct cell death caused by radiation leads to osteoporosis, bone resorption, pathological fracture and associated infection in a devitalized bone.

D. *Osteosarcomas and other primary bone malignancies*
- *Osteosarcomas* of jaw are rare lesions but have a very similar appearance to that seen elsewhere. The age of occurrence is 30-40 years and the prognosis is much better.

- Ewing's sarcoma has an epidemiology and appearance similar to that at other sites.

E. *Metastasis*
   - Four times more common in mandible (posterior esp.) than maxilla
   - Breast, kidney, lung, colon, prostate, thyroid.
     a. Localized lucent lesion
     b. Moth eaten lesion
     c,. Permeative lesion

F. *Direct invasion*
   - Squamous cell carcinomas. Salivary gland tumors and lymphomas can invade the dental sockets by direct invasion.

G. *Multiple myeloma*
   - Seen more commonly in mandible than metastasis.
   - 30% of all cases involve the mandible.
   - Skull >> mandible
   - Appearance is similar.

H. *Burkitt's lymphoma*
   - A condition occurring in maxillary bone/jaws of children in equatorial Africa
   - Probably Epstein-Barr virus
   - Leads to large soft tissue mass with involvement of all adjacent structures
   - New bone formation may be seen.

I. *Langerhan's cell histiocytosis*
   - Multifocal resorptions of periapical bone and may be also the tooth root
   - Children <5 years, most common
   - >50% of cases have jaw/dental involvement
   - Hand-Schüller-Christian disease is the condition most commonly forming such an appearance.

- Geographic skull and vertebra plana are other associated findings.

J. *Hyperparathyroidism*
  - Subperiosteal bone resorption (Lamina dura being one such bone area) is a pathognomonic sign of hyperparathyroidism.
  - Loss of lamina dura is always associated with changes in hand and feet, Brown's tumor, etc.
  - These, though specific, are poorly sensitive indicators of disease.
  - Now seen rarely due to early diagnosis and treatment.

K. *Fibrous dysplasia*
  - A homogenous, hyperdense, enhancing and greatly expansile lesion totaly replacing the normal bone.
  - Both polyostotic and monoostotic forms involve mandible and maxilla but monoostotic form involve maxilla slightly more.
  - Craniofascial fibrous dysplasia is a specific form involving >1 bone on one side.
  - Cherubism is a familial form of fibrous dysplasia involving predominantly the mandible but also the maxillary tuberosity.

L. *Ossifying fibroma*
  - Mandibular molar/premolar region of women in 3rd/4th decade.
  - Well-defined, well circumscribed, expansile.
  - Initialy lucent but later may become opaque.
  - If a lot of cementum is present then maybe known as cemento-ossifying fibroma.

M. *Cementoma-cemento-ossifying dysplasia*
  - Are periapical lucent lesion that may lead to floating tooth.
  - Cementoma is due to benign fibrous proliferation of periodontal membrane that later becomes ossified.

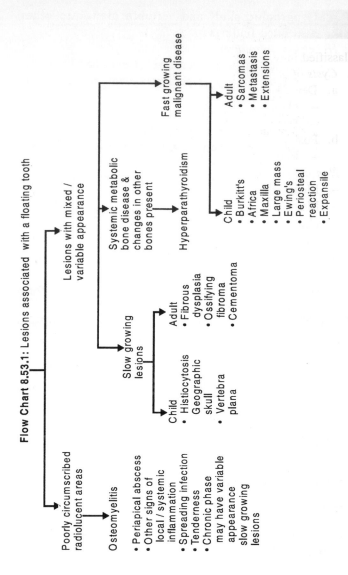

Flow Chart 8.53.1: Lesions associated with a floating tooth

Poorly circumscribed radiolucent areas

Osteomyelitis
- Periapical abscess
- Other signs of local / systemic inflammation
- Spreading infection
- Tenderness
- Chronic phase may have variable appearance slow growing lesions

Lesions with mixed / variable appearance

Slow growing lesions

Child
- Histiocytosis
- Geographic skull
- Vertebra plana

Adult
- Fibrous dysplasia
- Ossifying fibroma
- Cementoma

Systemic metabolic bone disease & changes in other bones present

Hyperparathyroidism

Fast growing malignant disease

Child
- Burkitt's
- Africa
- Maxilla
- Large mass
- Ewing's
- Periosteal reaction
- Expansile

Adult
- Sarcomas
- Metastasis
- Extensions

8.54 CYSTS OF JAW

Classified into

1. *Cysts of dental origin*
   a. Developmental
      - Odontogenic keratocyst (Primordial cyst)
      - Dentigerous cyst (follicular cyst)
   b. Postinflammatory
      - Radicular (apical) cyst.
2. *Non-dental/Developmental or fissural cyst*
   - Medial mandibular
   - Medial maxillary
   - Nasopalatine
   - Globulomaxillary
3. *Non-epithelialized bone cyst*
   - Simple bone cyst
   - Aneurysmal bone cyst.

ODONTOGENIC KERATOCYST

- Follow cystic degeneration, enamel arises before the tooth is formed so cyst replaces the tooth.
- More common in young men but seen in all ages.
- Cortex is thinned and axial view shows expansion in buccal - lingual plane.
- Most common in posterior mandible and usually monolocular.
- Usually keratinized and may react unless removed completely.

DENTIGEROUS CYST

- Cystic degeneration of enamel after formation but before eruption of tooth.

- Cyst related to crown of an unerupted tooth.
- Seen in adolescents and young adults.
- Permanent mandibular third molar and maxillary canine are affected.
- Usually unilocular.
- If multiple, may be associated with Gorlin syndrome.

RADICULAR (APICAL) CYST

- Most common jaw cyst.
- Lies directly upon the apex of a tooth.
- Follow inflammation of bulb and apical bone.
- Unilocular cyst with dense opaque margin continuous with lamina dura or at periphery of cyst. Within the cyst lamina dura is destroyed.
- Usually <1.5 cm and associated with carious teeth.
- It persist after dental extraction—Residual cyst.

Medial Mandibular

Medial Maxillary

- Similar in appearance to radicular cyst but with normal teeth.

Nasopalatine

- Usually seen due to failure of obliteration of nasopalatine ducts behind the central incisors.

Globulomaxillary

- These look like inverted pear and lie lateral of upper lateral incisor and canine, the roots of which are diverged.

Simple Bone Cyst

- Usually follow trauma and known as traumatic cyst.

- In young patients, in posterior aspect of body of Mandible.
- Diagnosis is usually histologic.

Aneurysmal Bone Cyst

- Not common in jaws.
- Diagnosis is histologic.

D/D

Location

1. Lateral
   More Common

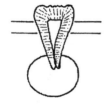 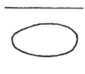

Radicular cyst
At apex of carious
tooth

Dentigerous cyst
Related to crown
of unerupted tooth
Fig. 8.54.1

Primordial cyst
Replacing the tooth

2. Medial/midline
   - Fissural or developmental
   - Usually rare

Cystic Lesions of the Jaw

Benign
Dental origin
Developmental

Odontogenic Keratocyst (Primordial Cyst)
- Monolocular cyst that form from cystic degeneration of tooth enamel before tooth is formed.
- Cyst replaces the tooth
- Common in young men and in posterior mandible.
- Cyst demonstrates expansion with cortical thinning.

Dentigerous Cyst (Follicular Cyst)
- Monolocular cyst related to the crown of unerupted tooth
- Common in adolescents/ young adults and the permanent mandibular third molar and maxillary canine are commonly affected
- Multiple such cysts are associated with Gorlin's syndrome.

Postinflammatory

Radicular Cysts (Apical)
- Unilocular cystic lesion associated with apex of a diseased tooth
- Dense sclerotic margins of the cyst are continuous peripherally with lamina dura but within the cyst lamina dura is destroyed.

Non-Dental

Developmental/Fissural Cysts
- These occur at sites of fusion of embryonic processes and include:
- Medial mandibular
- Medial maxillary
- Nasopalatine duct cyst
- Seen in 4th to 6th decade
- Asymptomatic cyst near anterior palatine papilla.
- Globulomaxillary cyst
- Seen between the lateral incisor and canine
- Nasolabial cyst arises in the soft tissues between the nose and upper lip with resorption of adjacent maxilla.

Nonepithelialized Bone Cysts

Simple Bone Cyst

Traumatic Cyst
- Seen in young patient following trauma
- Common in posterior part of body of mandible
- Are vaguely spherical but well-defined with thin sclerotic margin.
- May extend upwards displacing the vital teeth.

Aneurysmal Bone Cyst
- Well-defined multilocular expansile cystic lesion uncommonly seen in jaws.
- May be secondary to fibrous dysplasia.

Brown Tumors
- Seen in hyperparathyroidism
- Commonly involves mandible
- Arises as a cystic lesion unrelated to tooth.
- Associated loss of lamina dura.

Giant Cell Reparative Granuloma of Jaffe
- Soft tissue mass appearing like cyst with well-defined margin.
- Common between 7th yr and early 20's

Malignant
- Ameloblastoma
- Common in middle aged males in molar region of mandible
- Lesion are cystic, multilocular, expansile with thinning of cortex with peripheral satellite defects.

Giant Cell Tumor
- Multilocular cystic lesion with expansion
- Rare in the jaws.

Burkitt's Lymphoma
- Jaws are frequently affected which deformed face.
- Multilocular cystic destruction beginning around the roots of the tooth.
- A "sun ray" type periosteal reaction may be associated.
- Seen in childhood.

8.55 LOSS OF LAMINA DURA OF TEETH

Lamina dura is a layer of compact bone that lines the tooth socket and provides anchorage for the fibers of the periodontal membrane.

Causes

Generalized
1. Endocrine/Metabolic
   - Osteoporosis
   - Hyperparathyroidism
   - Cushing's syndrome
   - Osteomalacia
2. Paget's disease
3. Scleroderma

Localized
1. Infection
2. Neoplasms
   - Leukemia
   - Multiple myeloma
   - Metastases
   - Burkitt's lymphoma
   - Langerhan's cell Histiocytosis

Osteoporosis

- There is reduced bone mass of normal composition secondary to either osteoclastic (85%) or osteolytic (15%) resorption.
- Incidence is 7% of all women between 35-40 years and 1 in 3 women of greater than 65 years of age.

Hyperparathyroidism

- Loss of the lamina dura surrounding the roots of the teeth is an early manifestation of hyperparathyroidism, with alterations in the jaw trabecular pattern characteristically developing next. Not all teeth are affected.
- There is a decrease in trabecular density, and blurring of the normal pattern produces a "ground glass" appearance on the radiograph.

- With persistent disease, other osseous lesions develop, such as the so-called "Brown tumor" of hyperparathyroidism. The name of this lesion is derived from the color of the gross tissue specimen, which is usually dark reddish-brown due to the abundant hemorrhage and hemosiderin deposition within the tumor.
- Radiographically, Brown tumors are unilocular or multilocular well-demarcated radiolucencies, which commonly affect the mandible, clavicle, ribs and pelvis. They may be solitary, but more often are multiple. The long-standing lesions may produce significant cortical expansion.
- The value of loss of lamina dura as a radiodiagnostic sign is poor.
- All patients have hand changes, i.e. subperiosteal bone resorption.

Cushing's Syndrome or Hypercortisolism

- It results from a sustained increase in blood glucocorticoid levels. This can be due to either corticosteroid therapy or endogenous overproduction from the adrenal gland. Excess ACTH from a pituitary tumor also cause hypercortisolism and Cushing's disease.
- Associated osteoporosis is seen in the jaws. Pathological fractures of the mandible, maxilla or alveolar bone may occur.
- Lamina dura may be poorly visualized or absent.

Osteomalacia

- There is accumulation of excessive amounts of uncalcified osteid with bone softening and insufficient mineralization of osteid.
- There is poor visualization of the lamina dura.

Paget's Disease

- In the jaw, bone enlargement and sclerosis are usually seen.
- Irregular dense sclerotic patches may form on teeth, if any are present or merely in what had been the teeth bearing bone.
- Mandible usually remains normal, either jaw can become very large indeed.
- Infection is the commonest complication and may be the presenting lesion, especailly in the mandible.

Scleroderma

- Also called progressive systemic sclerosis, is a generalized disorder of connective tissue of unknown cause.
- Many of the diverse clinical manifestations in this disease are represented on radiographs as atrophy and calcification of soft tissue and bone resorption. Frequently the abnormalities predominate in the phalanges of the hand, although diffuse subcutaneous calcification, widespread periarticular calcification, and bone resorption are encountered at other sites, such as the mandible, the ribs and the clavicles. Joint alterations include erosive arthritis and intra-articular calcific collections.
- On radiographs, hand alterations include soft tissue resorption of the fingertips, subcutaneous calcification and bone destruction. Erosion of the phalangeal tufts leads to pencilling, sometimes with destruction of much or the entire distal phalanx.
- Thickening of the periodontal membrane and mandibular resorption may result in loss of the lamina dura and loosening of the teeth.
- Erosions may also occur on the superior aspect of multiple ribs. In the spine, paraspinal calcification may be evident.

- Joint involvement may be seen in the PIP and DIP joints, the first CMC joints, the elbow, the inferior radioulnar joints of the wrist, MCP and MTP joints, knee and hip.
- Incidence is lower than in the axial skeleton.

Burkitt's Lymphoma

- Occurs throughout the world but especially in equatorial Africa, where it accounts for 50% of all childhood malignancies.
- Jaws are frequently affected which deforme the face.
- Lesions are multifocal.
- Destruction of bone begins around the roots of teeth, which are then exfoliated.
- New bone formation in these lesions give a coarse, spiculated, sun ray appearance.

Langerhan's Sun Ray Histiocytosis

- LCH represents a spectrum of clinical disorders ranging from a highly aggressive and frequently fatal leukemia-like disease, affecting infants to a solitary lesion of bone.
- The presence of alveolar bone loss in young children with precocious exfoliation of primary teeth should suggest the possibility of LCH. LCH can also occur in adolescents and adults.
- Of the bones of the jaw, the mandible is the most frequently involved. The presenting signs usually include pain, swelling, ulceration, and loose teeth.
- Radiographically, the teeth often appear to be: floating in air" surrounded by large radiolucent regions. This is due to rapid alveolar bone loss.
- The term 'eosinophilic granuloma of bone' is used when

solitary lesion is found, but multiple lesions may develop later.
- Forming tooth-buds may be destroyed.

Infection
- Apical tooth abscess is the commonest cause of loss of lamina dura.
- Hyperemia and trabecular destruction are responsible.

Neoplasms

Leukemia
- Diffuse osteopenia is the commonest pattern, which is responsible for the poor visualization of lamina dura.
- Leukemic lines, which are the transverse radiolucent metaphyseal bands can be seen in the long bones.
- Associated periostitis of long bones are infrequently encountered.

Multiple Myeloma
- The incidence of jaw involvement in multiple myeloma averages about 15% and involvement of the mandible is commoner than in metastases.
- These lesions cause swelling of the jaws, pain, numbness, mobility of teeth, and pathologic fracture.
- Punched out lesions of the skull and jaw are characteristic radiographic findings.
- This malignancy is associated with diffuse osteoporosis which also contributes to the loss of lamina dura.

Metastases
- Overall, the most common primary site for metastases to the jaw is the breast. In men, the lung is the most common primary site for jaw metastases. The molar region of the mandible is the most common bony site for metastasis.

Flow Chart 8.55.1

Loss of lamina dura of teeth

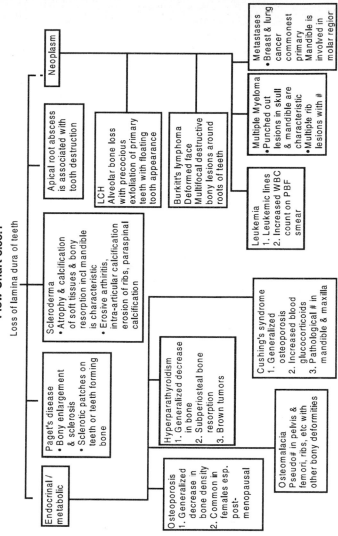

8.56 OPAQUE MAXILLARY ANTRUM

Traumatic	Inflammatory/ Infective	Neoplastic	Miscellaneous
Fracture	Sinusitis	Carcinoma	Fibrous dysplasia
Overlying Soft tissue Swelling	Allergy	Lymphoma	Cysts
Postoperative (Caldwell-LUC)	Pyocele (Rare)	Mucosal Polyp	Wegener's Granulomatosis
Epistaxis			Technical - (Overtilted view)
Barotrauma			Anatomical (Aplasia, Sloping antral wall)

Sinusitis

- Acute sinusitis produces an air-fluid level.
- Chronic sinusitis can be due to aspergillosis, mucomycosis, tuberculosis, and syphilis. Fungal sinusitis is commonly seen in diabetes mellitus. These produce hyperdense sinus secretions as seen on CT usually with bone destruction.

Cysts in Antrum

- *Mucous retention cyst*
  - Common complication of chronic sinusitis
  - Maxillary sinus is the commonest site.
  - Often arises in the floor.
  - Commoner than polyp but cannot be differentiated from it on imaging.
- *Dentigerous cyst*
  - It is related to the crown of the unerupted tooth.

- Expands into the floor of the antrum.
- Involved tooth may be displaced into the antrum.

Neoplasms

- *Polyps*
  - Complication of chronic sinusitis.
  - May extend up to the posterior choanae (antrochoanal polyp).
  - CT shows soft-tissue dense, minimally to mildly enhancing masses.
  - MRI reveals hyperintense masses on T2WI.
- *Carcinoma*
  - Associated bony destruction is seen.
  - Soft-tissue mass extending beyond the limits of the antrum.
  - Calcification seen in cases of squamous cell carcinoma.

Wegener's Granulomatosis

- Autoimmune disease.
- Usually presents at 40-50 years of age.
- Early mucosal thickening progresses to a mass with bone destruction.

Fibrous Dysplasia

- There is sclerosis of the facial bones with or without expansion (leontiasis ossea).
- Involvement of the face is usually asymmetrical.
- Involvement of the skull may be seen.

Disease	Bone destruction	Antral expansion	Hyperdense lesions on CT	Comments
Acute sinusitis	–	+/–	–	Air-fluid level
Chronic sinusitis	+/–	+/–	Usually +	Esp. in fungal and in inspissated secretions
Pyocele	–	+	–	Results from infected mucocele
Polyps/Cysts	–	+	–	Other stigmata of disease
Carcinoma	+	+	+	Associated soft tissue mass
Wegener's granulomatosis	+	–	–	Other stigmata of disease
Fibrous dysplasia	–	+/–	–	Ground-glass thickening of bone

8.57 THYROID LESIONS

Increase Uptake of Radiotracer

- Grave's disease.
- Toxic multinodular goiter.
- Toxic solitary nodule.
- Dyshormonogenesis.
- Hashimoto's thyroiditis.
- Following recovery from subacute thyroiditis or anti-thyroid drug therapy.

Grave's Disease

- It is very common cause of hyperthyroidism.
- The disease tend to occur in a younger age group than does toxic nodular goiter.
- The scan findings are quite characteristic. The radioiodine uptake is considerably elevated with 24 hours uptake values considerably in 60 to 80% range and sometimes higher.
- If dynamic range acquisition is performed following intravenous pertechnetate administration very intense flow to the thyroid will be seen.
- The distribution of tracer with in the thyroid is typically very homogenous.
- Routine thyroid imaging demonstrates an enlarged gland, that is usually rather symmetric. An enlarged pyramidal lobe is frequently present.

Toxic Multinodular Goiter

Toxic multinodular goiter is a common cause of hyperthyroidism in older individuals with a peak incidence in the fourth and fifth decades, which is later than that of Grave's disease.

The scan usually demonstrates irregular enlargement of the thyroid without a prominent pyramidal lobe.

- Tracer distribution with in the gland is very heterogenous with varying regions of uptake present.
- Frequently discrete hot and cold regions can be identified even in the presence of hyperfunctioning nodules, the remainder of the thyroid may not be suppressed because of the autonomy present with in it.

Hashimoto's Thyroiditis

It is a chronic inflammatory process of the thyroid
- F > M, may occur at any age, with peak incidence in fourth and fifth decades.
- The gland typically is enlarged with patchy traces distribution throughout the gland.

A prominent pyramidal lobe is frequently seen
- Hashimoto's thyroiditis commonly leads to hypothyroidism.
  Radioiodine uptake is variable, but is frequently low.
- In some instances, Hashimoto's thyroiditis is associated with thyrotoxicosis (called Hashitoxicosis) and they may demonstrate markedly increased radioiodine uptake.

Dyshormonogenesis: In the presence of defective thyroid hormone production.

Increased TSH Levels

Increase TSH levels may lead to adenomatous hyperplasia of thyroid, associated with hot thyroid nodule on thyroid scan
- These TSH dependent lesions will involute following administration of exogenous hormones.

Toxic Solitary Nodule

- It may be TSH dependent (adenomatous hyperplasia) or independent (adenoma).
- Adenomatous hyperplasia if associated with increased TSH levels.

Flow Chart 8.57.1

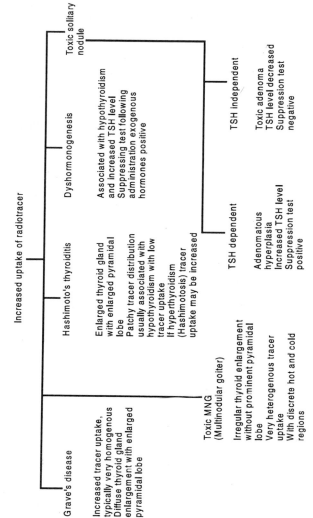

Increased uptake of radiotracer

Grave's disease

Increased tracer uptake, typically very homogenous Diffuse thyroid gland enlargement with enlarged pyramidal lobe

Toxic MNG (Multinodular goiter)

Irregular thyroid enlargement without prominent pyramidal lobe
Very heterogenous tracer uptake
With discrete hot and cold regions

Hashimoto's thyroiditis

Enlarged thyroid gland with enlarged pyramidal lobe
Patchy tracer distribution usually associated with hypothyroidism with low tracer uptake
If hyperthyroidism (Hashimotosis) tracer uptake may be increased

TSH dependent

Adenomatous hyperplasia
Increased TSH level
Suppression test positive

Dyshormonogenesis

Associated with hypothyroidism and increased TSH level
Suppressing test following administration exogenous hormones positive

Toxic solitary nodule

TSH independent

Toxic adenoma
TSH level decreased
Suppression test negative

- Toxic adenoma is associated with decreased TSH level, with partial or total suppression of remainder of gland.
- Rarely malignant thyroid nodule may show increased tracer uptake.

Hot Thyroid Nodule

- A hot nodule concentrates traces more rapidly than does the adjacent normal thyroid.
- They are seen in 8% of Tc 99m pertechnetate scans.

Causes

1. *Adenoma*
   a. *Autonomous adenoma*
      - Hot nodule
      - TSH independent.
      - Associated with decreased/normal TSH level
      - Patient can be hyperthyroid or/euthyroid
      - Partial or total suppression of remainder of gland.
   b. *Adenomatous hyperplasia*
      - Hot nodule
      - TSH dependent
      - Associated with increase TSH level secondary to defective thyroid hormone production.

Note: These nodules can be further evaluated by performing a suppression test. By administration of exogenous thyroid hormone.

- An autonomous nodule deep in the lobe will become visible as extranodular uptake is suppressed, and the nodule may be more easily palpable as the gland shrink.
- Any TSH-dependent lesion will involute with exogenous hormone administration. Although the nodule may not

be visible on scan, its diminution in size, or actual absence on palpation at the time of follow-up may be just as diagnostic. Those nodules that persist following suppression without activity present are treated as cold nodules.

2. *Thyroid carcinoma (extremely rare)*
   – Shows discordent uptake.

Note: Any hot nodule on Tc 99m scan must be imaged with I-123 to differentiate between benign or cancerous lesion.

Discordent Nodules

- Most cold nodules lack the ability to either trap or organify iodine. In a small percentage of tumors, however, the organification is blocked, but the trapping function is intact, such a nodule will be hyperfunctioning on Tc 99m pertechnetate scan and hypofunctioning on I-131 scan, which indicates reduced organification capacity.
- A nodule that is hot on technetium scanning reflecting trapping, but cold on iodine scanning because of absent organification, may represent either a benign or malignant lesion.
- Malignant
  – Follicular/papillary carcinoma
- Benign
  – Follicular adenoma/adenomatous hyperplasia.

Cystic Lesions of Thyroid

- *Thyroglossal duct cysts*
  – Appears in the midline along the migratory path of the embryonic thyroid gland anywhere from the foramen cecum at the base of the tongue to the lower neck.
- Characteristically moves with protrusion of tongue and swollowing.

– Usually cystic, these thyroglossal duct cysts can become infected and develop increased echogenicity but rarely develop thyroid papillary carcinoma.

– On CT most cyst are isodense to water, however, they may be hyperdense when there is high protein content.

– MR imaging—hypointense on T1WI and hyperintense on T2WI. When cyst contents are proteinaceous the cyst may be hyperintense on T1WI and intermediate to hyperintense on T2-WI.

– Characteristically shows thin peripheral rim enhancement of cyst well. Thick peripheral enhancement is unusual unless cyst is secondarily infected.

- *Simple Cyst*
  – True epithelial cysts are rare (<1% of all thyroid masses).
  – They are smooth-walled anechoic masses with posterior, acoustic enhancement.

Degeneration of Adenomatous Nodules

- Most cystic thyroid masses are degenerating adenomatous nodules.
- These are not true-epithelial lined cysts
- May contain bloody fluid, chocolate-colored fluid or xanthochromic fluid, depending on the age of the degeneration of the blood products.
- On USG-anechoic with thin walls and posterior acoustic enhancement.
- The presence of a 'Comet-tail sign' on USG has been said to be highly specific sign of benign colloid nodule.
- Low density on CT and hyperintense on T2WI and decreased or increased signal intensity on T1WI.

- Increased signal intensity on T1WI is related to the presence of hemorrhage, colloid or increased protein content.

Cystic Papillary Carcinoma

- Any cystic thyroid mass with a solid component must be approached with suspician for malignancy (especially papillary carcinoma) although a completely cystic nodule with uniformly thin walls is almost always benign.
- Cystic papillary carcinomas show a predominantly liquid content, with one or more solid, irregularly marginated projection in the lumen, each generally containing microcalcifications and central branching blood supply.

Thyroid Abscess

- Less common
  - Clinical features of fever, pain, tenderness.
  - US—ill-defined/well-defined hypo to anechoic lesion with thick irregular shaggy wall with internal debris.

COLD NODULES

- All nodular that cannot be demonstrated to function are considered cold.
- Causes
  A. *Benign tumor*
     - Non-functioning, adenoma
     - Cysts (11-20%)
     - Involutional nodule.
  B. *Inflammatory mass*
     - Focal thyroiditis
     - Granuloma
     - Abscess

Flow Chart 8.57.2

Cystic lesions of thyroid

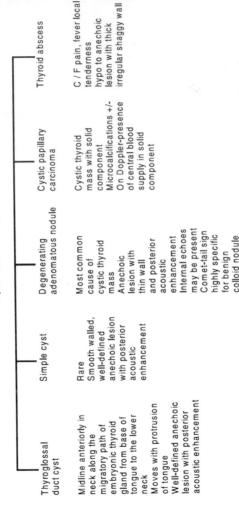

Thyroglossal duct cyst	Simple cyst	Degenerating adenomatous nodule	Cystic papillary carcinoma	Thyroid abscess
Midline anteriorly in neck along the migratory path of embryonic thyroid gland from base of tongue to the lower neck
Moves with protrusion of tongue
Well-defined anechoic lesion with posterior acoustic enhancement	Rare
Smooth walled, well-defined anechoic lesion with posterior acoustic enhancement	Most common cause of cystic thyroid mass
Anechoic lesion with thin wall and posterior acoustic enhancement
Internal echoes may be present
Comet-tail sign highly specific for benign colloid nodule	Cystic thyroid mass with solid component
Microcalcifications +/-
On Doppler-presence of central blood supply in solid component	C / F pain, fever local tenderness
hypo to anechoic lesion with thick irregular shaggy wall

C. *Malignant tumors*
  - Carcinoma
  - Lymphoma
  - Metastasis.

- All thyroid carcinomas will be cold, as will be lymphoma and metastatic disease. Many benign nodules, as enlisted above will also be cold. Because of the relative frequencies of these abnormalities, the vast majority of cold nodules are benign. Although the specificity of finding a cold nodule on scan is low, it does permit trial of the patient into a diagnostic pathway in which tissue diagnosis is needed to exclude the presence of malignancy. The true incidence of carcinoma in non-functioning nodules is difficult to determine, but probably lies somewhere near 6 to 20% range.

- However, in an attempt to provide more definitive diagnosis the following feature may be helpful.

- Ultrasound can easily identify a cystic lesion as a well defined anechoic lesion, with thin wall showing posterior acoustic enhancement. The presence of a Comet-tail sign on ultrasound has been said to be a highly specific sign of a benign colloid nodule.

- There are no specific imaging features to differentiate the varying inflammatory process that affect the thyroid gland. Acute suppurative thyroiditis is, rare, particularly affecting the children. It may be associated with fourth branchial cleft anomaly. The patient will present with painful thyroid swelling and fever. Abscess formation is common and the role of ultrasound is to confirm this, demonstrate it's boundaries and it's relationship to the major neck vessels.

- *Papillary carcinoma*
  - F>M, younger age group

- Slow growth with good prognosis
- USG characteristics
  - o Hypoechoic (90%)
  - o Microcalcification (85-90%)
  - o Hypervascular (90%) with widespread internal flow.
- Nodal metastasis (50-55%), which can show the same features as the primary lesion.
- Can be echofree, owing to serous cystic contents.
- Follicular carcinoma
  - F>M, older age group.
  - Non-specific feature that suggest follicular carcinoma are irregular tumor margins, a thick, irregular halo, and a tortuous or choatic arrangement of internal blood vessels on color or power Doppler.
- Sonograpic features of medullary carcinoma are similar to that of papillary carcinoma (low reflectivity, irregular margins, microcalcification and hypervascularity)
- *Anaplastic carcinomas* are often associated with papillary or follicular carcinomas, and presumbly represent a differentiation of the neoplasm. They tend not to spread via lymphatics, but are prone to local aggressive invasion of muscles and vessels. Low reflectivity and signs of invasion or encasement of large blood vessels and neck muscles are the most distinctive sonographic features of anaplastic carcinomas.
  - When they are not adequately imaged and staged with ultrasound, CT or MRI scans are performed to define the extent of the disease.

Lymphoma

- Acounts for about 4% of all thyroid malignancies.

- Mostly of non-Hodgkin's type, affects older female
- The typical finding is a rapidly growing mass which may cause symptoms of obstruction such as dyspnea and dysphagia.
- Seventy to eighty percent of cases arise from a pre-existing chronic thyroiditis (Hashimoto's disease), with subclinical or overt hypothyroidism.
- More commonly present as a solitary mass, but multiple nodules may be seen.
- On USG- lymphoma of thyroid appears as on echo-poor lobulated mass, that is nearly avascular. Large areas of cystic necrosis may occur, as well as encasement of adjacent neck vessels.
- Diffuse involvement may cause thyroid enlargement with little detectable abnormality, or a heterogenous pattern may be seen in the adjacent thyroid parenchyma due to associated chronic thyroiditis.
- There may be associated cervical lymphadenopathy.

Metastasis

- Metastatic disease involving the thyroid is uncommon.
- The common primary sites include melonoma, breast and renal cell carcinoma.

DECREASED OR NO UPTAKE OF RADIOTRACER

A. *Blocked trapping function*
  1. Iodine load (most common)
  2. Exogenous thyroid hormone (replacement therapy)
B. *Blocked organification*
  1. Antithyroid medication/goitrogenic substances
C. *Diffuse parenchymal destruction*
  1. Subacute/chronic thyroiditis
D. *Hypothyroidism*

Flow Chart 8.57.3

Cold nodule

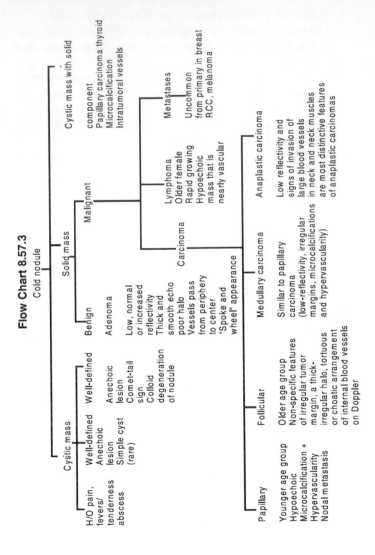

Cold nodule
├── Cystic mass
│   ├── H/O pain, fevers/tenderness abscess
│   └── Well-defined
│   ├── Well-defined Anechoic lesion Simple cyst (rare)
│   └── Anechoic lesion Comet-tail sign Colloid degeneration of nodule
├── Solid mass
│   ├── Benign
│   │   └── Adenoma
│   │   Low, normal or increased reflectivity
│   │   Thick and smooth echo poor halo
│   │   Vessels pass from periphery to center
│   │   "Spoke and wheel" appearance
│   └── Malignant
│   ├── Carcinoma
│   │   ├── Papillary
│   │   │   Younger age group
│   │   │   Hypoechoic
│   │   │   Microcalcification +
│   │   │   Hypervascularity
│   │   │   Nodal metastasis
│   │   ├── Follicular
│   │   │   Older age group
│   │   │   Non-specific features of irregular tumor margin, a thick-irregular halo, tortuous or choatic arrangement of internal blood vessels on Doppler
│   │   ├── Medullary carcinoma
│   │   │   Similar to papillary carcinoma (low-reflectivity, irregular margins, microcalcifications and hypervascularity)
│   │   └── Anaplastic carcinoma
│   │   Low reflectivity and signs of invasion of large blood vessels in neck and neck muscles are most distinctive features of anaplastic carcinomas
│   ├── Lymphoma
│   │   Older female
│   │   Rapid growing
│   │   Hypoechoic mass that is nearly vascular
│   └── Metastases
│   Uncommon from primary in breast RCC, melanoma
└── Cystic mass with solid
    component
    Papillary carcinoma thyroid
    Microcalcification
    Intratumoral vessels

1. Congenital hypothyroidism
2. Surgical/radioiodine ablation
3. Thyroid ectopia.

Iodine Load

*   Previous administration of iodine-containing medications is the most common extrinsic factor for decreased uptake of radiotracer. Extrinsic iodine administration will depress the thyroid uptake for a variable period, regardless of the thyroid's functional status.
*   If thyroid uptake is markedly reduced because of previous iodine exposure little diagnostic information can be obtained from the scan. Therefore all the patients should be screened prior to radioisotope administration.

Exogenous Thyroid Hormone

*   It is another frequent cause of decreased tracer uptake. In some cases, thyroid suppression scans are intentionally performed in the evaluation of nodules. At other times, however, unintentional thyroid suppression scans are likely to be performed, either because of patients confusion about discontinuing medication.
*   Administration of thyroid hormone (factitious hyperthyroidism).
*   Very rarely, functioning ectopic thyroid tissue, such as struma ovarii or functioning metastatic thyroid cancer will cause thyroid suppression.
*   Antithyroid drugs—Antithyroid drugs, such as
*   Propylthiouracil (PTU), or methimazole, block organification and will decrease radioiodine uptake.

However, pertechnetate uptake will not be affected and useful information can be obtained from Tc 99m scans in selected instances.

Subacute Thyroiditis

- Supposed to be caused by viral infection
- These patients usually present with a painful, tender and enlarged thyroid, and signs of hyperthyroidism are frequently present secondary to an outpouring of thyroid hormone into the blood) from the inflamed thyroid.
- The natural history is variable, but over the subsequent weeks to months, the hyperthyroid phase is succeeded by enthyroid and sometimes hypothyroid stages, before the gland recovers and function returns to normal.
- Initially the gland is inflamed and functions poorly with very low radioiodine uptake, as the patient progresses through the hypothyroid and recovery phases, the radioiodine uptake gradually increase to the normal range in some patients transiently rising above normal.

Congenital Hypothyroidism

- Scintigraphy is helpful by demonstrating the absence of thyroid tissue, which is the underlying problem in 30-40% of cases.
- Ectopic thyroid tissue may be seen in 40-50% of cases, most commonly seen as a nodule or mass at the base of the tongue.
- In the later case increased tracer uptake is present at the foramen caecum of the tongue and there is absence of the normal uptake in the neck.

Ectopic Thyroid

- Ectopic thyroid tissue may lie along the line of thyroglossal duct cyst or adjacent to it.
- The presence of ectopic thyroid tissue decreases tracer uptake in the normal thyroid gland. The ectopic thyroid tissue may co-exist with normal thyroid gland, and in same cases, the ectopic tissue may be the only functioning thyroid gland.

Flow Chart 8.57.4

Decreased or no tracer uptake

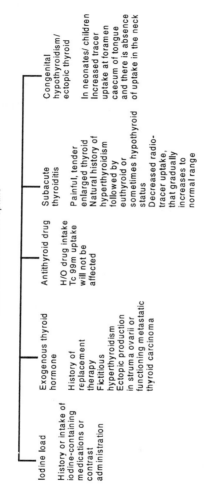

Iodine load	Exogenous thyroid hormone	Antithyroid drug	Subacute thyroiditis	Congenital hypothyroidism/ ectopic thyroid
History or intake of iodine-containing medications or contrast administration	History of replacement therapy Fictitious hyperthyroidism Ectopic production in struma ovarii or functioning metastatic thyroid carcinoma	H/O drug intake Tc 99m uptake will not be affected	Painful, tender enlarged thyroid Natural history of hyperthyroidism followed by euthyroid or sometimes hypothyroid status Decreased radio-tracer uptake, that gradually increases to normal range	In neonates/ children Increased tracer uptake at foramen caecum of tongue and there is absence of uptake in the neck

- Most commonly ectopic thyroid tissue presents in childhood as nodule or mass at the base of the tongue.

SOLID THYROID NODULE

A. *Benign*
   - Adenomatous hyperplasia (50%)
   - Follicular adenoma (20%)
   - Ectopic parathyroid adenoma
   - Hemorrhage/hematoma: Frequently associated with
     adenomas
   - Abscess
B. *Malignant*
   - Thyroid carcinoma
   - Lymphoma
   - Metastasis from breast, lung, kidney malignant
     melanoma.
C. *Hürthle cell tumors*

Adenomatous Hyperplasia

- Most commonly observed pathology of thyroid gland
- May be familial(disorders of hormonogenesis)
   - Iodine deficiency (endemic)
   - Compensatory hypertrophy (secondary to hypoplasia
     of one lobe or partial thyroidectomy).
- F>M: 3:1.
- May be diffuse or nodular.
- Diffuse hyperplasia results in enlargement of one on both
  lobes.
- Nodular hyperplasia is usually seen as multiple discrete
  nodules, varying greatly in number and size, separated
  by normal parenchyma.
- The typical hyperplastic nodule is of the same reflectivity
  as the normal gland, with a regular and complete peripheral
  halo, which is probably caused by perinodal blood vessels

and mild edema or compression of adjacent normal parenchyma.

Adenoma

- Adenomas represent 5-10% of all nodular diseases of the thyroid.
- F:M=7:1.
- A minority of adenomas are hyperfunctioning, develop autonomy, and may cause thyrotoxicosis (Plummer's disease).
- Follicular adenomas, which are much more frequently encountered than non-follicular adenomas, are true thyroid neoplasms, characterized by compression of adjacent tissue and fibrous encapsulation.
- Thyroid adenomas may be of low, normal or increased reflectivity usually with a thick and smooth peripheral echo-poor halo, owing to the fibrous capsule and blood vessels.
- Often vessels pass from the periphery to the center of the lesion, creating a "spoke and wheel" appearance.
  Malignant lesions are discussed with cold thyroid nodules.

Hürthle Cell Tumors

- Very rare
- They have been considered benign lesions in the past but may exhibit malignant characteristics with metastatic spread to lymph nodes and lung. This is seen more frequently (80%) in lesions measuring greater than 4 cm in diameter.
- These lesions are of mixed echogenicity on USG, usually solid and often ill-defined with no calcification.
- Currently no single ultrasound criterion can distinguish benign from malignant thyroid nodules with complete reliability.

However some features almost unique for benign goitrous nodules are:

- A thoroughly cystic appearance
- Moving Comet-tail artifact
- Fluid-fluid levels
- Widespread cystic appearance in isoechoic or highly echogenic nodules
- Highly reflective nodules
- A perilesional thin, uniform thickness, echo-poor halo
- Well-defined and regular margins
- Peripheral egg shell like or large coarse calcifications
- A perilesional blood flow pattern
- If most of these signs are found in a thyroid nodule the diagnosis of benign disease is highly reliable
- Conversely the possible ultrasound signs for malignancy are:
  - Low reflectivity
  - Irregular margins
  - Thick irregular halo
  - Intranodular blood flow pattern
  - Microcalcification
  - Hypervascularity
  - Invasion of vessels and adjacent structures
  - Vessel encasement
- The most reliable of these signs for detecting malignancy are microcalcification and the infiltration of structures adjacent to the thyroid gland.

Thyroid Calcifications

- Calcifications can be seen in both benign and malignant lesions of thyroid.

- Benign calcification are seen as stromal calcifications in adenoma or in patients with multinodular goiter.
- Benign calcifications are peripheral or egg shell like, usually coarse and scattered throughout the gland, unlike the clustered fine calcifications (Microcalcifications) which are more typical of malignant nodules.
- Microcalcifications (<1mm) occur in 54% of thyroid neoplasms, and are most commonly seen in papillary carcinoma of thyroid. Microcalcifications can also be seen in medullary carcinoma of thyroid.

9

Obstetrics and Gynecology

9.1 D/D BETWEEN BLIGHTED OVUM AND PSEUDOGESTATION OF ECTOPIC PREGNANCY

Blighted ovum		*Pseudogestation of ectopic pregnancy*
1. Uterine size	Usually normal	May be enlarged
2. Gestation sac with double decidual sac sign	Present	Absent
3. Yolk sac	+/-	Absent
4. Fetal node	Absent	Absent
5. Other criteria	GS size MSD >2 cm with no yolk sac MSD >2.5 cm with no fetal node Rate of increase in MSD <1 mm/day	Adnexal mass
6. Peritrophoblastic flow around uterus	Present (PSV > 21cm/sec)	Absent (Present around adnexal mass)

9.2 D/D BETWEEN ECTOPIC PREGNANCY, ABORTION IN PROGRESS (EARLY GESTATION) NABOTHIAN CYSTS

	Ectopic pregnancy	*Abortion in progress*	*Nabothian cysts*
1. Pregnancy test	+ve	+ve	−ve
2. Uterine size	May be increased	May be increased	Normal; cervix may be bulky
3. GS/double decidual sac sign in uterus	Absent	Present	Absent
4. Fetal node in uterus yolk sac	Absent	Present	Absent
5. Cervical os	Closed	Open	Closed
6. Adnexal mass	Present	Absent (Except for Corpus luteum cyst)	Absent

9.3 D/D BETWEEN PARTIAL MOLE, IUFD WITH HYDROPIC PLACENTAL DEGENERATION, TWIN PREGNANCY (MOLE AND FETUS)

	Partial mole	*IUFD with hydropic placental degeneration*	*Twin pregnancy*
1. Uterine size	Corresponds to dates	May be smaller for dates	Larger for dates
2. Placental appearance	Normal tissue with many small cysts (<15mm)	Normal tissue with few cystic lesion	One normal placenta and one with multiple cystic lesion

Contd...

Contd...

		Partial mole	*IUFD with hydropic placental degeneration*	*Twin pregnancy*
3.	Fetus (structurally)	Abnormal either blended /adjacent to placental tissue	Fetus and placenta seen separately	One normal fetus seen/2 fetal poles seen
4.	B-hCG levels	Highter than normal for GA	Lower than expected for GA	Very much higher for GA

9.4 D/D BETWEEN PELVIC MASSES, EXTRUDED FETAL PARTS WITH UTERINE PERFORATION; ECTOPIC PREGNANCY (POSTPARTUM/INTERVENTION)

		Pelvic abscess	*Extruded fetal parts*	*Ectopic pregnancy*
1.	Uterine size	Normal/ enlarged	Small for GA with breach in uterine wall	May be enlarged
2.	USG-appearance	Complex echogenic mass	Fetal bones with acoustic shadowing	Adnexal mass which is hetero-geneous
3.	B-hCG level	Falling titers	Falling titers/ normal for GA	Higher than GA
4.	Uterine Cavity	Empty/Pus	Fetal parts /Only Liquor	Pseudosac (Fluid in uterine cavity)

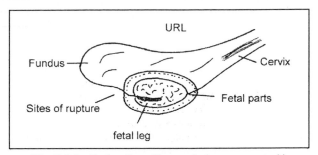

Fig. 9.4.1: Perforation of lower uterine segment with extension of fetal bones into cul-de-sac

9.5 D/D OF A PRESACRAL FETAL MASS

CAUSES

1. Sacrococcygeal teratoma.
2. Chordoma.
3. Anterior myelomeningocele.
4. Neurenteric cyst.
5. Neuroblastoma.
6. Sarcoma.
7. Lipoma.
8. Bone tumor.
9. Lymphoma.
10. Rectal duplication.

Differentiation between sacrococcygeal teratoma/anterior myelomeningocele and other presacral masses is easily achieved by biochemical tests as amniotic fluid alpha-fetoprotein and acetylcholinesterase levels are increased in the former two.

	Sacrococcygeal teratoma	*Anterior sacral myelomeningocele*
1. USG-Appearance	Soft tissue mass with calcified foci – Mixed and solid (85%) – Cystic (15%)	Soft tissue mass with nerve roots and spinal cord traversing the mass, devoid of any calcifications
2. Liquor volume	Polyhydramnios (2/3) Oligohydramnios (1/3)	Polyhydramnios
3. Fetal spine	Normal/destroyed	Defect in spine with widened spinal canal diameter
4. Location	Most commonly, dorsal to spine (47%); Presacral only in 10%	Presacral
5. Associated anomalies	NF-I; Marfan's syndrome, Partial sacral agenesis' imperforate anus, stenosis, tethered spinal cord, GU tract/colonic anomalies	Spinal dysraphism, sacral agenesis, dislocation of hip, hydronephrosis, Potter's syndrome imperforate anus, fetal hydrops, placentomegaly, curvilinear sacrococcygeal defect

9.6 FETAL NECK MASSES

CAUSES

1. Neural tube defects
   - Occipital cephalocele
   - Cervical
- Myelomeningocele
2. Cystic hygroma
3. Teratoma (Dermoid)

	Neural tube defects	*Cystic hygroma*	*Teratoma*
1. USG-Appearance	Soft tissue mass	Multiseptate, anechoic mass with thick midline septum	Complex mass containing echogenic components some with acoustic shadowing; predominantly solid on 10-31% and purely cystic in 9-15%
2. Skull and spine defects	Present	Absent	Absent
3. Other association	Brain anomalies	Chromosomal defects as Trisomy 21; Turner's syndrome, fetal hydrops; may be associated with fetal alcohol syndrome and multiple pterygium syndrome	Associated with thyroid gland

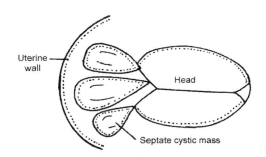

Fig. 9.6.1: Cystic hygroma

9.7 D/D OF FETAL RENAL CYSTIC DISEASES

	Multicystic dysplastic kidney (MCDK)	Obstructive cystic renal dysplasia	Autosomal recessive polycystic kidney disease (ARPKD)	Autosomal dominant polycystic kidney disease (ADPKD)
1. Renal size	Usually enlarged	Variable (normal, increased, decreased)	Enlarged	Enlarged
2. Reniform shape	May be deformed	May be deformed	Preserved	Preserved
3. Renal cyst	Multiple of variable size	Multiple in subcapsular region/cortex	May be seen, usually too small to be resolved US	May be seen, usually too small to be resolved by US
4. Dilated PC system	Absent	May be present	Absent	Absent
5. Laterality	Unilateral 80% Bilateral 20%	Usually Bilateral	Bilateral	Bilateral
6. Normal renal parenchyma	Absent	Usually present around the cyst with some cortical parenchyma	Present by/no CM differen-tiation	Present but no CM differen-tiation
7. Inheritance	Sporadic	NA	Autosomal recessive	Autosomal dominant (so one of the parent is affected)

Contd...

Contd...

	Multicystic dysplastic kidney (MCDK)	Obstructive cystic renal dysplasia	Autosomal recessive polycystic kidney disease (ARPKD)	Autosomal dominant polycystic kidney disease (ADPKD)
8. Association	Contralateral reveal abnormalities as UPJ obstruction, agenesis, hypoplasia, MCDK	Most commonly with urethral obstruction	With hepatic fibrosis, pulmonary hypoplasia, Jeune's syndrome, Meckel-Gruber syndrome	May be a part of VHL, tuberous sclerosis

9.8 D/D OF VARIOUS FETAL ANTERIOR ABDOMINAL WALL DEFECTS

	Gastros-chisis	Omphal-ocele	Limb body wall complex	Bladder/cloacal exstrophy
1. Location of defect	– Rt. para-umbilical	Midline cord insertion site	Lt. side lateral defect	Midline, infraumbilical
2. Size of defect	Small (2-4 cm)	Variable (2-10 cm)	Large	Variable
3. Covering membrane	Absent	Present	Present Contiguous with placenta, Umbilical cord absent	Variable

contd...

contd...

	Gastros-chisis	Omphal-ocele	Limb body wall complex	Bladder/cloacal exstrophy
4. Contents	Usually small bowel and at times large bowel, stomach and solid viscera	Usually liver but at times with bowel	Evisceration of abdominal viscera especially liver	Bladder wall evisceration with or without bowel
5. Bowel complication including thickening of wall and dilatation	Present	Absent (usually), Present with ruptured membrane	Absent	Absent
6. Cardiac anomalies	Rare	Common	Common	Uncommon
7. Other anomalies	Rare	Common (Related) to GUT, CNS, musculo-skeletal	Common –Limb defects –Internal organ malformation –Scoliosis –Craniofacial anomalies	GUT and spinal ano-malies
8. Chromosomal abnormalities		Common (Trisomy 13,18,21)	—	Variable

9.9 D/D BETWEEN RENAL CYSTS AND HYDRONEPHROSIS

		Renal cyst	Hydronephrosis
1.	Size	Variable	Uniform size
2.	Alignment	Non-specific	Aligned anatomically
3.	Communication	Absent	Communicate with dilated renal pelvis
4.	Shape	Round to oval	Tapering towards renal pelvis
5.	Reniform contour of kidney	May be distorted	Usually preserved
6.	Renal parenchyma	May be present/ absent depending on location	Present peripherally

9.10 D/D OF CYSTIC ADNEXAL MASSES

1. *Ovarian Causes*
   a. Physiologic ovarian cyst.
   b. Functional /retention cyst.
   c. Endometrioma.
   d. Dermoid cyst.
   e. Serous/Mucinous cystadenoma/cystadenocarcinoma.
   f. Hyperstimulation cysts.
   g. Massive ovarian edema.

2. *Tubal Causes*
   – Hydro/Pyosalpinx.

3. *Tubo-ovarian*
   – Abscess.
   – Ectopic pregnancy.

4. *Miscellaneous*
   – Peritoneal inclusion cyst.
   – Para-ovarian cyst.

contd...

9.11 D/D OF BENIGN AND MALIGNANT OVARIAN MASSES

	Benign	*Malignant*
1. Size	Small;<5 cm	Large;>10 cm
2. Contour	Well-defined with thin walls	Ill-defined with thick wall
3. Internal architecture	Cystic with thin septations	Solid/Complex with solid mural or papillary projections with thick septations
4. Doppler	Absent flow or high resistance flow nodules may be avascular	Vascular nodules with high resistance flow
5. Associated findings	—	Ascites; peritoneal implants

9.12 D/D OF CYSTIC ABDOMINAL MASSES

1. **Normal Ovaries**
   a. Normal Tubes
      i. Peritoneal inclusion cyst
         - USG-multiloculated cystic adnexal mass with intact ovary amide septations and fluid.
      ii. Para-ovarian (Paratubal cyst)
         - USG—Cystic
         - Mass frequently located superior to uterine fundus adjacent to ovary
   b. Abnormal Tubes
      - Hydro/Pyosalpinx
      - USG—Cystic tubular mass with somewhat folded configuration and well defined echogenic wall; anechoic contents in hydrosalpinx and echogenic debris seen in pyosalpinx.

2. **Abnormal Ovaries**
   a. Physiological
      • Cysts (Unilocular)
        − < 2.5 cm in diameter.
        − Sequential changes are most common.

Tubo-ovarian Abscess

• Complex multiloculated mass with irregular margins, variable septation with scattered internal echoes and DAS.

Functional Cysts

• (Unilocular), unilateral.
• >2.5 cm in diameter.
• Changes seen over few next MC.
• Low level reticular echoes may be seen in hemorrhagic cysts.
• Theca lutein cysts are bilateral multilocular cysts.

Massive Ovarian Edema

• Ovarian edema from partial or intermittent torsion.
• Large multicystic adnexal mass is seen on USG.

Endometrioma

• Unilocular asymptomatic cystic lesion with homogeneous low level echoes that rarely show significant changes with Menstrual cycles.

Dermoid

• Cystic anechoic to echogenic mass with dermoid plug, hair fluid/fat fluid level with foci of calcification.

Cystadenoma/Cystadenocarcinoma

• Uni/Multilocular/biunilateral cystic masses with thin/thick septations with mural nodules and low resistance flow in malignant masses with presence of ascites and peritoneal spread.

9.13 D/D OF NON-GYNECOLOGICAL PELVIC MASSES

These arise most commonly secondary to surgery involving either GIT and urinary tract.

DD of Postoperative Pelvic Mass

Abscesses	Hematoma	Lymphoceles/ Urinoma/Seroma
• Ovoid, anechoic masses with thick irregular wall with posterior acoustic enhancement with clinical symptomatology	• Spectrum of findings from anechoic to echogenic masses with DAS and variable appearance with time	• Cystic anechoic collection. • Fluid cytology helps in diagnosis

9.14 D/D OF NON-OVARIAN ADENEXAL MASS

a. Functional cysts
   – Follicular cyst.
   – Corpus luteal cyst.
   – Hemorrhagic cyst.
b. Ovarian remnant syndrome.
c. Paraovarian (Peritubal) cyst.
d. Peritoneal inclusion cyst.
e. Endometriosis.
f. PCOD.
g. Massive edema.

h. Inflammatory T-O mass.
i. Postoperative lymphocele, seroma, urinoma.
j. Bowel masses presenting as adenexal.

9.15 D/D OF OVARIAN MASSES

Ovarian Masses are Classified Histologically

1. *Epithelial Tumors:*
   - Serous
   - Mucinous
   - Mesonephroid(clear cell)
   - Endometrioid.
   - Brenner's.
   - Mixed.
   - Undifferentiated.
   - Unclassified.
2. *Sex Cord (Gonadal stromal) Tumors:*
   - Granulosa cell tumor, theca cell tumor.
   - Androblastoma (k/a Sertoli-Leydig cell tumor)
   - Gyndandroblastoma.
   - Unclassified.
3. *Lipid (lipoid) Cell Tumor:*
4. *Germ Cell Tumors:*
   - Dysgerminoma.
   - Endodermal sinus tumor.
   - Embryoma.
   - Polyembryoma.
   - Choriocarcinoma.
   - Teratoma
   - Mixed

5. *Gonadoblastoma*
   - Pure.
   - Mixed with dysgerminoma.
6. Soft tissue tumors
7. Unclassified.
8. Secondaries.
9. Tumor like conditions.

SALIENT FEATURES

A. Epithelial Tumors

- Constitute 95% of all malignant neoplasm of ovary.
- Most common are serous and mucinous cystadeno-carcinomas.
- Postmenopausal women.
- Spreads transcoelomically along the direction of ascitic fluid circulation:
  Right subphrenic and right paracolic gutters are early sites of spread.
  - Eighty five have peritoneal deposites at presentation.
  - Para-aortic and pelvic are the first lymph nodes to be involved. One of the few primaries to have splenic secondaries.

On USG

- First modality used to detect, confirm the presence, and characterize a pelvic mass. It's high sensitivity (97.3%) makes it an ideal screening tool in high-risk groups.
- Malignant masses are large, bilateral, complex, with thick walls, thick septa and have mural nodules. Conversly is true for benign.

On Color Doppler

- Increased abnormal neovascularity
  RI $\leq$ .4; PI $\leq$ 1 [but these are not highly specific sign]

On CT Scan

- Mainstay of preoperative assessment.
- The appearance is similar to that seen on USG. The solid component enhance on administration of IV contrast. Solid looking non-enhancing areas have either blood or thick mucin.Calcification is better detected.
- Spread to adjacent—Organ is well documented but distant and especially peritoneal spread is difficult to interpret. Conventional scanners detect less than 50% of metastases less than 5 mm.
- Peritoneal deposites may present as small focii of new peritoneal calcification, multiple nodular lesion in omental fat, omental cake, nodules surrounded by bowel loops and thickening along vessels and lymphatics.
- Pseudomyxoma peritoneii occurring due to rupture of mucinous tumors present as high density fluid loculi on the serosal surfaces of organ, indenting them.

On MRI

- Basic morphological features are same but it is better in determining the origin, characterization and landmasking the spread due to multiplanner capability and better soft tissue contrast.

B. Germ Cell Tumors

- 5-15% of ovarian malignancies.
- Seen in young and adolescent: Peak = 16-20 years mostly < 30 years.

- Most common pediatric ovarian tumor.
- Most common is dysgerminoma (the counterpart of seminoma).
- U/L, solid, well-defined, large (since aggressive). Dysgerminoma is multiloculated with vascular fibrous septa in between.
- Calcification seen in teratoma and dysgerminoma. Usually extends directly but metastasis to nodes, lung and liver is more common than epithelial tumors.

C. Stromal/Sex Cord Tumors

- 3-6% of ovarian malignancies.
- Most common is Granulosa cell tumors.
- Almost always malignant.
- Hormone (Estrogen) secreting.
- Postmenopausal or prepubertal age groups.
- Quite variable in appearance.

D. Metastasis

- 15% of all ovarian malignancies.
- Stomach, colon, breast, lung, gallbladder, pancreas.
- Krukenberg's tumor is a specific term used to describe a secondery having sarcomatous stroma interspered between mucin-secreting-Signet ring cells. Usually the primary site is stomach.
- Large, B/L, indistinguishable from primary.
- Presence of associated deposites in liver, lung are strong indicators that the ovarian mass is a secondary.
- Ovary is most common genital organ to recieve leukemic deposites.
- Maybe involved in diffuse non-Hodgkin's lymphoma.

Flow Chart 9.15.1
An Ovarian Mass Detected
Look for age

Young
i. *Incidental detection*
   Simple ovarian cyst

ii. *Acute presentation*
   – Torsion
   – Ruptured cyst
   – Hemorrhagic cyst
   – Massive edema
iii. *Presents with hormonal disturbance-PCOD*
iv. *Slowly growing mass*
   – Ovarian neoplasm mainly sex cord and germ cell tumors

Middle/Old
Apart from classification as in young differentiation between malignant and benign is more important

Features of Malignancy

1. RI $\leq$ 0.4.
2. PI $\leq$ 1.0.
3. Thick septa >3 mm.
4. Mural nodule.
5. Complex cyst.
6. Large size >10 cm.
7. Ascites.
8. Metastasis/peritoneal implants.

9.16 SONOGRAPHIC CLASSIFICATION OF ADENEXAL MASSES

SIMPLE CYST

Always Benign

1. Simple ovarian cysts.
   - Folicular cyst.
   - Corpus luteal cyst.
   - Hydrosalpinx.
   - Cystadenoma.
2. Non-gynecological
   - Of GI origin.
   - Bladder diverticulum.

Solid Masses

Benign

1. Pedunculated fibroid.
2. Torsion.
3. Brenners tumor.
4. Fibroma/thecoma.

Malignant

1. Germ cell tumor.
2. Endometrioid carcinoma.
3. Granulosa cell tumor.
4. Metastasis.

Non-gynecological

1. Lymphadenopathy.
2. Bladder tumor.
3. GI tumor.

COMPLEX CYST
Benign

1. Cyst with low level echoes.
   - Endometrioma.
   - Hemorrhagic cyst.
   - Cystadenoma.
2. Cyst with hyperechoic component
   - Cystic teratoma
3. Cyst with solid components.
   - Tubo-ovarian abscess.
   - Cystadenoma.
   - Cystic teratoma.
   - Fibrothecoma.
   - Peritoneal inclusion cyst.

Malignant

1. Mucinous/serous cystadenocarcinoma.
2. Clear cell carcinoma.
3. Endometrioid carcinoma.
4. Granulosa cell tumor.
5. Cystic teratocarcinoma.
6. Metastasis.

Non-gynecological

   - Abscess.
   - Hematoma.
   - Lymphocele.

MRI Classification of Adenexal Masses

A. LOW T1 + LOW T2   :   a. Leiomyoma
                                    b. Fibroma/thecoma.

B. LOW T1 + HIGH T2 : a. Functional cyst.
  b. Peritoneal inclusion cyst.
  c. Cystadenoma.
  d. Hydrosalpinx.

C. HIGH T1 : a. Dermoid
  b. Endometrioma.
  c. Hemorrhagic cyst.
  d. Proteinaceous material.

D. Heterogenous : a. Malignancies.
  b. Simple cyst with hemorrhage.
  c. Tubo-ovarian abscess.
  d. Ovarian torsion.
  e. Ruptured ectopic pregnancy.

9.17 D/D OF ABSENT INTRAUTERINE PREGNANCY WITH POSITIVE PREGNANCY TEST

CAUSES

1. Ectopic pregnancy.
2. Very early intrauterine Pregnancy.
3. Recent abortion.
4. Molar pregnancy/gestational trophoblastic neoplasia.

Salient Features

1. *Ectopic Pregnancy:*
   - *Specific Feature:* Live embryo in the adenexa.
   - *Non-specific feature* (Need β-hCG correlation)
     - Empty uterus.
     - Pseudogestational sac in uterus.

- Particulate ascites.
- Adenexal mass.
- Ectopic tubal ring.
- *Non-supportive features:*
  - Live intrauterine pregnancy.
  - Peritrophoblastic flow.
  - Intradecidual sign/double decidual sac sign.
- Slow rising β-hCG, i.e. doubling time <2 days.

2. *Very Early Intrauterine Pregnancy:*
- Pregnancy test becomes positive at approximately 23 days while the earliest sonographic sign of pregnancy, i.e. intradecidual sign is detected at approximately 25 days. During this window period of 2 days confusion may occur.
- It is always wise to screen after 72 hours in case of any confusion.

3. *Recent Abortion:*
In case of positive Pregnancy test with USG showing no intrauterine pregnancy serial monitoring of B-hCG should be done. In cases of abortion a falling titer is seen in maternal serum.

4. *Gestational Trophoblastic Neoplasia:*
Uterus is enlarged with cavity filled with multiple small vesicles and soft-tissue nodules. Fetal parts and myometrial invasion may or may not be seen. β-hCG levels are quite high.

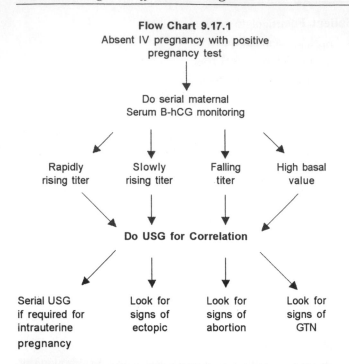

Flow Chart 9.17.1
Absent IV pregnancy with positive
pregnancy test

↓

Do serial maternal
Serum B-hCG monitoring

| Rapidly rising titer | Slowly rising titer | Falling titer | High basal value |

Do USG for Correlation

| Serial USG if required for intrauterine pregnancy | Look for signs of ectopic | Look for signs of abortion | Look for signs of GTN |

9.18 D/D OF THICKENED PLACENTA

CAUSES

1. Maternal diabetes.
2. Rhesus Iso immunization.
3. Fetal hydrops.
4. Triploidy.
5. Intrauterine infections.
6. Maternal severe anemia.
7. Fetal anemia.
8. Fetal hydrops.
9. Homozygous alpha-thalassemia.
10. Placental tumors.
11. Retroplacental/placental bleed.

Salient Features

- Placenta is called thickened when it measures > 4cm in thickness at the cord insertion.
- Most of the above causes are better evaluated by microscopic and biochemical evaluation of maternal blood.
- Karyotyping is an essential step in evaluation.
- USG has a corroborative role in evaluating structural abnormalities in above conditions, e.g. fetal hydrops chromosomal abnormalities.

Flow Chart 9.18.1

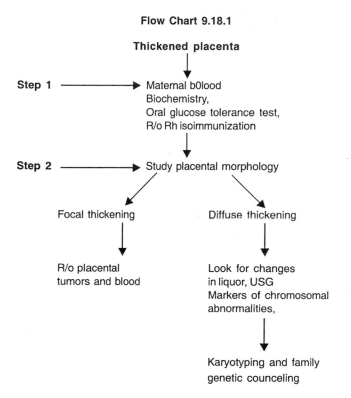

Thickened placenta

Step 1 → Maternal b0lood
Biochemistry,
Oral glucose tolerance test,
R/o Rh isoimmunization

Step 2 → Study placental morphology

Focal thickening

Diffuse thickening

R/o placental tumors and blood

Look for changes in liquor, USG Markers of chromosomal abnormalities,

Karyotyping and family genetic counceling

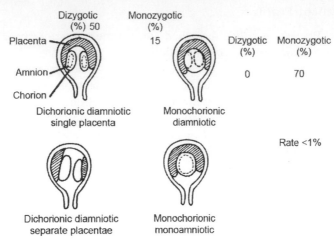

Fig. 9.18.1: Placenta and membranes in twin pregnancies

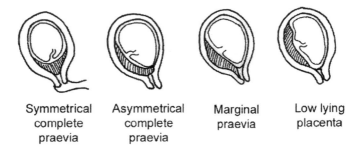

Fig. 9.18.2: Abnormalities of the placenta

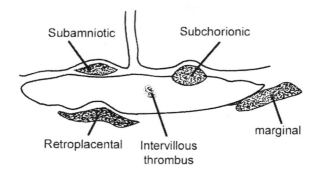

Fig. 9.18.3: Placental hemorrhage

9.19 ULTRASOUND SIGNS OF CHROMOSOMAL ABNORMALITY

**Generalized Signs
which are important even if isolated:**

1. Borderline ventriculomegaly.
2. Posterior fossa abnormality.
3. Cystic hygroma.
4. Nuchal fold thickness.
5. Nuchal translucency.
6. Atrioventricular septal defects.
7. Double outlet right ventricle.
8. Omphalocele.
9. Duodenal atresia.
10. Echogenic bowel.
11. Genitourinary abnormality.
12. Non-immune hydrops.

Important Specific Signs

Trisomy 21

1. Cystic hygroma.
2. Non-immune hydrops.
3. Nuchal thickening.
4. Hydrothorax.
5. Gut atresias.
6. Protruding tongue.
7. Cleinodactyly.
8. Increased distance between 1st and 2nd toes.

Trisomy 18

1. IUGR.
2. Single umbilical artery.
3. Cystic hygroma.
4. Microcephaly/dolichocephaly.
5. Mega cisterna Magna.
6. Omphalocele.
7. Renal dysplasias.
8. Rocker bottom feet.

Trisomy 13

1. Cyclopia.
2. Anophthalmia.
3. Cleft lip/palate
4. Low set deformed ear.
5. Holoprosencephaly.
6. Duplicated kidney.
7. Polydactyly.
8. Rocker bottom feet.

Triploidy

1. Early onset IUGR.

2. Myelomeningocele.
3. Agenesis of corpus callosum.
4. Micrognathia.
5. Sloping forehead.
6. Post axial Polydactyly/syndactyly.
7. Molar placenta.
8. Renal crtical cyst.

Turner's Syndrome

1. Cystic hygroma.
2. Non-immune hydrops.
3. Brachycephaly.
4. Small mandible.
5. Co-arctation of aorta.
6. Horse-shoe kidney.
7. Cubitus valgus.
8. Short stature.

Flow Chart 9.19.1

Approach to mother having USG signs of chromosomal abnormality

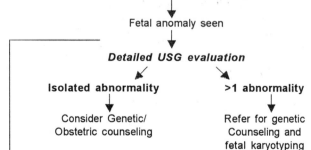

i.e. Head; Body; Extremities and thereby systematic evaluation of each part.

9.20 D/D OF ENLARGED UTERUS

CAUSES

1. Pregnancy
2. Leiomyoma
3. Carcinoma endometrium
4. Hemato/pyometria
5. Gestational trophoblastic neoplasia
6. Puerperal uterus
7. Ectopic pregnancy
8. Soft tissue sarcomas
9. Adenomyosis

Salient Features

- Most common cause of enlarged uterus in childbearing age is pregnant and puerperal uterus both of which may be evaluated by proper history and signs of pregnancy.
- In older females malignancy are an important consideration.
- In young congenitally malformed uterus hemato/pyometria may be seen.

Flow Chart 9.20.1
Clinically Enlarged Uterus

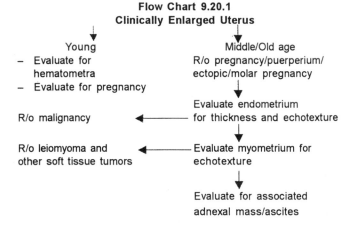

Young
- Evaluate for hematometra
- Evaluate for pregnancy

R/o malignancy

R/o leiomyoma and other soft tissue tumors

Middle/Old age
R/o pregnancy/puerperium/ectopic/molar pregnancy

Evaluate endometrium for thickness and echotexture

Evaluate myometrium for echotexture

Evaluate for associated adnexal mass/ascites

9.21 CYSTIC STRUCTURES IN FETAL ABDOMEN

CAUSES

1. Renal   – Multicystic dysplasia and other cystic diseases
                  – Hydronephrosis.
                  – Megacystis.
2. GI   – Duodenal obstruction.
                  – Jejunal obstruction.
3. Ovarian   – Simple cyst.
                  – Complex cyst associated with torsion.
4. Mesenteric cysts.
5. Hepatic cyst.
6. Pancreatic cyst.
7. Lymphangioma.
8. Urachal cyst.

Salient Features

- *Renal:* If multiple cysts with a distorted kidney and absent renal parenchyma are seen it suggests MCDK. If enlarged echogenic kidneys are seen it could be either ADPCKD or ARPCKD which are difficult to separate out by USG.
- *GI:* A double bubble sign with polyhydramnios shows duodenal obstruction while multiple air fluid levels indicate jejunal obstruction.
- *Ovarian:* 97% are benign functional cyst due to hormonal stimulation. These are simple cysts located eccentrically in pelvis with a normal GI and urinary system.
- *Megacystis* is caused by posterior urethral valves; urethral atresia /stricture; prune-belly syndrome; primary megacystis; cloacal malformation; megacystis-microcolon-intestinal-hypoperistalsis syndrome (MMIHS).

- *Meckel-Gruber Syndrome:* Polycystic kidney (100%); polydactyly postaxial (55%); occipital cephalocele (60-85%).
- Cystic lesions are usually indeterminate in appearance and correlation to associated features is helpful in final diagnosis.
- Cyst in association with echogenic bowel can be pancreatic cysts in cystic fibrosis.

Flow Chart 9.21.1

A Cystic Lesion Seen in Fetal Abdomen

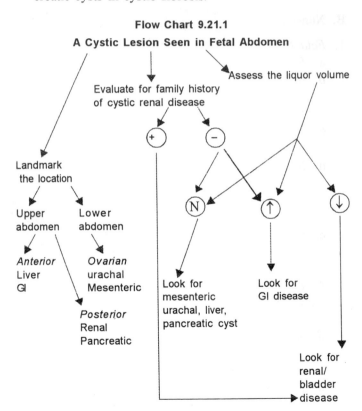

9.22   D/D OF FETAL HYDROPS

CAUSES

A. Immune Hydrops
 – Rh (D) incompatibility.
 – Other blood group antigens incompatibility, e.g. kell.

B. Non-immune Hydrops

1. *Fetal Causes:*
   a. *Idiopathic (15-20%)*
   b. *Infections*
      – CMV; HPVB19; Rubella; Coxsackie; Syphilis; Listeria; Toxoplasma.
   c. *Cardiovascular*
      – Malformations; arrhythmias; high output failure.
   d. *Neck/Thorax abnormalities*
      – Cystic hygroma; diaphragmatic; hernia; congenital cystic adenomatoid malformation; pulmonary sequestration.
   e. *Gastrointestinal abnormalities*
      – Cirrhosis; hepatitis;atresias; volvulus; meconium peritonitis.
   f. *Urinary tract abnormalities*
      – Congenital nephrotic syndrome; prune-belly syndrome; polycystic kidney.
   g. *Anemias*
      – Alpha-thalassemia; HPVB19 infections G-6-P deficiency; Twin-Twin Transfusion syndrome.
   h. *Chromosomal abnormality*
      – 45,X; Trisomy 13,18,21; Triploidy.

  i. *Genetic disorders*
   — Gaucher's; Hurler's; MPS; Sialoidosis; Achondroplasia; achondrogenesis; thanatophoric dysplasia; Jeune's dystrophy; Osteogenesis imperfecta; Arthrogryposis Multiplex Congenita; Pena-Shokier syndrome; Neu-Laxova syndrome;

2. *Maternal Causes:*
   — Severe diabetes.
   — Severe anemia.
   — Severe hypoproteinemia.
3. *Placental*
   — Chorioangioma.
   — Venous thrombosis.
   — Cord torsion, knot, tumor.

Salient Features

- Hydrops is defined as an abnormal accumulation of serous fluid in atleast two body cavities or tissues.
- *Sonographic features:*
   a. Ascites.
   b. Pleural effusion.
   c. Pericardial effusion.
   d. Subcutaneous edema.
   e. Placental edema.
   f. Alteration in arterial/Venous Doppler.
   g. Alteration in fetal well-being.
- Pseudoascites is a hypoechoic rim seen peripheraly in abdomen (<2 mm)due to muscle layer.
- Subcutaneous edema is best evaluated over the scalp and head.
- *Pattern of fluid collection helps in D/D:*

Immune hydrops	– Ascites first
Thoracic pathology	– Pleural fluid first
Anemia	– Ascites first
Meconium peritonitis	– Fluctuant ascites with echogenic bowel
Parvo virus infection	– Tense ascites with echogenic bowel

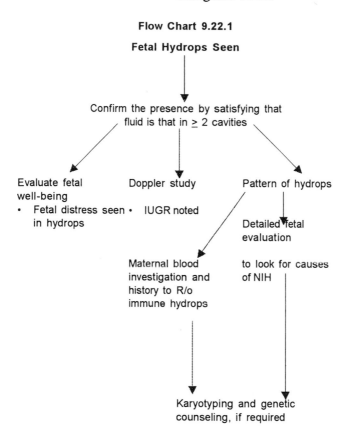

Flow Chart 9.22.1

Fetal Hydrops Seen

Confirm the presence by satisfying that fluid is that in ≥ 2 cavities

Evaluate fetal well-being
- Fetal distress seen in hydrops

Doppler study
- IUGR noted

Pattern of hydrops

Detailed fetal evaluation

Maternal blood investigation and history to R/o immune hydrops

to look for causes of NIH

Karyotyping and genetic counseling, if required

9.23   D/D OF FETAL BRAIN AND HEAD ABNORMALITIES

CAUSES

1. *Abnormalities of dorsal induction:*
   - Anencephaly
   - Encephalocele/iniencephaly.
   - Spina bifida/Chiari II malformation.
   - Caudal regression.
2. *Abnormalities of ventral induction:*
   - Holoprosencephaly.
   - Dandy-Walker malformation.
3. *Neuronal proliferation/differentiation:*
   - Macrocephaly.
   - Microcephaly.
   - Vascular malformations/tumors.
4. *Abnormalities of migration:*
   - Agenesis of corpus callosum.
   - Schizencephaly/lissencephaly.
   - Polymicrogyria/pachygyria.
5. *Aquired injuries:*
   - Porencephaly.
   - Aqueductal stenosis.
6. *Unclassified.*

Salient Features

- *Abnormalities are classified according to the time of their origin:*

Dorsal induction	– 4 th to 7 th week.
Ventral induction	– 5 th to 10 th week.
Neuronal proliferation and differentiation	– 2nd to 3rd month.

Neuronal migration   – 3rd to 5th month.
acquired injury   – 3rd to 4th month.

- *Anencephaly*
  - Absence of cranial vault, carebral hemispheres, diencephalic structures and their replacement by flattened amorphous neurovascular.
  - Mass known as area coxbiovasculosa.
  - Diagnosed earliest by confidence (100%) at 14th week
  - *Acrania:* Absent vault.
  - *Exencephaly:* brain matter is recognizable.
  - *Cranioschiasis:* Cranial abnormality with spinal dysraphism.
- *Encephalocele*
  - Is a pouch containing CSF, meninges and brain matter while cranial meningocele has no brain parenchyma.
  - 75% Occipital;13% frontal; 12% parietal.
  - Seen in Meckel-Gruber syndrome.
- *Lemon skull*
  - Bifrontal indentation is seen in 1% normal fetus, few dwarfism and spina bifida.
- *Strawberry skull*
  - A skull having reduced OFD, flattened occiput and pointed frontal area. Seen in trisomy 18.
- *Clover leaf skull*
  - Seen in thanatophoric dwarfism and craniosynostosis.
- *Ventriculomegaly*
  - Occipital horn >10 mm
  - Ventricle to choroid ratio>3 mm.
  - Anterior horns>20 mm (under 24 week)
  - VHR = 74% at 16 week

35% at 25 week.
- *Banana sign*
  - Compressed moulded cerebellum about brainstem, seen in spinal dysraphisms.

- *Iniencephaly*
  - A condition where occiput and cervical spine are involved together in dysraphism. Child is in a "stargazing" position and spinal segmentation abnormality is present.
- *Holoprosencephaly*
  - Results from incomplete cleavage and/or diverticulation of forebrain into cerebral hemispheres.
  - May be lobar, semilobar or alobar upon the severity of the disease.
  - Associated with midline facial defects.
- *Dandy-Walker malformation*
  - A condition where a malformed posterior fossa cyst communicating with fourth ventricle due to vermian agenesis and hydrocephalus is seen.
  - In D-W Varient less severe degrees of abnormality is seen.
- *Hydranencephaly* is the most severe degree of porencephaly or brain destruction where almost the whole of cerebral parenchyma is absent. Mostly due to early and total occlusion of supracleinoid carotids.
- *Schizencephaly*
  - Characterized by slits lined by gray-matter in brain parenchyma communicating brain surface to ventricles.
- *Lissencephaly (agyria)*
  - Abnormal neuronal migration from germinal matrix to surface leads to absence of convolution formation or formation of broad Gyri (Pachygyria)
- *Corpus callosum agenesis*
  - Callosal development occurs between 12 to 20 weeks. Any insult leads to total/partial lack of formation of this commissure.

- Frontal horns are Steer horn shaped with probst bundles lying medial to them.
- Colpocephaly and Sun-ray appearance of gyri radiating to ventricles is seen.

9.24 D/D OF BRAIN AND HEAD ABNORMALITY

1. *Anencephaly D/D amniotic band syndrome*
   1. Amputation of other parts.
   2. Membranes in liquor.
   3. Asymmetric cranial defects.
      D/D large encephaloceles.
2. *Encephaloceles*
   - D/D cystic hygroma.
   - D/D hemangioma.
   - D/D teratoma.
   - D/D scalp edema.
   - D/D branchial cleft cyst.
     All above do not have a cranial defect with protrusion of CSF, brain and meninges.
3. *Holoprosencephaly*
   - D/D severe hydrocephalus.
     1. Rim of parenchyma and vessels present.
        D/D hydranencephaly. Both above do not have associated facial defects.
4. *Dandy-Walker malformation*
   - D/D Varient (Dandy-Walker)
     1. Less severe anomaly and hydrocephalus.
   - D/D Arachnoid cyst.
     1. No communication to ventricles.
     2. No associated anomaly.

5. *Hydranencephaly D/D severe hydrocephalus.*
   – D/D alobar holoprosencephaly
   – D/D massive congenital subdural collection.
   – D/D postanoxic/infective encephalopathy.
     All above have thinned or injured brain parenchyma seen to varying degrees.

9.25   D/D OF THICKENED ENDOMETRIUM

CAUSES

1. Early intrauterine pregnancy/abortions.
2. Ectopic pregnancy.
3. Estrogen excess, e.g. polycystic ovary syndrome
4. Endometrial carcinoma/hyperplasia.
5. Endometrial polyp.
6. Hormonal replacement
   – Therapy in postmenopausal females.
7. Endometritis.

Salient Features

- Normal thickness   Phase
  3-5 mm   Proliferative
  Upto 14 mm   Secretory
- *Early Intrauterine Pregnancy*
  – With thickened endometrium and increased peritrophoblastic flow look for intradecidual and double decidual sac signs.
- *Ectopic Pregnancy*
  – Pseudogestation sac is an artefact due to minimal uterine collection with thickened endometrium under hormonal influence seen in these cases.

- *Endometrial Carcinoma*
  - In old ladies
  - < 4 cm thickness is N; 4-8 is equivocal and needs histopathological correlation while >8 mm is suggestive of malignancy. Associated myometrial invasion is seen in advanced cases.
- *Endometrial polyp* is a focal thickening seen best by sonohysterography, very minimal if any risk of malignancy is associated.
- *Endometrial hyperplasia* is said to occure when gland to stroma ratio exceeds that in normal proliferative endometrium. It is divided in hyperplasia with and that without cellular atypia. Nearly 1/4 progress to carcinoma if atypia is present. Occurs due to persistent hyperestrogenemia as in estrogen therapy, PCOD, granulosa/theca cell tumors, obesity and persistent anovulatory cycles. Endometrium appears thickened with few cystic areas.

Flow Chart 9.25.1

D/D of Thickened Endometrium

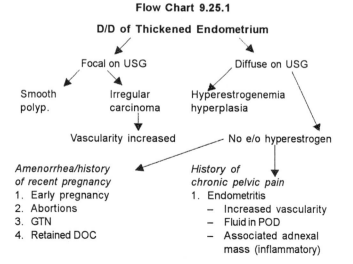

9.26 USG SIGNS IN ABORTIONS

ABORTION

(Fetal wastage before viability period)

Induced

- Legal.
- Illegal (Septic).

Spontaneous

1. Missed
2. Incomplete
3. Septic
4. Threatened
5. Inevitable
6. Complete

Salient Features

a. *Missed Abortion:* Usually between 8-14 weeks.
   - Dead fetus retained inside uterus for more than four weeks.
   - No fetal heartbeat with
     CRL > 5 mm (TVS)
     CRL > 9 mm (TAS)
   - Gestational age discordant to menstrual age.
   - Sac> 25 mm with no evidence of fetus.
   - Distorted sac configuration/shape.
   - Low down location.
   - Internal debris within the sac.

- discontinuous/irregular/thin (< 2 mm) peritrophoblastic reaction and inadequate flow.
- Subchorionic collections.

b. *Threatened Abortion:*
- First trimester bleed with a live fetus.
- Clinical triad of bleeding, cramp, closed cervix.
- 1/2 progress to spontaneous abortion, 1/2 develop normaly.

c. *Inevitable Abortion:*
- Gestational sac with fetus having become detached from implantation site and spontaneous abortion likely to occure in next few hours.
- Cervix is dilated.
- Abnormal shaped sac.
- Low lying sac.
- Collection suggestive of blood seen around the sac.
- Trophoblastic reaction unsatisfactory.

d. *Incomplete Abortion:*
- Consists basically of retained products of conception in the uterus.
- The product is usually heterogenous unidentifiable material and/or collection.
- Associated with bulky uterus and irregular endometrium.
- May lead to endomyo-metritis, DIC, septic shock.

e. *Septic Abortion:*
- Usually a consequence of illegal abortion.
- It is very important to look for any foreign body in the uterus/abdomen.
- Associated uterine perforation, signs of localized/diffuse abdominal sepsis and pelvic sepsis may be seen.

USG D/D of Abortions

Points	Missed	Incomplete	Inevitable	Threatened	Septic
1. Shape of GS	Crumpled non-identifiable	Irregular/ non-identifiable	Irregular	Well defined	±
2. Site of GS	US/LS	US/LS	L.S	U.S	US/LS
3. Collection around GS	Solid mass forms	±	+	±	+
4. Peritrophoblastic reaction and vascularity	Not present	Not present	Poor	Present	Not present
5. Status of fetus	Dead/non-identifiable	Dead/ non-identifiable	Dead	Live	Not present
6. Cervix	Closed	Partially open	Open	Closed	Closed
7. Abdomino pelvic signs of infection	Not present	Not present	Not present	Not present	Present

---

9.27 D/D OF FETAL CAUSES OF ABNORMALITY IN LIQUOR VOLUME

CAUSES

A. *Oligohydramnios:*
   – Fetal demise /IUD

- Renal/bladder abnormalities
  - PVU
  - Prune belly syndrome
  - ARPCKD
  - BRA
- IUGR
- Post dated pregnancy.

B. *Polyhydramnios:*
- Cardiovascular decompensation
- Diaphragmatic hernia
- Anencephaly/other severe cranial anomaly especially ONTD
- Obstructive malformations of GIT, e.g. TOF, duodenal stenosis/atresia
- Bone dysplasias.
- Neuromuscular abnormalities.
- Chromosomal abnormality, e.g. trisomy 18.

Salient Features

- Amniotic fluid assessment

	Single pocket	*AFI*
Oligohydramnios	<2 cm	< 7
Reduced	2-3 cm	7-10
Normal	3-8 cm	10-17
More than average	> 8-12 cm	17-25
Polyhydramnios	>12 cm	>25

- *Fetal demise:*
  - Fetal wastage after the time significant liquor production is seen leads to slow resorption of liquor.
  - Urine production status at 9 weeks and renal function starts at 11 weeks. At 12 weeks urine accumulates at the rate of 5 cc per day.

- *Signs of IUD are:*
  1. Spaldings sign
     - Overriding of skull bones.
  2. Gas in vessels.
  3. Some times associated hydrops.
  4. Extended limbs/lost tone.
  5. Absent-cardiac activity.
  6. Gas in abdomen.
- *IUGR:*
  - Weight of neonate below 10 percentile of the expected fetal weight for that age.
  - Usually detected after 32-34 weeks, i.e. the age of maximum fetal growth.
  - May be due to uteroplacental insufficiency that leads to asymmetric IUGR.
  - Asymmetric IUGR is early onset and leads to concordant reduction of all parameters.
  - Criteria for IUGR:

	Sensitivity	*Specificity*
– Advance placental grade	62%	64%
– FL/AC (increased)	34-49%	78-83%
– TIUV (decreased)	57-80%	72-76%
– Small BPD	24-88%	62-94%
– Slow increase in BPD	75%	84%
– Low EFW	89%	88%
– Decreased AFV	24%	98%
– Increased HC/AC	82%	94%
– Biophysical profile	<6 = Equivocal	
	<4 = Fetal compromise	

  - Doppler indices
  - Uterine artery -S/D >2.3, difference of the two sides >1, RI > .6
  - MCA –RI < .7

– Umbilical artery –RI – > .7
- *Post Dated Pregnancy/Large for Dates:*
  – When weight is > 90th percentile for the expected fetal weight.
  – also when weight >4000 gm.
  – Sonographic criteria.

LGA	Sensitivity	Specificity
– AD/BPD (increase)	46%	79%
– FL/AC (decrease)	24-75%	44-93%
– AFV increase	12-17%	92-98%
– Pondrel index increased	13-15%	85-98%
– High EFW	20-74%	93-96%
– Growth score increase	14%	91%
Macrosomia		
– FL increase	24%	96%
– AC increased	53%	94%
– High EFW	11-65%	89-96%
– BPD increased	29%	98%

– *Renal/bladder abnormality:* Any cause of reduction of urine formation as in renal (B/L) agenesis, ARPCKD or of obstruction to outlet of urine as in prune-belly syndrome, urethral atresia/stenosis, posterior urethral valve can lead to oligohydramnios. Look for signs of Megacystitis, i.e. UB >8 mm, hydronephrosis, i.e. Pelvis > 6 mm, abnormal renal parenchyma, dilated ureter and urethra.
- Polyhydramnios occurs when either increased production or decreased fetal Gullping of liquor is seen.
- *Cardiovascular decompensation:*
  Bradycardia – <100 BPM of >10 sec.
  Tachycardia – >180 BPM.
  PSVT – 180-300 BPM with conduction rate 1:1.
  Flutter – 300-400 BPM with conduction rate 2:1/4:1
  Fibrillation – >400 BPM

- *Diaphragmatic hernia:*
  Cystic areas in thorax with small abdomen. Absent fundic bubble, GB with portal vein pointing up.
- Double bubble and triple bubble sign of duodenal and jejunal ateresia should be looked for.
- Skeletal dysplasia, chromosomal abnormalities detection have been described elsewhere.

Flow Chart 9.27.1

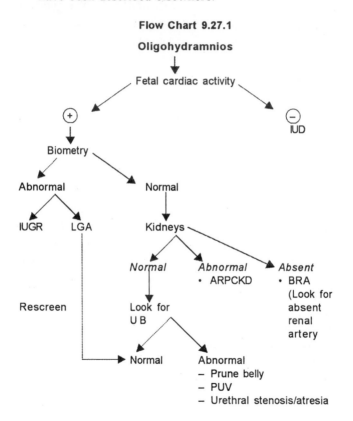

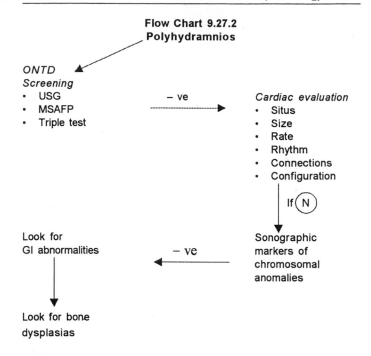

Flow Chart 9.27.2
Polyhydramnios

ONTD
Screening
- USG
- MSAFP
- Triple test

– ve →

Cardiac evaluation
- Situs
- Size
- Rate
- Rhythm
- Connections
- Configuration

If (N)

Sonographic markers of chromosomal anomalies

– ve ←

Look for GI abnormalities

Look for bone dysplasias

9.28 D/D GAS IN THE GENITAL TRACT

CAUSES

1. Fistula between genital tract and gastrointestinal tract
   - Congenital
   - Post-inflammatory, e.g. TB, Crohn's
   - Due to infiltrative, malignancies
2. Post-intervention
   - Hysterosalpingography
   - Hysteroscopy.

- Pervaginal examination.
- Tubal insufflation.
- Laparoscopy.
3. Gas forming infection
4. Post-traumatic

Salient Features

- Fistula between GUT and GIT occur most commonly due to inflammatory conditions like Crohn's disease and tuberculosis. In such cases it is usually the small bowel that communicates with uterus.

- Congenital fistulas occur between lower genital tract and terminal GIT leading to rectovaginal and rectouterine fistulas. These occur early during the course of development due to closely associated origin of both above.

- Malignancies of uterus, cervix, vagina, rectum, rectosigmoid and anal canal leads to fistula formation between them. Feculant material is also seen passing from genital tract.

- Contrast studies from both tracts are good for depiction of site of communication.

- MRI is fast picking up in demonstration of fistula.

- Gas forming anaerobic and gram-negative infections are usually uncommon but occur in cases of immuno-compromised, states as diabetes, AIDS, chemotherapy and systemic diseases.

- Trauma to genital tract may be due to vehicle accident, due to obstetric intervention or prolonged labors.

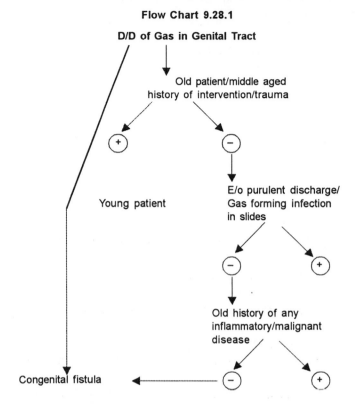

Flow Chart 9.28.1

D/D of Gas in Genital Tract

Old patient/middle aged
history of intervention/trauma

Young patient

E/o purulent discharge/
Gas forming infection
in slides

Old history of any
inflammatory/malignant
disease

Congenital fistula

9.29 D/D OF FETAL INTRA-ABDOMINAL CALCIFICATION

CAUSES

A. *Peritoneal:*
   - Meconuim peritonitis.
   - Plastic peritonitis with hydrometrocolpos.

B. *Tumors:*
 - Hemangioma.
 - Hemangioendothelioma.
 - Hepatoblastoma.
 - Metastatic neuroblastoma.
 - Teratoma.
C. *Infections:*
 - Toxoplasma.
 - Cytomegalovirus.

Salient Features

- *Meconium Peritonitis:*
  - Occures due to meconium exiting from the bowel lumen, due to perforation, causing sterile chemical peritonitis.
  - Perforation occurs due to valvulus, jejunal/ileal atresia, meconium ileus.
  - Immediately ascites occurs following which linear streaky or spotty calcification occurs.
  - Pseudocyst formation may also occur.
  - Calcified meconium balls in/out the lumen may also be seen.
- Infections like toxoplasma and CMV lead to calcifications in liver, spleen and also intracranial calcification.
- Hemangiomas may occur at multiple sites in fetal body and may be associated with calcification.
- Hemangioendothelioma and hepatoblastomas
  - Common fetal hepatic tumors which shows areas of specky linear calcification associated with vascular spaces showing high velocity Doppler shifts.
- Hepatoblastoma is the most common hepatic tumor (Primary) in young and nearly all present before the age

of five. Associated with hemihypertrophy, 11p13 chromosome and Beckwith-Wiedemann's syndrome. Serum AFP levels are almost always elevated. Shows lumpy calcification.

- Neuroblastoma is the most common neonatal tumor usually occurring in the adrenal gland. It is an echogenic mass, heterogenous in appearance. It commonly metastasizes to placenta, liver and subcutaneous tissues with the metastasis appearing echogenic calcified. Hydrops may commonly occure.

- Teratomas and dermoids are common fetal tumors occurring in retroperitoneal and gonadal locations most commonly. These show solid and cystic areas with areas of calcification.

Flow Chart 9.29.1
Intra-abdominal Fetal Calcification

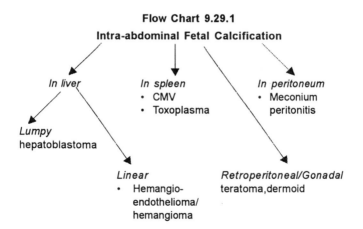

9.30   D/D OF FETAL THORACIC ABNORMALITIES

CAUSES

1. Pleural effusion.
2. Congenital diaphragmatic hernias.
3. Pulmonary hypoplasia.
4. Pulmonary sequestration.
5. Pulmonary cystic adenomatoid malformation.
6. Congenital bronchogenic cyst.
7. Bronchial/laryngeal atresia.
8. Thymic enlargment.
9. Cystic hygroma.
10. Teratoma.
11. Enteric cysts.
12. Neuroblastoma.

Salient Features

- Pleural effusion:
  - May be isolated or occur as a result of generalized fetal hydrops.
  - Fluid collects as a cresentric rim around lungs forming a 'Bat-Wing-appearance'of lungs floating in fluid.
  - *U/L*—CAM, diaphragmatic hernia, Sequestration, pulmonary hypoplasia.
  - *B/L* —infections, CHF, Turner's, Down's, pulmonary lymphangiectasia.
  - Long lasting larger effusions may lead to pulmonary hypoplasia.
  - May be treated by thoracocentesis.
- **Diaphragmatic Hernias:**
  A. *Bochdalek Hernia*
     - Posterolateral in location.

- Left>>right.
- Small intestine (88%), Stomach (60%),colon (56%), liver (51%),spleen (45%).
- Detected by sonography at 17 weeks.
- Mediastinal deviation seen by change in position and axis of heart.
- Hollow viscera may be seen with AC <5th percentile and polyhydramnios.
- Absence of GB in abdomen.
- Umbilical vein displaced up.

B. *Morgagni Hernia*
- Anteriorly behind the sternum.
- Right>>> left.
- Omentum,colon,liver, stomach, small bowel.
- May be covered by peritoneum and pleura or only pleura or none at all. If pericardium is also absent it lies in direct contact to heart.

C. *Eventration of Diaphragm*
- due to absent muscle fibers in the diaphragm.
- U/L asymptomatic.
- B/L may cause pulmonary hypoplasia.
- B/L associated with trisomy 13 and 18, CMV infection, Rubella infection and arthrogryposis multiplex congenita.

- **Pulmonary Hypoplasia**
  - *U/L*—rare, may be simulated by discordant rate of growth of both lungs. Due to thoracic masses.
  - *B/L*—commoner, due to restricted chest cage as in thanatophoric dwarfism, Jeune's asphyxiating dystrophy, achondrogenesis and all causes of early onset severe oligohydramnios.

- Chest area–heart area
$$\frac{\text{Chest area–heart area}}{\text{Chest area}} \times 100$$
is an accurate (85% sensitive and specific) in diagnosis, as correlated to age.

- **Cystic Adenomatoid Malformation**
  - Are hamartomas in lung divided by Adzich in Macroscopic (cysts>5 mm) and Microscopic (<5 mm)
  - Macroscopic type has better prognosis and is less commonly associated with hydrops.
  - Size of the mass may decrease over the times.
  - Has to be D/D from diaphragmatic hernia, bronchial cyst, cystic dilatation of esophagus, pericardial teratoma.

- **Pulmonary Sequestration**
  - Is a segment or part of lung not communicating at the usually bronchovascular tree.
  - Appear as solid echogenic masses inside (Intra-lobar sequestration) of the lung. Usually in basal parts.
  - Extralobar may occur inside the diaphragm, peri- cardium, hila, mediastinum.
  - in 50% malformations of sternum and diaphragm are seen but no major anomaly is seen.
  - D/D to diaphragmatic hernia, CAM and lobar emphysema.
  - A supplying vessel from aorta is the most confirmatory sign.

- Upto 27 weeks the thymus enlarges and appears as echogenic mass (from 14 weeks), after 27 weeks it becomes hypoechoic.

- *Cystic hygroma (lymphangiomas)* are cystic (Predomi- nantly) and solid dumb-bell masses extending in the mediastinum.

- Teratomas usually arise from pericardium and are surrounded by pericardial fluid (diagnostic point). Appearance is the same as in adults.
- *Neuroblastomas* are echogenic masses with echolucent centers lying in paravertebral area.
- Enteric cyst lined by GI mucosa are also seen in posterior mediastinum.

Flow Chart 9.30.1

D/D of Fetal Thoracic Abnormalities

Predominantly cystic
- Bronchogenic cyst → solitary
- Dilated esophagus
- Dilated bronchus
- CDH → peristalsis.
- Enteric cyst → posterior
- Meningocele → posterior
- Pericardial cyst

Predominantly solid
- CDH → significant Mediastinal shift
- Sequestration → vessel from aorta
- CAM (microcystic)
- Teratoma
- Hamartoma
- Ectopic kidney
- Eventration
- Intrathoracic spleen

Solid and cystic
- CDH → peristalsis.
- CAM → macrocystic
- Teratoma
- Cystic hygroma
- Eventration
- Neuroblastoma

Index

A

Abdominal mass in child 353
    gastrointestinal 353
    genital 354
    miscellaneous 354
    non-renal retroperitoneal 353
    renal 353
Abdominal mass in neonate 352
    genital 352
    renal 352
Abnormal digits 506
Abnormal shape, size and density
    of ribs 503
Abnormal skeletal maturation 418
Abnormal thumb 507
Abnormalities of bowel rotation
    357
    exomphalos 357
    extroversion of cloaca 358
    malrotation 357
    non-rotation 357
    paraduodenal hernias 358
    reverse rotation 358
Abnormalities of the placenta 1062
Abnormality related to clavicles
    500
    destruction of medial end of
        clavicle 500
    erosion or absence of outer end
        of clavicle 500
    penciled distal end of clavicle
        500

Abortion 1039, 1078
    incomplete abortion 1079
    inevitable abortion 1079
    missed abortion 1078
    septic abortion 1079
    threatened abortion 1079
Abscess typical imaging features
    670
Absent intrauterine pregnancy with
positive pregnancy test 1058
Acetabular sector angles 593
Achalasia 226
Achondrogenesis type I and II 426
Achondroplasia 420
Acquired cystic disease of kidney
    (ACKD) 682
Acquired cystic kidney disease 669
Acromelic dwarfism 528
Acromesomelic dwarfism 528
Acro-osteal changes 509
Acro-osteolysis 509, 564, 569
Acro-osteosclerosis 510
Acute arterial infarction 611
Acute cortical necrosis 620
Acute interstitial nephritis 622
Acute osteomyelitis 481
Acute pyelonephritis 613
Acute tubular necrosis 619
Acute urate nephropathy 624
Acyanotic heart disease 207
Acyanotic without shunt 208
Adamentinoma of long bones 547

Adrenal calcification 340
Adrenal mass 339, 735
    bilateral large adrenals 339
    unilateral adrenal mass 340
Adult orbital tumors 949
Aggressive fibromatosis 8
Air bronchogram 104
Air-fluid levels on chest X-ray 74
Alagille syndrome 320
Alternating radiolucent/dense
    metaphyseal bands 497
Alveolar microlithiasis 110
Alveolar shadowing 103
Ampulla of Vater 404
Anatomy of liver, bile ducts, and
    pancreas 390
Aneurysmal bone cyst 445
Angle of metatarsal heads 592
Ankylosing spondylitis 571
Ankylosis of interphalangeal joints
    517
Anterior indentation of
    rectosigmoid junction 308
Anterior scalloping of vertebral
    bodies 854
Anterior skull base lesion 788
Anterior vertebral body beaks 857
Aortic stenosis 193
Apert's syndrome 506
Aphthous ulcers 307
Appendicular skeleton 427
Arachnoid cyst 785, 816
Areas of decreased density 216
    fat 216
    gas 216
Arterial abnormalities 42
Arthritides 455
Arthritis involving spinal column
    571
Arthritis mutilans 515

Arthritis with demineralization 513
Arthritis with periostitis 513
Arthritis with preserved/widened
    joint space 514
Arthritis with soft tissue nodules
    514
Arthritis without demineralization
    513
Asbestosis 112, 134
Ascites 349
    causes 350
    radiographic signs 349
    technique 350
Asphyxiating thoracic dystrophy
    425, 528
Atlantoaxial subluxation 850
Atretic cephaloceles meningocele
    896
Atypical cysts 680
Avascular necrosis/osteonecrosis/
    aseptic necrosis 494

B

Ba-esophagogram 31
Bare orbit sign 829
Bare orbit/hypoplasia of greater wing
    of sphenoid 886
Barrett's exophagus 224
Basilar invagination 771
Benign and malignant ovarian
    masses 1048
Benign and malignant SPN 96
Benign prostatic hyperplasia 731
Berylliosis 112
Bilateral causes of
    hypertransradiancy 126
Bilateral large smooth kidneys 616
Bile duct variants 399
Bladder calculi 694

Bladder outflow obstruction 640
Blighted ovum 1038
Block vertebra 860
Blood clot 634
Bochdalek hernia 116
Boehler angle 586
Bone cyst 576, 589
    diaphysis 589
    epiphysis 589
    expansile unilocular cystic
        lesions 577
    metaphysis 589
    nonexpansile multilocular
        cystic lesion 576
    nonexpansile unilocular cystic
        lesions 576
Bone dysplasias-associated with
        multiple fractures 489
    increased density 489
    normal osseous density 489
    reduced density 489
Bone infarcts 539
Bone sclerosis associated with
        periosteal reaction 437
    idiopathic 438
    infective 437
    neoplastic 437
    traumatic 437
Bone within bone appearance 490
Brailsford Morquio syndrome 529
Brain and head abnormality 1075
Breast abscess 163
Breast calcifications 165
    benign calcification 165
        dystrophic calcification
            166
        egg shell calcification 165
        large rod-like calcification
            166

    milk of calcium 166
    popcorn calcification 166
    pseudocalcification 167
    skin calcifications 166
    tram tracks calcification
        166
    calcification suspicious for
        malignancy 167
Bright liver 321
Brodie's abscess 439, 544
Bronchial carcinoma 90
Bronchiolitis obliterans 124
Brown tumor of
    hyperparathyroidism 547
Bubbly bone lesions 443

C

Caffey's disease 438, 535
Calcaneal pitch 586
Calcification 174
    definitely benign 174
    possibly malignant 175
    probably benign 175
Calcification on chest radiograph
    72
Calcium pyrophosphate
    arthropathy 455
Campomelic dwarfism 426
Canada-Cronkhite syndrome 300
Cancellous bone 491
Caplan's syndrome 94, 148
Carcinoma 176
    primary features 176
    secondary features 176
Carcinoma of the esophagus 226
Carcinoma of the bladder 686
Carcinoma of the breast 164
Carcinoma prostate 535, 713, 732
    anatomy 713

categories 715
premalignant changes 715
staging 716
Cardiac calcifications 204
intracardiac 205
myocardial calcifications 205
pericardial calcifications 204
Cardiac valve calcifications 205
aortic valve 205
mitral valve 206
pulmonary valve 206
tricuspid valve 206
Cardiophrenic angle mass 150
Cardiovascular disorders 177
causes 177
collagen diseases 177
endocrine diseases 177
heart diseases 177
hemopericardium 178
inflammatory 177
malignancy 177
uremia 178
Carpal fusion 505
isolated 505
syndrome related 505
Carpenter syndrome 506
Causes of bilateral
hypertranslucency 128
Causes of osteomalacia 472
Causes of smooth esophageal
strictures 370
Caustic oesophagitis 371
Cavernous hemangioma 946
Cavitary lesions of lung 82
Cavitating pulmonary lesions 74, 76
Central skull base lesions 792
Cephaloceles 894
Cerebellar malformations 908
Cerebellopontine angle masses 794

Cervical abscess 5, 13
Cervical rib 11
Cervicothoracic hematoma 11
Characteristics of SPN 88
Chest wall-abnormalities 51
Childhood tumors metastasizing to
bone 441
Choledochal cyst 353
Chondroblastoma 444, 452, 546
Chondrocalcinosis 516
Chondrodysplasia punctata 421,
425, 527
Chondromyxoid fibroma 444, 452
Chordoma 818
Chronic active osteomyelitis 485
Chronic glomerulonephritis 603
Chronic pyelonephritis/reflux
nephropathy 605
Chronic tophaceous gout 460
Circumscribed radiolucent lesion
155
glactocele 155
lipoma 155
oil cyst 155
Cirrhosis 94
Classification of renal cysts 677
Clavicles 564
Cleidocranial dysostosis 564
Coal miner's pneumoconiosis 109
Coarse trabecular pattern of bone
439
Cobblestone duodenal cap 264
big polypoidal cap 264
carcinoma 265
Crohn's disease 264
lymphoma 265
small size cap 264
varices 265
Cock screw esophagus 364

Cold nodules 1025

Collagen disorders 131

Colonic polyps 295,298

    adenomatous polyps 295

    hamartomous polyp 296

    hyperplastic polyp 297

    inflammatory/postin-
        flammatory polyp 297

    nonadenomatous single polyps
        296

    Turcot's syndrome 295

Colonic strictures/narrowing 302

Common lytic bone lesions 465

Compact bone 491

Comparative features of sero-
    negative spondyloarthritides
    523

Compensatory hypertrophy 614

Complete opaque hemithorax 113

Complex sclerosing lesion 162

Congenital cystic eye 830

Congenital gallbladder anomalies
    400

    agenesis of gallbladder 400

    gallbladder ectopia 402

    hypoplastic gallbladder 401

    septations of gallbladder 401

Congenital heart disease 180

Congenital hernia 153

Cooley's anemia 757

Corrosives 225

Craniopharyngioma 813, 814

Cretinism 525

Crohn's disease 256, 412

    clinical features 413

    epidemiology 412

    pathogenesis and etiology 412

    radiologic findings 413

    risk factors 412

Cupping of metaphysis 498

Cushing's syndrome 555

Cyanotic heart disease 207, 776

Cyst of tunica albugenia 704

Cystic abdominal masses 1048

Cystic adnexal masses 1047

Cystic disease of kidneys 675

Cystic hygroma 41, 1043

Cystic lesions 943

Cystic lesions of thyroid 1023

Cystic mesenteric masses 310

Cystic structures in fetal abdomen
    1067

Cystosarcoma phylloides 158

Cysts of Jaw 1005

    cysts of dental origin 1005

    non-dental/developmental or
        fissural cyst 1005

    non-epithelialized bone cyst
        1005

D

Dandy-Walker complex 910

Dandy-Walker malformation 782

Demyelinating disorders 912

Demyelination 914

Dense vertical metaphyseal lines
    497

Dermatomyositis 219

Destruction of petrous bone (Apex)
    768

Diabetic osteomyelitis 484

Diaphyseal infarct 454

Diarthrodial joint 461

Differential diagnosis of abnormal
    nephrograms 711

Differential diagnosis of anterior
    mediastinal mass 32

    congenital and developmental
        anomalies 51

inflammatory and infectious 51

tumors 51

Differential diagnosis of esophageal carcinoma 234

advanced carcinoma 235

early esophageal carcinoma 234

Differential diagnosis of posterior fossa cysts 874

Differential diagnosis of skeletal lesion in nonaccidental injury 488

Diffuse hepatomegaly 314

Diffusely hypodense liver on NECT 326

Diffusely hypoechoic liver 321

Dilatation of pelvicalyceal system 612

non-obstructive 612

obstructive 612

Dilatation of pulmonary trunk 188

Dilated azygous vein 47

Dilated calyx 633

Dilated calyx and dilated ureter 631

with a narrow infundibulum 631

with a wide infundibulum 631

Dilated duodenum/obstruction of duodenum 265

congenital causes 265

extrinsic compression 265

inflammatory narrowing 265

intramural hematoma 265

miscellaneous 266

tumoral narrowing 265

Dilated esophagus 222

Dilated small bowel/jejunal and ileal obstruction 266

Dilated ureter 639

Dilated ureter and calyces 631

Discordent nodules 1023

Disuse osteoporosis 558

Down's syndrome 506, 858

Dumbbell-shaped long bones 426

Dwarfism 524

Dyschondrosteosis 421

Dysostosis multiplex 529

Dysphagia in adults 359

E

Ebstein's anomaly 121

Ectopic pregnancy 1039

Edematous breast 164

Elevation of diaphragm 62

bilateral 62

unilateral 62

Ellis-van Creveld syndrome 507

Empty sella 812

Enchondroma 444, 546

Endobronchial tumor 90

Enlarged femoral intercondylar notch 515

Enlarged left atrium 185

pressure overload 187

left atrial myxoma 187

mitral stenosis 187

secondary to left ventricular failure 187

volume overload 185

mitral regurgitation 185

Enlarged left ventricle 182

high output states 185

myocardial causes 185

pressure overload 184

aortic stenosis 184

coarctation of aorta 184

volume overload 182

aortic incompetence 184

mitral incompetence 184
patent ductus arteriosus 184
ventricular septal defect 182
Enlarged optic foramen 883
Enlarged right atrium 195
Enlarged right ventricle 196
Enlarged superior vena cava 204
Enlarged sylvian fissure/midline cranial fossa of CSF density 785
Enlarged uterus 1066
Enlarged vertebral body 863
Enlargement aorta 191
Enteropathic spondyloarthropathies 574
Enthesiopathy 517
Enthesitis 571
Eosinophilic enteritis 271
Erlenmeyer flask deformity 498
Erosion of medial metaphyses of proximal humerus 499
Esophageal carcinoma 229
clinical aspects 231
distribution 231
histology 230
pathology 230
predisposing factors 229
radiographic findings 232
routes of spread 231
Esophageal lesions 47
Esophageal lymphoma 227
Esophageal strictures 369
Esophagitis/esophageal ulcers 365
Esophagogram 224, 363
Evaluation of SPN 97
Ewing's sarcoma 442, 467
Excessive callus formation 489

Exogenous thyroid hormone 1031
Expanded pituitary fossa 819
Expansile bone lesion 543
Extension of thyroid masses 931
External acoustic masses 970
Extradural extramedullary lesion 991
Extraluminal intra-abdominal gas 342
abscess 342
gas in biliary tree 342
gas in bowel wall 342
gas in portal vein 342
gas in urinary tract 342
necrotic tumor 342
pneumoperitoneum 342
retroperitoneal gas 342
Extraparenchymal renal cysts
multilocular cystic nephroma 683
parapelvic cyst 682
perinephric cyst 683
Extruded fetal parts 1040

F

Fascial spaces in prevertebral region 928
Fatigue fractures 490
Fetal brain and head abnormalities 1072
Fetal causes of abnormality in liquor volume 1080
Fetal hydrops 1069
Fetal intra-abdominal calcification 1087
Fetal neck masses 1042
Fetal renal cystic diseases 1044
Fetal thoracic abnormalities 1090

Fetal/neonatal hepatic calcification 320
Fibrous tumors of pleura 153
Filling defect in the bladder 712
Floating tooth 1000
    causes 1000
    salient features 1000
Fluorosis 536, 763
Focal hypoattenuating lesions is spleen 329
Focal hypodense lesions on NECT liver 324
Focal pancreatic masses 338
Focal pancreatitis 331
Focal, hypoechoic, hepatic lesions 322
Forestiet's disease 574
Frayed metaphysis 498
Functional segmental liver anatomy 392
Fungal ball 695
Fusion of symphysis pubis 521

G

Gas in biliary tree 312
Gas in gastric wall 263
    cystic pneumatosis 263
    emphysematous gastritis 263
    interstitial gastric emphysema 263
Gas in portal venous 313
Gas in the genital tract 1085
Gas in urinary tract 641
    gas in bladder wall 641
    gas in kidneys and ureters 641
    gas inside the bladder 641
Gasless abdomen 347
Gastric adenocarcinoma 263
Gastric mass and filling defects 372

Gastrocolic fistula 381
Gaucher's disease 498
Generalized calcinosis 217, 220
    collagen vascular disorders 217
    idiopathic calcinosis universalis 217
    idiopathic tumoral calcinosis 217
Generalized increase in density of skull vault 760
    congenital 760
    endocrinal 760
    hematological 760
    idiopathic 760
    metabolic 760
    neoplasm 760
Generalized osteoporosis 552
Generalized osteosclerosis 429
Geode 544
Germinoma (Atypical teratoma) 817
Gout 456
Grave's disease 1019

H

Hair on end skull vault 774
Hajdu-Cheney syndrome 564
Hashimoto's disease 16
Hashimoto's thyroiditis 1020
Heel valgus 592
Helicobacter pylori 241
Hemangiomas 4
Hematemesis 358
    duodenal causes 359
    esophageal causes 359
    gastric causes 359
    vascular malformation 359
    visceral artery aneurysm 359

Hemolytic anemia 774
Hemophilia 456
Hemosiderosis 110
Hemothorax 142
Hepatic arterial anatomy 394
Hepatic calcification 315
Hepatic fissures 395
Hepatic tumors with vascular "scar"
    326
Herpes simplex encephalitis 917
Hiatus hernia 49
High resolution CT-pattern of
    parenchymal disease 149
Hilar enlargement 70
Histiocytosis X 109
Histoplasmoma 92, 108
HIV encephalopathy 918
Hodgkin's disease 8
Homozygos achondroplasia 426
Honeycomb lung 129
Honeycomb pattern 132
Horner's syndrome 14
Hot thyroid nodule 1022
Hurler's syndrome 529
Hürthle cell tumors 1035
Hydatid cyst 92
Hyperechoic splenic lesion 329
Hyperostosis frontalis interna 758
Hyperparathyroidism 473, 534,
    559
Hyperperfusion abnormalities of
    liver 325
Hyperthyroidism 556
Hypertranslucent lung field 128
Hypertransradiant lung field 120
Hypertrophic obstructive.
    cardiomyopathy 193
Hypertrophic osteoarthropathy
    486

cardiovascular 486
gastrointestinal 487
pleural 486
pulmonary 486
Hypervitaminosis—A, D 536
Hypochondroplasia 421
Hypogonadism 556
Hypophosphatasia 426
Hypopituitarism 525, 556
Hypopseudohypo and pseudopse-
    duohypoparathyroidism 534
Hypothyroidism 556

I

Idiopathic calcinosis universalis 219
Idiopathic hypercalcemia of infancy
    536
Idopathic tumoral calcinosis 219
Implantation dermoid 545
Infantile hypertrophic pyloric
    stenosis 348
Infection 140
Inferior rib notching 60
    bilateral 60
    unilateral 60
Inflammatory bowel disease 406
    clinical findings 408
    epidemiology 406
    etiology and pathogenesis 407
    findings 409
    radiologic findings 408
    risk factors 407
Inner ear masses 959
Intestinal obstruction in neonate
    356
    duodenal 356
    jejunal and ileal obstruction 356
Intra-abdominal calcification in
    neonate 358

extraluminal 358
intraluminal 358
Intradural extramedullary masses 984
Intrahepatic portal venous system 391
Intramedullary lesions 975
Intramural pseudodiverticulosis 364
Intraorbital calcification 954
Intraspinal masses 871
    benign lesions 940
    extradural masses 871
    intradural extramedullary 871
    intramedullary 871
    malignant lesions 939
Intrathoracic goiter 12
Invasive carcinoma 161
Invisible main pulmonary artery 178
    misplaced pulmonary artery 178
    underdeveloped main pulmonary artery 178
Iodine load 1031
Iron metabolism 405
Irregular esophageal strictures 371
Irregular/stippled epiphysis 492
IUFD with hydropic placental degeneration 1039
Ivory vertebral body 847

J

Japanese Society of Esophageal Disease 230
Joint tuberculosis 486
J-shaped sella 905
Juvenile osteoporosis 555
Juvenile polyposis 300
Juvenile rheumatoid arthritis 574

K

Kippel-Feil syndrome 860
Klebsiella penumoniae 93, 131
Krabbe's disease 922

L

Lacrimal gland tumors 951
Langerhan's cell histiocytosis 751, 1002
Large, smooth kidney 610
Laryngeal masses 939
Lateral pharyngocele 363
Lead 536
Leather bottle 376
Left to right shunts 193
Leiomyomas 226
Leontiasis ossia 758
Lèri's disease 438
Lèri-Weill disease 528
Lesions of thoracic inlet 1
    anatomy 1
    differential diagnosis 2
Lethal neonatal dysplasia 424
Leukemia 621
Leukodystrophies 921
Lhermitte-Duclos disease 910
Linear calcification of soft tissues 214
    arterial 214
    venous 214
    nerves 214
    ligamentous 214
Linitis plastica 376, 380
    common etiologies 377
        acids 378
        eosinophilic gastroenteritis 380
        granulomatous disease 378

lymphoma 378
   metastatic involvement 378
   radiation injury 378
   scirrhous gastric carcinoma 377
  differential diagnosis 376
   infection 376
   inflammation 376
   malignancy 376
   others 377
   trauma 377
  radiological appearance 377
   barium meal 377
   CT scan 377
   ultrasound 377
Lipoblastoma 7
Lipoma 6
Liposarcoma 14
Liver function tests 397
Lobar pneumonia 130
Localized air space disease 99
Localized hyperostosis of the skull 757
Localized increase in density of the skull vault 765
Localized lucent defect 84
Location of some common neoplasm/lesions 466
  diaphysis 467
  epiphysis 466
  metaphysis 466
Locations of tumors within bone 451
Long segment coarctation of aorta 193
Loose intra-articular bodies 514
Loss of lamina dura of teeth 1010
Loss of renal outline on plain film 644

Lucency in the skull vault—with surrounding sclerosis 754
Lucency in the skull vault—without sclerosis 749
Lucent bone lesion containing bone/calcium 464
Lucent lung lesions 83
  multiple lucent lung lesions 83
   cavities 83
   neoplasm 83
Lung abscess 93
Lung disease associated with honey combing 131
Lung tumors 66
Lutembacher's syndrome 207
Lymph 561
Lymphangiectasia 290
Lymphangioma 3, 13
Lymphoid tumors 951
Lymphoma 8
Lytic lesion in bone 543
Lytic lesion in digits 508

M

Macleod syndrome 124
Madelung deformity 504
Malabsorption 279
Malignant mesothelioma 142
Mammogram 158
Marchiafava-Bignami disease 919
Maroteaux Lamy syndrome 529
Mass of ilio-psoas compartment 386
Mass within cavity 75
Masses 961
Massively dilated stomach 260
Mastitis 165
Mastocytosis 537
Meckel-Gruber syndrome 507

Mediastinal masses 15
    anterior mediastinal masses
        16,36
        commonest tumors 17
        pleuropericardial cyst 19
        teratodermoid tumors 19
        thymic tumors 17
        thyroid tumor 16
    middle mediastinal masses
        21,38
        aortic aneurysm 21
        bronchogenic cyst 22
        lymph node enlargement
          21
        tortuous innominate artery
          22
        tracheal tumors 22
    posterior mediastinal masses
        22,45
        bochdalek hernia 24
        esophageal lesions 23
        hiatus hernia 23
        neurenteric cysts 24
        neurogenic tumors 22
        pancreatic pseudocyst 24
        paravertebral lesions 23
Mediastinal thymus 4
Medullary cysts 684
Medullary nephrocalcinosis 655
Medullary tumors 737
Megacolon in adult 305
Meig-Salmon syndrome 137
Melnick-needles syndrome 499
Mènètrier's disease 241
Mesomelic dwarfism 528
Mesomelic dysplasia 421
Metachromatic leukodystrophy
    921
Metastatic carcinoma 271

Metastatic lymph node mass 14
Metastatic lymph nodes 10
Metastatic tumors 946
Michels classification 394
Middle ear masses 965
    congenital 965
    inflammatory 965
    neoplastic 967
Miliary metastasis 109
Miliary shadowing 106,111
Miliary tuberculosis 108
Mitral stenosis 193
Mixed density lesions 156
    galactocele 156
    hematoma 156
    lymph node 156
Monoarthritis 512
Morgagni's hernia 36
Moth-eaten bone 467
MR changes in AVN 496
MRI in important hepatic lesions
    327
Mucinous cystadenoma 331
Mucolipidoses 427
Mucopolysaccharidoses and
    mucolipidosis 427
Multicystic dysplastic kidney 683
Multiple collapsed vertebrae 869
Multiple myeloma 618
Multiple pin point opacities 113,
    130
Multiple wormian bones 778
Myelosclerosis 537

N

Nabothian cysts 1039
Nasal cephaloceles, dermoids and
    gliomas 895
Nasopharyngeal masses 933

Neonatal and adult kidney 594
Neonatal dysphasia 362
Neonatal obstructive jaundice 318
Nephromegaly associated with
    cirrhosis, hyperalimenation and
    diabetes mellitus 624
Nerve sheath tumors 985
Neuroblastoma 9
Neurofibromas 7
Neurogenic tumors 48
Niemann-pick disease 498
Nodular appearance of small bowel
    278
Non-gynecological pelvic masses
    1050
Non-Hodgkin's disease 40
Non-ossifying fibroma 436, 453
Non-ovarian adenexal mass 1050
Non-visualization of a kidney 626
Nonvisualization of gallbladder on
    ultrasound 311
Normal diarthrodial joint 460
Normal hemodynamics parameter
    of liver 397
Normal ovaries 1048
Normal size of bile ducts 398
Normal size of liver 396
Normal values of prevertebral soft
    tissue 928

O

Obstructive uropathy 612
Occipital and parietal cephaloceles
    894
Ocular masses 952
Ollier's disease 420, 499
Opaque hemithorax 114
Opaque maxillary antrum 1016
Orbital hyperostosis 890

Orbital masses 943
Orbital meningiomas and
    schwannomas 945
Orbital pseudotumor 950
Orbital tumors 833
Ormonds disease 381
Osteoarthritis 455, 461
Osteoblastoma 435, 436, 538
Osteochondrodysplasias 524
Osteochondroma 453
Osteoclastic activity 469
Osteogenesis imperfecta 424
Osteoid osteoma 435
Osteolytic defect in the medulla 462
Osteoma 538
Osteomyelitis 539
Osteopenia 468, 552
Osteopetrosis 532
Osteopoikilosis 537
Osteoporosis 468
Osteosarcoma 538
Osteosclerotic metastasis 535
Ovarian masses 1051

P

Paget's disease 430, 536, 561, 757
Painless hematuria 741
    clinical features 743
    etiology 741
    pathology 743
Pancoast tumor 10, 14
Pancreas 402
    pancreatic development and
        anatomy 402
Pancreatic calcification 330
Pancreatic duct of Santorini 404
Pancreatic masses 331
Pancreaticobiliary junction variants
    400

Paranasal sinus masses 949
Parasitic calcification 215
    armilifer armillatus 216
    cysticercus cellulosae 215
    guinea worm 215
    loasis 215
Paravertebral lesions 47
Parenchymal pulmonary disease 180
Partial mole 1039
Pathologic lesions in terminal ileum 293
Pathological intracranial calcification 896
Patterns of bone destruction 451
Pediatric orbital tumors 943
Pelvic abscess 1040
Peptic stricture 223
Periarticular soft tissue calcification 217
    degenerative 217
    hypercalcemia 217
    idiopathic 217
    inflammatory 217
    neoplastic 217
    renal failure 217
Pericardial effusion 177
Periosteal reaction 478
    solitary and localized 478
Periosteal reaction in childhood 480
Periosteal reactions–types and conditions 474
    complex 477
    continuous 474
    interrupted 476
Periportal hyperechogenicity 323
Pertechnetate scan 46
Peutz-Jeghers syndrome 300

Pharyngeal/esophageal diverticula 363
Pituitary adenoma 810
Pituitary apoplexy 812
Placenta and membranes in twin pregnancies 1062
Placental hemorrhage 1063
Plain skiagram chest 122
Plantar calcaneal spur 516
Plasma cell granuloma 89
Platybasia 774
Pleural calcification 147
    common conditions 147
        asbestos inhalation 147
        old empyema 147
        old hemothorax 147
        silicosis 147
Pleural diseases 137
Pleural fluid 144
    radiological appearances of pleural fluid 144
Pleural lesions 145
Pleural masses 141
Pleural tumors 146
    benign 146
    malignant 146
Plummer-Vinson syndrome 226
Pneumatosis intestinalis 304
Pneumoconiosis 111
Pneumomediastinum 11, 64
    immunological 71
    inhalation 71
    vascular 71
Pneumonia 93
Pneumoperitoneum 343, 346
    causes 347
    etiology 344
    signs on a supine film 343
Pneumothorax 142

iatrogenic 142
spontaneous 142
traumatic 142
Poland syndrome 53, 506
Polycystic kidney disease 623, 681
    autosomal dominant polycystic
        kidney disease 681
    autosomal recessive polycystic
        kidney disease 681
Polyostotic fibrous dysplasia 545
Polyposis syndrome 301
Polysyndactyly syndrome 507
Polyvinyl chloride 568
Porencephalic cysts 785
Posterior fossa cysts and cysts-like
    masses 782
Posterior fossa neoplasm in
    childhood 820
Posterior scalloping of vertebral
    body 851
Postmenopausal osteoporosis 555
Pott's disease 485
Pott's spine 13
Presacral fetal mass 1041
Prevertebral soft tissue thickening
    928
Primary bone tumors 446
    aneurysmal bone cyst 446
    central chondrosarcoma 450
    chondroblastoma 447
    chondromyxoid fibroma 447
    enchondroma 447
    eosinophilic granuloma 449
    Ewing's sarcoma 449
    fibrosarcoma 449
    fibrous cortical defect 446
    giant cell tumor 448
    juxtacortical osteosarcoma 450
    malignant fibrous histiocytoma
        449
    monostotic fibrous dysplasia
        447
    multiple myeloma 450
    nonossifying fibroma 446
    osteoblastoma 448
    osteochondroma 448
    osteoid osteoma 448
    osteosarcoma 450
    polyostotic fibrous dysplasia
        447
    reticulum cell sarcoma 449
    simple bone cyst 446
Primary hepatic masses 317
Primary or secondary carcinoma
    153
Progeria 565
Proliferative/necrotizing disorders
    616
Prostate 724
    CT anatomy 726
    MR anatomy 726
    normal anatomy 724
    sonographic anatomy 725
Prostate and seminal vesicle cysts
    729
Prostatic agenesis/hypoplasia 729
Prostatic calculi 731
Prostatic cyst 729
Prostatic infections 730
Prostatic lesions 728
Protein deficiency 557
Protein losing enteropathy 292
Proteus 93
Protrusio acetabuli 519
    causes 519
Pseudoarthrosis 492
Pseudochondroplasia 421
Pseudogestation of ectopic
    pregnancy 1038

Pseudomass 163
Pseudopneumoperitoneum 345
Psoriatic arthritis 566
Pulmonary arterial hypertension 180
Pulmonary edema 99
Pulmonary hamartomas 89
Pulmonary thromboembolism 180
Pulmonary venous hypertension 201
Pycnodysostosis 565
Pyle's disease 499
Pyonephrosis 627

R

Radiation enteritis 273
Radiation esophagitis 228
Radiographic finding in degenerative, inflammatory and neuropathic arthritis 522
Radiologic characteristics of benign and malignant bone lesions 454
Radiologic differentiation of chest wall tumors 54
Radiotracer 1029
Rathke's cleft cyst 816
Reiter's syndrome 457
Relationship of metastatic lesions to the primary tumors 440
Renal artery stenosis (RAS) 652
Renal calcification 653
Renal cysts and hydronephrosis 1047
Renal mass 659
Renal osteodystrophy 534
Renovascular hypertension 648
Resorption of distal phalanges 510
Retroperitoneal fibrosis 381, 385
Retropharyngeal abscess 6

Rhabdomyosarcoma 947
Rheumatoid arthritis 455, 457, 558
Rhizomelic dwarfism 425
Rib lesions 501
Rib notching 502
    inferior margin 502
    superior margin 502
Right aortic arch 199
Ring enhancing lesions on CECT 824

S

Sacroiliitis 518
    isolated 505
    syndrome related 505
Sarcoidosis 43, 109, 567
Schistosomiasis 300
Schwannomas 7
Scimitar syndrome 153
Scleroderma 217, 225
Scleroderma/progressive systemic sclerosis (PSS) 567
Sclerosing adenosis 163
Sclerotic bone lesions 432, 540
    developmental 432
    vascular 434
Sclerotic lesions of bone 531
Scurvy 445
Secondary esophageal neoplasms 228
Sellar and suprasellar masses 810
Seminal vesicle calcification 708
    chronic infections 709
    differential diagnosis 708
        diabetes mellitus 708
    methods of investigation 708
        CT 708
        MRI 708
        plain X-ray 708
        USG 708

Senile osteoporosis 554
Septal lines 113
Septated bone lesions 467
    aneurysmal bone cysts 467
    chondromyxoid fibroma 467
    giant cell tumor 467
    hemangioma 467
    nonossifying fibroma 467
Serous cystadenoma 331
Sheet-like calcification in soft tissue
    219
Short limb skeletal dysplasia 420
    acromelic 422
    acromesomelic 421
    mesomelic 421
    rhizomelic 420
Short rib syndromes 426
Short rib-polydactyly syndrome
    507
Short spine dysplasias 528
Short spine skeletal dysplasia 423
    disease 423
        diastrophic dwarfism 424
        Kniest syndrome 424,426
        metatrophic dwarfism 424
        pseudoachondroplasia 423
        spondyloepiphyseal
            dysplasia 423
        spondylometaphyseal
            dysplasia 423
Sibson's fascia 1
Sickle cell anemia 774
Signs of esophagitis 365
Silicosis 108,112
Simple cyst typical findings 668
Sincipital and sphenopharyngeal
    cephaloceles 895
Situs 206

situs intermedius/ambiguous
    207
situs inversus 206
situs solitus-normal situs 206
Skeletal maturation disorders 418
    accelerated 419
        asymmetric 420
        generalized 419
        localized 419
    retarded 418
        chromosomal disorders
            418
        chronic ill health 418
        congenital syndromes 419
        endocrinal disorders 419
        miscellaneous 419
Skull base and cavernous sinus 788
Slice of sausage 156
Small aorta 193
Small intestinal stricture 269, 274
Small, irregular, kidneys 605
Small, smooth, bilateral kidneys 598
Small, smooth, unilateral kidney
    595
Smooth, small kidneys 594
Soft tissue density lesion 157
    circumscribed malignant lesions
        160
    fibroadenoma 158
    lymphoma 159
    metastasis 159
    papilloma 158
    phylloides tumor 158
    simple cyst 157
Soft tissue lesions 209
    acromegaly 209
    epanutin therapy 210
    infection/injury 210
    myxoedema 209

obesity 210
peripheral edema 209
Soft tissue ossification 211
    burns 212
    congenital myositis
        liposarcoma 211
    myositis ossificans 211
    ossificans progressiva 212
    paraplegia 212
    parosteal osteosarcoma 211
    surgical scar 212
    tumoral calcinosis 212
Solid thyroid nodule 1034
Solitary bone cyst 546
Solitary collapsed vertebra 866
Solitary dense metaphyseal band 496
Solitary dense vertebra 561, 563
Solitary pulmonary nodule 85, 86
Solitary radiolucent metaphyseal bands 496
Solitary sclerotic lesion with lucent center 439
Sonographic classification of adenexal masses 1056
Spiculated breast masses 161
Spinal column 571
Spleen 405
Splenic calcification 328
Splenomegaly 327
Staphylococcus aureus 93
Steinberg classification for AVN of hip 495
Streptococcus pneumoniae 131
Streptococcus pyogenes 131
Strictures in small bowel 268
Subarticular lytic bone lesion 455
Superior mediastinal masses 25
Superior mediastinum widening 26

differential diagnosis 25
Superior orbital fissure enlargement 828
Superior rib notching 55
    classification 55
    salient features 56
Suprasellar mass 803
    anterior 3rd ventricle/optic chiasmatic lesions 804
    infundibular lesions 803
    intrasellar lesions (pituitary) 803
    sphenoid sinus/cavernous sinus lesions 804
    suprasellar lesions 803
Suprasellar meningioma 814

T

Talocalcaneal angle 592
Target lesions in stomach 261
TBIDA scan 320
Temporal bone sclerosis 838
Tension pneumothorax 143
Teratoma 817
Tertiary contractions in esophagus 371
Testicular tumors 701, 707
Thanatophoric dwarfism 425, 527
Thickened duodenal folds 258
Thickened endometrium 1076
Thickened esophageal folds 236
    causes 236
        esophagitis 236
        lymphoma 236
        varices 236
        varicoid carcinoma 236
Thickened folds in small bowel 275
Thickened gallbladder wall 323
Thickened gastric 256

Thickened gastric folds 239
Thickened placenta 1060
Thickened small bowel 250
Thickened small bowel folds with
    gastric abnormality 278
Thickening of the skull vault 756
Thoracic aortic aneurysm 41
Thoracic outlet syndrome 12
Thumb printing in colon 306
Thymic cyst 4, 13
Thymic hyperplasia 27
Thyroid calcifications 1036
Thyroid carcinoma 9, 14
Thyroid lesions 1019
Toxic multinodular goiter 1019
Toxic solitary nodule 1020
Trabecular bone 211
Tram line calcification 620
Trauma 81
Trisomy 13, 507
Tuberculoma 91
Tuberculosis 43
Tuberculous spondylitis 6
Turcot's syndrome 301
Twin pregnancy 1039
Types of periosteal reaction 452
Typical carcinoma 160

U

Ulcer disease 246
Ultrasound signs of chromosomal
    abnormality 1063
Unilateral (localized) renal cystic
    disease 682
Unilateral pulmonary edema 99

Unilateral scarred kidney 606
USG signs in abortions 1078

V

Various fetal anterior abdominal wall
    defects 1045
Vascular anomalies 5
Vasculogenic lesions 944
Venous abnormality 42
Videocystometrography 696
Visual pathway glioma (VPG) 818

W

Waldeyer's tonsillar ring 8
Wegener's granulomatosis 93
Whipple's disease 286
Widening of symphysis pubis
    (Diastasis) 520
Widening/enlargement of presacral/
    retrorectal space 309
Wilm's tumor 353
Wisened old man 565
Wolf's syndrome 520
Wormian bones 762

X

Xanthogranulomatous
    pyelonephritis 613, 627

Z

Zellweger cerebrohepatorenal
    syndrome 493
Zenker's/pharyngoesophageal/
    hypopharyngeal diverticulum
    363
ZES and ulcer disease 241
Zollinger-Ellison syndrome 257